Medical Ethics

Medical Ethics

Edited by

R.S. Downie

Professor of Moral Philosophy,
University of Glasgow

Dartmouth
Aldershot • Brookfield USA • Singapore • Sydney

Published by
Dartmouth Publishing Company Limited
Gower House
Croft Road
Aldershot
Hants GU11 3HR
England

Dartmouth Publishing Company
Old Post Road
Brookfield
Vermont 05036
USA

British Library Cataloguing in Publication Data
Medical ethics. – (The international research library of
   philosophy)
   1. Medical ethics
   I. Downie, R. S. (Robert Silcock), 1933 –
   174.2

Library of Congress Cataloging-in-Publication Data
Medical ethics / edited by R.S. Downie.
        p. cm.— (The International research library of philosophy :
   v.)
   Includes bibliographical references.
   ISBN 1-85521-631-0
   1. Medical ethics. I. Downie, R. S. (Robert Silcock)
II. Series.
R724.M29272 1996
174'.2—dc20
                                                                    96-608
                                                                    CIP

ISBN 1 85521 631 0

Printed in Great Britain by Galliard (Printers) Ltd, Great Yarmouth

Contents

Acknowledgements

The editor and publishers wish to thank the following for permission to use copyright material.

American Psychiatric Association for the essay: Paul Chodoff (1976), 'The Case for Involuntary Hospitalization of the Mentally Ill', *American Journal of Psychiatry*, **133**, pp. 496–501. Copyright © 1976 The American Psychiatric Association. Reprinted by permission.

Appleton & Lange for the essay: P. Singer (1992), 'Xenotransplantation and Speciesism', *Transplantation Proceedings*, **24**, pp. 728–32. Copyright © 1992. Reprinted by permission of Appleton & Lange.

Blackwell Publishers for the essays: John Harris (1983), '*In Vitro* Fertilization: The Ethical Issues', *Philosophical Quarterly*, **33**, pp. 217–37; Mary Warnock (1983), '*In Vitro* Fertilization: The Ethical Issues (II)', *Philosophical Quarterly*, **33**, pp. 238–49; Laura M. Purdy (1989), 'Surrogate Mothering: Exploitation or Empowerment?', *Bioethics*, **3**, pp. 18–34; John Harris (1993), 'Is Gene Therapy a Form of Eugenics?', *Bioethics*, **7**, pp. 178–87.

BMJ Publishing Group for the essays: Raanan Gillon (1988), 'Euthanasia, Withholding Life-prolonging Treatment, and Moral Differences Between Killing and Letting Die', *Journal of Medical Ethics*, **14**, pp. 115–17; Brenda Almond (1988), 'Philosophy, Medicine and its Technologies', *Journal of Medical Ethics*, **14**, pp. 173–8; John Harris (1987), 'QALYfying the Value of Life', *Journal of Medical Ethics*, **13**, pp. 117–23; Carl Elliott (1995), 'Doing Harm: Living Organ Donors, Clinical Research and *The Tenth Man*', *Journal of Medical Ethics*, **21**, pp. 91–6; R.M. Hare (1986), 'Health', *Journal of Medical Ethics*, **12**, pp. 174–81; R.S. Downie (1993), 'The Ethics of Medical Involvement in Torture', *Journal of Medical Ethics*, **19**, pp. 135–7; R.M. Hare (1993), 'The Ethics of Medical Involvement in Torture: Commentary', *Journal of Medical Ethics*, **19**, pp. 138–41.

Commonweal Foundation for the essay: Daniel Callahan (1988), 'Vital Distinctions, Mortal Questions: Debating Euthanasia and Health-Care Costs', *Commonweal*, 15 July, pp. 397–404.

The Hastings Center for the essays: Carl Elliott (1992), 'Where Ethics Comes From and What to Do About It', *Hastings Center Report*, **22**, pp. 28–35. Copyright © The Hastings Center. Ruth Macklin (1991), 'Artificial Means of Reproduction and Our Understanding of the Family', *Hastings Center Report*, **21**, pp. 5–11. Copyright © The Hastings Center.

Journal of The Royal Society of Medicine for the essay: Bruce G. Charlton (1993), 'Public Health Medicine – A Different Kind of Ethics?', *Journal of the Royal Society of Medicine*, **86**, pp. 194–5.

Kluwer Academic Publishers for the essays: Albert R. Jonsen (1991), 'American Moralism and the Origin of Bioethics in the United States', *Journal of Medicine and Philosophy*, **16**,

Series Preface

The International Research Library of Philosophy collects in book form a wide range of important and influential essays in philosophy, drawn predominantly from English-language journals. Each volume in the Library deals with a field of inquiry which has received significant attention in philosophy in the last 25 years, and is edited by a philosopher noted in that field.

No particular philosophical method or approach is favoured or excluded. The Library will constitute a representative sampling of the best work in contemporary English-language philosophy, providing researchers and scholars throughout the world with comprehensive coverage of currently important topics and approaches.

The Library is divided into four series of volumes which reflect the broad divisions of contemporary philosophical inquiry:

- Metaphysics and Epistemology
- The Philosophy of Mathematics and Science
- The Philosophy of Logic, Language and Mind
- The Philosophy of Value

I am most grateful to all the volume editors, who have unstintingly contributed scarce time and effort to this project. The authority and usefulness of the series rests firmly on their hard work and scholarly judgement. I must also express my thanks to John Irwin of the Dartmouth Publishing Company, from whom the idea of the Library originally came, and who brought it to fruition; and also to his colleagues in the Editorial Office, whose care and attention to detail are so vital in ensuring that the Library provides a handsome and reliable aid to philosophical inquirers.

John Skorupski
General Editor
University of St. Andrews
Scotland

Introduction

Medical ethics or, as it is often called, bioethics or healthcare ethics, is of recent origin. Of course it is possible to point to passages in Greek writing and to occasional writings thereafter which deal with issues which are recognizably bioethical. But there is little doubt that the rumblings which became the explosion of writing on bioethics were first clearly heard in the US in the early 1960s. Something of the nature of that genesis is traced by Albert R. Jonsen in Chapter 1. There are three features of Jonsen's account to which I should like to draw attention. Firstly, bioethics arose out of public concerns, such as 'the selection of patients for chronic hemodialysis in Seattle in 1962'. Secondly, the cultural context in which it was formed was what Jonsen calls 'American Moralism' – a species of Calvinism. Thirdly, that particular sort of moralism encouraged the view that moral problems can be solved by applying principles whereby an ordering is given to complex medical and scientific facts.

Granted these features of bioethics as it emerged in the 1960s, it is easy to explain its appeal to moral philosophers. Moral philosophy in the post-war period was criticized for being arid, trivial and removed from the moral problems of real life. It was treated by philosophers as no more than the application of logical techniques to the analysis of moral language. This approach to moral philosophy was shaped by two assumptions: that moral philosophy must be sharply distinguished from anything empirical, and that it had no bearing on any first-order moral issues. Some philosophers were (and are) happy with these assumptions, but others felt that, if moral philosophy were to justify its centrality in a humane education, then it would need to engage more fully with the moral problems of real life. Bioethics had an obvious appeal to moral philosophers looking for a role in the shaping of their culture: it had an obvious first-order relevance, and discussion was conducted in a manner familiar to moral philosophers – in terms of principles. It is against this background that we are to understand Stephen Toulmin's essay, 'How Medicine Saved the Life of Ethics' (Chapter 2).

It is worth noting here – although the points are of sociological rather than philosophical interest – that there are two other reasons which encouraged philosophers to become involved with bioethics. The first is that, increasingly from 1980, university departments were obliged to seek funding from outside sources, and it is easier to obtain funding for projects with an obvious practical relevance. The second is that doctors were themselves perplexed as to when to use the new technology which had been created, and were increasingly challenged by patients and fund allocators to justify their decisions. They therefore appealed for help to philosophers in the belief (perhaps mistaken) that the latter had a special sort of expertise which would help them with their problems: if you need an analysis, then send the urine to the biochemist and the ethics to the philosopher.

However that may be, the historical origins of bioethics and the keen interest which moral philosophers began to show in the issues gave rise to a certain way of conducting bioethical discussion known as the 'four-principles' approach. This approach was given its definitive form in a work by James F. Childress and Tom L. Beauchamp entitled *The Principles of Biomedical Ethics*, first published in 1976. This approach dominated Anglo-American bioethics in the 1980s and has recently been stated, criticized and defended in a large edited work (Gillon, 1994), According to Gillon (p. xxii):

> ... the four principles plus scope approach claims that whatever your personal philosophy, politics, religion, moral theory or life stance, you will find no difficulty in committing yourself to four *prima facie* moral principles plus a concern for their scope of application. Moreover these four principles plus attention to their scope of application can be seen to encompass most if not all of the moral issues that arise in health care (I am increasingly inclined to believe that the approach can, if sympathetically interpreted, be seen to encompass *all* moral issues, not merely those arising in health care). The principles are respect for autonomy, beneficence, non-maleficence and justice. '*Prima facie*', a term introduced by the English philosopher W.D. Ross, means that the principle is binding unless it conflicts with another moral principle – if it does then you have to choose between them. The four principles approach does not claim to provide a method for doing so – a source of much dissatisfaction to those who suppose that ethics can be boiled down to a set of prioritized rules such that once the relevant information is fed into the algorithm (or computer) out will pop The Answer. What the principles plus scope *can* provide is a common set of moral commitments, a common moral language, and a common set of moral issues to be considered in particular cases, before coming to your own answer, using your preferred moral theory or other approach to choosing between these principles when they conflict. ...

The problem of scope is that of deciding to whom or to what we owe these *prima facie* moral obligations. For example, supposing we agree that we have a *prima facie* moral obligation to benefit people, we still have the problem of deciding who these people are and how much they should be benefited. Again, we must respect autonomy, but are children or the mentally deranged autonomous? What counts as an autonomous agent? For example, if a 14-year old boy refuses consent for a life-saving operation, does this count as an autonomous decision to be respected? If a 22-year old (or indeed a 62-year old) takes an overdose and leaves a note saying 'let me die', does this constitute an autonomous decision? These are issues of scope.

One question which will occur immediately to moral philosophers concerns the surprising absence of the principle of utility. The principle of justice, which is concerned with the distribution of resources, is included as one of the four because the distribution of resources is of current ethical concern (see Daniels, Chapter 33 and Harris, Chapter 34). But utility also is (at least) a principle of distribution, so why not include it as a fifth principle?

Defenders of the four-principles approach can offer two replies. The first is to depict the principle of utility simply as an extended version of beneficence. Indeed, historically, this was the way in which utility entered moral philosophy. An early exponent of the principle of utility (Francis Hutcheson 1694–1746) took the view that there are three kinds of (in his language) 'benevolence':

> Sometimes it denotes a calm, extensive affection, or good-will towards all beings capable of happiness or misery: sometimes, a calm deliberate affection of the soul toward the happiness of smaller systems of individuals; such as patriotism ... parental affection. ... Or, the several kind particular passions of love, pity, sympathy, congratulations. ... The first sort is above all amiable and excellent: it is perhaps the sole moral perfection of some superior natures ... (Hutcheson 1725, p. 88).

On this line, then, utility is simply benevolence or beneficence with a universal scope. The other reply is to think of the principle of utility as that which underlies the other four principles, which are simply expressions of utility in different circumstances. This line has the advantage of providing a (theoretical) decision-procedure when the four principles conflict. For some philosophers though it will have the general disadvantages of utilitarianism.

How are the four principles meant to work in the solving of bioethical problems? One way of seeing their function borrows from a general account of moral reasoning which was common in the period 1960–80. In this view, one of the four principles either itself features as a major premise in a moral argument or gives rise to more specific principles (or rules) which do feature. For example, the general principle that we ought to respect the autonomy of patients might plausibly be said to give rise to specific principles, for instance, that we ought to obtain consent for treatment, ought not to deceive a patient about his/her condition, ought to maintain confidentiality and so on. The minor premise was thought to be factual and the two premises combined were said to entail a practical conclusion. For example:

Major premise   It is wrong (one ought not) to deceive someone about a matter which is important for his future welfare.

Minor premise   Failure to disclose to Mr X the full facts about his disease deceives him about a matter important for his future welfare.

Conclusion   Therefore, it is wrong to fail to disclose to Mr X the full facts about his disease.

Debate about such arguments can be directed at either the minor premise (i.e. the alleged facts) or at the major premise (the principle, derived from 'respect for autonomy'). As far as the minor premise is concerned, it might be maintained that the alleged facts are inaccurate, mistaken, incomplete, not fully known or that they do not constitute a case to which the principle applies (scope). In the example given, it might be maintained that Mr X *was* told, or that he was too ill to take in what was said, or that it was not yet certain that he had the disease, or that a failure to go into the full facts (which he would not understand) did not really constitute a case of deception.

Dispute can also break out over the major premise (the principle). In the given case someone might defend the major premise by showing how it is derived from respect for autonomy which (it is hoped) we all accept. But an opponent might argue that disclosure of the full facts of his case might upset Mr X and so lead to a worsening of his disease, and thus claim that the principle of beneficence would forbid full disclosure. Once again there might be factual dispute over the minor premise – whether full disclosure would in fact lead to deterioration. Even if the facts were agreed, there might remain conflict between the two major premises: the principle of respect for autonomy and that of beneficence (or perhaps non-maleficence). This in turn might be resolved (if one were a utilitarian at heart) by arguing that greater general utility will result if doctors are believed to disclose the full facts rather than if they are thought sometimes to withhold information.

In discussions of this kind it is possible to spot the same sort of logical moves and fallacies as can be found in moral reasoning in many other spheres. But there is one sort of logical distinction commonly found in reasoning in bioethics which is of considerable philosophical interest: the distinction between doing and allowing or, as it is more usually called in the bioethics literature, the distinction between acts and omissions (see Quinn, Fischer and Ravizza, Gillon, and Callahan in Chapters 11, 12, 14 and 15 respectively). This distinction is drawn in a variety of contexts. For example, opponents of euthanasia sometimes argue that, whereas it is wrong to carry out an action with the intention of bringing about someone's death, it is not (necessarily) wrong to omit to perform an action (say, a resuscitation after a cardiac arrest) even if it is highly probable that such action would have prevented the death. The distinction between acts and omissions appeals to doctors, no doubt because there is a genuine psychological difference between doing something and omitting to do something. But many philosophers have attacked it as being morally irrelevant, on the grounds that one can be as morally responsible for what one chooses not to do as for what one actually does. There are many familiar articles in the bioethics and moral philosophy literature making this point (see Rachels, Chapter 13), though a spirited defence of the distinction appears in Callahan (Chapter 15).

The four-principles approach to reasoning in bioethics, which reigned supreme for many years, is now heavily under attack from several quarters. These attacks on the four principles in bioethics are sometimes derived from, influenced or paralleled by discussions of reasoning and, indeed, of philosophical method more generally. The syllogistic paradigm of practical reasoning handed down from Aristotle has been criticized along with the Kantian (or Calvinistic) idea of the centrality of principles in the moral life. An influential attack on the four-principles approach is provided by Clouser and Gert (Chapter 3).

Another line of criticism derives from a revival of the tradition of casuistry. The recent revival of casuistry derives in part from the influential book by Jonsen and Toulmin (1988). In his 'Casuistry as Methodology in Clinical Ethics' (Chapter 4), Jonsen develops his argument for construing bioethics on the model of casuistry. He points out that, from the time of Henry Sidgwick's *Methods of Ethics* (1877), moral philosophy has stressed theory at the expense of cases. Yet it is the problems of cases which interest physicians, making the analysis of cases the dominant feature of bioethics. Jonsen argues that it is more fruitful to use the methods of the casuists to analyse cases than it is to apply the abstract principles and theories of moral philosophy. He explains the techniques of casuistry in relation to three terms – morphology, taxonomy and kinetics – and illustrates these techniques by analysing a particular case.

The merits in casuistry, but also its problem of bias, are explained further by Loretta M. Kopelman in Chapter 5. She points out that 'the potential for bias arises at each stage of a case method of reasoning including in describing, framing, selecting and comparing of cases and paradigms. A problem of bias occurs because, to identify the relevant features for such purposes, we must use general views about what is relevant; but some of our general views are biased, both in the sense of being unwarranted inclinations and in the sense that they are one of many viable perspectives' (p. 71).

It should be noted that modern casuists are by no mean rejecting the use of principles; rather they are emphasizing the importance of the details of cases. The work of the modern casuists of bioethics would repay study by moral philosophers interested in the nature of moral reasoning.

Another line of criticism of the four-principles approach derives from feminist writers such as Carol Gilligan (1982), filtered through the growing literature on nursing ethics. Their general line is to the effect that an emphasis on principles represents a male view on ethics, including bioethics, whereas a feminist view should be based on virtues such as compassion, or on sentiment. In this approach to bioethics, the central concept becomes that of 'care', said to be what nurses do, as opposed to 'cure', what (male) doctors are said to try to do. The professional stereotypes and oversimplifications exemplified by this contrast are discussed by Jecker and Self in Chapter 6. Nevertheless, there is no doubt that discussions in the feminist/nursing literature do successfully identify a need for the concept of care, and also that ethics involves more than an appeal to principles.

The fact that there is more to ethics – considerably more – than can be encompassed in the 'four principles' is brought out in two essays in this volume by Carl Elliott. In Chapter 7, he indicates that our ethical judgments are an integral part of the culture to which we belong.

> [Ethics] is one thread in the fabric of a society, and it is intertwined with others. Ethical concepts are tied to a society's customs, manners, traditions, institutions – all of the concepts that structure and inform the ways in which a member of that society deals with the world. When we forget this, we are in danger of leaving the world of genuine moral experience for the world of moral fiction – a simplified, hypothetical creation suited less for practical difficulties than for intellectual convenience (p. 112).

To argue in this way is not of course to reject the four principles. Rather it is to insist that the interpretation of these principles in different cultural settings – Britain and America, say – will reflect the influence of many factors in addition to the purely ethical.

In Elliott's paper on organ donation (Chapter 35), he draws attention to the rich variety of concepts involved in our relationships with each other which cannot plausibly be reduced to four. The general point emerging from both essays is that 'moral theories trade in generalities and simplifications which make it easy to forget how particular and complicated our moral experience is' (p. 112). It is because of the recognition of the inextricable entanglement of ethical concepts with wider cultural institutions (which of course include medicine itself) that some thinkers have turned to hermeneutics as a way of helping the clinical ethicist. As has been implied, the conception of bioethics that prevails at the present time is that of applied ethics. The idea is that there are developed ethical theories or principles which can be applied to problems of clinical practice and generate solutions. But, as I have suggested, this view of moral reasoning is too abstract, too far removed from clinical practice. The solution proposed by Thomasma, Ten Have and Daniel (Chapters 8–10) is the hermeneutical one. According to Daniel, the nub of the hermeneutical approach is its emphasis on 'the concrete particulars of language and experience' (p. 160), rather than on the application of rules. Daniel sums up the hermeneutical approach in more detail in his conclusion:

> The emphasis on interpretation in the essays by Thomasma and Ten Have is salutary: it provides a ground for the discernment of spirit in the particularities of clinical experience and supports an ethic of caring in health care. The theory of hermeneutical clinical ethics will become a reflective practice if medical educators and clinicians can adapt several important operating ideas: (1) every clinical case is also ethical; (2) ethics is best learned through cases; and (3) accommodation between the value-free language of science and technology and the value-laden language of stories may be achieved through careful interpretation (p. 164).

It is also significant for philosophical ethics that Daniel is critical of Thomasma's discussion of various rules 'for interpreting the relative weights of principles and values' (Thomasma p. 130) and of Ten Have's 'rationalistic' call for 'a basic matrix identifying all fundamental characteristics of medicine's self-interpretation ... in a coherent framework' (p. 155). Daniel's view is that 'we probably need more projects like that of Robert Pirsig (1991) in his semi-autobiographical fiction *Lila*, an extended case study in which personal suffering is interpreted and creatively assuaged through the perspective of a "Dynamic Quality" that preserves the tension between conflicting moral codes' (p. 164).

One might conclude that if what is wanted is the raising of the ethical awareness of health-care students and clinicians, or the development of their hermeneutical skills (and therefore their own self-development as human beings), we should look more to the arts than to academic philosophy. It is in or through the arts, perhaps especially through literature, that skills in interpreting the particularities of experience – the minor premises – can be cultivated. I have tried to argue a case for this based on material compiled for the purpose (Downie 1994). An excellent illustration of the use of a story to provide insight into the ethical complexities of organ donation is provided in Chapter 35 by Elliott, as previously mentioned.

Nevertheless, the suggestions that clinical ethics is best learned through cases, and that the most sensitively articulated cases are to be found in the arts, is only half the truth. This is because clinical ethics is only half of what might reasonably be included within the remit of bioethics. There is a long list of special topics (of which I have included some representative examples) which, while they may be encountered in clinical practice, are also matters of public policy. Philosophers might be expected to make a contribution to the discussion of these (although even here they would first either have to overcome their squeamishness about empirical facts or work in conjunction with others who are knowledgeable on the facts). Part II of this collection is concerned with discussions of these topics.

Part II begins with a topic which is appropriate for the flexing of philosophical muscles – the distinction between doing and allowing (or acts and omissions), as already mentioned. The essays by Quinn and by Fischer and Ravizza bring out a striking difference between bioethics and mainstream philosophy. Even when the topic is the same – and the differences (moral and conceptual) between doing and allowing are crucial in discussing euthanasia, abortion and other problems – the treatment can be quite different. In particular, the emphasis in bioethics is increasingly on 'cases' or on fictional problems which are nevertheless realistic or compiled from clinical practice. The reason for this is that the aim in bioethics is to improve practice (as Aristotle put it, 'not knowing but doing') whereas, in mainstream moral philosophy, the aim is to provide theoretical or conceptual understanding. Mainstream moral philosophers are consequently happy to use a range of fantastical examples where the criterion is simply whether a particular example will assist in defining a conceptual boundary.

There is a second reason for the restriction of examples in bioethics to the realistic. It is that medical students, doctors and nurses must actually make decisions of the kind which moral philosophers only think about, and they therefore respond badly to far-fetched examples, thinking of them as displaying a lack of seriousness.

It is important, however, not to exaggerate the difference in aim of the bioethicist and the mainstream moral philosopher. If the goal of clinical ethics is to improve practice, the method will involve improving understanding, including the understanding of concepts and our moral language. We have already spoken of this in discussing the contribution to clinical practice of casuistry and hermeneutics. Conversely, although directed at the understanding of concepts, moral philosophy cannot but have an impact on moral practice since it affects the way in which moral problems are described.

The contention that the difference in aim of the moral philosopher and the bioethicist is really just one of emphasis is supported by a number of the essays in Part II. Gillon, Callahan,

Sprigge, Buchanan and Fulford (Chapters 14 to 17 and 32) all illustrate concerns which could be described in terms of their relevance either to philosophical theory or to the practice of medicine.

A widespread anxiety exists in relation to medical technology and where it is taking us. Brenda Almond's discussion in Chapter 18 of some of the general issues of medical technology is followed by a range of essays investigating new enterprises in the field. The contributions of John Harris and Mary Warnock (Chapters 19 and 20) date from the beginning of the 1980s since which time reproductive technology has developed rapidly. However, that many of the ethical issues remain unresolved is evidenced by Chapters 21 and 22 by Laura Purdy and Ruth Macklin who tackle the ethical problems of two different aspects of this new technology. Mary Anne Warren then discusses abortion, an ethical dilemma as old as the Hippocratic Oath. Peter Singer and Karen Dawson conclude this section on reproductive technology by considering the argument from potential which is frequently invoked in this context.

The ethics of the clinical trial is a specific problem of bioethics to which philosophical analysis can make a contribution. Hellman and Hellman state the ethical problem in Chapter 25 as follows: 'Researchers participating in such studies [randomized clinical trials] are required to modify their ethical commitments to individual patients and do serious damage to the concept of the physician as a practising, empathetic professional who is primarily concerned with each patient as an individual. Researchers using a randomized clinical trial can be described as physician-scientists, a term that expresses the tension between the two roles' (p. 373). Hellman and Hellman review various solutions, but conclude that 'techniques appropriate to the laboratory may not be applicable to humans. We must develop and use alternative methods for acquiring clinical knowledge' (p. 377). This is a forthright conclusion with which many researchers would disagree.

A special problem in clinical trials is that of 'equipoise', the ethical requirement that the researcher be in genuine uncertainty about the relative merits of two possible treatments. In Chapter 26, Freedman proposes a revision to the definition of 'clinical equipoise', making it applicable to uncertainty about a treatment within the expert medical community, rather than being simply felt by an individual researcher.

In Chapter 27, Peter Singer examines some ethical aspects of another problem in medical research – the use of animals. His central thesis is that 'if an animal feels pain, the pain matters as much as it does when a human feels pain – if the pains hurt just as much. *Pain is pain*, whatever the species of being that experiences it' (p. 386). Using powerful though very straightforward arguments, Singer challenges the view that human beings have some innate value superior to that of animals. He places 'speciesism' in the same category as 'racism' and 'sexism'; all exemplify the principle that might is right.

The development of medical technologies has thus both stimulated the public imagination and created public anxiety. The latter arises from the belief that scientific expertise in the mastery of nature, especially human nature, might have outstripped ethical controls.

In particular the ethics of genetic manipulation creates considerable unease in the public mind. One source of fear is the belief that gene manipulation is a form of eugenics, a term which conjures up images of the Nazi regime. In Chapter 28, John Harris discusses whether it is plausible to regard gene manipulation as a form of eugenics.

Psychiatry is a branch of medicine which, for obvious reasons, has always fascinated philosophers. As far as the ethics of psychiatry is concerned, one perennial problem involves the involuntary hospitalization of the mentally ill, a procedure which tends to be deplored by liberals. This is discussed by Chodoff in Chapter 29. However, even competent patients can be irrational and thereby create problems, as analysed by Brock and Wartman in Chapter 30. In Chapter 31, Carl Elliott raises the problems of the possibility and desirability of achieving scientific objectivity in psychiatry, and in Chapter 32, Fulford *et al.* illustrate this difficulty in the context of Soviet psychiatry.

Another specific issue in bioethics, acute in all developed countries, is that of resources and value of life. Norman Daniels discusses one aspect of this in Chapter 33, followed by John Harris' investigation into the use of QALY (Quality Adjusted Life Year). In Chapter 35, Carl Elliott brings out the moral complexities which can slip through the broad meshes of economic and philosophical theory when applied to health care problems.

Health is a puzzling concept. Attempts to reduce it to biological or to sociological terms fail because, as R.M. Hare points out in Chapter 36, its content is not entirely descriptive. K.W.M. Fulford argues in Chapter 37 that illness can be interpreted as a bridge between the biological concepts of disease and the social conceptions of health.

Medical ethics tends to be individualistic, deriving from the problems of the doctor-patient relationship. Public health tends to be omitted from ethical discussion (except in relation to AIDS). Bruce Charlton points out in Chapter 38 that public health also requires ethical scrutiny.

The torture endemic in many societies raises the question of whether the medical profession should in any way be involved. My Chapter 39 was a contribution to a conference on the subject, to which R.M. Hare critically responded.

In conclusion it should be noted that in some instances these essays are written by philosophers and in some by doctors alone or in conjunction with philosophers. In other words, bioethics is an area in which there is genuine interdisciplinary work.

References

Childress, James F. and Beauchamp, Tom L. (4th ed., 1994), *The Principles of Biomedical Ethics*, Oxford: Oxford University Press.

Downie, R.S. (1994), *The Healing Arts: An Oxford Illustrated Anthology*, Oxford: Oxford University Press.

Gilligan, Carol (1982), *In a Different Voice: Psychological Theory and Women's Development*, Cambridge, Mass.: Harvard University Press.

Gillon, Raanan (ed.) (1994), *The Principles of Health Care Ethics*, Chichester: John Wiley.

Hutcheson, Francis (1725), *An Inquiry Concerning the Original of Our Ideas of Virtue or Moral Good* in R.S. Downie (ed.) (1994), *Francis Hutcheson: Philosophical Writings*, London: Dent, Everyman Library.

Jonsen, Albert R. and Toulmin, Stephen (1988), *The Abuse of Casuistry: A History of Moral Reasoning*, Berkeley, University of California Press.

Pirsig, Robert (1991), *Lila: An Inquiry into Morals*, New York: Bantam Books.

Sidgwick, Henry (1877), *Methods of Ethics*, London: Macmillan.

Part I
Methods of Medical Ethics

[1]

ALBERT R. JONSEN

AMERICAN MORALISM AND THE ORIGIN OF BIOETHICS IN THE UNITED STATES

ABSTRACT. The theology of John Calvin has deeply affected the American mentality through two streams of thought, Puritanism and Jansenism. These traditions formulate moral problems in terms of absolute, clear principles and avoid casuistic analysis of moral problems. This approach is designated American moralism. This article suggests that the bioethics movement in the United States was stimulated by the moralistic mentality but that the work of the bioethics has departed from this viewpoint.

Key Words: bioethics, Calvinism, casuistry, Jansenism, moralism, moral principle, Puritanism

I. AMERICAN MORALISM

In November, 1989, Dr. James Mason, Assistant Secretary for Health at the Department of Health and Human Services rejected the recommendations of an ad hoc committee established to study the use of human fetal tissue for transplantation therapy of Parkinsonism and Diabetes. The committee had extensively studied the ethical aspects of the proposed procedure and, while recognizing certain serious problems, concluded that such a use could be considered ethically acceptable. Dr. Mason, to whom Secretary Sullivan had delegated final authority on this issue, rejected the committee's report. When he did so, he stated that his decision was "a matter of heart and of mind as well" (New York Times, 1989).

Dr. Mason's words, undoubtedly sincere, reveal much about bioethics in the United States. In using the words, "a matter of heart", and in adding almost as an afterthought, "and of mind as well," he inadvertently recalled a moral tradition that runs wide and deep, although in our days, quite silently, through American culture. I name that tradition 'American moralism'. I will describe

---

Albert R. Jonsen, Ph.D., Professor and Chairman, Department of Medical History and Ethics, School of Medicine, University of Washington, Seattle, Washington 98195, U.S.A.

The Journal of Medicine and Philosophy 16: 113–130, 1991.

it, identify its historical and doctrinal roots and suggest how it at first fostered the movement we call bioethics and then became increasingly uncomfortable with it. My thesis is supported more by rough intuition than by refined research, but I believe that research would support intuition. Anyone who would undertake the research would have to look more attentively at the history of the ideas I will sketch here, be more careful about the concepts I outline and search out more thoroughly the texts that relate the events and ideas at the origins of bioethics in the decade between 1965–75, which I take as the formative decade of bioethics in the United States. This research, for the most part, remains to be done. In its absence, I will follow my intuition and set off on a rather bold, perhaps rash, exposition of my thesis about American moralism and bioethics.

I first propose what I take to be an uncontroversial premise: cultures have discernibly unique moralities, in the sense of explicit and implicit beliefs about the values that should inform personal and communal life. The designation, definition and emphases on these values differ from culture to culture in varying degrees and at different times. In recent years, historians and anthropologists have used the French term *mentalité* to describe communal ways of thinking about and seeing the world. American moralism is the *mentalité* of persons whose views and values have been formed within the historical culture of this country. It is, so to speak, American culture's matrix morality, that is, the deep source in which a certain way of thinking and feeling about the moral life is engendered and nourished.

The meaning I attribute to moralism is best explained by an historical and doctrinal excursus. In general, by moralism I mean a form of moral thought and expression nurtured within the religious tradition of Calvinism. Calvinism is, of course, the theology of the Swiss Reformer of the 16th century, John Calvin (Calvin, 1960). But it is far more than the intellectual creation of that one man: his thought has streamed out into many religious traditions and even into secular thought about politics and economics, as sociologist Max Weber and historian R.H. Tawney attempted to demonstrate years ago (Weber, 1958; Tawney, 1926). The influences of Calvinism are profound and widespread. In America, Calvinism set down its roots in New England, where the Puritan settlers intended to establish their 'City upon a Hill', in accord with the interpretation of Biblical precepts that they learned from John Calvin's Institutes and from his example in Geneva. The Puritans were dissenters from the Anglican Church who favored Calvin's version of Christian belief. The influence of Puritan theology and polity on American life is commonly acknowledged. A recent newspaper article on the wave of abstinence from tobacco, drinking, and other noxious substances contained the phrase, "Each is a thread in the skein of Puritanism that has always run through American life" (New York Times, 1990). But the influence of Calvinism on the American *mentalité* goes far beyond this popular attribution of asceticism to the Founding Fathers. Those influences have been the object of a vast scholarly literature (Miller, 1962; Morgan, 1963).

There is another, less familiar Calvinism in American life. It appeared on these shores almost two centuries after the Puritan settlements. The Irish immigrants who came to the United States in great numbers after the 1830s brought the Roman Catholic version of Calvinism, known in Catholic theology as Jansenism (Abercrombie, 1938). Different as were the Puritan fathers and their Protestant descendants from the Irish immigrants and their Catholic children, both were marked by the tone and tenor, if not the content of the theology of John Calvin. Both profoundly influence the way in which Americans view the moral life. Both shaped the *mentalité* I call American moralism.

It is impossible in a short essay to explicate fully the doctrinal and historical complexities of Calvinism, Puritanism, and Jansenism. Permit me a rapid summary (which may, I fear, offend scholarly historians and theologians). In the 17th century, the Puritans, dissenters from Anglican ecclesiastical governance and influenced strongly by Calvinist theology, settled New England. The history and the mentality of the Puritan settlers has been extensively described. Its foremost historian, Perry Miller, describes the Puritans' intent as "a society founded by men dedicated in unity and simplicity to realizing on earth eternal and immutable principles, and which progressively became involved with fishing, trade and settlement." (Miller, 1962, p. 40). The clash between "eternal and immutable principles" and involvement with "fishing, trade and settlement" set a theme for American moralism that has persisted through this country's history.

The Puritan response was not to advise retreat from the world of secular activities, but to plunge into it with pure hearts. A clear, unambiguous perception of God's Commandments and an unquestioning voluntary dedication to their observation would protect believers from contamination as they moved to subdue nature and society to the Divine Governance. This serene confidence found its intellectual counterpart in the moral philosophy taught at New England's first institution of higher learning, Harvard. The tenets of that moral philosophy were: "empirical and introspective study of human nature would lead to absolute standards and norms for human conduct ... immutable divine law was as discoverable in ethics as in physics" (Fiering, 1981, p. 7)

The moral philosopher Samuel Clarke profoundly influenced American moral philosophy, proclaiming that "the created world ... reveals inherent moral truths directly to man ... this order is so logically fixed that God himself cannot but act and command in accord with it ... only an imperfect and depraved understanding of the order, a will corrupted by particular interest or affection" would lead the believer astray (Fiering, 1981, p. 297). Of course, depraved understanding and corrupt affections beset the human race, radically broken by sin. The will, or as was usually said, 'the heart' must be continually purified. In the 18th century, the first Great Awakening, presided over by the religious genius, Jonathan Edwards, summoned Americans to this purity of heart and dedication of life. Again, clear and unambiguous moral Commandments were uttered; deep, affective response was demanded. It was less a matter of teaching people what they did not know than of reinforcing dedication to what was already known. In Edwards' words, "the informing of the understanding is all in vain any further than it affects the heart" (Edwards, 1959, II, pp. 96, 106). Here are the words that echoed in the subconscious (or the superego) of Secretary Mason.

Interrupted briefly by the Revolutionary War, the religious awakening revived in the first decades of the 19th century under the inspiration of Charles Finney. The revival meeting, at which manifest truths about salvation and morality were preached in vigorous and emotional terms and utter personal dedication was demanded, was the predominant method. As Miller wrote, "The dominant theme in America from 1800 to 1860 was the invincible presence of the revival technique ... the revival ... was a central mode of this culture's search for national identity ... the task was to ascertain the sins of the community that needed reforming ... to save the western migration from barbarism (Miller, 1965, pp. 6, 7, 13). Again, after the Civil War, revivalism, in many new forms, swept the country, presided over by Dwight Moody and Billy Sunday. The earlier fundamentalism, largely derived from Calvinist theology and Scottish Common Sense philosophy, preserved an intellectual heritage, in which reflection, guided by rightly ordered affection, revealed an immutable order of divine providence and moral truths. In this third period, fundamentalism ceded to the profoundly emotional, anti-intellectual religious sentimentalism that today goes by the name 'fundamentalism'. In this form, fundamentalism displays an overwhelming emphasis on soul-saving, personal experience and individual prayer. To Dwight Moody, "most ideas seemed divisive and hence all but the least controversial were to be avoided" (Marsden, 1980, pp. 120, 43).

This quick, superficial history reveals a pattern. From the earliest settlement of North America to the present day, a powerful moral tradition has shaped the culture. That powerful tradition begins as a Puritan application of Calvinist doctrine to the situation of the new world and develops as the insistent affirmation of clear, distinct moral principles, derived from the nature of things in which God's will was perceived, and accepted by an affective, singleminded dedication of the heart. The most prominent evangelist of the second Awakening, Charles Finney, affirmed that "everybody can agree upon the intellectual proposition. The only difference is that some grasp them with the heart and others with the mind ... 'holy angels and devils apprehend and embrace intellectually the same truths, yet how differently they are affected by them'" proclaimed Finney (Miller, 1965, pp. 25–26).

However, America is more than the Protestant tradition flowing from the Puritans to the modern Fundamentalists. Immigrant Catholicism provides its own moral culture. Strangely enough, it parallels the Calvinist tradition in spirit, if not in specifics. The first generation of American Catholics brought an English spiritual tradition to these shores, but rapidly, in the first decades of the 19th century, an immigrant clergy, many of them fleeing from the French Revolution, brought with them a spiritual and moral doctrine that was marked by Jansenism, a Catholic cousin of Calvinism. Calvin and Cornelius Jansen, a Belgian theologian, both found their spiritual inspiration in the theology of St. Augustine and both exploited the fideistic, voluntaristic, pessimistic notions of the greatest of the Western Church Fathers. The followers of Jansen denied Calvinist sympathies, but could not deny the similarity of concepts, logic and inclinations that joined them to the Huguenots. "The type of piety that developed out of Jansenism," says the New Catholic Encyclopedia, "was inflexibly rigoristic ... Jansenists were excessively moralistic and held that humanity had to be kept in check by penitential rigor" (New Catholic Encyclopedia, 1967, Vol. 7, p. 825). A bitter theological and political battle raged over Jansenism in the French speaking countries and in Rome and, even after Roman authorities formally condemned the doctrine, it lingered deeply in the spirituality and theology of French Catholicism. Belgian missionaries brought it to the United States in the first decades of the 19th century.

Jansenism came in full force, however, with the waves of Irish immigrants from the 1820s until after the Civil War. Irish clergy, unable to be educated in British dominated Ireland, attended seminaries in France and Belgium (and to a lesser degree in Spain, which promoted its own brand of rigorism). The first seminary allowed to open in Ireland after the Ascendancy, St. Patrick's at Maynooth, was staffed by many professors educated at Louvain, where the University had always been sympathetic to Jansenism. In the very first year of its operation, (1796) the faculty at Maynooth were warned by Roman authorities not to admit any liberal opinions in moral theology, repudiating "the excessive and wanton liberality of some in laying down the rules of morality, so that the mildness and suavity of evangelical charity shall never be disassociated from the salutary severity which is characteristic of Christian teaching" (Ellis, 1971, p. 19). The use of a text by a rigorist theologian was required. The liberal opinion that was to be repudiated was known as 'probabilism', a doctrine despised by Jansenists even though permitted by the magisterium of the Church. Probabilism was the rule that allowed a person who is troubled in conscience about the right course of action to choose to act on any well founded opinion that is 'probably' correct. The Jansenists insisted that this led to moral laxity and that conscience must be guided by the 'certain' or, at least, 'more probably' correct opinion (Jonsen and Toulmin, 1988).

The Seminary at Maynooth sent a steady stream of missionaries to the Irish in America. John Tracy Ellis, dean of Catholic historians, writes, "if many of those of Irish birth or background in the United States continued ... to display a strain of Jansenism in their thinking on moral issues such as problems concerned with sex ... it was no mystery where the ideas had taken their rise"

(Ellis, 1971, pp. 21, 22). They had taken their rise in Irish seminaries staffed by clergy trained in Jansenist leaning institutions on the continent. They came, as well, from the thousands of nuns whose spiritual guidance and religious rules were dictated by those male clergy. When in 1857 American Bishops established a seminary in Europe, in order to attract European clergy to serve in the United States, and to which promising young Americans could be sent for a European education, they situated it at the University of Louvain, fountainhead of Jansenistic theology.

In the last half of the 19th century, American Catholicism embraced the techniques of revivalism that had long prevailed in Protestant fundamentalism. Groups of priests, specially trained in pulpit oratory, travelled from parish to parish, conducting 'retreats' or 'missions' at which powerful emotional appeals were made to convert sinners and revive religious fervor. A historian of the movement writes, "The stern moral code encouraged by the revival promoted an individual morality that blended with the evangelical thrust of the Catholic revivalism. Morality, not dogma, right doing, not correct believing, was the thrust of the revival method ... preachers impressed upon people what must be done, or more often, what must be avoided in order to gain salvation ... revivalists sought a change of heart, not a change of opinion" (Dolan, 1978, pp. 111–112). Thus, at the same time in American life, Protestants and Catholics, who otherwise wished nothing more than to be distinct from each other, were engaged in the similar program: the encouragement of moralism, rigid in content and emotive in tone.

At the risk of some misunderstanding, this *mentalité* can be called moral fundamentalism. (The misunderstanding would arise if moral fundamentalism were identified exclusively with modern popular religious fundamentalism: it does appear there, but is much broader in meaning and in influence.) A moral fundamentalism relies on, and continually recalls the fundamental moral principles. Indeed, it is loath to depart very far from them. The similarities between Protestant and Jansenist moral fundamentalism are many. For our purposes, the most important are the insistence on clear, unambiguous moral principles, known to all persons of good faith. Both deny the possibility of moral paradox or irreconcilable conflict of principles. Fundamentalism cannot accept the possibility of Kierkegaardian moral conflict, for the Righteous God cannot command, as He seems to have commanded Abraham, to obey and, at the same time, to do a moral evil. Conflict must be explained as only apparent, never as real paradox. Both fundamentalisms avoid, as much as possible, detailed examination of exceptions to principles and rules. Exception to principle may come from an occasional, 'miraculous' suspension of divine command, but more likely is a symptom of sinful weakness of will. Probabilism, the doctrine that a moral problem can be understood in diverse ways and that differential moral judgments can be offered, is repudiated. Casuistry, the technique of moral analysis of particular cases, is despised in Calvinism and converted into legalism in Jansenist Catholicism. Both have a strong tendency to lump complex moral problems into simple, overarching ideas and to link together issues which, viewed from a more discerning viewpoint, appear distinct. For example, contraception and abortion are inextricably linked in Jansenist thinking; sex education and pornography are equated in Protestant fundamentalism.

I have spoken primarily about the moral forms of Calvinism and Jansenism: they both proclaimed that moral truths were clear, discernable to all of pure heart; they both affirmed absolute moral principles, from which any departure must be counted as sinful, making little or no room for justifiable exception. The actual content of those principles varied: both traditions heralded the Ten Commandments as dominant. Indeed, John Calvin had incorporated his entire moral theology under the rubric of the Decalogue: all moral action can be subsumed under a 'Thou shalt' or, more suitably, 'Thou shalt not'. Both cherished strictly ordered plans of life. Both were obsessed by sexuality. Both attacked intemperance by proposing, not temperance, but abstinence. Both promoted to absolutist moral status certain virtues, such as patriotism. In the long history of these traditions, the moral inflexibility sometimes achieved moral victories of great note – Abolitionism, untempered by concern for social and economic consequences, was a Calvinist moral victory; other battles urged by moral absolutism, such as Prohibition, were miserable moral defeats. (Both these episodes in American moral history are, of course, more complicated than this simplistic evaluation conveys.)

Moralism is absolutist in the etymological sense, namely, it tends to remove (*absolvere*) a moral problem from the actual circumstances of moral action. It seeks to shake the pure and sublime principle free of the dross of living situations. The principles are correct in themselves and must be affirmed: exceptions and excuses must not be considered because such consideration would distract from the principle itself. Indeed, as Calvin himself once noted, casuistry is to be condemned because its consideration of a variety of exceptions and excuses, "deepens anxiety" (Calvin, 1960, III, pp. iv, 17).

In fact, the theological father of both fundamentalisms displayed an attitude that prevails even in his most remote progeny. One of his sympathetic biographers has described that attitude: "he tended to feel uneasy if he could not organize his understanding of the world by dividing phenomena neatly into antithetical categories: black and white, darkness and light, we and they, insiders and outsiders ... he relieved his fear of the abyss by cultural constructions, boundary systems and patterns of control that might help him recover his sense of direction ... his moralism found expression in his characteristic vocabulary of order and disorder, purity and contamination" (Bouwsma, 1988, pp. 43, 48, 49). American moralism also sees the world in antithetical categories and seeks boundary systems and patterns of control that will affirm order against disorder. This is a moralism that fits the experience of a people settling in a new land, moving into the western wilderness, immigrating to a strange country among religious and ethnic strangers, affirming individual liberty and social cohesion at the same time.

It might be suspected that one of the favorite ethical arguments in current usage, 'the slippery slope' derives from, or is at least congenial to, American moralism. This argument, closely inspected, seems to assert that while the actual case or issue at hand might be morally acceptable, analogous cases would not be, and thus, the actual case must be prohibited. The move from the actual to the analogous case comes, not through logical or conceptual connections, but from the weakness of will of persons, who are very unlikely to resist the temptation to perform the unacceptable, once the acceptable is allowed them. This distrust of human moral strength is profoundly Jansenistic and Calvinistic.

I am proposing that the confluence of these two streams, flowing from the same source in Calvinist-Augustinian thought, have watered the ground of American culture. The crop that they produce is a strain of moral thinking that deeply believes in clear, unambiguous moral principles, in the ability of common sense to grasp those principles, when common sense is not clouded by self-

Albert R. Jonsen

interest, in the importance of the observance of these principles for the common good of the community. However, the stream beds through which coursed these great rivers of thought are now quite dry: they are, in effect, like the deep canyons of the Southwest, traces of waterways that indelibly mark the landscape.

This metaphor suggests that contemporary American culture is unaware of the sources of its moralism, although the marks made by those sources are manifest. Even aspects of the American moral *mentalité* that seem remote bear its marks. The Paterfamilias of American liberal thought, John Locke, was not immune from the reach of Calvin's thought (Dunn, 1969). Even that quintessential American ethic, pragmatism, was touched by it. One author, entitling his intellectual biography of eight eminent American thinkers, *Puritans and Pragmatists*, finds "a degree of continuity, some elements of underlying unity in the varied and always idiosyncratic thought of these men" – men as different as Jonathan Edwards and John Dewey, John Adams and William James (Conkin, 1968, p. v).

In modern America, moral behaviors seem to represent the widest pluralism; the rigidity of the Calvinist and Jansenist heritage seems to have dissolved into vague tolerance for all but the most outrageous violations. Indeed, an argument can be made that American moralism has been so thoroughly repudiated that nothing remains of it but ridicule. Many would affirm that, far from being moral fundamentalists, modern Americans are moral vagrants, wandering far from any fixed principles. So they may be. However, I believe that the moralism generated by those deep traditions survives in the form, if not the content of the American mentality. Behind our moral vagrancy lives the vague memory of the land of firm and fundamental principles. The recent upsurge of interest in ethics in all aspects of American life flows, I think, in the rivers beds cut by the old traditions.

We have recently seen a resurgence of the old religious fundamentalisms. The moral majority, and their like, emerged to prominence. The stream beds cut by the Calvinist and Jansenist floods begin to fill again. Even apart from this resurgence, we must recognize that everywhere in our culture, even where it is most secular, we can find the remnants of this deep fundamentalism: we may speak of a 'secular fundamentalism'. This describes the same absolutism, the same dichotomous world of good and bad, right and wrong, but shorn of its religious rationale and of its religious sanctions. The fundamentalism of Calvin, the Awakenings and Jansenism had as its rationale what Calvin himself called "the first use of the law," namely, to convict men of their failure to live up to the righteousness of God. It is, he wrote, "a mirror ... in which we see our iniquity" and are driven to repentance (Calvin, 1960, II, VII, p. vii). Such a use of the law demands absolute adherence; it can brook no exceptions or excuses. Secular fundamentalism is equally as rigid but without the religious rationale: it is rigidity that has lost its meaning. Religious fundamentalism was also sanctioned by God's reward and punishment. One could win heaven or deserve hell; no middle place was available (Jansenists, being Catholics, could stop over in purgatory, but only for peccadillos, of which there were not many). Secular fundamentalism retains the ominous seriousness of obedience to the law, but lacks the sanctions of eternal reward and punishment. It is, then, a secular morality, a secular fundamentalism: law, rule and principle detached from religious rationale and sanction.

II. AMERICAN MORALISM AND BIOETHICS

What has this to do with bioethics in the United States? I maintain that the original interest in bioethical issues grew out of American moralism. I do not mean that contemporary fundamentalism had anything to do with the emergence of bioethics: it essentially ignored these issues with the exception of abortion and contraception. I do mean that the remnants of American moralism as they form the characteristic way Americans think about morality had a great deal to do with the origins of bioethics.

The response of American moralism is stimulated by the innovative and the unfamiliar: how is this new thing or this new thought to be drawn into the ordered and clear structure of moral principles? If the world reveals moral truth to the conscientious (the secular substitute for the devout) observer, what does this new thing in the world tell us of moral order? Where is it to be subsumed under the plan of clear and unambiguous principles? Obviously, the ambiguity of the new is intolerable and must be reduced to the clarity of the familiar and accepted.

The actual history of the emergence of bioethics in the United States remains to be written. In the absence of that record, we can start the history where we choose. The options are multiple: the selection of patients for chronic hemodialysis in Seattle in 1962, the initiation of heart transplants in 1969, Beecher's accusation of unethical research in 1966 or the revelation of the Tuskeegee and Willowbrook experiments in 1972. Clearly, the interest was strong enough to support the foundation of the Hastings Center in 1969 and the Kennedy Institute in 1970.

Certainly, one crucial event was the publication of Paul Ramsey's *Patient as Person* in 1970 (Ramsey, 1970). That book gave a text, arcane and turgid, but passionate and reasoned, to the emerging concerns. Properly, the book was written by a man steeped in the theology of Calvin and Edwards and revealed a mind as anxious as Calvin's to bring order to the new chaotic features of contemporary medical science. Ramsey was more comfortable with the title 'moralist' than the new fangled 'ethicist'. His concerns were clearly within the stream of American moralism: he sought principles to bring clarity into confusion and, while admitting room for exceptions, made that room as narrow as possible (Ramsey, 1968). The biblical concept of covenant was as important to him as a theme of moral order as it was to his Puritan ancestors. Although Paul Ramsey was a moral theologian of great sophistication, he rarely moved far from his base in American moralism.

A second event of importance was one in which I played a personal role. I was asked to serve on the Totally Artificial Heart Assessment Panel, formed by Dr. Theodore Cooper, Director of the National Heart and Lung Institute in 1972. This was the first formal acknowledgement of the nascent bioethics movement by the Federal Government. The Panel was asked to assess the "ethical and moral implications of the totally implantable artificial heart" then under study at the Institute and in several research institutions (National Heart and Lung Institute, 1973). I have described the process of this Panel and my own contribution to it elsewhere (Jonsen, 1973). For our purposes here, however, only one point is relevant: the search for 'ethical and moral implications' of this and of other new technologies was likely to diverge from American moralism. Questions were latent in the problem of the artificial heart that required something more than application of principles. The totally implantable heart was powered by an implanted nuclear power device. It was not easy, for example, to find a moral formula that would help in balancing the benefits of several years of continued life for the recipient of the heart against the risks of radiation induced cancer to other unassociated persons.

The Artificial Heart Assessment Panel was followed by a second, major investment of the Federal Government in bioethics. Congress established the National Commission for the Protection of Human Subjects of Biomedical and Behavioral Research. In the wake of several alleged abuses of subjects by researchers, the Congress directed the Commission to devise ways to protect the rights and welfare of the subjects of research. Among the Congressional mandates was the instruction to study the "principles governing biomedical research". The Commission responded to that instruction by producing the Belmont Report in which the ethical principles of beneficence, respect for autonomy and justice were applied to the activities of research (National Commission, 1978).

As a Commissioner, I participated in the formulation of that Report (in fact, its first draft was formulated at a small gathering of Commissioners and consultants in my study in San Francisco). Today, I am skeptical of its status as a serious ethical analysis. I suspect that it is, in effect, a product of American moralism, prompted by the desire of Congressmen and of the public to see the chaotic world of biomedical research reduced to order by clear and unambiguous principles. Fortunately, however, the Commission realized that, despite the statement of principle, the problems posed by doing research in an ethical manner went beyond principle. They were essentially casuistic: requiring a method and mechanism for inspecting each problem on its own terms. Thus, the Commission endorsed the Institutional Review Board as the casuistic forum in which principles would be tested against special circumstances. The IRB is by far more important ethically than the Belmont Report.

A similar reflection could be made on the President's Commission for the Study of Ethical Problems in Medicine, on which I also served. Among the many problems studied by that Commission, one must suffice to illustrate my thesis. The Commission was satisfied that sound ethical analysis demonstrated that no moral obligation could be imposed to provide life support for persons in the clinical condition called "Persistent Vegetative State" (President's Commission, 1983). We believed that this conclusion would be readily accepted by professionals, by the public and by the law. Indeed, it was in the first few cases to come to public attention. However, in the last several years, the matter has become controversial, primarily over the question of the withdrawal of nutrition and hydration. Yet, the ethical reasoning developed to justify the original proposition remains unchallenged in concept and in logic. Ethical argument has encountered American moralism.

The incident with which this essay opened, namely, Dr. Mason's rejection of the deliberations of the ad hoc committee on fetal tissue transplantation now comes into focus. Dr. Mason responded to a message from his 'heart'. I'm sure he did not appreciate the Augustinian, Calvinist, Edwardian and Jansenist undertones of his expression. Still, his decision echoed American moralism. There are clear and unambiguous principles touching all aspects of life. They are known not by the intellect but by the heart. As such, they are profoundly personal, although, strangely, open to all conscientious persons in the moral community. This is American moralism. The reports of the committees, on the other hand, were the products of ethics, an intellectualist, casuistic exercise that dissolved the clarity of principle and appreciated exceptions and consequences over unbreachable rule and immutable value. Thus, Dr. Mason was listening in his conscience to the advice of Jonathan Edwards, "the informing of the understanding is all vain any further than it affects the heart".

I am suggesting that the original impetus for bioethics came from an American moralism that sought to bring the chaos of the new scientific medicine into the order of moral principle. However, the task of doing this fell into the hands of persons who had studied philosophy and theology in quite a different tradition than Calvinist fundamentalism and Jansenist Catholicism. The small group of scholars in the first generation of bioethicists were sceptics within the culture of moralism. They were the intellectuals whom the old fundamentalists so mistrusted. The moral philosophers and moral theologians who became the first bioethicists had read logical positivists, pragmatists, utilitarians and existentialists. Protestant theologians among them were disciples of the Niebuhrs and readers of Kierkegaard. Catholic theologians were struggling free of the legalism and authoritarianism that had entrapped Catholic moral theology. Clarity of method was more salient an issue than clarity of principle; moral ambiguity was more respectable a stance than moral certitude (Fr. Richard McCormick's first major contribution was a small book entitled *Ambiguity in Moral Choice*) (McCormick, 1973). While in the beginning, the misfit was not noted, it has become slowly manifest. Today, the ethical analysis of the moral philosophers and theologians who do bioethics is much more likely to produce 'probabilistic' opinions, that is, a range of options that enjoy greater or less probability in terms of the strength of rational argument and logic that support them. This is dismaying to American moralism. The recent collapse of the attempt to establish a Congressional Bioethics Commission and the failure to have reestablished the Ethics Advisory Board may be symptoms of the misfit. The work of ethicists can no longer be expected to uphold the clear and unambiguous principles of American moralism. Those who affirm these principles can only suffer from Calvinist anxiety in the presence of those more likely to allow exceptions than to uphold principles. They suffer from the pervasive effect of American moralism which is, at certain points, unshakably resistant to the intellectual analysis of the devils, the bioethicists.

III. THE 'DEVILS' OF BIOETHICS EDUCATION

It is, of course, those devils who teach bioethics to medical students and to physicians and nurses. Despite the popularity of their courses and lectures, are they not going against the grain of the American *mentalité*? How does their activity in the classroom and on the podium fit in with American moralism? As I noted above, very few of these bioethicists preach the American moralism or even think in its format. Most of them are 'ethicists', who are more comfortable with complexity, qualifications and hypotheses than with laws and rules. Still, many who teach modern bioethics will encounter the remnants of moralism in themselves and in their students.

The remnant of moralism in the mind of the American bioethicists is the insistent lure of principles. Since bioethics began to take shape as a discipline, its scholars adopted a peculiarly American approach to ethical analysis, namely, the application of a few clear and distinct principles to the problems of bioethics. Autonomy, beneficence, non-maleficence and justice became the bioethicists' distant echoes of the Calvinist's Decalogue. These principles were law-like statements that presumably were comprehensive, covering all moral questions that could arise. In effect, when the bioethicists 'applied' these principles to cases, they became crypto-casuists, appreciating the circumstances and the constraints of the situation as much as, if not more than, the principle. Yet, it has been difficult to persuade the bioethicists that casuistry is an alternative approach to moral problems that, while not dispensing with principle, insists that principle prove itself in the case. Similarly, other 'looser' approaches to moral life, relying on 'virtues' rather than principles, have not been much appreciated.

Moralism shows itself in the students in several ways. Every teacher of ethics is aware that the contemporary American student is a convinced, but unreflective, moral relativist. The first task in any ethics course is to argue the students out of that unreflective relativism. The relativism comes, in my opinion, from the impression that hardly anyone today puts much credence in moral absolutes. If there are no moral absolutes, then all moral opinion is relative (whatever that is supposed to mean). This sort of thought represents the ruins of American moralism: a view that maintains that morality can *only* consist of absolutes. The teacher of ethics will continually hear students contrast 'ethics' with 'pragmatism' or utilitarianism'. In order for anything to rank as 'ethical', it seems, no room for calculations, predictions, qualifications, exceptions, etc., can be allowed!

If the teacher of bioethics wishes to convey the methods of casuistry, he or she runs the perils of reinforcing this unreflective relativism. The student who equates morality with absolute principles is likely to see any ethical analysis that respects exceptions and exemptions as immorality or at least 'situationism' (which is, in effect, amorality). The remnants of American moralism makes the teaching of modern medical ethics both welcome and difficult. The deep (and often deeply buried) conviction that life, personal and professional, ought to be morally serious is a remnant of moralism. Its echo in the American spirit renders us ready to listen to those who can expound on the implications of that moral seriousness. On the other hand, the belief that morality is a structure of law-like commands, rules and principles, rather than a tissue of maxims, circumstances, motives, intentions and habits, makes it difficult to expound on the moral seriousness in anything more than generalities. Everyone quickly learns to affirm the principle of autonomy, the clearest principle and the favorite of most students; very few learn to modulate that principle in relationship to beneficence and justice and in the light of virtues such as compassion and appreciation of moral solidarity. We have been brought to bioethics by American moralism; we must discover how to exploit its moral strength without being trapped in its moral bonds.

REFERENCES

Abercrombie, N.: 1936, *The Origins of Jansenism*, Oxford University Press, Oxford.

Bowsma, W.J.: 1988, *John Calvin, A Sixteenth Century Portrait*, Oxford University Press, New York.

Calvin, John: 1960, *Institutes of the Christian Religion*, Westminster Press, Philadelphia.

Conkin, P.: 1968, *Puritans and Pragmatists*, Dodd, Mead, New York.

Dolan, J.: 1978, *Catholic Revivalism. The American Experience 1830–1900*, University of Notre Dame Press, Notre Dame, Indiana.

Dunn, John: 1969, *The Political Thought of John Locke. An Historical Account of the Argument of the Two Treatises of Government*, Cambridge University Press, London.

Edwards, Jonathan: 1959, *Religious Affections*, in J. Smith (ed.), *The Works of Jonathn Edwards*, Yale University Press, New Haven, Connecticut.

Ellis, J.T.: 1971, 'The formation of the American priest: A historical perspective', in J.T. Ellis (ed.), *The Catholic Priest in the United States*, St. John's University Press, Collegeville, Minnesota.

Fiering, N.: 1981, *Moral Philosophy at 17th Century Harvard*, University of North Carolina Press, Williamsburg.

Jonsen, A.R.: 1973, 'The totally implantable artificial heart', *Hastings Center Report* 3, 1–4.

Jonsen, A.R. and Toulmin, S.E.: 1988, *The Abuse of Casuistry*, University of California, Berkeley and Los Angeles.

McCormick, R.A.: 1973, *Ambiguity in Moral Choice*, Marquette University Press, Milwaukee, Minnesota.

Marsden, G.M.: 1980, *Fundamentalism in American Culture*, Oxford University Press, New York.

Miller, Perry: 1962, *The New England Mind*, Harvard University Press, Cambridge, Mass., 2 vols.

Miller, Perry: 1965: *The Life of the Mind in America*, Harcourt, Brace, New York.

Morgan, E.S.: 1963, *Visible Saints. The History of a Puritan Idea*, New York University Press, New York.

National Commission for the Protection of Human Subjects of Biomedical and Behavioral Research: 1978, *The Belmont Report. Ethical Principles and Guidelines for Research Involving Human Subjects*, Government Printing Office, Washington, D.C.

National Heart and Lung Institute: 1973, *The Totally Implantable Artificial Heart*.

130   *Albert R. Jonsen*

Legal, Social, Ethical, Medical, Economic and Psychological Implications. A Report of the Artificial Heart Assessment Panel, Department of Health, Education and Welfare, Washington, D.C.

The New York Times: 1990, 'Words to survive life with: None of this, none of that', May 27.

The New York Times: 1989, 'Ban extended on research using fetal tissue', November 2.

New Catholic Encyclopedia: 1967, 'Jansenism', McGraw-Hill, New York.

President's Commission for the Study of Ethical Problems in Medicine: 1983, *Deciding to Forego Life Sustaining Treatments*, The Government Printing Office, Washington, D.C.

Ramsey, P.: 1968, 'The case of the curious exception', in G.H. Outka and P. Ramsey (eds.), *Norm and Context in Christian Ethics*, Scribner's, New York.

Ramsey, P.: 1970, *The Patient as Person*, Yale University Press, New Haven, Connecticut.

Tawney, R.H.: 1926, *Religion and the Rise of Capitalism*, Harcourt, Brace, New York.

Weber, Max: 1954, *The Protestant Ethic and the Spirit of Capitalism*, Scribner's, New York.

[2]

HOW MEDICINE SAVED THE LIFE OF ETHICS

Stephen Toulmin

During the first 60 years or so of the twentieth century, two things characterized the discussion of ethical issues in the United States, and to some extent other English-speaking countries also. On the one hand, the theoretical analyses of moral philosophers concentrated on questions of so-called metaethics. Most professional philosophers assumed that their proper business was not to take sides on substantive ethical questions but rather to consider in a more formal way what kinds of issues and judgments are properly classified as moral in the first place. On the other hand, in less academic circles, ethical debates repeatedly ran into stalemate. A hard-line group of dogmatists, who appealed either to a code of universal rules or to the authority of a religious system or teacher, confronted a rival group of relativists, and subjectivists, who found in the anthropological and psychological diversity of human attitudes evidence to justify a corresponding diversity in moral convictions and feelings.[1]

For those who sought some 'rational' way of settling ethical disagreements, there developed a period of frustration and perplexity.[2] Faced with the spectacle of rival camps taking up sharper opposed ethical positions (e.g. toward premarital sex or anti-Semitism), they turned in vain to the philosophers for guidance. Hoping for intelligent and perceptive comments on the actual substance of such issues, they were offered only analytical classifications, which sought to locate the realm of moral issues, not to decide them.

Two novel factors contributed to this standoff by making the issue

265

III: The future of ethics

of subjectivity an active and urgent one. For a start, developments in psychology – not least, the public impact of the new psychoanalytic movement – focused attention on the role of feelings in our experience and so reinforced the suspicion that moral opinions have to do more with our emotional reactions to that experience than with our actions in it [3]. So, those opinions came to appear less matters of reason than matters of taste, falling under the old tag, *quot homines. tot sententiae*. This view of ethics was strengthened by the arguments of the ethnographers and anthropologists, who emphasized the differences to be found between the practices and attitudes of different peoples rather than the common core of problems, institutions, and patterns of life that they share. To cap it all, the anthropologist Edward Westermarck took over Albert Einstein's term 'relativity' from physics and discussed the moral implications of anthropology under the title of *Ethical Relativity* [4].

Between them, the new twentieth-century behavioral and social sciences were widely regarded as supporting subjectivist and relativist postitions in ethics; this in turn provoked a counterinsistence on the universal and unconditional character of moral principles; and so a battle was joined which could have no satisfactory outcome. For, in case of substantive disagreement, the absolutists had no further reasons to offer for their positions: all they could do was shout more insistently or bring up heavier theological guns. In return, the relativists could only turn away and shrug their shoulders. The final answers to ethical problems thus came, on one side, from unquestioned principles and authoritative commands; on the other, from variable and diverse wishes, feelings, or attitudes; and no agreed procedure for settling disagreements by reasonble argument was acceptable to both sides.

How did the fresh attention that philosophers began paying to the ethics of medicine, beginning around 1960, move the ethical debate beyond this standoff? It did so in four different ways. In place of the earlier concern with attitudes, feelings, and wishes, it substituted a new preoccupation with situations, needs, and interests; it required writers on applied ethics to go beyond the discussion of general principles and rules to a more scrupulous analysis of the particular kinds of 'cases' in which they find their application; it redirected that analysis to the professional enterprises within which so many human tasks and duties typically arise; and, finally, it pointed philosophers back to the ideas of 'equity,' 'resaonableness,' and

How medicine saved the life of ethics

'human relationships,' which played central roles in the *Ethics* of Aristotle but subsequently dropped out of sight [5, esp. 5.10.1136b30–1137b32]. Here, those four points may be considered in turn.

THE OBJECTIVITY OF INTERESTS

The topics that preoccupied psychologists and anthropologists alike during the first half of the twentieth century were foreign to the concerns of physicians, and they tended to distract attention from those shared features of human nature which define the physiological aspects of human medicine and so help to determine the associated ethical demands. To begin with, the novel anthropological discoveries that exerted most charm over the general public were those customs, or modes of behavior, which appeared odd, unexpected, or even bizarre, as compared with the normal patterns of life familiar in modern industrial societies. The distinctive features of unfamiliar cultures (rain dances, witch doctors, initiation ceremonies, taboos, and the like) captured the imaginations of general readers far more powerfully than those which manifested the common heritage of humanity: the universal need to eat and drink, the shared interest in tending wounds and injuries, and so on. Theoretically, likewise, field anthropologists focused primarily on the differences among cultures, leaving the universals of social structure to the sister science of sociology. In their eyes, the essential thing was to explain the modes of life and activity typical of any culture in terms appropriate to that particular culture, not in terms brought in from outside with the anthropologist's own cultural baggage.

As a result, the whole field of medicine was something of a stumbling block to anthropology. If one studied the procedures employed in handling cases of tuberculosis among, say, pygmies in the Kalahari Desert, it might well turn out that they did not recognize this affliction as being, by Western standards, a true 'disease.' In that case it might – anthropologically speaking – be inappropriate to comment on their procedures in medical terms at all. On the contrary, witch doctoring must be appraised in 'ethnomedical' terms, by standards adapted to the conception of witch doctoring current inside the culture in question.

267

III: The future of ethics

For those who were concerned with the internal systematicity of a given culture, this might be an acceptable method. In adopting it, however, one was obliged to set aside some of the basic presuppositions of the modern Western (and international) profession of medicine: notably, the assumption that human beings in all cultures share, in most respects, common bodily frames and physiological functions. While the epidemiology of, say, heart disease may in some respects be significantly affected by such cultural factors as diet, the evils of heart disease speak no particular language, and to that extent the efficacy of different procedures for dealing with that condition can be appraised in transcultural terms.

So, the *cross*-cultural study of epidemiology and kindred subjects – what may be called 'comparative medicine' – has to be distinguished sharply from the *intra*cultural study of 'ethnomedicine.' The latter is concerned with the attitudes, customs, and feelings current within exotic cultures in the face of those afflictions that we ourselves know to be diseases, whether or not the people concerned so perceive them. The former, by contrast, is concerned with the treatments available in different countries or cultures, regardless of the special attitudes, customs, or feelings that may cluster around those conditions locally, in one place or another. Fieldworkers from the World Heath Organization, for instance, are concerned with comparative medicine and are not deterred from investigating the links between, say, eye disease and polluted water supplies just because members of the affected community do not recognize these links. The central subject matter of medicine thus comprises those objective, universal conditions, afflictions, and needs that can affect human beings in *every* culture, as contrasted with those relative, subjective conditions, complaints, and wishes that are topics for anthropological study in *any given* culture.

Now we are in a position to see how needlessly moral philosophers thrust themselves into the arms of the 'ethical relativists' when they adopted anthropology as their example and foundation. An ethics built around cultural differences quickly became an ethics of local attitudes. The same fate overtook those philosophers who sought their example and foundation in the new ideas of early twentieth-century psychology. For they were quickly led into seeing ethical disagreements between one human being and another as rooted in their personal responses to and feelings about the topics in debate; as a result, questions about the soundness of rival moral

How medicine saved the life of ethics

views were submerged by questions about their origins.

Contrast, for instance, the statement, 'She regards premarital sex as wrong *because* her own straitlaced upbringing left her jealous of, and censorious toward, today's less puritanical young' – which offers us a psychological account of the causes by which the ethical view in question was supposedly generated – with the statement, 'She regards it as wrong because of the unhappiness which the current wave of teenage pregnancies is creating for mothers and offspring alike' – which states the interests with which the view is concerned and the reasons by which it is supported. Modeling ethics on psychology thus once again diverts attention from genuine interests and focuses them instead on labile, personal feelings.

The new attention to applied ethics (particularly medical ethics) has done much to dispel the miasma of subjectivity that was cast around ethics as a result of its association with anthropology and psychology. At least within broad limits, an ethics of 'needs' and 'interests' is objective and generalizable in a way that an ethics of 'wishes' and 'attitudes' cannot be. Stated crudely, the question of whether one person's actions put another person's health at risk is normally a question of ascertainable fact, to which there is a straightforward 'yes' or 'no' answer, not a question of fashion, custom, or taste, about which (as the saying goes) 'there is no arguing.' This being so, the objections to that person's actions can be presented and discussed in 'objective' terms. So, proper attention to the example of medicine has helped to pave the way for a reintroduction of 'objective' standards of good and harm and for a return to methods of practical reasoning about moral issues that are not available to either the dogmatists or the relativists.

THE IMPORTANCE OF CASES

One writer who was already contributing to the renewed discussion of applied ethics as early as the 1950s was Joseph Fletcher of the University of Virginia, who has recently been the object of harsh criticism from more dogmatic thinkers for introducing the phrase 'situation ethics.'[3] To judge from his critics' tone, you might think that he was the spokesman for laxity and amorality, whereas he belongs, in fact, to a very respectable line of Protestant (specifically, Episcopalian) moral theologians. A main influence on him in his

III: The future of ethics

youth was Bishop Kenneth Kirk, whose book on *Conscience and Its Problems*, published in 1927 [9], was one of the few systematic works by an early twentieth-century Protestant theologian to employ the 'case method' more usually associated with the Catholic casuists. Via Kirk, Fletcher thus became an inheritor of the older Evangelical tradition of Frederick Dennison Maurice.[4]

Like his predecessors in the consideration of 'cases of conscience,' Kirk was less concerned to discuss conduct in terms of abstract rules and principles than he was to address in concrete detail the moral quandaries in which real people actually find themselves. Like his distinguished predecessors – from Aristotle and Hermagoras to Boethius, Aquinas, and the seventeenth-century Jesuits – he understood very well the force of the old maxim, 'circumstances alter cases.' As that maxim indicates, we can understand fully what is at stake in any human situation and how it creates moral problems for the agents involved in it only if we know the precise circumstances 'both of the agent and of the act': if we lack that knowledge, we are in no position to say anything of substance about the situation, and all our appeals to general rules and principles will be mere hot air. So, in retrospect, Joseph Fletcher's introduction of the phrase 'situation ethics' can be viewed as one further chapter in a history of 'the ethics of cases,' as contrasted with 'the ethics of rules and principles'; this is another area in which the ethics of medicine has recently given philosophers some useful pointers for the analysis of moral issues.

Let me here mention one of these, which comes out of my own personal experience. From 1975 to 1978 I worked as a consultant and staff member with the National Commission for the Protection of Human Subjects of Biomedical and Behavioral Research, based in Washington, D.C.; I was struck by the extent to which the commissioners were able to reach agreement in making recommendations about ethical issues of great complexity and delicacy.[5] If the earlier theorists had been right, and ethical considerations really depended on variable cultural attitudes or labile personal feelings, one would have expected 11 people of such different backgrounds as the members of the commission to be far more divided over such moral questions than they ever proved to be in actual fact. Even on such thorny subjects as research involving prisoners, mental patients, and human fetuses, it did not take the commissioners long to identify the crucial issues that they needed to

How medicine saved the life of ethics

address, and, after patient analysis of these issues, any residual differences of opinion were rarely more than marginal, with different commissioners inclined to be somewhat more conservative, or somewhat more liberal, in their recommendations. Never, as I recall, did their deliberations end in deadlock, with supporters of rival principles locking horns and refusing to budge. The problems that had to be argued through at length arose, not on the level of the principles themselves, but at the point of applying them: when difficult moral balances had to be struck between, for example, the general claims of medical discovery and its future beneficiaries and the present welfare or autonomy of individual research subjects.

How was the commission's consensus possible? It rested precisely on this last feature of their agenda: namely, its close concentration on specific types of problematic cases. Faced with 'hard cases,' they inquired what particular conflicts of claim or interest were exemplified in them, and they usually ended by balancing off those claims in very similar ways. Only when the individual members of the commission went on to explain their own particular 'reasons' for supporting the general consensus did they begin to go seriously different ways. For, then, commissioners from different backgrounds and faiths 'justified' their votes by appealing to general views and abstract principles which differed far more deeply than their opinions about particular substantive questions. Instead of 'deducing' their opinions about particular cases from general principles that could lend strength and conviction to those specific opinions, they showed a far greater certitude about particular cases than they ever achieved about general matters.

This outcome of the commission's work should not come as any great surprise to physicians who have reflected deeply about the nature of clinical judgment in medicine. In traditional case morality, as in medical practice, the first indispensable step is to assemble a rich enough 'case history.' Until that has been done, the wise physician will suspend judgment. If he is too quick to let theoretical considerations influence his clinical analysis, they may prejudice the collection of a full and accurate case record and so distract him from what later turn out to have been crucial clues. Nor would this outcome have been any surprise to Aristotle, either. Ethics and clinical medicine are both prime examples of the concrete fields of thought and reasoning in which (as he insisted) the theoretical rigor of geometrical argument is unattainable: fields in which we should

271

III: The future of ethics

above all strive to be *reasonable* rather than insisting on a kind of *exactness* that 'the nature of the case' does not allow [5, 1.3.1094b12–27].

This same understanding of the differences between practical and theoretical reasoning was taken over by Aquinas, who built it into his own account of 'natural law' and 'case morality,' and so it became part of the established teaching of Catholic moral theologians. As such, it was in harmony with the pastoral practices of the confessional [12, D.3, Q.5, A.2, Solutio]. Thus, Aquinas's own version of the fundamental maxim was framed as an injunction to the confessor – 'like a prudent physician' – to take into account *peccatoris circumstantiae atque peccati*, that is, 'the circumstances both of the sinner and of the sin.' Later, however, the alleged readiness of confessors to soften their judgments in the light of irrelevant 'circumstances' exposed them to criticism. In particular, the seventeenth-century French Jesuits were attacked by their Jansenist coreligionists on the ground that they 'made allowances' in favor of rich and high-born penitents that they denied to those who were less well favored. And, when the Jansenist Arnauld was brought before an ecclesiastical court on a charge of heterodoxy, his friend Pascal launched a vigorous counter attack on the Jesuit casuists of his time by publishing the series of anonymous *Lettres provinciales* which from that time on gave 'casuistry' its unsavory reputation.[6]

By taking one step further, indeed, we may view the problems of clinical medicine and the problems of applied ethics as two varieties of a common species. Defined in purely general terms, such ethical categories as 'cruelty' and 'kindness,' 'laziness' and 'conscientiousness,' have a certain abstract, truistical quality: before they can acquire any specific relevance, we have to identify some actual person, or piece of conduct, as 'kind' or 'cruel,' 'conscientious' or 'lazy,' and there is often disagreement even about that preliminary step. Similarly, in medicine; if described in general terms alone, diseases too are 'abstract entities,' and they acquire a practical relevance only for those who have learned the diagnostic art of identifying real-life cases as being cases of one disease rather than another.

In its form (if not entirely in its point) the art of practical judgment in ethics thus resembles the art of clinical diagnosis and prescription. In both fields, theoretical generalities are helpful to us only up to a point, and their actual application to particular cases demands, also, a human capacity to recognize the slight but signifi-

How medicine saved the life of ethics

cant features that mark off, say, a 'case' of minor muscular strain from a life-threatening disease or a 'case' of decent reticence from one of cowardly silence. Once brought to the bedside, so to say, applied ethics and clinical medicine use just the same Aristotelean kinds of 'practical reasoning,' and a correct choice of therapeutic procedure in medicine is the *right* treatment to pursue, not just as a matter of technique but for ethical reasons also.

In the last decades of the nineteenth-century, F.H. Bradley of Oxford University expounded an ethical position that placed 'duties' in the center of the philosophical picture, and the recent concern of moral philosophers with applied ethics (most specifically, medical ethics) has given them a new insight into his arguments also. It was a mistake (Bradley argued) to discuss moral obligations purely in universalistic terms, as though nobody was subject to moral claims unless they applied to everybody – unless we could, according to the Kantian formula, 'will them to become universal laws.' On the contrary, different people are subject to different moral claims, depending on where they 'stand' toward the other people with whom they have to deal, for example, their families, colleagues, and fellow citizens [13].

As the modern discussion of medical ethics has taught us, professional affiliations and concerns play a significant part in shaping a physician's obligations and commitments, and this insight has stimulated detailed discussions both about professionalism in general and, more specifically, about the relevance of 'the physician/patient relationship' to the medical practitioner's duties and obligations.[8]

Once embarked on, the subject of professionalism has proved to be rich and fruitful. It has led, for instance, to a renewed interest in Max Weber's sociological analysis of vocation (*Beruf*) and bureaucracy, and this in turn has had implications of two kinds for the ethics of the professions. For, on the one hand, the manner in which professionals perceive their position as providers of service influences both their sense of calling and also the obligations which they acknowledge on that account. And, on the other hand, the professionalization of medicine, law, and similar activities has exposed practitioners to new conflicts of interest between, for example, the individual physician's duties to a patient and his loyalty to the profession, as when his conduct is criticized as 'unprofessional' for harming, not his clients, but rather his colleagues.

273

III: The future of ethics

In recent years, as a result, moral philosophers have begun to look specifically and in greater detail at the situations within which ethical problems typically arise and to pay closer attention to the human relationships that are embodied in those situations. In ethics, as elsewhere, the tradition of radical individualism for too long encouraged people to overlook the 'mediating structures' and 'intermediate institutions' (family, profession, voluntary associations, etc.) which stand between the individual agent and the larger scale context of his actions. So, in political theory, the obligations of the individual toward the state was seen as the only problem worth focusing on; meanwhile, in moral theory, the difference of status (or station) which in practice expose us to different sets of obligations (or duties) were ignored in favor of a theory of justice (or rights) that deliberately concealed these differences behind a 'veil of ignorance.'[9]

On this alternative view, the only just – even, properly speaking, the only moral – obligations are those that apply to us all equally, regardless of our standing. By undertaking the tasks of a profession, an agent will no doubt accept certain special duties, but so it will be for us all. The obligation to perform those duties is 'just' or 'moral' only because it exemplifies more general and universalizable obligations of trust, which require us to do what we have undertaken to do. So, any exclusive emphasis on the universal aspects of morality can end by distracting attention from just those things which the student of applied ethics finds most absorbing – namely, the specific tasks and obligations that any profession lays on its practitioners.

Most recently, Alasdair MacIntyre has pursued these considerations further in his new book, *After Virtue* [16]. MacIntyre argues that the public discussion of ethical issues has fallen into a kind of Babel, which largely springs from our losing any sense of the ways in which *community* creates obligations for us. One thing that can help restore that lost sense of community is the recognition that, at the present time, our professional commitments have taken on many of the roles that our communal commitments used to play. Even people who find moral philosophy generally unintelligible usually acknowledge and respect the specific ethical demands associated with their own professions or jobs, and this offers us some kind of a foundation on which to begin reconstructing our view of ethics. For it reminds us that we are in no position to fashion individual lives for

How medicine saved the life of ethics

ourselves, purely *as individuals*. Rather, we find ourselves born into communities in which the available ways of acting are largely laid out in advance: in which human activity takes on different *Lebensformen*, or 'forms of life' (of which the professions are one special case), and our obligations are shaped by the requirements of those forms.

EQUITY AND INTIMACY

Two final themes have also attracted special attention as a result of the new interaction between medicine and philosophy. Both themes were presented in clear enough terms by Aristotle in the *Nicomachean Ethics*. But, as so often happens, the full force of Aristotle's concepts and arguments was overlooked by subsequent generations of philosophers, who came to ethics with very different preoccupations. Aristotle's own Greek terms for these notions are *epieikeia* and *philia*, which are commonly translated as 'reasonableness' and 'friendship,' but I shall argue here that they correspond more closely to the modern terms, 'equity' and 'personal relationship' [5].

Modern readers sometimes have difficulty with the style of Aristotle's *Ethics* and lose patience with the book, because they suspect the author of evading philosophical questions that they have their own reasons for regarding as central. Suppose, for instance, that we go to Aristotle's text in the hope of finding some account of the things that mark off 'right' from 'wrong': if we attempt to press this question, Aristotle will always slip out of our grasp. What makes one course of action better than another? We can answer that question, he replies, only if we first consider what kind of a person the agent is and what relationships he stands in toward the other people who are involved in his actions; he sets about explaining why the kinds of relationship, and the kinds of conduct, that are possible as between 'large-spirited human beings' who share the same social standing are simply not possible as between, say, master and servant, or parent and child [5].

The bond of *philia* between free and equal friends is of one kind, that between father and son of another kind, that between master and slave of a third, and there is no common scale in which we can measure the corresponding kinds of conduct. By emphasizing this

III: The future of ethics

point, Aristotle draws attention to an important point about the manner in which 'actions' are classified, even before we say anything ethical about them. Within two different relationships the very same deeds, or the very same words, may – from the ethical point of view – represent quite different *acts* or *actions*. Words that would be a perfectly proper command from an officer to an enlisted man or a straightforward order from a master to a servant, might be a humiliation if uttered by a father to a son, or an insult if exchanged between friends. A judge may likewise have a positive duty to say, from the bench, things that he would never dream of saying in a situation where he was no longer acting *ex officio*, while a physician may have occasion, and even be obliged, to do things to a patient in the course of a medical consultation that he would never be permitted to do in any other context.

With this as background, we can turn to Aristotle's ideas about *epieikeia* ('reasonableness' or 'equity'). As to this notion, Aristotle pioneered the general doctrine that principles never settle ethical issues by themselves: that is, that we can grasp the moral force of principles only by studying the ways in which they are applied to, and within, particular situations. The need for such a practical approach is most obvious, in judicial practice, in the exercise of 'equitable jurisdiction,' where the courts are required to decide cases by appeal, not to specific, well-defined laws or statutes, but to general considerations of fairness, of 'maxims of equity.' In these situations, the courts do not have the benefit of carefully drawn rules, which have been formulated with the specific aim that they should be precise and self-explanatory: rather, they are guided by rough proverbial mottoes – phrases about 'clean hands' and the like. The questions at issue in such cases are, in other words, very broad questions – for example, about what would be *just* or *reasonable* as between two or more individuals when all the available facts about their respective situations have been taken into account [17–19]. Similar patterns of situations and arguments are, of course, to be found in everday ethics also, and the Aristotelean idea of *epieikeia* is a direct intellectual ancestor of a central notion (still referred to as 'epikeia') in the Roman Catholic traditions of moral theology and pastoral care [11].

In ethics and law alike, the two ideas of *philia* ('friendship' or 'relationship') and *epieikeia* (or 'equity') are closely connected. The expectations that we place on people's lines of conduct will differ

How medicine saved the life of ethics

markedly depending on who is affected and what relationships the parties stand in toward one another. Far from regarding it as 'fair' or 'just' to deal with everybody in a precisely *equal* fashion, as the 'veil of ignorance' might suggest, we consider it perfectly *equitable*, or *reasonable*, to show some degree of partiality, or favor, in dealing with close friends and relatives whose special needs and concerns we understand. What father, for instance, does not have an eye to his children's individual personalities and tastes? And, apart from downright 'favoritism,' who would regard such differences of treatment as unjust? Nor, surely, can it be morally offensive to discriminate, within reason, between close friends and distant acquaintances, colleagues and business rivals, neighbours and strangers? We are who we are: we stand in the human relationships we do, and our specific moral duties and obligations can be discussed in practice *only* at the point at which these questions of personal standing and relationship have been recognized and taken into the account.

CONCLUSION

From the mid-nineteenth century on, then, British and American moral philosophers treated ethics as a field for general theoretical inquiries and paid little attention to issues of application or particular types of cases. The philosopher who did most to inaugurate this new phase was Henry Sidgwick, and, from an autobiographical note, we know that he was reacting against the work of his contemporary, William Whewell [20, 21]. Whewell had written a textbook for use by undergraduates at Cambridge University that resembled in many respects a traditional manual of casuistics, containing separate sections on the ethics of promises or contracts, family and community, benevolence, and so on [22]. For his part, Sidgwick found Whewell's discussion too messy: there must be some way of introducing into the subject the kinds of rigor, order, and certainty associated with, for example, mathematical reasoning. So, ignoring all of Aristotle's cautions about the differences between the practical modes of reasoning approprite to ethics and the formal modes appropriate to mathematics, he set out to expound the theoretical principles (or 'methods') of ethics in a systematic form.

By the early twentieth century, the new program for moral philosophy had been narrowed down still further, so initiating the

III: The future of ethics

era of 'metaethics.' The philosopher's task was no longer to organize our moral beliefs into comprehensive systems: that would have meant *taking sides* over substantive issues. Rather, it was his duty to stand back from the fray and hold the ring while partisans of different views argued out their differences in accordance with the general rules for the conduct of 'rational debate,' or the expression of 'moral attitudes,' as defined in *metaethical* terms. And this was still the general state of affairs in Anglo-American moral philosophy in the late 1950s and the early 1960s, when public attention began to turn to questions of medical ethics. By this time, the central concerns of the philosophers had become so abstract and general – above all, so definitional or analytical – that they had, in effect, lost all touch with the concrete and particular issues that arise in actual practice, whether in medicine or elsewhere.

Once this demand for intelligent discussion of the ethical problems of medical practice and research obliged them to pay fresh attention to applied ethics, however, philosophers found their subject 'coming alive again' under their hands. But, now it was no longer a field of academic, theoretical, even mandarin investigation alone. Instead, it had to be debated in practical, concrete, even political terms, and before long moral philosophers (or, as they barbarously began to be called, 'ethicists')[10] found that they were as liable as the economists to be called on to write 'op ed' pieces for the *New York Times*, or to testify before congressional committees.

Have philosophers wholly risen to this new occasion? Have they done enough to modify their previous methods of analysis to meet these new practical needs? About those questions there can still be several opinions. Certainly, it would be foolhardy to claim that the discussion of 'bioethics' has reached a definitive form, or to rule out the possibility that novel methods will earn a place in the field in the years ahead. At this very moment, indeed, the style of current discussion appears to be shifting away from attempts to relate problematic cases to general theories – whether those of Kant, Rawls, or the utilitarians – to a more direct analysis of the practical cases themselves, using methods more like those of traditional 'case morality.' (See, e.g., the discussion in a recent issue of the *Hastings Center Report* of the moral issues that are liable to arise in cases of sex-change surgery [23, pp. 8–13].)

Whatever the future may bring, however, these 20 years of interaction with medicine, law, and the other professions have had

How medicine saved the life of ethics

spectacular and irreversible effects on the methods and content of philosophical ethics. By reintroducing into ethical debate the vexed topics raised by *particular cases*, they have obliged philosophers to address once again the Aristotelean problems of *practical reasoning*, which had been on the sidelines for too long. In this sense, we may indeed say that, during the last 20 years, medicine has 'saved the life of ethics,' and that it has given back to ethics a seriousness and human relevance which it had seemed – at least, in the writings of the interwar years – to have lost for good.

NOTES

This paper is one outcome of a research project undertaken in collaboration with Dr. Albert R. Jonsen, of the University of California at San Francisco, with the support of a grant from the National Endowment for the Humanities, no. RO–0086–79–1466.

*Committee on Social Thought, Department of Philosophy and Divinity School, University of Chicago.

1 For a further exploration of the standoff, see [1].
2 It was, in fact, just this problem which presented itself to me when I wrote my doctoral dissertation [2].
3 Just how much of a pioneer Joseph Fletcher was in opening up the modern discussion of the ethics of medicine is clear from the early publication date (1954) of his first publications on this subject [6–8].
4 It was Albert Jonsen who drew my attention to the work of Kenneth Kirk and his great forerunner, the mid-nineteenth-century Evangelical teacher, F.D. Maurice [10]. For further discussion consult A.R. Jonsen [11].
5 The work of the national commissions generated a whole series of government publications – mainly reports and recommendations on the ethical aspects of research involving research subjects from specially 'vulnerable' groups having diminished autonomy, such as young children and prisoners. I have written a fuller discussion of the commission's work for a forthcoming Hastings Center book on the 'closure' of disputes about matters of technical policy. As a member of the commission, A.R. Jonsen was also struck by the casuistical character of its work, and this led to the research project of which this paper is one product.
6 The *Lettres provincales* were published periodically, and anonymously, in 1656–57, but it did not take long for their authorship to be discovered, and they have remained perhaps the best-known documents on the

III: The future of ethics

subject of 'case reasoning' in ethics. The intellectual relationships between the vigorous attack on the laxity of the Jesuits' case morality contained in the *Lettres* and the larger program of seventeenth-century philosophy deserves closer study than it has yet received.

7 For the word 'casuistry,' see the entry in the complete *Oxford English Dictionary*, which revealingly points out how many English nouns ending in 'ry' (e.g., 'Sophistry,' 'wizardry,' and 'Propery') are dyslogistic. It seems to be no accident that the earliest use of the word 'casuistry' cited in the *OED* dates only from 1725 – i.e., after Pascal's attack on the Jesuit casuists. This helps to explain, and confirm, the current derogatory tone of the word.

8 See Bledstein's discussion [14, p. 107] of the nineteenth-century confusion between codes of ethics and codes of etiquette within such professional societies as the American Medical Association.

9 I borrow this phrase a trifle unfairly from John Rawls [15], but I have argued at greater length in [1] that *any* unbalanced emphasis on 'universality' divorced from 'equity' is a recipe for the ethics of relations between strangers and leaves untouched those important issues that arise between people who are linked by more complex relationships.

10 Once again, the *Oxford English Dictionary* has a point to make. It includes the word 'ethicist' but leaves it without the dignity of a definition, beyond the bare etymology, 'ethics + ist.'

REFERENCES

1 Toulim, S. The tyranny of principles. *Hastings Cent. Rep.* 11:6, 1981.
2 Toulmin, S. *The Place of Reason in Ethics*. Cambridge: Cambridge University Press, 1949.
3 Stevenson, C.L. *Ethics and Language*. New Haven, Conn.: Yale University Press, 1944.
4 Westermarck, E. *Ethical Relativity*. New York: Harcourt Brace, 1932.
5 Aristotle. *Nicomachean Ethics*.
6 Fletcher, J. *Morals and Medicine*. Princeton, N.J.: Princeton University Press, 1954.
7 Fletcher, J. *Situation Ethics*. Philadelphia: Westminster, 1966.
8 Fletcher, J. *Humanhood*. Buffalo, N.Y.: Prometheus, 1979.
9 Kirk, K. *Conscience and Its Problems*, 1927.
10 Maurice, F. *Conscience: Lectures on Casuistry Delivered in the University of Cambridge*, London, 1872.
11 Jonsen, A.R. Can an ethicist be a consultant? In *Frontiers in Medical Ethics*, edited by A. Abernathy. Cambridge: Bollingen. 1980.
12 Aquinas, Thomas. *Commentarium Libro Tertio Sententiarum*.
13 Bradley, F. *Ethical Studies*. London, 1876.

How medicine saved the life of ethics

14 Bledstein, B. *The Culture of Professionalism*. New York: Norton, 1976.
15 Rawls, J. *A Theory of Justice*. Cambridge, Mass: Harvard University Press, 1971.
16 MacIntyre, A. *After Virtue*. South Bend, Ind.: Notre Dame University Press, 1981.
17 Davis, K. *Discretionary Justice*. Urbana: University of Illinois Press, 1969.
18 Newman, R. *Equity and Law*. Dobbs Ferry, N.Y.: Oceana, 1961.
19 Hamburger, M. *Morals and Law: The Growth of Aristotle's Legal Theory*. New Haven, Conn.: Yale University Press, 1951.
20 Sidgwick, H. *The Methods of Ethics*, Introduction to 6th ed., London and New York: Macmillan, 1901.
21 Schneewind, J. *Sidgwick's Ethics and Victorian Moral Philosophy*. Oxford and New York: Oxford University Press, 1977.
22 Whewell, W. *The Elements of Morality*, 4th ed. Cambridge: Bell, 1864.
23 Marriage, morality and sex change surgery: four traditions in case ethics. *Hastings Cent. Rep.*, August 1981.

[3]

K. DANNER CLOUSER AND BERNARD GERT

A CRITIQUE OF PRINCIPLISM

ABSTRACT. The authors use the term "principlism" to refer to the practice of using "principles" to replace both moral theory and particular moral rules and ideals in dealing with the moral problems that arise in medical practice. The authors argue that these "principles" do not function as claimed, and that their use is misleading both practically and theoretically. The "principles" are in fact not guides to action, but rather they are merely names for a collection of sometimes superficially related matters for consideration when dealing with a moral problem. The "principles" lack any systematic relationship to each other, and they often conflict with each other. These conflicts are unresolvable, since there is no unified moral theory from which they are all derived. For comparison the authors sketch the advantages of using a unified moral theory.

Key Words: bioethical principles, medical ethics, moral theory, principlism

I. INTRODUCTION AND OVERVIEW

Throughout the land, arising from the throngs of converts to bioethics awareness, there can be heard a mantra "...beneficence...autonomy...justice..." It is this ritual incantation in the face of biomedical dilemmas that beckons our inquiry.

In the last twenty years the field of biomedical ethics has expanded in an unprecedented way. The numbers of persons involved, its acceptance as an important field, the myriad university courses, the ubiquitous workshops and conferences, and the plethora of articles, books, and journals have exceeded all expectations. In response to this enormous demand for training in ethics, there have appeared countless books, workshops, and courses that package the theories and methods of ethics, making them readily available to more people in a shorter time.

K. Danner Clouser, Ph.D., Professor of Humanities (Philosophy), The Pennsylvania State University College of Medicine, The Milton S. Hershey Medical Center, Hershey, Pennsylvania 17033, U.S.A.
Bernard Gert, Ph.D., Stone Professor of Intellectual and Moral Philosophy, Dartmouth College, Hanover, New Hampshire 03755, U.S.A.

The Journal of Medicine and Philosophy 15: 219–236, 1990.

The major strategy in the most influential of these responses is the deployment of "principles" of biomedical ethics. Conceptually, as diagrammed for example by Beauchamp and Childress (1983), the principles are located just below theories and just above rules. The general notion is that principles follow from moral theories and, in turn, generate particular rules that are then used to make moral judgments. Brandishing these several principles, adherents to the "principle approach" go forth to confront the quandaries of biomedical ethics.

We believe that the "principles of biomedical ethics" approach (hereinafter referred to as "principlism") is mistaken and misleading. Principlism is mistaken about the nature of morality and is misleading as to the foundations of ethics. It misconceives both theory and practice. By no means do we wish to impugn the many significant moral insights of the proponents of principlism. Our quarrel is not so much with the content of the various "principles" as it is with the use of "principles" at all. We consider this to be crucial and not just a matter of philosophical style. Our focus is on philosophical point: the conceptual or systematic status of "principles" as used in principlism.

Our bottom line, starkly put, is that "principle", as conceived by the proponents of principlism, is a misnomer and that "principles" so conceived cannot function as they are in fact claimed to be functioning by those who purport to employ them. At best, "principles" operate primarily as checklists naming issues worth remembering when considering a biomedical moral issue. At worst "principles" obscure and confuse moral reasoning by their failure to be guidelines and by their eclectic and unsystematic use of moral theory.

It is important that the nature of this article be understood at the outset. We are criticizing a highly influential trend in biomedical ethics, and our focus is on that trend and not on its perpetrators. That is, though we illustrate our points by citing several authors, our mission is not to refute this or that author but rather to show why a certain way of thinking about morality is wrong-headed. Citing chapter and verse of individual authors on individual points, and then defending our interpretations, would detract significantly from the thrust of our major points about a trend which is not author specific, but which is exemplified in various aspects and parts by many authors and editors.

II. THE USELESSNESS OF "PRINCIPLES"

Though principlism is widely prevalent, we will cite only two particular texts to illustrate our points. One is William Frankena's *Ethics* (1973), and the other is Beauchamp and Childress's *Principles of Biomedical Ethics* (1983). Though he does not specifically deal with biomedical ethics, we chose Frankena because he seems to be the progenitor of this approach. And we chose Beauchamp and Childress, because theirs is by far the most influential book exemplifying principlism.

A. Our General Claim

Our general contention is that the so-called "principles" function neither as adequate surrogates for moral theories nor as directives or guides for determining the morally correct action. Rather they are primarily chapter headings for a discussion of some concepts which are often only superficially related to each other. When, for example, we are told that a particular case calls for the application of the principle of beneficence, this can mean that the case involves either (1) the utilitarian ideal of promoting some good, or (2) the moral ideal of preventing some harm or removing some harm, or (3) some duty which is morally required. This use of "principles" bears no similarity to principles that "summarize" theories, e.g., as used by Rawls and Mill. Rawls' principle of justice and Mill's principle of utility or principle of liberty are directives toward a moral resolution of particular cases. The principles of Rawls and Mill are effective summaries of their theories; they are shorthand for the theories that generated them. However, this is not the case with principlism, because principlism often has two, three, or even four competing "principles" involved in a given case, for example, principles of autonomy, justice, beneficence, and nonmaleficence. This is tantamount to using two, three, or four conflicting moral theories to decide a case. Indeed some of the "principles" – for example, the "principle" of justice – contain within themselves several competing theories.

Classically, a principle embodies the moral theory (or part thereof) that spawned it; it is used by itself to enunciate a meaningful directive for action. "Do that act which creates the greatest good for the greatest number", "Maximize the greatest amount of liberty compatible with a like liberty for all". The thrust of the directive is clear; its goal and intent are unambiguous. Of course, there are often ambiguities and differing interpretations with respect to how the principle applies to a particular situation. But the principle itself is never used with other principles that are in conflict with it. Furthermore, if a genuine theory has more than one general principle, the relationship between them is clearly stated, as in the case of Rawls' two principles of justice. Unlike principlism, we are not given a number of conflicting principles and then told to pick whatever combination we like.

By contrast, for proponents of principlism "principles" seem primarily to name important aspects of morality, and, as such, a principle functions mainly as a check list of considerations. When we read their chapters discussing a principle, we get a description of several ways in which the authors think beneficence or autonomy or justice is a relevant moral consideration; we do not get a specific directive for action. Partly, that is because each "principle" includes quite disparate moral matters, unrelated by systematic considerations.

Why do we make so much of the fact that in principlism the "principles" provide no systematic guidance? After all, the proponents of principlism would simply say, "Principles are complicated directives. When we say 'apply the principle of beneficence', we mean consider those points that we discuss in our chapter on the principle of beneficence". In other words, they would say that "the principle of beneficence" is shorthand for their discussion of beneficence. But in that case there is really nothing to be "applied". In effect the agent is being told "think about beneficence and here's thirty pages of distinctions and deliberations to get you started", and that is very different from being told, e.g., "Do that act which will create the greatest good for the greatest number". At best the agent may be reflecting on the relevance of beneficence to the current problem, but he is only deceiving himself if he believes that he has some useful guideline to apply.

There are two problems with an agent's being deceived about whether or not he has a principle that can be applied. One is that the principles are assumed to be firmly established and justified. A person feels secure in applying or in presuming to apply them. The other problem is that an agent will not be aware of the real grounds for his moral decision. If the principle is not a clear, direct imperative at all, but simply a collection of suggestions and observations, occasionally conflicting, then he will not know what is really guiding his action nor what facts to regard as relevant nor how to justify his action. The language of principlism suggests that he has applied a principle which is morally well-established and hence *prima facie* correct. But a closer look at the situation shows that in fact he has looked at and weighed many diverse moral considerations, which are superficially interrelated and herded under a chapter heading named for the "principle" in question.

The agent meanwhile may have "applied" other competing "principles" as well, e.g., autonomy and justice, to the same case. This actually amounts simply to thinking about the case from diverse and conflicting points of view. By "applying" the "principles" of autonomy, beneficence, and justice, the agent is unwittingly using several diverse and conflicting accounts rather than simply applying a well-developed unified theory. It is risky to be doing the former while believing one is doing the latter. A unified moral theory reflects the unity and universality of morality. While it does not eliminate all moral disagreement, it does show what is responsible for that disagreement, e.g., that it is a disagreement about the facts, or about the ranking of different goods and evils, or whatever.

Using principles in effect as surrogates for theories seems to us to be an unwitting effort to cling to four main types of ethical theory: beneficence incorporates Mill; autonomy, Kant; justice, Rawls; and nonmaleficence, Gert. Presenting the matter as so many principles suggests that the principles have been integrated into one unified theory, whereas the exact opposite is true. The four main theories are reduced to four principles from which agents are told to pick and choose as they see fit, as if one could sometimes be a Kantian and sometimes a Utilitarian and sometimes something else, without worrying whether the theory one is using is adequate or not.

B. Our Thesis Illustrated with Frankena

It is necessary to see some real examples of principlism. But we wish to reiterate our earlier caveat that we use aspects of individual authors only illustratively. An early and influential example can be seen in William Frankena's *Ethics* (1973). Frankena gives great prominence to the principle of beneficence. He finds it to be presupposed by the principle of utility (which principle he ultimately rejects) and ranks it, along with the principle of justice, as one of the two basic principles of all morality.

But precisely what are his principles of beneficence and of justice? What directive is the moral agent following when he "applies" one of these principles? In reality what we have are two basic types of ethical theory – utilitarian and deontological – presented as if they were simply two principles of a single moral theory. Yet there is no attempt to work out that single theory so it would actually incorporate both types of consideration into a coherent whole. We do not deny that both consequences (utilitarianism) and rules (deontology) are essential features of morality. Rather our point is that it is not sufficient simply to say they are essential, but one must also *show how* they are related to each other.

Frankena gives several descriptions of the principle of beneficence, treating them as if they were identical, thus committing what we call "the fallacy of assumed equivalence". When he first mentions that the principle of utility presupposes another more basic principle (namely, beneficence), he characterizes it as "that we ought to do good and to prevent or avoid doing harm" (p. 45). Later, on the same page, he describes it as "that of producing good as such and preventing evil". In still another place he says that the principle "tells us to do good and to eschew evil and eliminate evil" (p. 53). He further complicates the "principle" (p. 47) by saying that, even if it is not required, it is a "desirable" and "important" part of morality!

In his most systematic attempt to spell out the principle of beneficence Frankena cites four directives: (1) one ought not inflict evil, (2) one ought to prevent evil, (3) one ought to remove evil, (4) one ought to promote good (p. 47). He expresses uncertainty as to whom and for whom they are binding. And he suggests that very likely they are arranged in descending order of priority, such that directive #4 may not even be a duty. Though he does not define duty, he clearly does not use it in the ordinary sense, where it is restricted to duties imposed by roles, professions, circumstances, etc. Furthermore he entertains the possibility that there should be a fifth directive which would settle conflicts among the other four. It would read "do what will bring about the greatest balance of good over evil". Overall it should be clear that in presenting the principle of beneficence he is really presenting a substitute for a moral theory rather than putting forth either a well worked out theory or a useful action-guide.

How can Frankena's principle be "applied"? "Not inflicting evil" is very different from "preventing evil", and "promoting good" is significantly different from them both. Several persons being told to apply the principle of beneficence to a situation could each end up doing very different things. There are two significant observations concerning this state of the "principle". One is that the "principle" itself is not capable of determining what action should be taken. There must be other factors (intuitions, rules, theories, or whatever) that are surreptitiously and otherwise influencing the agent's decision making. The other observation is that the four or five different "directives" of the principle need justification which is not provided. They are not tied together systematically by an underlying theory whose supporting arguments could then be explicitly assessed and from which moral rules could be derived to apply to real cases.

Frankena's principle of justice (the other one of the twosome on which he bases all of morality) exemplifies the same difficulties we have seen with beneficence (pp. 51–54). Again it fails to be a straightforward action-guide. He holds what he calls the "equalitarian" view of distributive justice. This commits us to the *prima facie* obligation of treating people equally. But of course it is impossible to treat everyone equally. Thus, he presents various modifications. Treat them equally according to morally relevant similarities and dissimilarities – that is, as he says, "the ones that bear on the goodness or badness of people's lives", such as abilities, interests, and needs (p. 51). It is still an impossible principle to follow. Given that there are billions of people, could we really treat every person equally with respect to their abilities, interests, and needs – to name only three of the presumably large reservoir of matters "that bear on the goodness or badness of people's lives"? And we are not helped on this score by the additional modification: we have to make only the same *relative* contribution to the goodness of each of their lives. Relative to what? Ability? Interest? Need? Merit? And this is further modified by his saying that this proportional distribution of goodness takes place "once a certain minimum has been achieved by all" (p. 51). There is no explanation of where that modification came from, what justifies it, or how we can know when it obtains.

226   K. Danner Clouser and Bernard Gert

According to Frankena, the principle of justice may on occasion be overridden by the principle of beneficence (which itself has internal conflicts) but there is no formula for determining those occasions (p. 51). We suspect that he fails to recognize that he has no theory, and so does not recognize that a theory needs to specify how it is to be applied. As with his principle of beneficence, his principle of justice is also of no practical use in determining action. If a person claimed to have decided on a line of action simply by virtue of applying either of these principles or some combination of them, we would know that he was mistaken and that he had unwittingly employed other beliefs, intuitions, rules or whatever in order to make that decision. It is generally acknowledged that any adequate moral theory must incorporate considerations about consequences, about rules, about impartiality, etc. But it is not an adequate moral theory simply to say that all of these kinds of considerations must be included. That is all that principlism does. Rather, an adequate theory must show how all of these considerations should be integrated.

C. Our Thesis Illustrated with Beauchamp and Childress

The same type of conceptual confusions can be found in what is surely the most popular of all biomedical ethics textbooks, Beauchamp and Childress's *Principles of Biomedical Ethics* (1983).[1] The authors enunciate four basic principles, each of which illustrates the problems that we have been delineating. Consider their principle of beneficence. For Beauchamp and Childress beneficence is a duty "to help others further their important and legitimate interests" (1983, p. 149); it is morally required (p. 148). The "principle" explicitly prescribes at least two very different kinds of action: (1) to prevent and remove harm, and (2) to confer benefits. These are both included in the general duty of beneficence. Additionally, there seem to be other subprinciples buried in the general "principle". Some are genuine duties to help, which accrue by virtue of special relationships and roles, whereas others are triggered by needs and one's ability to meet those needs, though without clear limitations on the scope of such obligations. All these are included in *"the* principle of beneficence". Clearly, this "principle" is simply a chapter heading under which many superficially related topics are discussed; it is primarily a label for a general concern with consequences. But by

A Critique of Principlism   227

being called a principle, it avoids the kind of fundamental questioning that a theory would undergo.

Beauchamp and Childress are obviously sensitive to and articulate about many nuances of morality. But our focus here is on the lack of a systematic account of the "principles" themselves and of the relationships between the "principles". At best, the "principles" function as hooks on which to hang elaborate discussions of various topics that are sometimes only superficially related. When they refer to a principle, in effect they are saying, "go read the chapter on beneficence, justice, autonomy, or non-maleficence and take all those diverse considerations into account when thinking about the situation". To regard all of those diverse considerations as "a principle", and to treat them as such is, as we have described, to be misled both practically and theoretically.

The Beauchamp and Childress "principle of justice" manifests our point even more than their other "principles". There is not even a glimmer of a usable guide to action. There is a discussion of the concept of justice and about various well-known and conflicting accounts of justice, yet there is no specific action-guide stated. Nevertheless, they refer to a principle of justice as though it is something we ought to apply to moral situations. It is clearly not a guide to action, but rather a checklist of considerations that should be kept in mind when reflecting on moral problems. Not being the kind of classical principle that summarizes a theory and yields specific action-guides, it is deceptive in purporting to have conceptual status and systematic validity. Their "principle" is neither derived from a theory nor does it provide a usable guide to action.

III. PRINCIPLISM: SYSTEMATIC CONSIDERATIONS[2]

A. Lack of Systematic Unity and Some Consequences

The points we want to raise are rarely if ever addressed in the literature. Therefore it is important that we make clear what our focus is. It is that principlism lacks systematic unity, and thus creates both practical and theoretical problems. Since there is no moral theory that ties the "principles" together, there is no unified guide to action which generates clear, coherent, comprehensive, and specific rules for action nor any justification of those rules.

For example, Beauchamp and Childress (1983) list five conditions necessary in order for a general duty of beneficence to become a specific duty of beneficence to another person (p. 153). But whence these conditions? Are they integrated into a moral theory? And what precisely is the relation between the general duty of beneficence and the specific duty of benevolence? On what is the general duty of beneficence founded? The authors suggest some possibilities, but not really in an argued, systematic way. They recommend reciprocity as a good possibility, but they toss in Rawls' "duty of fair play" for good measure (pp. 155–6).

In principlism each discussion of a "principle" is really an eclectic discussion that emphasizes a different type of ethical theory, so that a single unified theory is not only not presented, but the need for such a theory is completely obscured. Rather we are given a number of insights, considerations, and theories, along with instructions to use whichever one or combination of them seems appropriate to the user. But what is needed is that which tells us what actually is appropriate in a consistent and universal fashion. Certainly the "principles" themselves, as portrayed by principlism do not do so. Rather, it is a moral theory that is needed to unify all the "considerations" raised by the "principles" and thus to help us determine what is appropriate.

When an author does not put forward a theory explicitly, he does not subject himself to the same standards of rigor as one who does. Neglecting to do serious ethical theory in favor of making general observations about various principles can lead to some unfortunate arguments. Principlism, in failing to operate within an overall unified moral theory, defaults to eclectic, *ad hoc* "theories" which ultimately obfuscate moral foundations and moral reasoning.

Given space limitations, one example will have to suffice. Consider the argument for and some of the consequences of making beneficence a moral requirement, that is, a duty. (Autonomy would be an even better example, but its problems are so extensive as to deserve a separate article.) How could benefiting others ever become a moral duty required of everyone? After all, systematic considerations would convince us that impartiality is an essential feature of moral requirements. But the "duty" of beneficence cannot be impartially followed. That is, it is impossible for us to do good toward everyone, impartially, all the time.

Nevertheless, Beauchamp and Childress, for example, argue

that beneficence is a requirement, duty, or obligation, and not an ideal or supererogatory moral act. Their reason seems to be: "if there is a competing duty of confidentiality, beneficence may outweigh it" (p. 155). But that suggests what must surely be false, namely, that only a duty can outweigh another duty, and that a supererogatory act or moral ideal cannot outweigh a duty. Ergo, beneficence must be a duty, and not merely supererogatory. However, consider some heroic act in which one puts himself at considerable risk and which everyone regards as supererogatory. If the harm that one is preventing is a significant harm for many people, then one would be right to do it even if it involved causing some minor harm to others. In harming others one is violating a moral rule (or, as Beauchamp and Childress would say, the principle of nonmaleficence), yet, as in this example, that violation is outweighed by the moral ideal or supererogatory act. Our point is that a comprehensive and unified theory which gave an account of the support for moral ideals and their relation to the morally required would have avoided this line of reasoning.

Another unfortunate consequence of the conceptual mistake of making beneficence a requirement is that it obscures the role that real duties play. Real duties must be distinguished from what is morally required of all those subject to morality. Making beneficence morally required and calling it a duty distorts the essence of moral requirements (i.e., impartiality) and misleads as to the nature of real duties, which are created by special relationships and roles. Beauchamp and Childress do extensively address specific relationships and roles in connection with duties, but they are not able to give an adequate account of these in terms of principles. That is, for example, there is no systematic moral explanation of the relationship between the "general duty of beneficence" and customs, standards of practice, and codes such that we could morally evaluate the various duties established by virtue of these relationships and roles.

Taking what is properly the moral *ideal* of helping others (and hence not morally required), and lumping it under a "principle" of beneficence along with genuine duties (which *are* required), e.g., the duty of health care professionals to help their patients, leads to confusion and misunderstanding. The confusion basically results from treating beneficence as if it were morally required just as noninterference with the freedom of others is morally required. But only in the context of a comprehensive and unified theory would the significant difference in their moral status become clear. We believe that this conceptual mistake is the result of having no comprehensive moral theory, whose absence is barely noticed because of the flurry of attention and deference given instead to "principles".

A universal moral theory can systematically accommodate and account for the significance of particular circumstances. For example, if we understood the philosophical foundation for "Do Your Duty" as a universal moral rule, we would then understand how duties would be more precisely and appropriately fashioned for particular roles, times, and places. An adequate moral theory would set limits on what health professionals are allowed to do; however, it would also acknowledge that their duties cannot be completely determined *a priori*, but instead must be based on the relevant customs and practice of a particular culture. Just as morality sets limits on when one is morally required to obey the law, so morality sets limits on when health care professionals are morally required to follow the standard custom and practice in treating patients. And just as, within these limits, the law often determines what one is morally required to do, so within the limits of morality, custom and practice often determine how a health care professional is morally required to act. Thus, there is no incompatibility at all between a single unified moral theory and the acceptance of a difference in the duties of health care professionals based upon different customs and practices. Indeed, it is the theory that is necessary to indicate what is relevant and to set limits; it guides one through the endless variations in customs and circumstances.

B. Relativism: The Anthology Syndrome

Beauchamp and Childress accompany their account of moral reasoning with a diagram:

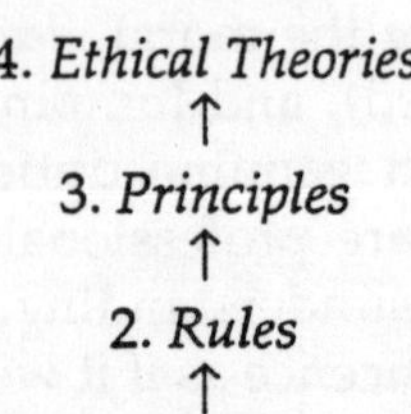

4. *Ethical Theories*
↑
3. *Principles*
↑
2. *Rules*
↑
1. *Particular Judgments and Actions*

A Critique of Principlism 231

"According to this diagram, judgments about what ought to be done in particular situations are justified by moral rules, which in turn are justified by principles, which ultimately are justified by ethical theories" (p. 5). Admitting that their diagram "may be oversimplified", they nevertheless claim that "its design indicates that in moral reasoning we appeal to different reasons of varying degrees of abstraction and systematization" (p. 5).

The authors give no argument for this account of moral reasoning. We suspect that they give no argument because none exists to support the role of principles in the hierarchy they propose. We believe that giving principles a significant role in moral reasoning is not only mistaken, but it also has unfortunate practical and theoretical consequences.

We had earlier seen a kind of relativism embodied by their "principles". Each principle seemed to have a life and logic of its own, as well as a number of internal conflicts. This relativism seems to be endorsed by their diagram having *theories* at the top of the hierarchy rather than a single unified ethical theory. This same kind of ethical relativism is endorsed by almost all anthologies in medical ethics, as well as in all other areas of applied and professional ethics. These anthologies (as well as most courses) almost invariably start by providing brief summaries of some standard ethical theories, e.g., utilitarianism, Kantianism, and contractualism. Next, the inadequacies of each of these theories are pointed out. There is no attempt to repair or remedy these defects, nor to present readers with a theory that they can actually use in solving the problems that are presented in the main body of the book (or course). Rather, the theories are either completely ignored and each problem is dealt with on an *ad hoc* basis, or the student is told to apply whatever inadequate theory he thinks is most useful in dealing with the problem at hand. Often he is told to apply several different, inadequate theories to a given problem, using whatever part of each theory seems most appropriate. This is an extraordinary way to proceed. It is difficult to imagine any respectable discipline proceeding in a similar fashion. Having acknowledged that all of the standard theories are inadequate, one is then told to apply them anyway, and even to apply competing theories, without any attempt to show how the theories can be reconciled.

In effect, the "anthology" approach is that of principlism. The proponents of principlism claim to derive principles from several different theories, none of which they judge to be adequate, and then they urge the student or health care professional to apply one or more of these competing principles to a given case. There is no attempt to show how or even whether these different principles can be reconciled. There is no attempt to show that the different theories, from which the principles are presumably derived, can be reconciled, or that any one of the theories can be revised so as to remove its defects and inadequacies. In the case of Beauchamp and Childress, this strongly suggests that there are several competing but equally good sources of final justification. And since "ethical theories" are at the very top of their hierarchy of justification, there would seem to be no way to adjudicate between them. This relativism is supported by their inadequate account of what an ethical theory is: "*theories* are bodies of principles and rules, more or less systematically related. They include second-order principles and rules about what to do when there are conflicts" (p. 5).

C. Morality vs. Moral Principles

An adequate ethical theory should not be just some more or less systematically related set of principles and rules. Rather it should provide an explanation of our moral agreement and disagreement; it should organize our moral thinking; it should tell us what is relevant to a moral judgment. In formulating theory we start with particular moral judgments about which we are certain, and we abstract and formulate the relevant features of those cases to help us in turn to decide the unclear cases. Simply to use the phrase "ethical theory" to refer to some historical examples of theories, e.g., those of Kant and Mill, which everyone recognizes to be inadequate, makes ethical theory irrelevant to practical moral reasoning. Thus in principlism, although "ethical theories" are at the top of the hierarchy of justification, it is no surprise that they play no role whatsoever in practical moral reasoning. Instead, as we have seen, moral "principles" are *de facto* the final court of appeal.

The appeal of principlism is that it makes use of those features of each ethical theory that seems to have the most support. Thus, in proposing the principle of beneficence, it acknowledges that Mill was right in being concerned with consequences. In proposing the principle of justice, it acknowledges that Rawls was right

A Critique of Principlism   233

in being concerned with the distribution of goods. In proposing the principle of autonomy, it acknowledges that Kant was right in emphasizing the importance of the individual person. In proposing the principle of nonmaleficence, it acknowledges that Gert was right in emphasizing the importance of avoiding harming others. But there is no attempt to see how these different concerns can be blended together as integrated parts of a single adequate theory, rather than disparate concerns derived from several competing theories.

An adequate moral theory is one that will encompass all the major thrusts of each "principle", showing how they are related to each other. It will explain both our moral agreement and disagreement, and show which disagreements can be settled and which cannot, and why. This theory will resemble in part various historical ethical theories, because it will incorporate those aspects of each theory which made that theory seem so plausible. Thus, an adequate theory will include as essential to morality (1) a concern with consequences, (2) a concern with how these consequences are distributed, (3) acknowledgment of the importance of the individual, and (4) the centrality of prohibitions against harming individuals. But more than this, it will show how these features are related to each other, integrating them into a clear, coherent, and comprehensive system that can actually be used to solve real moral problems that arise in medicine and other fields.

Insofar as an adequate moral theory has any unacceptable conclusions, it will, like scientific theories, be revised. For an ethical theory, properly understood, is not an historical relic, created at a given time and frozen in that form for eternity. It is an ongoing attempt to explain and justify our common moral intuitions. An adequate moral theory should provide a description of morality, i.e., of the moral system that is actually used by thoughtful people in making judgments about what to do in particular cases. Such a theory will be complicated, but, after all, morality is a very complex phenomenon, and we can hardly expect a theory that explains it to be statable in one sentence slogans.

The value of using a single unified moral theory to deal with the ethical issues that arise in medicine and all other fields, is that it provides a single clear, coherent, and comprehensive decision procedure for arriving at answers. All of those dealing with the problem can communicate easily with one another; they will agree on what the relevant features of the case are, and how changes in

234   *K. Danner Clouser and Bernard Gert*

those features can change the decisions that should be made. This
does not require that they always arrive at the same decision, for
they may rank the different values involved somewhat differently.
But even then, they will know precisely where they disagree and
why. And even if the theory provides an unacceptable answer,
one can go back to the theory and attempt to revise it. Contrariwise, with principlism, disagreements are often not only
unresolvable, but one often does not even know what the basis of
the disagreement is or what change in facts would produce
agreement. Furthermore, an unacceptable answer is of no value to
principlism, since there is no theory to revise accordingly.

An adequate account of morality would see morality as a public
system that applies to all rational persons. By "a public system"
we simply mean a system that is understandable and acceptable
to all those to whom it applies, e.g., as the rules of a game form a
public system which is understandable and acceptable to all those
who play the game. Since morality applies to all rational persons,
it must be understandable and acceptable to all rational persons.
The moral theory, in turn, would justify the moral system (which
tells us how to make moral judgments) by showing why morality
would be supported by all impartial rational persons. It would
provide an explicit description of the various parts of the moral
system: (1) the moral rules, e.g., "Don't kill", "Don't deceive",
"Keep your promise", and "Do your duty", for which punishment
for unjustified violations is appropriate, (2) moral ideals, such as
relieving pain and preventing death, for which punishment for
failure to follow is inappropriate, unless such a failure is also a
violation of a duty, (3) the procedure for determining when a
violation of a moral rule is justified, which would include an
explicit statement of what counts as morally relevant features,
several of which would be the harms caused, avoided, and
prevented by violation. And, finally, (4) a moral theory would
explain the disagreement about the scope of morality, i.e., whether
the moral rules protect only actual moral agents or whether it has
a wider scope, including, e.g., some or all potential moral agents,
namely infants and fetuses, and some or all sentient beings such
as nonhuman mammals.

This account of a moral theory is obviously more complex than
that presented by many historical ethical theories. But in one
respect it is simpler than the account offered by Beauchamp and
Childress: there is neither room nor need for principles between

A Critique of Principlism 235

the theory and the rules or ideals which are applied to particular cases. Rather, one applies the relevant rules and ideals and then, after taking into account all of the morally relevant features, one decides whether or not it is justified to violate a particular moral rule. The decisive question in determining whether or not to violate the rule is whether or not one would advocate that this kind of violation be publicly allowed, i.e., whether one would allow this kind of violation to be part of the public moral system. Although this resembles Kant's Categorical Imperative, it is significantly different. It captures the impartiality that is an essential part of morality without leading to the absurdities that Kant's theory does. And, just as important, in determining the *kind* of action, it takes into consideration the action's foreseeable consequences, thus capturing the concern with consequences that is the strongest feature of Utilitarianism – but without leading to the absurdities of Utilitarianism. We believe that this kind of theory does accurately describe the kind of moral reasoning that thoughtful people go through when they make moral judgments in particular cases. An excellent example of such a unified theory is Bernard Gert's *Morality: A New Justification of the Moral Rules* (1988).

D. And Finally

We believe, in the sense given to "principle" by Frankena and by Beauchamp and Childress, that for all practical and theoretical purposes there are no moral principles. Rather, for the former it is merely a way of combining some aspects of utilitarian and deontological theories without actually working out how they can be combined. For the latter, moral principles seem primarily to be chapter headings, which pen together superficially related topics. Although we find their discussions of these individual topics often to be extremely well done, we think that grouping them together under the heading of their "principles" gives a misleading account of moral reasoning.

Invocations of these principles leads to *neglect* of (1) the theories from which the principles supposedly are derived, (2) the individual rules and ideals that apply to the particular case, (3) the procedure that should be used in applying the rule to the particular case, and (4) the statement of the particular duties of a profession. And, most importantly, by invoking several

236   *K. Danner Clouser and Bernard Gert*

"principles" they implicitly deny the unity of morality. As John Stuart Mill says in the first chapter of *Utilitarianism*,

...there ought either to be some one fundamental principle or law at the root of all morality, or if there be several, there ought to be a determinate order of precedence among them; and the one principle, or the rule for deciding between the various principles when they conflict, ought to be self evident (paragraph #3).

We do not concur with Mill's implication that there has to be agreement about the answer to all moral questions, but we do accept that everyone must agree on the procedure to be used in deciding moral questions.

NOTES

[1] A third edition of *Principles of Biomedical Ethics* was published in mid-1989. Nevertheless we have continued to cite the second edition for two reasons. At this time it is more likely that readers will have copies of and be familiar with the second edition thus making reference checking more convenient. And secondly, not pursuing the third edition underlines our emphasis on not criticizing individual authors but rather on criticizing a conceptual "gestalt" which we see manifested in various forms and places, and the second edition is sufficient for that.

[2] Two other authors in this issue make charges similar to ours. Both Baruch Brody and Ronald Green note the insufficiency of principles: conflicts among, and unclarity within them, and of lack of a unifying theory. Brody emphasizes the difficulty in application with respect to scope, conditions for applying, etc. and the lack of a more fundamental theory (pp. 165–169). Whereas he concludes that we need to improve the principles, we argue that they have no role whatsoever within a unified moral theory whose derived rules are the proper and sufficient guides to action. Green not only notes that a fundamental moral theory is missing in the approach of Beauchamp and Childress but also claims that biomedical ethics in general has avoided serious attention to basic theoretical issues in ethics (pp. 187–190).

REFERENCES

Beauchamp, T.L., and Childress, J.F.: 1983, *Principles of Biomedical Ethics*, second edition, Oxford University Press, New York.

Brody, B.A.: 1990, 'Quality of scholarship in bioethics', this issue, pp. 161–178.

Frankena, W.: 1973, *Ethics*, second edition, Prentice-Hall, Englewood Cliffs, New Jersey.

Gert, B.: 1988, *Morality: A New Justification of the Moral Rules*, Oxford University Press, New York.

Green, R.M.: 1990, 'Method in bioethics: a troubled assessment', this issue, pp. 179–197.

[4]

CASUISTRY AS METHODOLOGY IN CLINICAL ETHICS

ALBERT R. JONSEN

*Department of Medical History and Ethics, University of Washington School
of Medicine SB-20, Seattle, WA 98195, USA*

ABSTRACT. This essay focuses on how casuistry can become a useful technique of
practical reasoning for the clinical ethicist or ethics consultant. Casuistry is defined, its
relationship to rhetorical reasoning and its interpretation of cases, by employing three
terms that, while they are not employed by the classical rhetoricians and casuists,
conform, in a general way, to the features of their work. Those terms are (1) morphology,
(2) taxonomy, (3) kinetics. The morphology of a case reveals the invariant structure of
the particular case whatever its contingent features, and also the invariant forms of
argument relevant to any case of the same sort: these invariant features can be called
topics. Taxonomy situates the instant case in a series of similar cases, allowing the
similarities and differences between an instant case and a paradigm case to dictate the
moral judgment about the instant case. This judgment is based, not merely on application
of an ethical theory or principle, but upon the way in which circumstances and maxims
appear in the morphology of the case itself and in comparison with other cases. Kinetics
is an understanding of the way in which one case imparts a kind of moral movement to
other cases, that is, different and sometimes unprecedented circumstances may move
certain marginal or exceptional cases to the level of paradigm cases. In conclusion,
casuistry is the exercise of prudential or practical reasoning in recognition of the
relationship between maxims, circumstances and topics, as well as the relationship of
paradigms to analogous cases.

Key words: casuistry, clinical ethics, rhetorical reasoning

INTRODUCTION

Cases are the common coin of medical ethics. They are exchanged incessantly
and worn smooth in argument. Karen Ann Quinlan, Elizabeth Bouvia, Baby Doe
and Baby M are cases of large denomination. The dominate the public discussion and scholarly analysis of certain major problems, such as forgoing life
support, assisted suicide and discriminatory treatment and surrogacy. But every
hospital, clinic and service has its own well known cases that have stimulated
local debate about ethical issues. The literature of medical ethics is a collection
of cases, real and fictitious, around which analyses of autonomy, beneficence,
non-maleficence and justice circle.

These analyses are presumably ethical, that is, they seem to draw upon the
concepts and logic of moral philosophy (and to a lesser extent, of moral
theology). However, it is not always clear how the theoretical content of moral

Theoretical Medicine **12**: 295–307, 1991.

philosophy fits together with the concrete content of cases. Partly, unclarity in moral issues is attributable to the complex nature of such issues and the disparity of principles and values espoused in a pluralistic society. But the unclarity is also partly due to the history of recent moral philosophy. Since the mid-19th century, Anglo-American moral philosophy has eschewed cases in favor of theory. Henry Sidgwick's *Methods of Ethics* (1877) set the tone for subsequent studies in moral philosophy. He wrote:

The development of Ethics has been much impeded by the preponderance of practical considerations. Although Aristotle said, "the end of our study is not knowledge but conduct", it is still true that the peculiar excellence of his own system is due to the pure air of scientific curiosity in which it has been developed. It would seem that a more complete detachment of the scientific study of right conduct from its practical application is to be desired [1].

For over a century, the literature of moral philosophy has followed Sidgwick's lead. Careful analysis of basic concepts and language of moral discourse and reasoning have been its major products. In particular, concern about the logic of comprehensive theories, predominantly utilitarianism in its various forms, has been the prominent interest of moral philosophers. Until recently, moral philosophers have ignored the moral dilemmas and perplexities of actual personal, institutional and social life. In the 1960's, moral philosophers began to be exercised by the burning issues of the day: the war in Southeast Asia, racial discrimination, poverty and, above all, by the ethical implications of rapidly developing medical technology [2]. Now that some philosophers have discovered these 'actual' problems, they sometimes wonder about the relevance of their theories to problematic situations. Those who have become 'ethicists' in medicine, dealing with cases of foregoing life support, refusals of needed treatment, confidentiality, and so on, seem to be living in a land remote from their intellectual heritage in moral philosophy [3,4].

Standard textbooks on bioethics devote considerable attention to the fitting of theory to cases. Certain of these books concentrate on the theory and move to the cases, others preface the discussion of cases with an exposition of theory. Those bioethicists who are deeply engaged in what is called 'clinical ethics' frequently devise a method for the analysis of cases. Often enough, those methods make only slight reference to ethical theory. Only recently have these scholars in clinical ethics moved to a serious effort to justify their clinical methods in a more formal manner. Thus, at present, the theoretical moral philosophers are engaged in moving down from theory to practice, the clinical ethicists move from practice to method.

In this essay I will describe the method that appeals to me as the most suited to practical discourse about ethical problems. It is a method with a long history and, in recent times, an unsavory reputation. It is called "casuistry". Casuistry can be defined as

the interpretation of moral issues, using procedures of reasoning based on paradigms and analogies, leading to the formulation of expert opinion about the existence and stringency of particular moral obligations, framed in terms of rules or maxims that are general but not universal or invariable, since they hold good with certainty only in the typical conditions of the agent and circumstances of action [5].

This definition is quoted from *The Abuse of Casuistry*. In that book, Stephen Toulmin and I reviewed the history of the casuistic method, which had its origins in Stoicism and the writings of Cicero and flourished with particular vigor during the 15th and 16th century in the writings of Roman Catholic and Anglican moral theologians. Our purpose in that book was to dispel the disrepute that clings to the name 'casuistry' and to reveal its relevance for moral philosophy, particularly as that discipline reflects on practical problems of life. The reader is referred to that book for a fuller explanation of much that follows in this essay.

However, this essay takes a step that was not taken in the book. Toulmin and I did not specify in any detail the exact features of casuistry as a technique for clinical ethics. We only laid the groundwork for so doing. In the present essay, then, I shall become more explicit about how casuistry can become a useful technique of practical reasoning for the clinical ethicist or ethics consultant. We point out in *The Abuse of Casuistry* that classical casuistry was not closely associated with any ethical theory. By this we meant that, although its practitioners worked within the conceptual framework of 'natural law', they used rather indiscriminately forms of reasoning compatible with most modern ethical theories. Indeed, the classical casuists, as well as the moral philosophers of the past, did not seem to have any refined concept 'theory' as part of their intellectual armamentarium. In view of that feature of classical casuistry, this essay will not attempt to fit casuistry to ethical theory in any of its forms. This does not imply that ethical theory is useless, but that its influence on casuistry is remote.

Toulmin and I also maintain that the form of reasoning constitutive of classical casuistry is rhetorical reasoning. It seems rash to try to dispel the disrepute of casuistry by proposing that casuistry is rhetorical, for the modern reader is likely to think even less of rhetoric, which is daily derided in political campaigns, than of casuistry. However, the modern reader knows almost nothing of the rhetoric that dominated the intellectual life of western culture for many centuries. That rhetoric, which served as the backbone of education, was elucidated in Aristotle's *Rhetoric* and the works of Cicero and Quintillian, works rarely read today even by scholars. The casuists knew these authors well and found in them a method of reasoning or, better, of arguing, that was suited to cases. They were aware that practical reasoning has rules of logic that differ from the logic of scientific reasoning. These rules were set out by the authors of

298   ALBERT R. JONSEN

antiquity in their 'rhetorics' rather than their 'logics' [6,7].

For purposes of this essay, I will explain casuistry, its relationship to rhetorical reasoning and its interpretation of cases by employing three terms that do not actually appear in the classical rhetoricians and casuists, but do conform, in a general way, to the major features of their work. Those categories I call (1) morphology, (2) taxonomy, and (3) kinetics. For simplicity's sake, I will refer throughout to a particular case, known to readers of the bioethics literature as Debbie's case:

A resident in obstetrics is called late at night to see a young woman whom he does not know. On reviewing her chart he sees that she is in the terminal stages of ovarian cancer. Entering her room, he notes her emaciated state and obviously great pain. She pleads, "let's get this over". The resident administers a heavy dosage of morphine and Debbie dies within an hour of the respiratory depression induced by the morphine [8].

MORPHOLOGY

A case, derived from the Latin verb "cadere", is literally an event or a happening. Cicero defined a case as "constructed out of statements about certain persons, places, times, actions and affairs" [9]. These statements constitute what the classical rhetoricians and casuists called 'the circumstances'. They listed them in a standard way as 'who, what, when, where, why, how and by what means'. However, the circumstances, literally, 'what surrounds or stands around', stand around the center of the case. That center is constituted of certain maxims, brief rule-like sayings that give moral identity to the case. A maxim was, for the rhetoricians, 'maxima sententia', a leading or important proposition. Sometimes they referred to them as 'gnomoi' or wise sayings, because they seemed to distill, in a pithy way, experience reflected upon by wise men.

Thus, in Debbie's case, the circumstances are the roles of physician and patient, the terminal nature of the patient's illness, her mental and physical distress, the import of her request, the doctor's drawing up of 10 mgs of morphine, the lateness of the hour, etc. These are the descriptive elements of the narrative, the story. The maxims that come to mind might be, 'competent persons have a right to determine their fate', 'the physician should respect the wishes of the patient', 'relieve pain', 'thou shalt not kill', 'give the patient no deadly poison, even if requested' (Hippocratic Oath). These maxims provide the 'morals' of the story. For most cases of interest, there are several morals, because several maxims seem to conflict. The work of casuistry is to determine which maxim should rule the case and to what extent. To what extent means under what constellation of circumstances, for certain changes of circumstances will lead to another maxim emerging as more significant. 'Circumstances', say the casuists, 'make the case'. This appears to mean that the selection of the

CASUISTRY IN CLINICAL ETHICS 299

appropriate maxim to rule the case is profoundly dependant upon the circumstances. When we speak about a principle or maxim being 'weighty', we use a metaphor that might have appealed to the imagination of the classical casuists rather differently than to ourselves. For us, weighty principles are heavy in their own right: autonomy, for example, ranks high in the panoply of moral principles. For the classical casuist, a maxim would accumulate weight from the circumstances that hung from it in a particular case.

This interplay of circumstances and maxims constitute the structure of a case. Thus, we can speak of the morphology or the perception of form and structure. But there is more than circumstances and maxims when the case is laid out for analysis. There is also the structure of moral argument or the logic of moral reasoning appropriate to the case under discusssion. Toulmin first described that structure in his *Uses of Argument* [10] and he and I recognized its relevance to casuistry. This logic is not at all similar to the logic of scientific reasoning. Rather it is an invariant pattern of reasoning in which certain claims are related to grounds, warrants, backing and modal qualifiers. The claim consists of a judgment that this person should or should not perform a specific action, e.g., 'I, the resident physician, should help this woman to die'. The grounds, which are usually introduced by a 'because' statement, set out the factual circumstances in which the claim is made, e.g., 'because she is suffering great pain and is requesting help'. The warrants are the maxims that justify the claim in those circumstances, e.g., 'it is a physician's duty to relieve pain and to be respectful of the wishes of the patient'. The backing consists of those more elaborate, theoretical arguments that support the warrants, e.g., the doctrine of autonomy. Finally, most cases will bring to mind certain qualifiers that usually begin with a term like 'unless' or 'provided that'. In Debbie's case, the qualifier might be 'unless she is mentally incompetent at this time', or 'provided that there are no other ways to relieve her pain'. Obviously, the logic of the argument can be set out in different ways, with different claims, warrants, grounds and qualifiers. Thus, the claim 'I should not help Debbie to die', would be surrounded by different grounds, warrants, etc. This pattern constitutes the structure of practical discourse.

Practical discourse also has what might be called a substructure which is an important part of the morphology of the case. Any argument contains a sample of one or more standard and invariant patterns of discourse, that is, an argument about causality, or about sequences, or about priority or about contingency, etc. These arguments have invariant patterns that can, and must be used, in any substantive argument. For example, whenever one is proposing that event a caused event b, one must show that a preceded b temporally, that a was in contact with b, that b could not have occurred unless a had occurred. All discourse about causality must review these points, and so with discourse about sequence, priority, etc.

These invariant structures of argument were called by the rhetoricians, 'topics' or 'loci' which literally means 'places' and the term came into English as 'commonplaces'. (Unfortunately, this term is taken to refer to pithy, common sense and rather boring propositions.) The rhetoricians recognized general topics, such as the ones described above, and special topics, areas of discourse used in particular enterprises. These topics provided familiar ground amidst the variable, complex circumstances of particular cases. Regardless of the specific content of the case (the circumstances), the forms of argument called topics remained invariant.

In Debbie's case, for example, the question 'Did the doctor cause Debbie's death?' is not about physical causality alone, but about moral causality. Certain points must be covered in order to make the case for or against his moral accountability. Among these points, intention is always relevant. In Debbie's case, the resident's intention, whether to kill or to assuage pain, must be reviewed, since he used a means, morphine, which will do both. Is he killing or merely helping her to be more comfortable and only allowing her to die? The causists' distinction between direct and indirect killing was crafted for this situation. This distinction, and its larger formulation as the so called Principle of Double Effect, has fallen into disfavor with philosophers in recent years. However, that disfavors stems, I believe, from thinking of the distinction as a principle rather than as a general topic, an invariant form of argument that fits within any discourse about moral accountability and moral causality.

The rhetoricians also recognized that different fields of activity had their own 'special topics'. For example, in politics, it is necessary to discuss authority, sovereignty, the public good, representation, etc.; in business, it is necessary to discuss investment, profit, productivity, etc. Regardless of the particular political system or commercial activity, these special topics have an invariant structure and variable content. Clinical-ethical activity has its proper special topics, the invariant constituents of that form of discourse. These consist of statements about the medical indications of the case, about the preferences of the patient, about the quality of the patient's life and about the social and economic factors external to the patient, but affected by the case. Mark Seigler, William Winslade and I originally proposed these as a means of analysis of a clinical case in our book, *Clinical Ethics* [11]. I now believe that they represent the special topics of clinical medicine, always relevant to the clinical decision and with an invariant structure, although a variable content. Thus, in Debbie's Case, the medical indications state her prognosis and current clinical condition; the preferences note her request and its basis in competent or incompetent judgment; quality of life describes her intractable pain and hopeless future; external factors comprise such matters as the homicide laws, the secrecy of the case, the apparent acquiescence of a present relative, etc.

The morphology of a case reveals the invariant structure of the particular case, whatever its contingent features, and also the invariant forms of argument relevant to any case of this sort. The first task of the casuist is to discern this structure. To modify the metaphor, the casuist must 'parse' the case, getting below the surface of the story to the grammatical structure of argument from grounds to claim through warrant and to the deeper grammar of the topics that underlie that argument.

TAXONOMY

Debbie's case represents one instance of a type. In all cases that fall under this type, physicians presumably bring about in some way the death of their patients. The type can be given a general name such as 'euthanasia'. The questions will always bear on whether the doctor has the right or duty to act in this way, whether the patient has the right to request the doctor to so act, whether the patient or the doctor is the responsible agent, and what conditions or circumstances of competence, pain, terminality, etc., should obtain. All cases that fall under the type are alike in some respects and different in others.

One of the crucial steps in the casuistic method is the lining up of cases in a certain order. This might be called the taxonomy of cases; "taxis" is the Greek word meaning the drawing up or marshalling of soldiers in a battle line. Just as an Athenian general might place his strongest and most aggressive soldiers in the forefront of the battleline, so the casuist seeks out those cases, within the type, that demonstrate the most obviously, unarguably wrong (or right) instance. This would be a case in which the circumstances were clear, the relevant maxim unambiguous and the rebuttals weak, in the minds of almost any observer. The claim that this action is wrong (or right) is widely persuasive. There is little need to present arguments for the rightness (or wrongness) of the case and it is very hard to argue against its rightness (or wrongness). Think, for instance, of gratuitous care of the impoverished sick or, conversely, sexual abuse of children or of the Holocaust. Such cases can be paradigms, a word that literally means 'an example' and was used in that sense by the ancient rhetoricians who considered them an indispensable element of moral reasoning.

Once the morphology of Debbie's case is set out, it is possible to construct the taxonomy to which it belongs. The most obviously relevant taxonomy is the lineup of cases that deal with killing. The alternative proposal that the relevant taxonomy is care for the patient might be briefly entertained but would probably be dismissed by most commentators as question begging. The taxonomy about killing starts with the clearest sort of case in which the maxim, 'thou shalt not

302   ALBERT R. JONSEN

kill' meets little or no opposition from contrary maxims or confounding circumstances. Thus, the case of unprovoked killing of one person by another seems an appropriate paradigm. Next in the taxonomy belong cases of provoked killing of different sorts, such as self-defense against a direct, lethal attack, preemptive defense, etc. At some point in this taxonomy, the question will be raised, 'Is it permissible to kill someone who requests you to do so?'. The instant case of 'physician assisted euthanasia' will find its place here in the taxonomy and be ready for an analysis of the relevant similarities and differences that lead to a judgment of justifiable or unjustifiable killing.

Debbie's case stands in a line that might begin with a case about a competent, lucid patient with terminal illness requesting his or her personal physician to administer a lethal drug. Debbie's case differs in several circumstances, namely her lucidity is questionable, the physician did not know her or much about her condition. These differences might lead someone to judge that while the paradigm was ethically appropriate, the action in Debbie's case was not. However, the immediate paradigm has to stand in its own lineup. This lineup extends back to the most basic paradigm: the killing of one human being by another. Taken in this naked form, without qualifications, it is almost impossible to imagine anyone approving. (Why that is so is a matter for moral theory.)

As one elaborates the basic paradigm, certain circumstances can be envisioned that raise the possibility of a justifiable killing: self-defense, defense of others, being the most obvious. These circumstances move away from the paradigm step by step and, as they do, the question is raised in each case whether the circumstances are changed enough to admit maxims other than, say, 'thou shalt not kill' as a rebuttal: for example, 'each person has the right to his own life'. These cases, then, are analogous to the paradigm. The euthanasia cases fit into that taxonomy by asking whether the circumstances of, say, competent request, intractable pain or terminal illness, are sufficient to allow an exception to the maxim in the basic paradigm. If so, the claim in the euthanasia cases would be, 'thou shalt not kill, except when requested to do so by a suffering, terminally ill, competent patient'.

The taxonomy of cases is crucially important in casuistry. It puts the instant case into its moral context and reveals the weight of argument that might countervail a presumption of rightness or wrongness. The fact that exceptions to the prohibition against killing remain very close to the protection of self and others (even in the disputable exception of warfare and capital punishment) suggests that killing to relieve pain might be an inadequate candidate. On the other hand, it might be suggested that the taxonomy is wrong; euthanasia should not be seen as an act of killing but an act of mercy. This puts the case into another taxonomy and requires that some paradigm of mercy, say, saving threatened life, be the starting place of the reasoning by analogy.

CASUISTRY IN CLINICAL ETHICS 303

In bioethics, paradigm and analogy has provided a clear line of reasoning about the problem of foregoing life support. The determination of death by brain criteria initiates the taxonomy: there is no obligation to continue to treat medically a dead body. Next come those cases in which the patient has irretrievably lost consciousness and exists in a persistent vegetative state. These circumstances radically diminish the obligation to provide medical care, particularly forms of technological support, such as respirators. Cases of diminished mental capacity, such as senility, raise the presumption that certain forms of life support might be omitted, but others remain obligatory. At the beginning of the taxonomy, moral consensus prevails; as the analogous cases are lined up, more disagreement appears. Claims that persons in persistent vegetative state can be deprived of medically mediated forms of nutrition and hydration are open to debate. Claims that a mentally retarded person might be deprived of ordinary forms of care, such as a simple operation, are widely repudiated.

A taxonomy makes clear that an instant case is not unique. It allows the differences between the instant case and the paradigm case to dictate the judgment about moral propriety. The judgment is based, not on a principle or a theory, but upon the way in which circumstances and maxims appear in the morphology of the case itself and in comparison with similar cases.

KINETICS

I borrow the term "kinetics" from classical physics as I borrowed the term "morphology" from classical biology. I mean by it an understanding of the way in which one case imparts a kind of moral movement to other cases, as a moving billiard ball imparts motion to the stationary one it hits. In casuistry, the motion is a shift in moral judgment between paradigm and analogous cases, so that one might say of the paradigm, 'this is clearly wrong' and of an analogous case, 'but, in this case, what was done was justified, or excusable'.

The kinetics of casuistry is not mechanical, as is its counterpart in physics. One renown casuist was called by his modern biographer, "a marvellous moral computer" ([12], p. 126), but he was an aberration, representing the decay of casuistry. Quite the contrary of mechanical or mathematical reasoning, casuistry is in essence prudential reasoning, or, as Aristotle described it, phronesis, that is, practical wisdom. This sort of reasoning is cultivated by critical reflection upon human experience and upon the human condition. In casuistry, the reflection bears upon the relation between maxims and circumstances: the former are appreciated as valid, but limited rules for the good conduct of life; the latter report the actual conditions of living through a particular situation.

304   ALBERT R. JONSEN

The circumstances of human life are, of course, mutable, but at the same time, they are embedded in important social institutions that are, if not immutable, at least relatively stable. The prudent person has the knack of recognizing that following this or that maxim, in these or those circumstances, contributes to the support of strengthening of the relevant social institutions or that, contrariwise, certain actions will undermine or modify the institution in certain ways. Similarly, actions are embedded in personal ideals, revealing or obscuring them. The prudent person also appreciates the way in which certain actions, under certain circumstances, correspond to the ideals that he or she credits. In both the social and personal realm, prudent judgment apprehends the fit of maxims and circumstances. It is interesting to note that moralists as different as the Greek sceptics and H. Richard Niebuhr used the term "fitting" as an expression of moral approbation. Aristotle's well known notion 'equity' is, in Greek, a cognate of 'the fitting'.

Another metaphor frequently used in moral discourse speaks of reasons being 'weighty' and of 'balancing considerations'. Again, moral kinetics comes into play, since these metaphors suggest that claims can be moved up and down, from right to wrong, by adding certain 'considerations' to the scale of reasoning. In reading the classical casuists, one finds that cases frequently turn on whether a sum of money is large or small, an act of aggression slight or violent, a promise about a serious or frivolous matter. The introduction of these 'quantities' into moral reasoning is crucial to casuistry. On the contrary, quantifiable circumstances are rather an embarrassment to moral theory: it is very difficult to deal with 'a little utility' or 'a certain amount of autonomy'. As we mentioned above, the weight of principles is a metaphor that is heard differently by the casuists and by the moral theorist.

The import of these 'quantified' circumstances of each case is that prudent judgment must discern the relevance of a maxim in the light of the matter under consideration. In the traditional debate about truth-telling, for example, any disparity between thought and word was, in theory, a lie. But jokes are often made up of such disparities and to banish joking from life seems extreme. Thus, the 'jocose lie' of tradition was a prudent accommodation: it recognized that, in the circumstances of fun, the purpose of truthtelling, namely, the preservation of trust in a community was not at stake.

In Debbie's case, the degree of her lucidity, the extent of her pain and of its intractability to palliation, the scope of the resident's familiarity with her case, are all crucial features in reaching a conclusion about the morality of the action. Each of these is susceptible of greater and less and the only way of judging 'how great, and how less' comes from the wisdom of experience. Similarly, the case is sorted into a taxonomy of killing or of helping, not because one knows the dictionary definition of both, but because one understands the meaning of taking a life or helping another in suffering. This knowledge is not deduced from principles but learned from reflective experience.

The kinetics of casuistry must now take on Debbie's case. In the historical taxonomy about killing, no general exception had been allowed for voluntary request or permission. However, certain marginal cases troubled the casuists. For example, the classical case of the general who asks his officers to kill him lest in weakness he betray secrets to the enemy or the more modern case of the trapped driver in a burning truck who asks the police to shoot him. The kinetics of casuistry asks whether in these conditions, voluntary request or permission can rebut the strong presumption in favor of maintaining the maxim, 'thou shalt not kill'. When opinion was divided among authorities, either course of action could be sanctioned, although if the death of another was the consequence of one of them, the more strict opinion had to be respected. Thus, the traditional casuists, regardless of their speculative opinion on these marginal cases, would probably have advised that permitted killing was immoral. Possibly, they might have tolerated killing the truck driver in view of the certain immanence of his death by fire.

In Debbie's case, however, the modern casuist must go further. The division of opinion among the classical casuists about the marginal cases would lay more in such questions as whether death would be immanent and inevitable and whether alternatives were available than in the mere fact of permission or request. Today, as distinguished from the age of classical casuistry, much greater weight is given to maxims that support personal autonomy. Thus, the kinetics of this case might move in two different directions. The most likely one for the clinical ethicist to take would be to challenge the competency of the requester who is in great pain and depression, as well as to question the adequacy of the physician's knowledge and involvement in the case. Taking this course, the weight of the maxim of personal autonomy is not itself denied; the circumstances for the exercise of an autonomous choice are questioned. A second approach that the casuist might take is to explore the implications of a physician accepting voluntary euthanasia requests even in appropriate circumstances. This approach admits the importance of autonomous choices, but suggests that the implications of honoring them in the matter of euthanasia must be carefully examined: Are these implications so negative as to provide a rebuttal to the maxim of autonomy? This approach is a form of the so-called 'slippery slope' response.

Debbie's case is resolved casuistically with ease. The casuist need not move to more theoretical considerations about the principle of autonomy. Staying at the level of the case, the casuist can note that defects in the voluntary nature of the request and the adequacy of the physician's involvement are sufficiently serious that no exception to the dominance of the maxim against killing is

306   ALBERT R. JONSEN

justified. The resident was wrong to administer the morphine in a lethal dose. Almost all commentators on the case came to this conclusion [13]. Even the one ethicist who defended the morality of euthanasia in exceptional cases (a properly casuistic argument) disapproved of the resident's action in Debbie's case [14].

CONCLUDING REMARKS

We said above that the kinetics of casuistry is prudence or practical wisdom. The casuist will be able to scan or parse the case, revealing its structure of claim, maxim, grounds, rebuttals. Casuistry will be able to locate the case in a taxonomy of cases, recognize the similarities and differences and appreciate the shift from moral certainty to moral doubt. Above all, casuistic reasoning is prudential reasoning: appreciation of the relationship between paradigm and analogy, between maxim and circumstances, between the greater and less of circumstances as they bear on the claim and the rebuttals.

Mention of the 'prudent or wise person' inevitably invokes an image of the sage or guru, immersed in his or her own profound insights and occasionally uttering an oracle. This is, of course, an exaggerated picture. The prudent person can be quite ordinary, but is marked by 'common sense' joined to experience and linked to ideals that makes possible good judgment. The ethicist must be at least that sort of person. In addition, the ethicist must be educated in the issues of his or her field. Such education consists, in great part, in knowing the cases. Knowing the cases means familiarity with the circumstances, maxims and arguments that make each case unique and, at the same time, make it fit into a taxonomy. If there is any sense in which an ethicist can rightly be called an expert, it is because he or she has the knack of doing this well and of showing others how to do it.

REFERENCES

1. Sidgwick H. *Methods of Ethics*. London: Macmillan, 1877.
2. Toulmin SE. How medicine saved the life of ethics. *Perspect Biol Med* 1982; 25:736–50.
3. Murray TH. Medical ethics, moral philosophy and moral tradition. *Soc Sci Med* 1987; 25:637–44.
4. McCullough LB. Methodological concerns in bioethics. *J Med Philos* 1986; 11:17–37.
5. Jonsen AR, Toulmin SE. *The Abuse of Casuistry*. Berkeley: University of California Press, 1988.
6. Vickers B. *In Defense of Rhetoric*. Oxford: Clarendon Press, 1988.
7. Ryan E. *Aristotle's Theory of Rhetorical Argumentation*. Montreal: Bellarmine Press, 1984.

CASUISTRY IN CLINICAL ETHICS 307

8. Anonymous. It's over, Debbie. *JAMA* 1988; 259:272.
9. Cicero MT, *De Inventione*. [Transl HM Hubbell]. Cambridge, MA: Harvard University Press, 1949.
10. Toulmin SE. *The Uses of Argument*. Cambridge: Cambridge University Press, 1969.
11. Jonsen AR, Siegler M. Winslade WJ. *Clinical Ethics*. New York: Macmillan, 1986.
12. Dunoyer E. *L'Enchiridion Confessariorum del Navarro*. Pamplona: n p, 1957.
13. Gaylin W, Kass LR, Pellegrino ED, Siegler M. Doctors must not kill. *JAMA* 1988; 259:2139–40.
14. Vaux KL. Debbie's dying: mercy killing and the good death. *JAMA* 1988; 259:2140–41.

[5]

CASE METHOD AND CASUISTRY: THE PROBLEM OF BIAS

LORETTA M. KOPELMAN

Department of Medical Humanities, East Carolina University School of Medicine, Greenville, NC 27858–4354, USA

ABSTRACT. Case methods of reasoning are persuasive, but we need to address problems of bias in order to use them to reach morally justifiable conclusions. A bias is an unwarranted inclination or a special perspective that disposes us to mistaken or one-sided judgments. The potential for bias arises at each stage of a case method of reasoning including in describing, framing, selecting and comparing of cases and paradigms. A problem of bias occurs because to identify the relevant features for such purposes, we must use general views about what is relevant; but some of our general views are biased, both in the sense of being unwarranted inclinations and in the sense that they are one of many viable perspectives. This reliance upon general views to determine relevancy creates additional difficulties for defenders who maintain that case methods of moral reasoning are not only useful, but more basic, reliable or prior to other forms of moral reasoning. If we cannot identify the case's relevant features and issues independently of our general views or biases, we need further explanation about why a case method or casuistry should be viewed as prior to or more basic or reliable than other forms of moral reasoning. Problems of bias also arise for other methods of reasoning. In medical science, case reviews are regarded as an unreliable way to form generalizations, and methods such as clinical trials are used to address bias.

Key words: applied ethics, case method, casuistry, ethics, medical ethics bias, clinical trials

1. INTRODUCTION

In using a case method of reasoning, people compare the similarities and differences between particular situations (cases) to seek guidance or rules about what to believe or how to act. Assessing and comparing particular situations serve as an increasingly popular way to try to address moral problems and establish generalizations about how we ought to act. In medical science, however, generalizations based only upon case reviews garner suspicions because we know that our unintended biases infect how we describe situations, collect data, interpret results and use the resulting information. In what follows I raise similar concerns about the use of case reviews in moral reasoning, arguing that we need to address problems of bias in order to use case methods to reach morally justifiable conclusions. I hope that this will advance improvements of this important form of moral reasoning, just as concerns about bias in medical

Theoretical Medicine 15: 21–37, 1994.
© 1994 *Kluwer Academic Publishers. Printed in the Netherlands.*

science prompted the development of clinical trial methodologies.

A case method presupposes that we can solve our quandaries and disputes by matching cases to morally unambiguous situations where we agree about what we ought to do (core cases, exemplars, or paradigms). It also assumes that we generally agree about what cases are morally unambiguous and when disputed situations are adequately similar to the core cases [1–9].

Casuists employ a special form of a case method to solve moral disputes and quandaries; as Jonsen and Toulmin state, casuistry also "requires institutions that provide the locus for and lend support to the uniquely casuistical way of approaching moral problems" ([1], p. 388). They define casuistry as,

the interpretation of moral issues, using procedures of reasoning based on paradigms and analogies, leading to the formulation of expert opinion about the existence and stringency of particular moral obligations, framed in terms of rules or maxims that are general but not universal or invariable, since they hold good with certainty only in the typical conditions of the agent and circumstances of action ([2], p. 297).

An analogy may help introduce case method forms of moral reasoning and show how they are different, for example, from a deductive method. Novice art students learn how to mix colors by comparing them to colors that they know how to mix and to paradigms (like cobalt blue and magnesium blue). To gain expertise, they must be able to see where the color belongs in relation to others, something which cannot be taught to the color-blind. The standard colors are paradigms fixed within an artistic tradition. Mixing colors is a practical activity, learned by doing. Students can engage in this practical activity successfully without any knowledge of abstract color theories of physics.

Those employing a case method also compare particular situations and learn to "see" important resemblances and differences between actual situations. They, too, use paradigms in moral reasoning and view ethics as a practical activity we learn about from doing [1–9]. Morality, like mixing paint, is seen as rooted in action.

Advocates of a case method or casuistry seek to compare and refine our intuitions (our spontaneous beliefs) about moral situations and problems. These advocates hold that by using a case method or casuistry, we can improve our intuitions about how we ought to act, what things are virtuous or vicious, what actions merit approval or disapproval or how to use moral language [1, 12].

Some [1–3, 5, 7–9, 12] but not all [6] defenders of case methods regard practical decisions about cases as more basic than, prior to, or more reliable than moral theories, maxims, rules or principles. Once conceived, however, theories can have a limited role in giving us direction when we lose our way. [7,9] For example, Jonsen uses an analogy where "... the bicycle is like a practical judgment, [and] the hot-air balloon is like ethical theory" ([9], p. 14) and writes: "The balloon of theory can give us orientation of mind and exhilaration of moral imagination. However, we are not tethered to the balloon; we do not need it for moment to moment directions through ethical problems. The balloon is an occasional extravagance. The bicycle is daily transportation and exercise" ([9], p. 16). He argues that, "The weight of any ethical consideration comes, not from the principles or maxims invoked, but from the more fact-like considerations that are piled onto practical judgment" ([9], p. 15).

Bambrough also favors building up moral rules from particular cases, but offers a different response than Jonsen about the role of theory. Bambrough finds the notions of foundations problematic in all areas of knowledge, and challenges views that moral justification and deliberation are entirely different from other kinds of cognitive activities. He argues that higher standards are set in ethics than in science, unfairly creating higher expectations about our use of paradigms, deliberations, theories and justifications for ethics than science [7]. Bambrough agrees with Wittgenstein, Peirce and Hume that the roots of our reasoning are in the human fabric. If we look at how children learn about manners and morals, we find no theories or supreme principles operative but difficulties, problems and solutions that are a part of the "going concern" of living a human life. We may explore roots, but "Digging down to the roots is at the same time exploring the garden and fields, thickets and jungles, in which human life is lived." ([8], p. 43)

Questions about the meaning and use of "paradigm" and "theory" have been an important part of the discussion of the role of a case method or casuistry [1-13]. I propose to set them aside for this discussion and focus upon issues of bias.

The thesis of this paper is that to use our shared understanding of cases to reach morally justifiable conclusions, we must acknowledge and deal with problems of bias in describing, framing, comparing and using cases or paradigms. Problems of bias arise because we cannot identify what count as relevant features for such purposes unless we have general views about what is relevant; but some of our general views are biased, both in the sense of being unwarranted and in the sense that they may represent one-sided perspectives. The need to use our general views to determine what is relevant in describing, framing, selecting or comparing cases or paradigms, creates additional problems for some defenders of casuistry or case methods [1–3, 5, 7–9, 12] who maintain that case methods are more basic, reliable or prior to other forms of moral reasoning.

For example, Bambrough identifies a core, central or paradigm case: "My proof that we have moral knowledge consists essentially in saying, 'We know that this child, who is about to undergo what would otherwise be painful surgery, should be given an anaesthetic before the operation. Therefore, we know at least one moral proposition to be true'" ([7], p. 15). He knows this more certainly, he continues, than any premise, theory or principle advanced to confirm or suggest otherwise.[1]

Even if we agree with Bambrough that this is a morally unambiguous or core case, it does not show that our decisions about cases are more basic, reliable or prior to formation of our rules, maxims, principles or theories. If we ask why we share this understanding of the matter, we might reply that it is wrong to inflict unnecessary pain. Our view of the case supports and is supported by this maxim. Suppose we discover that the life-saving operation cannot be postponed and that the pain killers cannot be used for the child. We then conclude that we should go ahead because this is not a case of unnecessary pain. Our judgment about cases is not prior to our rules, for example, if we learn the meaning of rules, maxims, principles and theories as we learn how to think about cases [10].

I will begin with some remarks about bias, and then try to show how the problem of bias arises for case method and casuistry. I also discuss how analogous problems of bias in case review and theory construction arise in medical science, where clinical trial methodology was devised to deal systematically with it. Bias is also a difficulty for other methods of moral reasoning [3, 10–13], but I do not explore this.

2. BIAS

Centuries ago people used the word "bias" to described roads that inclined to one shoulder and bowling balls that spun to one side when thrown. We still use it to describe the disposition of woven fabric to pull to one side when stretched. Over time "bias" came to have a figurative meaning, referring to the "one-sidedness" of people's judgments [14]. Our beliefs, values, fears, hopes, traditions, training, goals, and so on, "pull" or "incline" us to certain views or attitudes, giving a "spin" or "slant" to our estimates and evaluations, sometimes despite our best efforts to the contrary.

Different figurative uses of bias are distinguishable. First, "bias" means *unwarranted inclinations*, or those judgments, dispositions, or belief systems that interfere with any form of careful reasoning because they are untested or unreasonable [15,16]. These unwarranted inclinations slant how we describe situations, compare cases, apply laws, use maxims, employ principles, or collect and use data. Personal beliefs, hopes, fears, prejudices, and so on, often distort reasoning because our beliefs are wrong, our judgments unwarranted and our sentiments misdirected or uncritical. Our religion, profession, society or tradition can also misdirect us through doctrinaire biases; we condemn these inclinations when they, for example, cause us to deny people opportunities based on race, religion or gender. Scientific investigators' enthusiasms about particular hypotheses can also cause them to introduce bias unintentionally by selective observations, promoting "favorable" responses, or other uncritical methods of observation, collection, interpretation or use of data. Nonrepresentative samples can lead investigators to make faulty generalizations. The elaborate system of safeguards used in science to protect against bias, do not always work [10, 15–22]. Such unintended bias is, of course, distinct from intentional bias in collecting or using data [15].

Second, some use "bias" to refer to *special perspectives* that dispose us to one-sided reasoning [15–16]. Special points of view may slant how we describe situations, compare cases, apply laws, use paradigms, employ principles, or collect and use data. For example, because of their special perspectives, doctors, malpractice attorneys and third-party payers may regard different features of a patients' medical records as noteworthy, good or interesting. Such slants are understandable but dispose us to cite certain features as important or reach certain judgments. Third, some even refer to any of our *goals*, such as dispositions to seek justice or truth, as "biases" [16]. If such use is warranted (and I have doubts that it is), then some biases are even good. I will not use "bias" in this way when considering how bias may be a problem for kinds of moral reasoning known as case method or casuistry. In what follows, I will use *bias* to mean our *unwarranted inclinations* or *one-sided perspectives* that dispose us to certain judgments, and *the problem of bias* to mean the difficulties with careful reasoning caused by such biases.

3. CASE METHOD

Jonsen[2] identifies three stages of moral reasoning using case review to solve moral quandaries [2]. I assume that Jonsen's characterization of the case method is acceptable to those advocating its use. In the first stage we should identify what the case and its relevant features are including the moral problems embedded therein. That is, we identify the situation's salient features or "core," as well as the moral issue it exemplifies. In the second stage we should compare the case to other cases, including paradigms. Finally, we should use analogies to decide how the cases "fit" various paradigms. Problems of bias, I argue, arise at each of these three stages of the moral reasoning, even if we assume that the persons using a case method are reasonable and informed people of good will.

3.1. Identification of the case and issues

To illustrate that our biases affect how we pick out cases, their relevant features and what problems we think they exemplify, imagine people presenting three accounts of the same events to an institutional ethics committee meeting:

26   LORETTA M. KOPELMAN

Case A. Baby W's parents want her to continue to have maximal treatment in the neonatal intensive care unit, where she has spent her entire four months of life. The doctors and nurses object because they view such treatment as futile and inhumane. The baby, they believe, is dying and these painful interventions will needlessly, and without benefit, prolong her suffering. Moreover, the neonatal intensive care unit is crowded, care is costly, and others are being denied admission. The parents threaten to sue if treatments are stopped.

When the case is presented in this way, most of us would agree that the case's relevant features concern devising fair procedures to overrule surrogates who demand futile, costly and painful procedures for patients. This case might lead us to consider getting a court order to stop inhumane treatment, or to reexamine some of our policies about surrogate consent, malpractice, physicians' right to refuse to provide care they believe harmful, or the differences between rights to refuse and to demand medical treatments.

Case B. Our agreement about the nature of the problems exemplified in Case A and what to do, however, presupposes we have framed the case in a way that captures the relevant features. Let us suppose that the doctors, nurses, and ethics committee members have ignored certain information that Baby W's family considers important. They argue that the reason they want her treated is because their extended family is coming from other parts of the world to be together for Baby W's death. This gathering has great symbolic meaning to them and so they beg that the treatments be briefly continued. The treatment is futile to prolong Baby W's life beyond a few weeks or months, but not futile for the different goal of having the family gather and grieve.

Deliberately omitting this information seems to show bias, because this material could transform our view of the situation, what is relevant for discussion, and the problems exemplified. We might now see the problems differently: as whether a treatment that is futile for prolonging life more than a few weeks or months could be provided for a short time as long as it did not cause unnecessary suffering or risk other's well-being; or as what constitutes compassionate treatment of a family in such distress; or as why the doctor, nurses, and committee members were biased in their original presentation and unsympathetic in deciding what was relevant to the discussion.

Case C. Now suppose that the family confronts the members of the ethics committee, doctors, and nurses charging them with bias because they ignored the information that the family wants the treatments continued until their relatives gather for the death of Baby W. The doctors, nurses and committee members respond that they are not biased because Baby W's parents have been saying this for two of the four months that Baby W has been in the hospital. The parents, they believe, are using this as an excuse to get the high technology treatments they refuse to believe are futile and inhumane.

CASE METHOD   27

In an actual consultation, these various views described as Cases A, B, and C would quickly emerge. Informed and impartial persons of good will would probably come to a shared understanding of what the case is and the problems it exemplifies. In an actual consultation, however, other biases might arise from activities or procedures that are harder to identify, including: who has access to the committee, how committee members are appointed, what procedures are followed, when the meeting is held, the order of business, who collects the information and presents it, who decides whether the results are recorded in the chart, who is introduced by first names and by "doctor," and so on.

Making sound moral judgments about actual cases presupposes accurate and pertinent information. Yet, real cases have ragged edges and what we pick out as "the case" can unintentionally introduce bias. In framing a case, we have to sift material, assign it importance, and decide what further information we need. Whether intentionally or not, we bring a variety of goals and values to our encounters with people and this is reflected in how or in what way we use cases. We are not passive in listening to or formulating cases. Training, profession, socio-economical backgrounds, or even prejudices may uncritically affect what we take to be relevant about the problem exemplified or plausible solutions about what ought to be done. Biased personal beliefs and attitudes, as well as professional and other points of view, then, can come into play in framing cases and determining what problem is exemplified.

Cases A, B and C show that a small change in the descriptions of events radically alters our views of "the case" and "the problems" it exemplifies. In different areas of the world, general views about someone's race, sex, religion, ethnic background or wealth would also affect decisions about whether treatments should be given to a certain baby. But one does not have to look across cultures to find disagreements stemming from our general views about how to identify the relevant features of a case or the problems it exemplifies. For example, general views about abortion cause some of us to "view" a thirteen-year old's decision to abort following a rape to be a prudent decision, while others "see" the choice as compounding the evil. Even without articulated general views, we may have strongly held but different intuitions. For example, some of us "saw" the Rodney King beating by police as a clear case of police brutality; others "saw" the police defending the public against the criminal element. Thus, a problem for those defending a case method of moral reasoning or casuistry is to identify how we can reach general agreement in our selection of information or how to frame controversial cases in a way that neutralizes the effects of bias.

28   LORETTA M. KOPELMAN

3.2. Comparing Cases

We make comparisons for some purpose and from some point of view, so additional problems of bias can arise in the second facet of case method reasoning. First, since people are interested in different issues, they may seize upon different comparisons as important. Medical students, for example, objected that one of their instructors created prejudicial attitudes toward African-American patients because all his teaching slides illustrating venereal diseases were of African-American people. The physician protested that he had no intention of insulting any group but had merely selected his best illustrations of the diseases. He changed his slides, however.

Second, the range of comparisons can affect decision making about a particular case. For example, suppose that we agree for the sake of argument that Story C captures the relevant features of the situation under review. The hospital attorney wants to protect the hospital from potentially bad publicity and save herself long court days. Consequently, she stresses the inconvenience and poor chances of getting a court order to stop life-saving treatment of a baby over parental objections. By telling vivid but selective stories about legal cases where hospitals futilely opposed families, the hospital lawyer encourages the committee not to seek a court order.

The kind of cases we use in making comparisons, then, can promote views uncritically. For example, defenders of paternalism in medicine, in their desire to promote the duties of beneficence, may focus on cases where professionals need to intervene on behalf of incompetent or impaired people, or to protect them from irresponsible surrogates. Opponents of paternalism, in contrast, may only focus on cases where competent people are being manipulated or coerced by others. Both excesses illustrate that the case(s) we pick for comparison can lead to informal fallacies of reasoning. Such methods minimize the need to address difficult problems about how to distinguish competence from incompetence, or trace the limits of paternalism and self-determination.

Third, the order in which cases are presented may powerfully influence belief. A case history about a needy patient with Acquired Immunodeficiency Syndrome (AIDS) can build empathy for all patients with this disease. On the other hand, a vivid but unsympathetic story about someone with AIDS can destroy support for them. Worse still, once people form their views based upon atypical cases, aggregate data may not change their opinions. In one study, two lively but non-representative case histories led people to form views which summaries of twenty well documented and representative cases could not dispel [19].

Such evidence showing that a vivid case may be more influential than the aggregate data in influencing our thoughts and judgments should give us concern in how we select, use and compare cases. The cases we use in our comparisons, then, incline people to certain views or conclusions. The type, range and order of cases we pick can distort reasoning because they reflect biased general views.

3.3. Using Analogy and Paradigm

The third stage of moral reasoning in case method involves using analogies to decide how the cases "fit" various paradigms. This method presupposes that we agree upon the core cases and how this helps us resolve disputes, especially for controversial situations.[3] One problem for those using a case method is that we do not always agree upon what cases are paradigms or how disputed cases relate to them. Even when there is wide agreement about core cases[4], moreover, we need to understand why such agreement serves as a basis for picking out exemplars or justifying moral choices. It requires something more than mere consistency between moral judgments, or between moral judgments or certain rules, maxims or paradigms [23]. Consistency offers no assurance of reliability, since people's judgments, maxims, rules or paradigms can be systematically and consistently biased. Nazi prison guards may have been consistent in their rules and judgments, yet immoral.

Second, suppose that we agree upon certain paradigm cases based upon our shared understanding. If the paradigm is noncontroversial (it is bad for a youth gang to kill a kind and helpless elderly man in an unprovoked attack), it may not be helpful at the very point one needs help – in solving controversial cases. The marginal cases are often complex and controversial because they do not fit paradigms. If one picks a complex and controversial case as a paradigm, we are likely to disagree about whether or how it serves as a paradigm.

One of the most widely used films in bioethics is *Please Let Me Die* [24]. Dax Cowart is the central character and the film was made ten months after an accident that left him severely burned. He does not want painful life-saving treatments or to live the life of a burn victim. His physicians and mother refuse to accept his decision, and seek a psychiatric consultation to have him declared incompetent. They want to continue to treat him over his objections. The film raises the question of whether Dax is competent to refuse life-saving treatment. Although the film does not indicate this, he is eventually found competent by two psychiatrists.

This is a complex and controversial case. To many of us who use this film in bioethics teaching, this story is a paradigm of a competent person being forced to have treatments he does not want. To others it is a paradigm of doctors and a mother refusing to abandon someone to a terrible decision. Some even view Cowart as a paradigm of what the competent person is like. If you think most adults are competent, this is mistaken since Cowart is exceptionally smart and well-educated. Most competent people could not discuss options, alternatives and theories like Cowart.

Reaching agreement about what cases to use as core cases, then, does not necessarily show that they *ought* to be agreed upon as core cases or illuminate what they are core cases of. Moreover, agreement about core cases does not show what criteria should be used to adopt core cases, or solve the problem of how to deal with marginal cases.

The fact that we sometimes have great difficulty reaching agreement, however, is not a decisive criticism of this or any other method. We hope that we can in time agree upon how disputed cases relate to established paradigms. We presume that we may discover implicit assumptions or attitudes that merit further examination and stand in the way of our reaching an agreement. There are areas of dispute, however, where we seem to lack similar intuitions even after this is done. For example, some of our disagreements about euthanasia, abortion, war, and the use of animals seem to resist our best efforts to reach agreement.

Finally, to compare cases, we have to abstract what is relevant or irrelevant, and determine how cases are alike or different from each other or from some paradigm. This creates difficulties for those who claim that "cases are prior to principles and theories" ([5], p. 16), because the classification of cases is a theoretical activity in at least one important meaning of "theory" [15]. For example, if we pick a complex situation as a paradigm, we may disagree about what it exemplifies because of our general views. If we pick a simple case, we may agree about what it exemplifies, but disagree about how to use in complex situations. The burden of proof is upon defenders, then, to clarify how the use of case methods can be more basic, reliable or prior to general views or theories that may shape judgments about what is relevant in describing, framing, selecting or using cases or paradigms.

4. CASUISTRY

In their defense of casuistry, Jonsen and Toulmin[1–2] try to address many of the problems of bias mentioned herein. They argue that morally sensitive and informed people can be identified by their communities, institutions and practices and encouraged to develop shared understanding of paradigms, how relevant features are selected for comparison, what constitutes adequate comparisons, why decisions are not purely local, and whose intuitions are reliable. Do Jonsen and Toulmin's appeals to community and intuitionism account for our shared understanding of core cases or how we compare these cases to others? Let us consider their use of these two means of defending casuistry.

4.1. Communities

Jonsen and Toulmin argue that experts construct paradigms within institutions or communities and that these paradigms generate maxims, norms, middle level principles, rules of thumb, or definitions. These, in turn, help us solve problems in a reliable way. One uses the facts of the case along with appropriately established paradigms, maxims, norms, middle level principles, definitions, or rules to arrive at practical moral solutions. While the solutions are contingent, they are accumulated within a community accounting for why, when consistent, a community becomes increasingly confident that they have reached a firm foundation for morality. As we compare cases, we see if we want to reevaluate our time-tested judgments. The less we are inclined to do this, the more secure we can be that these judgments are correct. Because cultures share methods of internal self-criticism, this approach avoids cultural relativism and dogmatism. Casuistry, Jonsen and Toulmin argue, enables us to override our preconceived notions or theories, and to employ insight and conscience. These are a correctable source of moral knowledge.

Casuistry is not simply the review of cases, according to Jonsen and Toulmin; rather it requires institutions to support this unique approach. It needs experts working within traditions who have learned how to identify the salient features of a case, the most important problems and the appropriate comparisons. Jonsen and Toulmin claim that even though those who work in applied ethics share no common single institution, they can share enough so that they become experts of sorts in evaluating, organizing, and applying these paradigms to new situations.

Jonsen and Toulmin model their version of casuistry upon the Roman Catholic tradition, where informed conscience, discernment and expertise is developed within a community or tradition. "The dialogue and debate consists in the critical application of paradigms to new circumstances, but those 'paradigms' were the collective possession of people ... who had education, the opportunity and the expertise to reflect on the differences raised by new cases and to argue them through among themselves" ([1], p. 335).

To illuminate the importance of discernment, charity and equity in using a case method, Jonsen and Toulmin offer an example in the last chapter of their book. As we shall see, however, this discussion inadvertently illustrates difficulties with their attempt to use communities and their experts to account for our shared understanding of core cases and how to apply them.

In the last chapter of *The Abuse of Casuistry* [1], Jonsen and Toulmin argue that extremists on both sides of the abortion debate fail to acknowledge relevant

32   LORETTA M. KOPELMAN

differences between early and late term abortions. The extreme conservative
holds that there is no morally relevant difference between killing a zygote and
an eight month old fetus, and both are impermissible. The extreme liberal sees
no difference either, but concludes abortion is always permissible. In the
following passage, Jonsen and Toulmin maintain that liberal and conservative
extremists both ignore relevant similarities and differences.

During the nine months from implantation to birth, the embryo develops in ways that are
relevant to the nature of its moral standing; and it requires a certain obstinacy or
obtuseness to deny any morally significant differences exist between a newly formed
zygote and a fetus in the eighth month ... Only people whose minds are too firmly made
up to reconsider the complexities of the abortion issue can say in advance that none of
these changes has any possible relevance to the matter ... before we take a "principled"
stand toward particular cases of abortion, charity and equity require that we be informed
about the circumstances of the particular case ([1], pp. 336,337).

As moderates on abortion, Jonsen and Toulmin claim the liberal and conservative extremists are blinded by their general views and lack charity and equity.
But, the conservatives and liberals also claim it is they alone who are truly
charitable and equitable, and identify the relevant features embedded in the
situation. The conservative finds a developing human life most significant, the
liberal sees the woman's right to decide what happens to her body as most
important, and the moderate sees an important value conflict requiring compromise.

Jonsen and Toulmin's intuitions about what is relevant, charitable and
equitable, therefore, do not settle the abortion debate. Moreover, the debate is
not always solved by appealing to casuistry within a well-established tradition.
The Roman Catholic tradition is well-established and has used casuistry for
centuries, yet Jonsen and Toulmin disagree with its official abortion position.

If we can know that traditions and their appointed experts may be wrong, then
institutions and their experts cannot entirely account for our shared understandings about core cases and how to use them. Since we can determine that
institutions and their experts sometimes misidentify core cases or mistakenly use
methods of casuistry, we need a further account for the source of our shared
understandings about the core cases and how to use them. Ironically, Jonsen and
Toulmin inadvertently show this with the very institution upon which they
model their approach to casuistry, raising questions about the reliability of
institutions and their experts to escape systematic error. Moreover, we know
from our committee meetings, courts and legislative bodies that experts do not
always agree about how to view specific cases even within well-established
traditions.

4.2. Intuitionism

Jonsen and Toulmin agree that we may sometimes want to reconsider our intuitions about what ought to be done or about which cases are similar. This is not surprising since we sometimes reconsider what we seem to see or feel as well. The novice art student may also have to struggle to see how colors are similar or different. They argue, however, that we use intuition to decide about cases, compare them, select our paradigms and rules, alter our maxims, and allow exceptions. We decide this based upon how well they fit our "true moral perception" and "the ability to see" when, for example, tolerance or strictness is the better course ([1], p. 327). Jonsen and Toulmin, then, use "intuition" to mean something more than our spontaneous beliefs; they use it as a source of a true or reliable insight about morality.

One difficulty is that appealing to what one believes to be "true moral perceptions" in itself offers no justification for the claim of these intuitions being true [25–26]. Such "true" intuitions may only reflect our sincerely held prejudices. We cannot test our differing intuitions on controversial cases; yet, we know that some cannot be correct since we often have incompatible intuitions about important issues like abortion, euthanasia, war, and so on. Appeals to our true feelings show sincerity but are unhelpful when we disagree. Where the cases are controversial, our appeals to intuition alone will not advance the discussion or convince others. As Jonsen and Toulmin themselves point out, neither the sincere beliefs of the conservatives nor those of the liberals on abortion convince the other group [1].

Second, even if we suppose that our intuitions about one case are correct, this would not necessarily be helpful in dealing with other more controversial cases. Jonsen and Toulmin agree that there is no single path from the paradigm to judgments about other cases. We can make mistakes systematizing and correcting our insights, or stating and defending reasons why cases are the same or different.

To summarize, I have tried to show how problems of bias occur in case review. The classification and use of cases require prior decisions about what features are relevant. Bias can arise in describing what we take the case to be, stating the problem exemplified, choosing the cases used for comparison, and identifying the paradigms we select. Jonsen and Toulmin's appeals to community or intuitionism do not appear to solve these problems of bias.

34   LORETTA M. KOPELMAN

5. BIAS AND GENERALIZATIONS

I have focused upon how bias arises in case reviews in moral reasoning and casuistry because this is an important method which we need to improve. I do not mean to suggest, however, that bias is either more or less of a problem for this method of reasoning than others. There are good discussions of how bias arises in using moral principles [1, 3, 12], about how we may select and use moral theories to bolster views uncritically [3, 11], and about systematic bias in traditions committed to other forms of rational enquiry such as in science [10, 20–22]. An instance of the problem of bias in another form of reasoning that is particularly relevant to our discussion about case reviews and bias, concerns problems of bias when trying to establish generalizations from case reviews in medical science.

For example, a series of case reports appeared following a 1965 publication where Jacobs and her associates reported an association of the genetic condition XYY with possibly deviant behavior [27]. About 0.1% of males have the XYY chromosome pattern, but she found the frequency of XYY males increased four times (.25) in penal institutions and increased 2–4% in penal mental institutions. Case reports appeared in the psychiatric literature supporting the view that the extra Y chromosome is associated with violent, aggressive or antisocial behavior. Consequently, lawyers argued that their XYY clients were not responsible for their violent crimes because their genetic hard-wiring meant they could not do otherwise. In the end, the association with aggressiveness was discredited by means of a careful retrospective study which examined the records of a whole population of XYY males, not just those who were seeing psychiatrists. Their increased conviction rate was attributed to greater incidence of learning disabilities, impulsiveness and lower intelligence, but not to aggressiveness [25].

In reaction to the dangers of generalizing from case reports, investigators try to develop methods to eliminate bias. One of the most used and respected of these methods is the double-blind, placebo controlled randomized clinical trial methodology [17]. These trials are prospective studies where patients are divided into different groups, or study-arms, by a chance mechanism (such as random numbers). A control group receives standard care or a placebo (an inert preparation such as a sugar pill), and one or more treatment groups gets special care. The group assignments are kept from patients and therapists until after the trial. This design helps eliminate bias in several ways. Since physicians do not know in which treatment arm patients are enrolled, their beliefs or hunches about the different treatments will not affect their estimates of outcomes or endpoints. Since patients do not know if they are receiving a placebo or an active substance, the results are uncontaminated by their expectations (the

CASE METHOD 35

placebo effect). Randomization also helps eliminate bias. The goal of randomization is to distribute individual characteristics (such as age, health, wealth, education, habits, beliefs, and practices) among study-arms in order to minimize their effects. This procedure helps assure that outcomes reflect the different modes of care, and that the results can be generalized.

Despite such efforts, critics continue to expose systematic bias. For example, there are often strict eligibility criteria excluding certain groups from clinical trials. Often they exclude women and children [21–22]. If treatments are only tested on men, the generalizations from the data are restricted since it is not clear how they affect women or children.[5]

To conclude, case methods of reasoning are effective and important, but to use them to reach morally justifiable judgments, we need to address problems of bias in using cases. In exploring the sort of bias that distorts moral reasoning in casuistry or the use of a case method, I have offered no reason to believe bias is a greater problem here than in other kinds of reasoning or for other methods of moral inquiry. The problem of bias should not cause us to stop using case reviews in moral reasoning any more than in medical science. This discussion of the problem of bias is not meant to strike a devastating blow against case reviews in moral reasoning, but to show the need to address certain difficulties or admit certain limitation with case methods. Many people have argued persuasively that ethical reasoning needs to be rooted in particular human activities, and that comparisons of situations is an important method of moral reasoning. To use this method as a means to reach morally defensible conclusions, however, we need, as best we can, to justify that we have eliminated bias in describing, framing, selecting, and comparing cases and paradigms.

ACKNOWLEDGEMENT

I wish to thank Albert Jonsen, Ed Erde, Peter Williams, Carl Elliott, David DeGrazia, Robert L. Holmes, and Richard McCarty for helpful comments on various drafts of this paper.

NOTES

[1] Bambrough argues that moral knowledge can be defended against skepticism with arguments that parallel those used to defend knowledge of the external world against skepticism [7].

[2] Jonsen calls these three categories morphology, taxonomy, and kinetics [2].

[3] Different views might rely upon some theory of human nature, divine revelation or authority from some institution. Each view has well known problems, but each is designed to try to solve the problem of the obvious diversity in our cultures and

36   LORETTA M. KOPELMAN

institutions about what considerations are central and why their judgments are not purely
local [13].
[4] An important area of empirical research would be to determine to what extent we agree
about central cases and criteria for identifying adequate similarities of cases to the
paradigms.
[5] One reason that women are routinely excluded is that they might become pregnant and
the fetus could be harmed by an experimental drug. Barring women from participating in
trials just because they might become pregnant, however, denies them the same access to
new and promising therapies as men, and may place fetal interests ahead of theirs as a
matter of public policy. Dr. Bernadine Healy, then director of the National Institutes of
Health (NIH) has been critical of "[d]ecades of sex-exclusive research." ([22], p. 275)
She argues that excluding women from studies causes sex bias in the management of
certain illnesses and ignores women's unique medical problems.

REFERENCES

1. Jonsen, AR, Toulmin, S *The Abuse of Casuistry: A History of Moral Reasoning*,
   University of California Press, Berkeley: 1988.
2. Jonsen, AR Casuistry as methodology in clinical ethics. *Theor Med* 1991; 12:
   295–307.
3. Hoffmaster B. Philosophical ethics and practical ethics: Never the twain shall meet.
   In Hoffmaster B, Freedman B, & Fraser G, eds., *Clinical Ethics: Theory and
   Practice*. Clifton, New Jersey: Humana Press, 1989: 201–230.
4. Juengst ET. Casuistry and the locus of certainty in ethics. *Med Hum Rev* 1989; 3:
   19–27.
5. Klinefelter DS. How is applied philosophy to be applied? *J Soc Phil*, 1990; Spring:
   16–26.
6. Downie R. Health care ethics and casuistry, *J Med Ethics* 1992; 18: 61–22, 66.
7. Bambrough R. *Moral Skepticism and Moral Knowledge*. London: Routledge and
   Kegan Paul, 1979.
8. Bambrough R. The roots of moral reasoning. In: Regis E Jr ed. *Gewirth's Ethical
   Rationalism*. Chicago: University of Chicago Press, 1984: 39–51.
9. Jonsen AR. Of balloons and bicycles; or, the relationship between ethical theory and
   practical judgment. *Hastings Center Report*, (Sept-Oct)1991: 14–16.
10. Kuhn TS. *The Structure of Scientific Revolution*. 2nd Ed. Chicago: University of
    Chicago Press, 1970.
11. Holmes R. The limited relevance of analytic ethics to the problems of bioethics. *J
    Med Phil* 1990 15(2): 143–159.
12. Toulmin S. The Tyranny of Principle, *Hastings Center Report* 11, 1981: 31–38.
13. Williams B. *Ethics and the Limits of Philosophy*, Cambridge: Harvard University
    Press, 1985.
14. *Oxford English Dictionary*. Bias; Vol. 1, 1991; 844–845.
15. Durbin PT. Theory, *Dictionary of Concepts in the Philosophy of Science*, Westport,
    CT: Greenwood Press, 1988: 320–322.
16. Paul R, Rudinow J. Bias relativism and critical thinking, *J Thought* 1988; 23,
    Fall/Winter: 125–138.
17. Kopelman LM. Consent and randomized clinical trials: Are there moral or design
    problems?, *J Med Phil* 1986; 11: 317–345.
18. Kopelman LM. Moral problems in psychiatry. Veatch RM, ed. *Medical Ethics*
    (1989). Boston: Jones and Bartlett, pp. 253–290.
19. Anderson CA. Abstract and concrete data in perseverance of social theories: When
    weak data lead to unshakable beliefs *J Exp Soc Psych* 1983; 19; 93–108.

CASE METHOD 37

20. Harding S, O'Barr, JF. *Sex and Scientific Inquiry*, Chicago: Chicago University Press, 1987.
21. Dresser R. Wanted: single white male for medical research, *Hastings Center Report* 22 (January/February); 1992: 24–29.
22. Healy B. The yentl syndrome. *New Engl J Med* 1991; 325: 274–276.
23. Daniels N. Wide reflexive equilibrium and theory acceptance in ethics, *J Phil* 1979; 76: 256–282.
24. *Please Let Me Die*: Department of Psychiatry, Galveston: University of Texas, 1973.
25. Frankena WK. *Ethics*. 2nd ed., New York: Prentice Hall: 1973.
26. Nowell-Smith PH. *Ethics*, Oxford: Basil Blackwell, 1957.
27. Kopelman LM Ethical controversies in medical research: The case of XYY screening, *Perspectives in Biology and Medicine* 1978, 196–204.
28. Kopelman LM What is applied about applied ethics? *J Phil Med* 1990; 15(2): 199–218.

[6]

NANCY S. JECKER AND DONNIE J. SELF

SEPARATING CARE AND CURE: AN ANALYSIS OF HISTORICAL AND CONTEMPORARY IMAGES OF NURSING AND MEDICINE*

ABSTRACT. This paper provides a philosophical critique of professional stereotypes in medicine. In the course of this critique, we also offer a detailed analysis of the concept of care in health care. The paper first considers possible explanations for the traditional stereotype that caring is a province of nurses and women, while curing is an arena suited for physicians and men. It then dispels this stereotype and fine tunes the concept of care. A distinction between 'caring for' and 'caring about' is made, and concomitant notions of parentalism are elaborated. Finally, the paper illustrates, through the use of cases, diverse models of caring. Our discussion reveals the complexity of care and the alternative modes of caring in health care.

Key Words: caring, curing, gender identity, nursing ethics, professional ethics

Care as a central organizing concept is a relative newcomer to moral theory (Blum, 1988; Kittay and Meyers, 1987; Noddings, 1984, 1987, 1989; Pearsall, 1986) and moral development theory (Gilligan, 1982, 1986; Gilligan and Wiggins, 1987; Lyons, 1983). However, its roots in American nursing trace back to nursing's early history. In the late nineteenth century, Florence Nightingale thought medical therapeutics and 'curing' were of less importance to patient outcome and willingly left this realm to the physician. Caring, the arena she considered of greatest importance, she assigned to the nurse (Reverby, 1987a, 1987b).[1]

Although nurses and physicians entertain a more sophisticated picture of their professions today, the image of caring as the exclusive province of nurses continues to influence public perceptions. Because patients exert influence over professionals' self-perceptions, patients' attitudes have the potential to strengthen and reinforce traditional stereotypes, obstruct efforts to re-define

---

Nancy S. Jecker, Ph.D., SB 20, Department of Medical History and Ethics, School of Medicine, University of Washington, Seattle, Washington 98195, U.S.A.

Donnie J. Self, Ph.D., Department of Humanities in Medicine, Texas A & M, College Station, Texas 77843, U.S.A.

The Journal of Medicine and Philosophy 16: 285–306, 1991.

 Nancy S. Jecker and Donnie J. Self

professional relationships and provide political fuel for traditional hierarchies. In this way, the idea that 'doctors cure and nurses care' continues to exercise a pervasive influence on health professionals' self-images and inter-professional relationships. In addition to these practical consequences, the care-cure division easily can produce a lack of philosophical clarity regarding the concept of care itself. In particular, dissociating the labor of physicians from the realm of care narrows our understanding of care, while treating nursing work as an exclusive care paradigm encourages one-dimensional thinking about care.

This essay provides a philosophical critique of professional stereotypes in medicine. In the course of this critique, we also offer a detailed analysis of the concept of care in health care. More precisely, our aims are to (1) identify factors that contribute to viewing care as the exclusive province of nurses; (2) fine tune the concept of care by exploring alternative forms of care; and (3) illustrate, through the use of cases, diverse models of caring.

GENDER-BASED EXPLANATIONS OF PROFESSIONAL STEREOTYPES

In a popular text on nursing ethics, Andrew Jameton observes that "Physicians are...said to focus on the *cure* function, while nurses focus on the *care* functions" (1984, p. 10). Jameton goes on to explain that nurses are expected to perform such functions as follow hospital procedures, report significant incidents and mishaps to supervisors, and organize work on wards and hospital departments. Presumably, physicians order procedures, make medical decisions and take charge of wards and departments. What are the origins of this apparent division of labor? Why does the perception that nurses, and only nurses, perform care functions remain with us? Since nursing and medicine are largely gender segregated professions, the answers to these questions may lie as much in gender-related tendencies as in the histories of nursing and medicine.

One explanation for this apparent division is suggested by Gilligan and Pollak (1989). They report that the association of danger with intimacy is a more salient feature in the fantasies of men than of women. In their study, men projected more danger into situations of close, personal affiliation than situations of impersonal achievement. For example, male subjects expressed "a fear of being caught in a smothering relationship or humiliated by rejection or deceit" (1989, p. 246). Females, by contrast, perceived more danger in situations of impersonal achievement than situations of personal affiliation. For instance, females "connected danger with the isolation that they associated with competitive success" (1989, p. 246). If male and female attitudes toward attachment and separation do cluster in the way this study suggests, this indicates one fairly obvious explanation for care and cure stereotypes in the health professions. Female nurses would tend to cultivate skill at caring activities, because these activities involve the intimacy and close personal affiliation that women, as a group, prefer. Curing activities would, on the whole, be shunned by nurses, because such activities involve forms of impersonal achievement that women, as a group, find threatening. The opposite tendency should occur in medicine, a male dominated profession, namely: physicians would be likely to stress scientific and technical achievement, while down playing patient contact and physician-patient relationships.

Consistent with the above line of reasoning is a second possible explanation. According to this second account, the detached objectivity of scientific fields generally, and medical science in particular, discourages many women from excelling at them. Keller maintains that the goal of post-enlightenment science has been a method of perception that affirms empirical reality, while denying subjectivity (1985). This method of knowing implies a purely mechanical view of persons and objects: "no longer filling the void with living form," scientists in the modern age "learned to fill it with dead form" (Keller, 1985, pp. 69–70). In our culture, such a view of self and world is, according to Keller, pervasively associated with masculinity (1985, p. 71).

If Keller is correct about both the association between science and objectivity and the association between objectivity and masculinity, her analysis sheds light on the alleged cure-care division. Following Keller's analysis, once scientific medicine became the dominant mode of medicine in this country, a method of perception that denied the significance of subjectivity took hold. Such an approach focused attention on patients' physical signs and symptoms, while down playing the significance of their subjective preferences, feelings and experiences. The masculine image this method portrayed in the culture induced males to practice medicine, but encouraged women to assume healing roles that fit better the culture's idea of femininity.

A third explanation of professional stereotypes in nursing and medicine also appeals to gender stereotypes. This explanation holds that our culture associates ethics and humanism with femininity rather than masculinity. For example, ethics and values frequently are referred to as being learned at mother's knee. Morantz-Sanchez (1985) traces this association between ethics and femininity to the early nineteenth century. She argues that during this time, the popular image of women shifted from the biblical and puritan idea of an innately sexual temptress to the idea of women as naturally passionless, spiritual and moral. When women were no longer seen as "the inheritors of Eve's questionable legacy" (Morantz-Sanchez, 1985, p. 22), their prudery confined the social roles they were qualified to fill. In particular, women were judged unqualified to enter the medical profession because, unlike men, they could not restrain their natural sympathies as a physician must. For example, women could not be brought into the dissecting room and undergo other rigors of medical training without destroying their innate moral sensibilities.

Referring to the modern tradition, Jameton makes the point that it is "women [not men who] have carried the humane tradition in modern western cultures: they educate children, soften the blows of the world, nurture others and humanize modern life. Nursing and medicine have reified this stereotype" (1987, p. 67). Jameton also notes the long standing tradition of ethics in the female dominated profession of nursing, and the comparatively weaker and more recent tradition of ethics in medicine. According to Jameton, since 1900 not a single decade has passed without publication of at least one basic text in nursing ethics. Moreover, in its very first volume (1901), *The American Journal of Nursing* published an article on ethics. In the 1920s and 1930s, the *Journal* carried a regular column of ethics cases. In addition to ethics publications, ethics courses have a long history in nursing: they were included in the first formal training programs for nurses. In medicine, by contrast, the tradition of ethics teaching in a sustained and consistent manner is much more recent. It was not until the 1970s that medicine incorporated a significant formal ethics curriculum into medical school classes, and even then "it resulted in large part from outside pressures" (Jameton, 1987, p. 67). Assuming Morantz-Sanchez's and Jameton's historical analyses are correct, they illuminate another possible source of

Separating Care and Cure 289

professional stereotypes. If our culture associates ethical concern and response with femininity, one would expect females in general to gravitate toward roles that call upon these abilities. Men who wished to enter the health care profession would fill other roles.

It should be noted that all of the above explanations take for granted the idea that American nursing and medicine are gender segregated professions. This assumption is historically accurate, since a generation or more ago over ninety per cent of medical students and physicians were white men (Relman, 1989), and nursing has long been dominated by women. Yet despite this historical precedence, today more men are becoming nurses and women are much more likely to enter the medical profession. In 1972, for example, 1,694 men graduated from American nursing schools, a fourfold increase over 1963, and in 1981 the number of men graduating from R.N. programs jumped to 3,492 (Rowland, 1984). Since women continue to dominate nursing, it is not surprising that overall they occupy more high-level administrative and supervisory positions than men. Yet, the percentage of male nurses who have reached administrative or supervisory positions is much larger than the percentage of female nurses who have reached administrative or supervisory positions (Rowland, 1984). Thus men who do enter nursing are more likely to be in positions where their presence and influence is felt.

Likewise, in the American medical profession, the percentage of female applicants and matriculants to medical school began to rise abruptly in 1970–1971. The number of applications from men, which had been rising steeply, reached a peak in 1974–1976 and has been falling ever since (Relman, 1989). Although few women serve on medical faculty (Eisenberg, 1989), and women are underrepresented in positions of power in academic institutions and as leaders in medical organizations (Levinson, Tolle, Lewis, 1989), their presence in medicine is growing and their influence in shaping medicine's professional identity is increasing.

For these reasons, the above explanations of professional stereotypes are incomplete as they stand. A more complete account would need to explain recent changes in the gender constitution of each profession, perhaps by appealing to shifts in the culture's gender ideals. For example, new gender ideals for men may lie behind changes currently underway in the medical profession. For example, the Association of American Medical

290 *Nancy S. Jecker and Donnie J. Self*

Colleges has substantially revised its Medical College Admission Test (MCAT) to place greater emphasis on 'humanistic' skills in selecting physicians; the American Board of Internal Medicine has requested directors of residency programs to assess compassion, respect for patients and integrity in candidates for board certification; and the American Medical Association recently embarked on a major quality assurance initiative which will include research into attributes of 'interpersonal exchange' (Nelson, 1989). Alternatively, a fuller explanation might uncover ways in which traditional gender attitudes persist, despite greater integration of men in nursing and women in medicine. For example, despite greater numbers of male nurses, the American nursing profession is still overwhelmingly female: ninety seven per cent of the total nurse population is female (American Nurses' Association, 1987). Moreover, the majority (56.3 per cent) of men cite employment availability as their reason for entering nursing, while most women (62.1 per cent) cite interest in people (Rowland, 1984). This suggests that practical economic considerations, rather than a desire to enter a caring role, are more frequent motives among men. Furthermore, the fact that more men are entering nursing may simply indicate that more men are willing to challenge prevailing stereotypes, rather than indicating that these stereotypes and the expectations associated with them no longer apply. Evidence for this is that males who become nurses are more likely than female nurses to be viewed as gay or asked why they do not become doctors (Rowland, 1984). Male nurses also report greater difficulty than female nurses in telling others of their occupational choice: in one study, only sixty-six percent felt comfortable doing so, as compared with eighty-three percent of women (Rowland, 1984). Finally, although more men are choosing nursing, gender segregation reportedly persists between nursing specialties. Men's highest priorities after graduation are jobs in critical or acute care settings, whereas women prefer pediatric and public health fields (Rowland, 1984). In one study of nursing students, male students preferred, in rank order: emergency nursing, then outpatient, intensive care, medical-surgical, psychiatric, and coronary care nursing, and lastly, anesthesia. By contrast, female students ranked pediatric nursing first, then public health, medical-surgical, obstetrics/maternity, and psychiatric nursing (Rowland, 1984).

Separating Care and Cure 291

HISTORICAL EXPLANATIONS OF PROFESSIONAL STEREOTYPES

Another kind of explanation for the cure-care division has less to do with hypothesized gender differences and more to do with the unique histories of the nursing and medical professions. First, the history of nursing, and its domestic roots in particular, may shed light on the association of nursing with care. Although historians sometimes ignore these roots and begin the history of nursing with the introduction of formal training programs for nurses in the 1870s, a growing number of revisionist historians reject this approach. For example, Reverby makes the point that American nursing "did not appear *de novo* at the end of the nineteenth century...[instead,] nursing throughout the colonial era and most of the nineteenth century took place within the family" (1987a, p. 5). O'Brien also finds the roots of nursing "deep in the domestic world of the family" (1987). And Starr maintains that "care of the sick was part of the domestic economy for which the wife assumed responsibility. She would call on the networks of kin and community for advice and assistance when illness struck" (1982, p. 32, 1982).

According to these historians, the history of American nursing begins prior to the 1870s. During this earlier period, mothers, daughters and sisters nursed their families at home, sometimes aided by female neighbors who called themselves 'professed' or 'born' nurses and had previous experience caring for their own families (O'Brien, 1987, p. 13). So long as the locus of nursing remained domestic, its primary task was the nurturing of loved ones through ongoing feeding, clothing, bathing and comforting.

Increasingly, the nurturing tasks in which home-based nurses engaged during the colonial era were set apart from the responsibility of their physician counterparts. First, the medical manuals that domestic nurses consulted drew a sharp line between "what could be accomplished by a loving mother and nurse and what needed the skilled consultation of a physician" (O'Brien, 1987, p. 13). The popular 18th century book, *Domestic Medicine*, assured readers that physicians need be consulted rarely, and that most people underestimate their own abilities and knowledge (Buchanan, 1778). Second, the very fact that nurses lived with their patients and constantly were immersed in the practical activity of caring for them, meant that their job took on a distinctive character. In contrast to nurses, physicians made house calls or were visited by patients in offices. Patients were not primarily relatives, but neighbors and town's people. The physician's job was to offer expert advise or perform specific medical procedures, while nurses carried out physicians' instructions. Thus, physicians used their presumed expertise to direct the caring process, while nurses who lived with patients carried out the actual tasks of ongoing care.

According to this account, the association of American nursing with care traces back to the time when nurses' chief task was caring for sick offspring in the home. Later in the nineteenth century, when nurses left the domestic front to care for patients in hospitals and during wartime, and when they attended the first professional training schools, these early domestic roots continued to shape nursing's identity. In these new locations, nurses' roles continued to include traditional domestic tasks, such as bed making, feeding and hygiene. Thus, a significant emphasis of early training programs was on practical skills. Later educational reforms which sought to introduce scientific content into the nursing curriculum stirred heated debate, attesting to the continued influence of the domestic tradition on the nursing profession.

While American nursing was linked intimately with caregiving activities, American physicians achieved professional status and identity by fashioning a separate sphere. Given the association between caring and 'women's work', physicians surely had little incentive to identify their own professional function as caring. As Benner and Wrubel note, "caring is devalued because caring is associated with women's work and women's work is devalued and most often unpaid" (1989, p. 368). During the colonial era, physicians had only part time medical practices. They earned a livelihood performing other tasks, such as clergy, teaching and farming (Conrad and Schnieder, 1990). Not until the nineteenth century did medicine become a full time vocation, but during this period its dangerous and often unsuccessful therapies undermined its prestige. According to Starr, "while some physicians were seeking to make themselves into an elite profession with a monopoly of practice, much of the public refused to grant them any such privileges" (1982, p. 31). In addition, physicians were fiercely competitive with homeopaths and other medical sects for a share of the medical market. Thus, much of American medicine's early history was characterized by repeated efforts to gain repute and professional standing. The first state licensing laws, which granted to physicians with special training and class sole authority to practice medicine, were repealed during the Jacksonian period (Starr, 1982). Later in the nineteenth century, with the formation of the American Medical Association, physicians were finally successful in their efforts to professional-ize medicine and control medical markets. Medicine was credited with the decline in incidence and mortality of diseases, such as leprosy, malaria, small pox and cholera, thereby increasing the public's faith in its healing powers. During the latter part of the nineteenth century, the rise of scientific medicine ushered in significant progress and ensured the continued prestige and dominance of the medical profession.

The early history of American medicine suggests a possible explanation for the association of medicine with cure, rather than care. The presence of fierce competition and marginal status during its early years forged a mission for medicine that focused on achieving cultural authority and an elite status for its prac-titioners. Efforts to gain authority and status required physicians to stand apart from laypersons and develop exclusive modes of language, technique and theory. This put physicians at odds with activities, such as patient empathy and care, that call upon abilities of engagement and identification with others. The scien-tific paradigm that became the language and practice of medicine further reinforced a separation between physician and patient. This paradigm pictured the human being as a machine, and disease as an objective entity that interfered with the human being's mechanical functioning. Such a perspective implied that the 'ghost in the machine' was superfluous to the healing process.

RETHINKING THE CONCEPT OF CARE

Having considered several possible explanations for the associa-tion of nursing with care, and medicine with cure, we need to consider next whether these common stereotypes are justified. To address this question, we now turn to a critical analysis of the concept of care. To begin with, it should be noted that the very idea of separating care from cure assumes that these ideas are distinct and non-overlapping. An alternative view sees caring as part of the very meaning of curing. According to this view, physicians who cure also care. Interestingly, the *Oxford English*

294   *Nancy S. Jecker and Donnie J. Self*

Dictionary supports this interpretation of cure. Cure comes from the Latin word "curare" meaning "to care for, take care of". Cure refers to "care, heed, concern; to do one's (busy) care, to give one's care or attention to some piece of work; to apply one's self diligently". This definition renders the idea of a physician who cures without caring unintelligible. A person who heals a wound, or otherwise restores a patient to health, cures only if this outcome is the result of devoted caring.

On this reading, although curing entails applying one's care to some one or thing, caring does not imply curing. Thus, physicians can and often do *care* for patients, while suspending attempts to *cure* them. This occurs, for example, when physicians withdraw medical treatments they judge futile, while continuing palliative measures. Hauerwas notes the practical importance of acknowledging the possibility of caring *without* curing. Physicians who fail to recognize the possibility of caring without curing might attempt futile therapies, based on the false belief that efforts to cure patients are all they have to offer.

The *Oxford English Dictionary* distinguishes two distinct senses of care. First, care means "a burdened state of mind arising from...concern about anything...mental perturbation", and "serious or grave mental attention, the charging of the mind". In this first sense, to "have a care" or "keep a care" is to be in a subjective state of concern about something. Second, care refers to "oversight with view to protection, preservation, or guidance; hence to have the care of". In this second sense, care implies an activity of looking out for or safeguarding the interests of others.

We shall designate the first sense of care, 'caring about'. Caring about indicates an attitude, feeling, or state of mind directed toward a person or circumstance (Hauerwas, 1978, p. 145). To assert that 'My nurse cares about me' or that 'Everyone ought to care about the environment' refers to care in this first sense. The second sense of care involves the exercise of a skill, with or without a particular attitude or feeling toward the object upon which this skill is exercised. We shall refer to this as 'caring for'. For example, we use care in this sense when we say that 'Nurse Jones is caring for your mother' or 'The mechanic down the street offered to take care of my car'. Caring in both senses is a relational term, referring to an attitude or skill directed to someone or something. One's concern about others may be more or less deep, and one's skill at caring for others may display more or less ability. Thus, we refer to the quality of caring to describe how deeply one feels, or how good or poor one is at caring for another. Whereas caring about can occur at a distance from its object, caring for usually requires direct contact with the one who is cared for. Excellence at caring for particular patients typically requires repeated contacts and skill in ascertaining each patient's particular needs. Thus, an expert caregiver learns "through repeated experience with patients...to perceive the particular rather than the typical, care becomes individualized rather than standardized and planning becomes anticipatory of change rather than simply responsive to change" (Benner and Wrubel, 1989, p. 382).

Applying these definitions of cure and care to the medical setting enables us to say that a health professional who cares *about* a patient makes a cognitive or emotional decision that the welfare of the patient is of great importance. Caring about requires keeping the patient's best interest in the forefront of mind and heart. By contrast, a health professional who cares *for* a patient engages in a deliberate and ongoing activity of responding to the patient's needs. Caring for, executed in an exemplary or excellent way, involves deciphering the patient's particular condition and needs. This calls upon verbal skills of questioning and listening and requires attending to and translating non-verbal cues. Caring for thus requires cultivating a capacity to understand others' subjective experiences. Understood in this light, caring for draws upon and teaches a way of knowing that involves "awareness of the complexities of a particular situation" and "inner...resources that have been garnered through experience in living" (Benoliel, 1987). The source of this knowledge tends to be participation in relationships with others and observation of others' actions, rather than verbal debate and conversation or the reading of texts (Benner, 1983). Knowledge in this form is practical and interpersonal (Schultz and Meleis, 1988). In the case of unconscious or mentally compromised patients and infants, caring for especially draws upon a person's skill at interpreting gestures, postures, sounds, grimaces, eye scans and bodily movements (Jecker, 1990a). For instance, through intimate engagement, a daughter who serves as a caretaker for a disoriented elderly parent may be able to decipher what counts as pain and comfort, or boredom and interest to the parent. Evidence is gleaned through partaking in daily rituals, such as bathing and feeding, and interpreting the parent's responses.

                      Nancy S. Jecker and Donnie J. Self

Caring *about* does not imply caring for. For example, a ward supervisor may care deeply about her patients, without being engaged in the activity of caring directly for them. Nor does caring *for* entail caring about. For instance, one who skillfully cares for patients may be meticulous in her efforts to interpret patients' needs, without actually caring about patients: she may regard them as just one more puzzle to be solved, excel at caring for its own sake, or simply seek to impress colleagues or a boss.

While it is fairly easy to tell who cares *for* a patient, it can be exceedingly difficult to construe who cares *about* a patient. Some professionals may prefer colleagues and supervisors to think they care about their patients, even if they in fact are preoccupied with other matters. Others may learn to cover up the fact that they do care about patients. For example, the idea of masculinity to which some aspire discourages outward expressions of care and concern for others. It would be difficult to gauge whether males who express masculinity in this way care about their patients. Still others may appear uncaring because they learn deference in conflict. For example, women or nurses who are taught to follow orders blindly may appear not to take a genuine interest in their patients. Historically, nurses were instructed to discharge medical orders in an obedient, unquestioning manner (Jameton, 1987), but this expectation does not necessarily entail the absence of caring about.

EXAMPLES OF CARE

In order to bring the concept of care into sharper focus, it is useful to review cases in which individuals exhibit care in different ways. In the course of this review, we shall consider in more detail the protective qualities associated with different kinds of care and the positive and negative forms these qualities can take.

1. Case One: Caring For and About a Patient

I was taking care of a 40-year old female who had been hospitalized for 3 months in another hospital and came to our hospital the day before to have her abdominal fistulas corrected. The night before I met her, the bag collecting her fistula drainage fell off three times and was reapplied the same way each time by her former nurse due to the patient's insistence that nothing else works. Her skin was very excoriated in spots and tender. When I removed the leaking bag I noticed that the problem was that she had a large crease between two recessed fistulas. I attempted to reapply it to avoid these. She was resistant to my suggestions, and protested my efforts to replace the bag. So I told her that she should trust me because I've had numerous similar situations with which I've had positive outcomes. I pointed out that if the bag was not replaced to avoid the fistulas it would continue to fall off and her pain and discomfort would only increase. She reconsidered. I told her that I was sure I could get a bag to stay on her for at least 24 hours, if not more. She said she'd love that to happen and told me I could do what I wanted (Benner, 1984, pp. 138–139).

In this first case, a nurse appears to care both for and about a patient. Each effort calls upon a distinct set of responses. Caring *for* manifests itself in the activities of removing the leaking bag, locating the problem in adhering it to the patient's skin and replacing the bag. Caring *about* is shown by the *manner* in which the nurse cares for the patient, a manner which expresses concern and involves efforts to reassure and gain the patient's confidence.

Notice too the nurse's response to her patient's initial resistance. This response exhibits the nurse's ability to persuade a recalcitrant patient that a certain procedure (replacing the bag) is in the patient's best interest and that she can execute this procedure successfully. A different response would have been simply to say, 'you *must* let me do this'. The difference between these two responses reveals alternative forms of parentalism (Taylor, 1985). In the medical setting, parentalism is an attempt to justify performing (or omitting) an action that is contrary to a patient's expressed wishes, yet judged to be in a patient's best interest. Were the nurse in this situation to respond to the refusal of treatment by saying 'that's my final word', she would illustrate a kind of parentalism that justifies medical actions by presuming to abrogate a patient's *rights*. An alternative mode of parentalism invokes a morality of *responsibility*, rather than rights (Taylor, 1985; Ruddick, 1989). Here, one appeals to the patient's self-interest and personal responsibility, rather than invoking one's own authority to override the patient. For example, the nurse in case one displays this latter kind of parentalism by effectively laying out for the patient the consequences that attach to different alternatives:

 Nancy S. Jecker and Donnie J. Self

replacing the bag properly ensures that it will adhere; not doing so may result in the bag falling off and so heighten the patient's pain and discomfort. In this way, the patient is led to choose between taking responsibility for safeguarding her own interests, or behaving in a less responsible fashion.

Parentalism that is based on promoting the patient's sense of personal responsibility elicits our powers of practical persuasion, and it is often cultivated by those who care *for* others. This is because those charged with caring for others are more often in the position of having to gain other's cooperation. Those who care about, but not for, may need only to confirm in their *own* mind that a certain course of action is justified.

Both kinds of parentalism can be instantiated in positive and negative ways. For example, parentalism that fosters the patient's sense of responsibility can be a positive force. However, this kind of parentalism can also deteriorate into a manipulative tool, for example, when it is used merely to produce guilt in patients, block the expression of patient's feelings, or manipulate patients to acquiesce to decisions they do not prefer in order to gain petty conveniences for caregivers (Taylor, 1985).

The other form of parentalism, that appeals to the health professional's rights and authority over the patient, can represent both positive and negative approaches as well. Negative expressions include a doctor or nurse who knowingly assumes greater authority than she is morally entitled to claim. Or negative parentalism occurs when the justified exercise of authority is conjoined with callousness, e.g., bullying a patient or giving patients orders in an abrupt or cruel fashion. By contrast, an example of positive parentalism of this sort is overriding the rights of someone that one is close to in order to protect that person's interests. Hardwig, for example, notes that in the context of close personal relationships, parentalistic behavior is often warranted and failing to show parentalism can signal a failure to fulfill special responsibilities (Hardwig, 1984). Elsewhere (Jecker, 1989, 1990b, 1990c), it is argued that the responsibilities of individuals in close relationships are different and often greater than the responsibilities that exist between acquaintances or strangers. If this approach is correct, then whether or not abrogating others' rights is justified in the health care setting depends, in part, upon whether particular health professionals stand in close relationships with their patients. Between virtual strangers, interference with others for their own good is less often desirable and more apt to overstep moral boundaries between persons.

2. Case Two: Caring For, but Not About a Patient

A demented thirty year old man had AIDS for eight months. His final admission to our hospital was prompted by the development of large decubitus ulcers. On the ward his oral intake was minimal, and the attending physician instructed me to administer parenteral nutrition. I didn't like taking care of this patient. I kept thinking that he had brought this fate upon himself by his gay lifestyle. Gays repulsed me, and I was unable to feel any compassion for this fellow. I also found his medical problems disgusting and resented the fact that caring for him exposed me to life threatening risks. The patient had copious diarrhea; the decubiti were oozing fluids; and administering parenteral nutrition was complicated by high, spiking fevers that twice necessitated removal of the central line (Cooke, 1986).

In case two a nurse is involved in caring *for* a patient. Caring for is manifest in the activities of treating the patient's ulcers and administering parenteral nutrition. Although the nurse is engaged in the activity of caregiving, her negative feelings about the patient suggest that she lacks an attitude of caring *about* the patient. Mustering such an attitude would require the nurse to reject or subdue her negative responses to the patient. On the other hand, particular nurses will always dislike particular patients, and subduing negative feelings will not necessarily change or mitigate bad feelings. Attempting and failing to reduce negative feelings may simply compound a nurse's difficulties by festering guilt or lowering self-esteem. Where dislike for patients is likely to persist, it is important to keep separate the ideas of *dislike* and *disrespect*. A nurse who dislikes a particular patient may still express respect toward the patient as a fellow human being, for example, through her ongoing activity of caring *for* the patient. Thus, although the nurse may not care *about* the patient, she can still regard the patient in a positive manner and express this regard in action.

300 *Nancy S. Jecker and Donnie J. Self*

3. *Case Three: Caring About, but Not For a Patient*

A twenty-seven year old model was admitted to the emergency room after an automobile accident that caused multiple fractures and burns over sixty-five per cent of his body. Glass had penetrated both eyes so severely as to leave him blind, although a good chance for survival existed. In the emergency room, the patient was met by friends who candidly told him that his physician expects that his life can be saved. Later when I, the physician, met with the patient to discuss treatment, the patient bluntly told me that he had enjoyed a life in which he had identified with his body and physical pleasure and abilities. He had few intellectual or other interests. On these grounds, he flatly refused treatment and asked me to keep him comfortable. My only concern was to promote this patient's welfare. I had seen many burn patients begin with a negative attitude toward treatment and then undergo a change of heart. Based on these experiences, I decided to order aggressive treatment and arranged for a psychiatric consult (Brody and Engelhardt, 1987, pp. 327–328).

The third case is about a physician who cares about a patient, but may not be engaged, in an ongoing way, in caring for the patient. For example, the physician orders burn treatments, but may not be the one who actually will provide these treatments to the patient. Unlike the nurse in case one, the physician in this case does not need to gain the patient's cooperation immediately. Moreover, the physician expresses parentalism by appealing to her authority and presumed superior knowledge to justify overriding the patient's wishes. The justification she gives for this is the silent refrain: "I know better; I've seen many burn patients in this situation change their mind". A different kind of parentalism would involve persuading the patient, as well as herself, of the wisdom of continued treatment. The alternative response intends to justify an action *to the patient* through iteration of the consequences of different choices. By contrast, the physician in case three seeks to justify the action mainly *to herself*. Thus her reasoning is 'silent' and she does not attempt negotiation of a solution agreeable to the patient.

Separating Care and Cure 301

4. Case Four: Caring Neither For nor About a Patient

I supervise a ward of terminally ill cancer patients. I deliberately avoid getting emotionally involved with these patients because I realize it would be terribly depressing. Fortunately, most of my responsibilities involve management of nurses, paper work and general organization, so I by and large can steer clear of patients and families. Most of the time, I limit my contact with nursing staff while eschewing patient contact. This enables me to direct my energy toward problems I can solve effectively and prevents me from feeling overwhelmed and powerless about dying patients.[2]

The nurse in this last case does not assume the responsibility of caring *for* patients. Nor does she display an attitude of caring *about* patients on her ward. Instead, she strives to maintain a neutral or indifferent stance. Presumably, such a stance affords her a sense of control in an otherwise emotionally charged environment.

FORMS OF CARE IN HEALTH CARE PROFESSIONS

The foregoing analysis of the concept of care places us in a better position to consider traditional stereotypes with a critical eye. In rethinking the idea that 'doctors cure and nurses care', it is helpful to be aware of four possible models of caring. These models parallel the cases discussed above:

1. Health professionals who care for and about their patients,
2. Health professionals who care for, but not about their patients,
3. Health professionals who care about, but not for their patients,
4. Health professionals who care neither for nor about their patients.

In the first model, health professionals care for and about patients. Since caring for is an ongoing and deliberate activity, a health professional whose patient contact is limited to brief visits or to discrete medical interventions, such as taking vital signs, does not fit the first model. Rather, to care in the sense defined by the first model a health professional must both carry out the tasks required to provide health care to the patient and possess an attitude of being concerned about what happens to the patient.

302   *Nancy S. Jecker and Donnie J. Self*

The difference between the first and second models of caring is that in the second it does not ultimately matter much to the professional what happens to patients. Nonetheless, it would be misleading to say that the second professional 'does not care'. After all, the second kind of health professional cares *all the time*: he or she is an ongoing caregiver, even though she lacks an attitude of caring *about* patients. This lack may impede her ability to care for patients, but (as noted above), it need not.

Similarly, it would be misleading to state that health professionals whose caring exemplifies the third model 'do not care'. Such professionals (who care about but not for their patients) may think about patients with great frequency, pray for their recovery and be deeply moved to witness it. These kind of professionals do indeed care, but their care is more remote by virtue of being removed from the immediate context of the patient. This does not imply that caring *about* is 'intellectual' or 'cold', but it does represent a more abstract mode of caring.

The grounds for saying that a health professional 'does not care' can only be that the professional cares neither for nor about patients. In the fourth model, health professionals do not care in either sense. An *uncaring* health professional is neither a caregiver nor concerned about the welfare of patients. Multiple factors may contribute to health professionals' lacking an attitude of caring about patients. In the cases discussed in the previous section, the absence of caring is prompted, in part, by feeling superior, being emotional indifferent, needing control, blaming the patient for the disease and disliking the patient. Caring neither for nor about patients often will be an unacceptable role for health professionals. Yet it also may represent a legitimate coping tool, for example, when one's responsibilities are experienced as overwhelming and the need to distance oneself emotionally is felt forcefully.

It is now time to ask how the above models can serve to deepen our understanding of nurses' and physicians' professional roles. To begin with, it is never correct to hold that nurses who function as caregivers do not care. Caring, in the sense of *caring for*, is an inextricable part of their role. The history of nursing is *essentially* a history of caring in this sense. In the colonial era, home-based nurses always cared in the sense of caring *for* family members. Nursing also has a caring tradition in the sense of caring *about* patients. As noted earlier, the first training programs for nurses sought to cultivate moral virtues, including devotion to the welfare of patients.

Despite the historical tradition of care by nurses, there are, and always have been, nurses who do not care much *about* patients in general, or *about* particular patients they nurse. Moreover, as more and more nurses become engaged in administrative and supervisory roles, they may do less caring *for* patients. On these grounds, it is misleading to accept the traditional stereotype that 'nurses care'. This stereotype obscures the fact that over time nursing has changed in its stratification and fields of specialization. These changes have meant that in some areas nurses have less direct patient contact and are less engaged in caring *for* patients. In addition, the traditional stereotype obscures the fact that there always have been nurses who do not care *about* patients.

Turning to physicians, a similar cautionary note is in order. Although some physicians may be less likely to care for patients, and so less likely to exemplify the first two models of caring, many physicians obviously care profoundly *about* patients. Moreover, physicians are a diverse group. In a university hospital, medical students or residents-in-training may seek or be delegated a considerable amount of caring for responsibilities, while attendings or senior staff may assume very little. Likewise, in health maintenance organizations, physician assistants and nurse practitioners may be utilized to perform a majority of caring for activities. By contrast, in private practices, physicians may undertake most of the caring for responsibilities. Such physicians may establish ongoing relationships with each patient over several years, e.g., monitoring medications, performing regular check-ups and treating minor emergencies. However, regardless of whether physicians care directly *for* patients, they usually assume a stance of caring *about* patients. Attempting to *cure* a patient is ordinarily an expression of a physician's caring about the patient. It is unfortunate, as well as confusing, then, to assume that doctors cure, as *opposed* to care. Thus, to the extent that the care-cure distinction informs our present thinking, it wrongly denies to the medical profession a caring role and unfortunately clouds our conception of the complexities of nursing care.

CONCLUSION

In closing, this paper has intended to take a careful look at professional stereotypes in nursing and medicine. Doing so required

304 *Nancy S. Jecker and Donnie J. Self*

clarifying the concept of care and articulating different models of caring. That the concept of care is multiform and the models of caring many should attune us to the dangers of buying into popular stereotypes. Holding tenaciously to traditional stereotypes can prevent us from seeing the evidence that both medicine and nursing are caring professions and both men and women care for and about their patients.

Appreciating the richness of the concept of care also should infuse new energy into research on care in health care and professional settings. The following are suggested research topics that merit further consideration. (1) How can cure and care be joined and integrated into the curriculum of both nursing and medical schools? (2) Is care a virtue? If so, under what circumstances might it deteriorate into a vice? Is care ever a duty or obligation? (3) Is caring a way of knowing? How do cure and care relate to both scientific and intuitive forms of knowledge? (4) What is the proper balance between cure and care in developing an ethic for specific patient groups, such as the elderly, the terminally ill and the chronically ill? Although answering these questions is a tall order, our analysis shows the importance and promise of further research in this area.

NOTES

* We wish to thank Sara T. Fry, Albert R. Jonsen and an anonymous reviewer of this journal for valuable comments. A version of this paper was presented at a University of Maryland School of Nursing conference on Ethics and Nursing Practice in May of 1990 and at a conference on The Politics of Caring held at the Emory University Institute for Women's Studies in October of 1990.

[1] Throughout this paper, we will use the terms 'care' and 'caring' interchangeably. There may be important shades of meaning unique to each term, but exploring this is beyond the scope of the present inquiry.

[2] Whereas the previous cases are drawn from the medical ethics literature, we could find no cases in the literature to illustrate the fourth model. We believe this is significant if it represents a lack of attention to the ethical problems of health care workers who exemplify this model.

REFERENCES

American Nurses' Association: 1987, *Facts About Nurses*, American Nurses' Association, Kansas City, Missouri.

Benner, P.: 1983, 'Recovering the knowledge embedded in clinical practice', *Image: Journal of Nursing Scholarship* 15, 30–41.

Benner, P.: 1984, *From Novice to Expert: Excellence and Power in Clinical Nursing Practice*, Addison-Wesley Publishing Company, Menlo Park, California.

Benner, P., and Wrubel, J.: 1989, *The Primacy of Caring*, Addison-Wesley Publishing Company, Menlo Park, California.

Benoliel, J.Q.: 1987, 'Response to 'toward holistic inquiry in nursing: A proposal for synthesis of patterns and methods', *Scholarly Inquiry for Nursing Practice: An International Journal* 1, 147–152.

Blum, L.A.: 1988, 'Gilligan and Kohlberg: Implications for moral theory', *Ethics* 98, 472–491.

Brody, B.A., and Engelhardt, H.T.: 1987, *Bioethics: Readings and Cases*, Prentice-Hall, Englewood Cliffs, New Jersey.

Buchanan, W.: 1778, *Domestic Medicine, The Third American Edition*, John Trumbull, Boston.

Conrad, P., and Schneider, J.W.: 1990, 'Professionalization, monopoly, and the structure of medical practice', in P. Conrad and R. Kern (eds.), *The Sociology of Health and Illness: Critical Perspectives, Third Edition*, St. Martin's Press, New York, pp. 141–147.

Cooke, M.: 1986, 'Ethical issues in the care of patients with AIDS', *Quality Review Bulletin*, October, 343–346.

Eisenberg, C.: 1989, 'Medicine is no longer a man's profession', *New England Journal of Medicine* 321, 1542–1544.

Gilligan, C.: 1982, *In a Different Voice: Psychological Theory and Women's Development*, Harvard University Press, Cambridge, Massachusetts.

Gilligan, C.: 1986, 'Remapping the moral domain: New images of the self in relationship', in T.C. Heller, M. Sosna, and D.E. Wellbery (eds.), *Reconstructing Individualism: Autonomy, Individuality, and the Self in Western Thought*, Stanford University Press, Stanford, California, pp. 237–252.

Gilligan, C., and Wiggins, G.: 1987, 'The origins of morality in early childhood', in J. Kagan and S. Lamb (eds.), *The Emergence of Morality in Young Children*, University of Chicago Press, Chicago, pp. 277–305.

Gilligan, C., and Pollak, S.: 1989, 'The vulnerable and invulnerable physician', in C. Gilligan, J.V. Ward, and J.M. Taylor (eds.), *Mapping the Moral Domain*, Harvard University Press, Cambridge, Massachusetts, pp. 245–262.

Hardwig, J.: 1984, 'Should women think in terms of rights?', *Ethics* 94, 441–455.

Hauerwas, S.: 1978, 'Care', in W.T. Reich (ed.), *The Encyclopedia of Bioethics*, Free Press, New York, Vol. 1, 145–150.

Levinson, W., Tolle, S., and Lewis, C.: 1989, 'Women in academic medicine', *New England Journal of Medicine* 321, 1511–1517.

Jameton, A.: 1984, *Nursing Practice: The Ethical Issues*, Prentice-Hall, Englewood Cliffs, New Jersey.

Jameton, A.: 1987, 'Physicians and nurses: A historical perspective', in B.A. Brody and H.T. Engelhardt, *Bioethics, Readings and Cases*, Prentice-Hall, Englewood Cliffs, New Jersey, pp. 66–73.

306   *Nancy S. Jecker and Donnie J. Self*

Jecker, N.S.: 1989, 'Are filial duties unfounded?' *American Philosophical Quarterly* 26, 73–80.

Jecker, N.S.: 1990a, 'The role of intimate others in medical decision making', *The Gerontologist* 30, 65–71.

Jecker, N.S.: 1990b, 'Conceiving a child to save a child: Reproductive and filial ethics', *The Journal of Clinical Ethics* 1, 99–103.

Jecker, N.S.: 1990c, 'Anencephalic infants and special relationships', *Theoretical Medicine* 11, 333–342.

Keller, E.F.: 1985, *Reflections on Gender and Science*, Yale University Press, New Haven, Connecticut.

Kittay, E.F., and Meyers, D.T. (eds.): 1987, *Women and Moral Theory*, Rowman and Littlefield, Totowa, New Jersey.

Lyons, N.P.: 1983, 'Two perspectives: On self, relationships, and morality', *Harvard Educational Review* 53, 125–145.

MacIntyre, A.: 1987, 'How virtues become vices', in B.A. Brody and H.T. Engelhardt (eds.), *Bioethics: Readings and Cases*, Prentice-Hall, Englewood Cliffs, New Jersey, pp. 100–101.

Morantz-Sanchez, R.M.: 1985, *Sympathy and Science: Women Physicians in American Medicine*, Oxford University Press, New York.

Nelson, A.R.: 1989, 'Humanism and the art of medicine: Our commitment to care', *Journal of the American Medical Association* 262, 1228–1230.

Noddings, N.: 1984, *Caring: A Feminine Approach to Ethics and Moral Education*, University of California Press, Berkeley.

Noddings, N.: 1987, 'Do we really want to produce good people?', *Journal of Moral Education* 16, 177–188.

Noddings, N.: 1989, *Women and Evil*, University of California Press, Berkeley.

O'Brien, P.: 1987, 'All a woman's life can bring: The domestic roots of nursing in Philadelphia, 1830–1885', *Nursing Research* 36, 12–17.

Pearsall, M. (ed.): 1986, *Women and Values*, Wadsworth Publishing Company, Belmont, California.

Relman, A.: 1989, 'The changing demography of the medical profession', *New England Journal of Medicine* 321, 1540–1542.

Reverby, S.: 1987a, 'A caring dilemma: Womanhood and nursing in historical perspective', *Nursing Research* 36, 5–11.

Reverby, S.: 1987b, *Ordered to Care: The Dilemma of American Nursing*, Cambridge University Press, New York.

Rowland, H.S.: 1984, *The Nurse's Almanac, 2nd edition*, Aspen Systems Corporation, Rockville, Maryland.

Ruddick, S.: 1989, *Maternal Thinking*, Beacon Press, Boston.

Schultz, P.R., and Meleis, A.I.: 1988, 'Nursing epistemology: Traditions, insights, questions', *Image: Journal of Nursing Scholarship* 20, 217–221.

Starr, P.: 1982, *The Social Transformation of American Medicine*, Basic Books, New York.

Taylor, S.G.: 1985, 'Rights and responsibilities: Nurse-patient relationships', *Image: Journal of Nursing Scholarship* 17, 9–13.

Hastings Center Report, July-August 1992

One of the most alarming aspects of describing an ethical problem, and of hearing it described by others, is discovering just how many ways it can be done. How a moral problem is described will turn on an array of variables: the role and degree of involvement in the case of the person who is describing it, the person's particular profession or discipline, her religious and cultural inheritance—indeed, with all of the intangibles that have contributed to her character. What is more, the description any person offers will also vary—notoriously—according to whether an ethical decision has been made or is still to come, whether that decision is now judged to be a sound one or a poor one, whether the consequences were intended or unforeseen.

Consider a relatively common case: a middle-aged man with multisystem organ failure, poor but not hopeless prognosis, now incompetent, experiencing what seems to be considerable pain, whose family is faced with the decision about whether to continue his medical treatment. Think of the possible alternatives to the brief and inadequate description I have offered here. A clinician will describe the patient's medical problems, his hospital course, his treatment, his laboratory work, and so on. A moral philosopher will be less interested in the medical details of the case than she will the moral ones, and her description will be constructed from a vocabulary of terms such as autonomy, justice, and beneficence, and the patient's goals, values, and wishes. The patient's wife will describe not a "case," but a continuing chapter in her life. A chaplain, social worker, nurse, or hospital administrator will offer still another description, as will the patient's daughter, his minister, his friends, his colleagues, and his enemies. The perceptions of each of these will change as the patient's story unfolds: what seemed to be minor decisions at one time now appear disastrous; incidents that might have been overlooked now seem to be portents. And any description offered will reflect whether the patient is in a Tel Aviv teaching hospital, a Heidelberg *Krankenhaus*, or a Chicago V.A. facility.

Perhaps the most frustrating feature of describing a moral problem is the gulf between moral description and moral experience. No description, it seems, can do justice to the realities of our moral problems.[1] It is extraordinarily difficult, if not impossible, to capture the countless subtleties that go into the

Where Ethics Comes from and What to Do about It

by Carl Elliott

The practical difficulty with applying ethical theories to particular problems is that ordinarily people pay little attention to theories when they make moral decisions. Instead, we are guided by our ethical beliefs, which are primarily the result of cultural factors beyond our reach—factors subject to rational scrutiny and to change, but largely out of our control.

perceptions and judgments of each person involved: the hopes, fears, prayers, guilt, pride, and remorse; the conflicting emotions that accompany irrevocable decisions; the self-imposed pressure to carry through with an action once a decision has been made. Much of what goes into actual moral choices remains unarticulated. To express these things, even to perceive them consciously, requires a talent possessed by few of us other than novelists and poets.

A second problem comes from the realization that in describing a given case, one has done much of the ethical work already. A person's moral judgment is reflected in what he chooses to include in a description: whether he mentions that the patient's wife has visited her critically ill husband only twice over the past three weeks, whether he reports a bed shortage in the ICU, if he notes that the patient's children stand to inherit the dying man's estate, how he describes the patient's prognosis, whether he brings up the option of palliative care, if he notes that the nursing staff feels strongly that treatment should be stopped, whether he mentions that the patient was an IV drug abuser. One of the most interesting and disturbing discoveries to be made in a medical ethics case conference is how one's moral intuitions change as each player in the drama says his piece, as another perspective is added to one's own. One begins to suspect that it is self-deception to think any descrip-

Carl Elliott is research fellow, faculty of medicine, University of Natal, Durban, South Africa.

Carl Elliott, "Where Ethics Comes from and What to Do about It," *Hastings Center Report* 22, no. 4 (1992): 28-35.

Hastings Center Report, July-August 1992

tion free of ideology, to believe that any viewpoint can approximate that of an impartial spectator.

A third problem is that to make sense of a particular case, one must have some sort of conceptual framework in which to place it. This conceptual framework structures one's perception of the case. Medical students know this as well as ethicists; it is only with time, as more patients are encountered and filed within certain conceptual categories, that one begins to understand how to think about particular cases— what to ask, what to examine, what is relevant and what is not. But concepts of necessity involve generalities, not particulars, types of cases, not individual ones. We swap precision for simplicity. As Nigel Barley says, "Generalizations always tell a little lie in the service of a greater truth."[2] But if general, conceptual frameworks are psychologically essential in ethics, they also make it easy to overlook those aspects of our moral experience that are not easily generalized. Let me mention only a few examples: in theory, it is often said that moral concerns override other concerns, but in practice, one can often readily understand their being overridden themselves, perhaps by practical considerations. In theory, it seems that moral dilemmas can be solved, but in practice they often cannot. In theory, we speak of beings who rationally choose what they believe to be the best action, but in practice, we find ourselves making irrational decisions, under the sway of seemingly inscrutable desires. In theory, guilt is an emotion that we feel (or rationally should feel) when we have acted wrongly, but in practice, we sometimes feel guilty when we have done nothing at all. Indeed, a caricature history of ethics could be written merely by cataloguing various attempts to make our moral experience more intelligible by describing it in terms of something else: moral goodness can be defined in terms of happiness; our moral sense is like our physical senses; moral judgments are like expressions of approval or disapproval. All this is not to imply, I hasten to say, that all theories are caricatures. Such an implication would itself be a caricature. I only point out that moral theories trade in generalities and simplifications which make it easy to forget how particular and complicated our moral experience is.

Implicit in these problems is a tension between, on the one hand, the ethics of description (and consequently of theory), and on the other, the experience of making ethical judgments in concrete cases. The ethics of description and theory seems necessary to make sense of such a wide range of cases, but as with narrative fiction and reality, moral description differs from our actual moral experience. To make sense of ethical problems we must impose some sort of artificial order on the story we tell, whether we do it in terms of a narrative, or ethical principles, or a medical case history. The order imposed on it affects how we respond to it; thus we treat differently the cases we have heard described and those we have actually experienced. In fact, not even those cases we experience at first hand are innocent of theory; our moral judgments change with how we describe the case to ourselves. Joan Didion puts this well:

> We look for the sermon in the suicide, for the social or moral lesson in the murder of five. We interpret what we see, select the most workable of the multiple choices. We live entirely, especially if we are writers, by the imposition of a narrative line upon disparate images, by the "ideas" with which we have learned to freeze the shifting phantasmagoria which is our actual experience.[3]

For those who make a living by talking and writing about ethics, it is often easy to forget that ethics never came in flavors of deontology and consequentialism; the principles of justice and autonomy and utility are not intrinsic properties of ethical problems. When we speak of ethical principles—or more fashionably, of a communitarian or a narrative ethics—we do so because we find these useful ways of thinking about ethics; they are self-standing conceptual systems by which we can impose some sort of order upon ethical problems. But in reality, ethics does not stand apart. It is one thread in the fabric of a society, and it is intertwined with others. Ethical concepts are tied to a society's customs, manners, traditions, institutions—all of the concepts that structure and inform the ways in which a member of that society deals with the world. When we forget this, we are in danger of leaving the world of genuine moral experience for the world of moral fiction—a simplified, hypothetical creation suited less for practical difficulties than for intellectual convenience.

Theory and Practice

It is sometimes thought that the job of applied ethics is to apply normative ethical theories to particular practical problems. Recent years have seen growing dissatisfaction with such an approach, and the reason is simple: it does not work. The problems are becoming increasingly well rehearsed.[4] In the first place, as there is no shortage of ethical theories, one must be able to adjudicate among rival theories to decide which to apply to any given ethical problem. This can be difficult, especially when intuition does not incline us in a particular direction. When we do have strong moral intuitions, they are usually concerned with a particular case, and not with a theory. Moreover, theories are tested not only against moral intuitions; they are also tested against other theories. As moral theories present problems arising

Hastings Center Report. July-August 1992

out of their own internal tensions—how to mediate between conflicting moral principles; how to account for exceptions to principles—adjudicating between rival theories is usually done by appeal to tests such as clarity, economy, comprehensiveness, and coherence. But while it is obviously easier to understand and apply theories that are clear, economical,

---

The conflict here is one between tidiness and truth; we want our theories to be simple and elegant, but also true, and the only measure of the "moral truth" of a theory seems to be our own inconsistent, untidy moral intuitions.

---

comprehensive, and coherent, it is not at all plain why we should expect a moral theory to measure up to such tests, when our own moral beliefs are often genuinely unclear, uneconomical, noncomprehensive, and incoherent. To put it rather bluntly, the conflict here is one between tidiness and truth; we want our theories to be simple and elegant, but also true, and the only measure of the "moral truth" of a theory seems to be our own inconsistent, untidy moral intuitions.

But the most trying problem for ethical theorists is how we should understand the equilibrium in a particular case between our moral intuitions and the mandate of an ethical system. On the one hand, ethical theories are supposed to corroborate and justify our moral judgments, but on the other, particular judgments are also supposed to count against theories. That is, theorists expect particular moral judgments to be backed up by principles and theories, but it may also be considered a failing for a theory if that theory yields an especially counterintuitive judgment. Most of us would consider it sufficient to dismiss a given ethical theory, for example, if it told us that betraying one's friends and torturing the innocent were morally obligatory. Yet why do ethical theories justify some moral judgments and not others? How are we to decide if the theory counts against the judgment, or the judgment against the theory? Our problem is understanding this practical check on ethical theory. For clearly, if a given problem does in fact yield moral disagreement, then any theory that does its job will be counterintuitive for someone, in generating a judgment that runs squarely against that person's sincerely held moral beliefs.

The practical difficulty with applying ethical theories is that ordinary people pay little attention to theories when they make their moral decisions. Moral decisions are, of course, often influenced by

theories of one sort or another, but this influence is usually indirect rather than explicit. (I myself refer to no systematic moral theories or doctrines in making moral judgments, but I have no illusions that these judgments are independent of the fact that I grew up as a Presbyterian in South Carolina.) What is more, the rules for moral argument in the ethics of theory seem to differ from the rules that carry weight in the ethics of ordinary life. In theory, one is likely to be criticized for making illogical jumps and deriving illegitimate conclusions. In ordinary life one persuades, cajoles, jokes, threatens, coerces, reminds, harasses, begs, and forgives. One tells stories, makes analogies, sermonizes, moralizes, holds grudges, and gets righteously indignant. This is not to say that one never behaves this way in academic ethics, of course—or that all forms of moral argument are equally valid. But one need only compare the discussion of an ethical issue in a medical journal, a theology journal, and a philosophy journal to see that even in the circumscribed world of American academe, and even in the subculture thereof that has devoted itself to discussing ethics, there are strikingly different methods of ethical argument. And the differences between the conduct of moral argumentation in ordinary experience and in academic ethics presents certain barriers to the academic who is concerned with influencing practical decisions. It is difficult to say how a theory can be applied, or even whether it should be applied, if it is alien not only in content but in structure to the way that people are accustomed to making their moral choices.

What, then, accounts for the attractiveness of moral theories? For clearly, a notion so deeply entrenched in moral philosophy cannot be entirely useless. One obvious answer is the theories' psychological appeal. This is not just to say that most of us seem to have some sort of ground-level preference for simple explanations, though there is probably some truth to that. It is also that we need to impose some degree of order on our moral judgments, and theory gives us that order. We do not need order to the degree conventionally required of a moral theory, but it would be psychologically impossible to have a completely random, unrelated, orderless set of moral judgments. We speak and think in terms of concepts, and concepts impose at least a minimal degree of order on our moral experience.[5]

But another reason for the appeal of moral theories, one that moral antifoundationalists tend to overlook, is the extent to which moral theories are genuinely helpful. Simplifying a complicated case to "autonomy versus beneficence" does tell a little lie (many little lies, in fact), but we should not ignore the truth in that simplification—or its usefulness. I can still recall the startling clarity that emerged out of the seeming chaos of numberless cases when I learned to classify them in certain ways: autonomy and beneficence, beneficence and truth-telling, acting and refraining. The simplifications eventually crumble, but it is only because the cases have first been simplified that a critique of simplification is possible. What is more, the truths carried by these simplified ways of seeing often help to sort out the problems in these cases; they capture and summarize the kinds of intuitions that we (at least we in the West) often come to when we think about such problems. It may not help a doctor "solve" an ethical problem to know that it exemplifies a conflict between beneficence and autonomy, but it does often help her to clarify her own thoughts about the matter—not least because it orders and focuses a wide range of disparate intuitions.

And finally, we should not forget theory's rhetorical power. Even if a moral theory is not the sort of thing that can be rigidly "applied," it is one of the tools of rational persuasion, and thus powerful fuel for moral argument. The consistency of a moral theory may point out inconsistencies in conventional moral thinking, which may in turn result in real changes in moral values. (Think of natural rights theory and the French and American Revolutions, or, to take a more recent example, Peter Singer's application of utilitarianism to animals.) Where we go wrong, on the other hand, is in beginning to expect more from a moral theory than it can provide.

Choosing Ethics

When we analyze ethical problems, we are able to choose the ethical principles, values, and beliefs that we think should apply to that problem and govern its resolution. Thus we sometimes tend to see ethics not as an intrinsic part of a society, but as some sort of abstract system to be imposed upon, chosen by, or rejected by a society. The temptation to think of ethics in this way can be especially strong in the United States, where one is likely to encounter individuals with moral beliefs varying over a wide range. Ethics becomes a microcosm of politics, and the question, What shall I do? becomes instead, What is the best moral system for us to have?

In some cases this approach is fine—if, for instance, the question to be addressed is what sort of policy we want in general for our society, and if this is a question about which we are genuinely undecided. And it would be foolish to think that the ethical decisions of individuals in particular cases do not influence the moral values of other individuals, and thus of society in general. The question of how a particular moral judgment will affect the course of moral thinking in a society is always a legitimate one to consider. This is why, in the previously mentioned

case, it is appropriate not only to consider what would be the morally best course of action, but also whether that course of action reflects the sort of policy one would like to see influencing similar decisions elsewhere. The objections of some writers to active euthanasia reflect these sorts of concerns: they recognize that euthanasia may well be the best course of action in some few, individual cases, but fear that disastrous consequences would result if active euthanasia were a widely endorsed policy.

But in other situations the notion that ethics can be chosen might be quite misleading. We do not—we cannot—choose our moral beliefs at will, and consequently a society has only very limited and indirect control over the moral values it embraces. Here the contrast between morality and politics is helpful, because political structures, when they are not tyrannical, are to some extent the product of willful control. In a democratic society we can change our laws, policies, and (less easily) our political institutions. Our moral values, on the other hand, are primarily the result of cultural factors beyond our reach. They are subject to rational scrutiny, to be sure, and also subject to change, but, like the broader aspects of character of which moral values are a part, they are largely out of our control.

The point here is that although they are often concerned with the same problems, questions about personal moral values differ fundamentally from questions about political and institutional policy. And while ethical theories are often genuinely helpful in addressing political and institutional questions, they are much less helpful in particular cases. The reason, of course, is that while we make policy, we do not make our values. We can quite easily choose the sort of principles we think should guide general policy about, say, the allocation of scarce medical resources, or about abortion, but we cannot choose,

> We do not—we cannot—choose our moral beliefs at will, and consequently a society has only very limited and indirect control over the moral values it embraces.

at least not in the same way, to change people's values, nor can we simply choose the values upon which our own decisions about policy are made. Values are rooted much deeper than that.

Thus it is at least in some sense misguided, even futile, to call for a new "ethics," as seems to be increasingly common nowadays—be it a communitarian ethics, a return to premodern virtue, a narrative ethics, a family or a citizen ethics—if what is

Hastings Center Report. July–August 1992

intended by such calls is an actual change in our society's moral values." To be sure, sometimes this is not what is intended; what is meant by a new ethics is sometimes a new ethical *theory*, a call for writers and consultants in ethics to pay attention to forgotten or overlooked values. But often, it seems, the point of a call for a new ethics is to promote in moral agents some new value or new way of thinking about values—to effect real change in the values of a society. And while one small step toward changing moral values is to criticize them and call attention to new ones, we cannot simply return to an Aristotelian world view, or adopt a communitarian ethics. Such sweeping changes in a society's moral values come about only with broader changes in a society's way of life—its traditions, political institutions, family structures, and so on—changes that occur, to a disturbing degree, as a consequence of events that are rarely planned, and often undesired.

Calling for society to adopt new moral values is one way of responding to moral pluralism, as a diversity of values might be the barrier to agreement. A similar and more common way of responding is to construct moral theories that treat individuals as abstractly as possible, appealing to the broadest and most general values that they share, and then constructing a theory on the foundations of these shared values. People are replaced by rational deliberators, bundles of pure will. The solution to moral disagreement is to construct a theory based on principles to which all rational persons can agree, and which will in turn yield conclusions to which they must also agree, if they are rational and consistent.

However, while this may well be an adequate approach to political (policy, institutional, legal) differences, where the aim is a minimal degree of cooperation necessary for peaceful coexistence,

---

> Contemporary moral debate often seems to overlook the fact that ethics can be a very intimate affair; it involves not only respecting rights, but also such things as gratitude, hurt feelings, embarrassment, and love.

---

moral agreement requires more than a theory, and it requires more than peaceful coexistence. Contemporary moral debate often seems to overlook the fact that ethics can be a very intimate affair; it involves not only respecting rights, but also such things as gratitude, hurt feelings, embarrassment, and love. These things are deeply intertwined with culture and individual character. Policy and law set boundaries for human behavior, but because morality is bound up so tightly with family ties and cultural inheritance, with character, communication, and self-perception, moral agreement requires shared values above a basic minimum. It also requires shared institutions, cultures, and traditions. Moral differences are usually settled not by simply blunting individual differences, but by becoming individuals more like each other. (For all of the hostility United States nationalism understandably arouses abroad, it at least serves this effect: it provides shared ideals that individuals of wildly divergent cultural backgrounds can embrace.)

Concepts and Disagreement

It is often taken for granted that the moral concepts of a society should reflect some underlying standards of order. If they do not, it is up to those who work in ethics to point out the disorder (incoherence, inconsistency) and perhaps to work at correcting it, for this lack of order is at the root of moral disagreement. For instance, when in *After Virtue* Alasdair MacIntyre argues that moral language is in a "state of grave disorder"(p. 2), he cites the existence of widespread, apparently irresolvable moral disagreement as evidence. "The most striking feature of contemporary moral utterance is that so much of it is used to express disagreements; and the most striking feature of debates in which these disagreements are expressed is their interminable character"(p. 6). MacIntyre goes on to suggest that the reason for the disordered state of moral discourse is that we have inherited the conceptual fragments of a multitude of moral traditions, concepts which have been severed from those traditions that grounded them.[7]

Part of the appeal of MacIntyre's account of moral language stems from the extent to which it is obviously true: moral disagreement grows as traditions change and as individuals of divergent cultural traditions come to live together. But part of its appeal also comes from the way it plays upon the tacit assumption, widely shared among writers in ethics, that moral beliefs and values in a society should reflect standards of order of the sort we expect in a moral theory—consistency, coherence, simplicity, and so on—with the result being that disorder becomes a phenomenon that needs explanation.

But what sort of order should we expect in our moral language? Or perhaps even more importantly, what is it for a moral language to be in a state of disorder? Surely it does not mean that individuals in a society have moral beliefs that are inconsistent with each other, or that conflict with the moral beliefs of others; in the West, anyway, this seems historically to have been a fairly constant feature of moral discourse. MacIntyre compares the state of contemporary moral discourse to that of a society which,

Hastings Center Report. July-August 1992

through some catastrophe, has lost all knowledge of the content and methods of science, and whose scientific discourse must therefore struggle along with the remnants of scientific knowledge and methods left from the old society. The image of a disordered language of morality called up by MacIntyre's scenario resembles that described by Paul Auster in his novella, *The City of Glass*, where the world, once in the state of Eden, has collapsed into confusion, leaving in disarray the language that describes it:

> Nature became detached from things; words devolved into a collection of arbitrary signs; language became severed from God. . . .
>
> For our words no longer correspond to the world. When things were whole, we felt confident that our words could express them. But little by little things have broken apart, shattered, collapsed into chaos. And yet our words have remained the same. They have not adapted themselves to the new reality. Hence, every time we try to speak of what we see, we speak falsely, distorting the very thing we are trying to represent.[8]

But surely this state of affairs, in which language has somehow remained static while the world has changed and in which human beings can barely understand each other, is not the state of contemporary moral language. Whatever moral disagreement we find in society, contemporary moral discourse allows for communication among individuals with minimal confusion as to what is *meant* when a moral judgment is expressed. When I say that active euthanasia is wrong, you may disagree, but you understand what I mean. In fact, disagreement of this sort, far from being evidence of a disordered language of morality, *presupposes* understanding between speaker and hearer about what is meant when a moral judgment is expressed. Before I can disagree with your judgment that active euthanasia is wrong, I must know what you mean when you say it.

Yet the point at which MacIntyre's account goes awry contains an important clue to the extent to which we should expect order in our moral language. We should not expect our moral language to reflect the underlying standards of order we might expect of a moral theory—the standard that insists all of our moral beliefs be consistent with each other and with those of others, formulable in principles for behavior upon which all rational persons would agree. Rather, we should expect our language to meet the minimal standards of order that would allow communication and understanding among those who use it.

How much order will this be? Quite a lot, as it turns out—and this will place limits on the extent of our moral disagreement. For a moral term such as

humane, cruel, wrong, or *perverse* to gain currency in our language, speakers must understand what the term means. That is, they must understand that using the word to describe actions or persons reflects a certain *attitude* on the part of the speaker. Not "just" an attitude, of course, but an attitude of a certain sort, carrying all of the baggage we normally attach to moral terms, such as extreme importance, certain characteristics related to universalizability and objectivity, and so on.

Agreement as to what moral words *mean* places some constraints on the things to which they can be *applied.* My understanding of what is meant by *kind* or *cruel* is determined by the sorts of things to which these words are applied by the broader community of speakers. If there were not at least some minimal overlap as to the sorts of things to which this community of speakers applies the words *cruel* and *kind,* I would be unable to learn what these words meant. Mutual understanding of the word *cruel* would be impossible if one person applied it to the practice of causing needless pain, another used it to designate the practice of punishing and rewarding only people who deserve it, and a third used it to describe self-sacrifice in the service of one's fellows. Of course, because moral words do reflect attitudes that differ from one person to the next, we will not always have *complete* agreement about what actions of persons the words should be applied to. But we must have some minimal amount of agreement about certain paradigm examples of cruelty or kindness or perversity, or else moral words would cease to be tools of communication.[9]

It is not always easy, however, to see just how moral concepts are tied to a way of life, especially when that way of life is one's own. Clifford Geertz offers an instructive example from Balinese life with the concept of *lek,* which is occasionally translated as "shame," but which Geertz says is probably closer to "stage fright." However, to understand what the Balinese mean by *lek,* one must also have some understanding of the Balinese concept of the self. The Western notion of the self (or at least what is sometimes called, somewhat disparagingly these days, the Enlightenment concept of the self) is roughly circumscribed, independent, free, self-governing, and (more or less) rational. The Balinese notion of the self, says Geertz, is quite different; in contrast to the independent individualism of the Western self, in Bali "anything idiosyncratic, anything characteristic of the individual merely because he is who he is physically, psychologically, or biographically, is muted in favor of his assigned place in the continuing, and, so it is thought, never-changing pattern that is Balinese life." A person is identified by various labels: birth order, caste titles, kinship markers, sex

Hastings Center Report, July-August 1992

indicators. These identify him as "a determinate point in a fixed pattern, as the temporary occupant of a particular, untemporary, cultural locus." In Bali, says Geertz, life is theater. As such, "it is dramatis personae, not actors, that endure; indeed it is dramatis personae, not actors, that in the proper sense, really exist."[10]

Lek, then, is not just shame; it is the fear of exposure, that fear that "the public performance to which one's cultural location commits one will be botched and that the personality—as we would call it but the

---

If you want to understand America, you must first understand baseball.

Balinese, of course, not believing in such a thing, would not—of the individual will break through to dissolve his standardized public identity." Geertz says: "When this occurs, as it sometimes does, the immediacy of the moment is felt with excruciating intensity and men become suddenly and unwillingly creatural, locked in mutual embarrassment, as though they had happened upon each other's nakedness."[11]

The point here, of course, is that a moral concept such as *lek* cannot be understood apart from the Balinese concept of selfhood, which cannot be understood apart from Balinese ritual life, which cannot be understood apart from the Hindu, Buddhist, and Polynesian religions of Bali, and so on. Moral concepts are interwoven into the tapestry of a life. Oddly enough, this is easier to see by looking at another culture than by looking at one's own. We look at Bali through American eyes, with American values; but to look at American life requires that we do it with equipment made from the very stuff we are trying to judge.

I once heard it said (I cannot recall where) that if you want to understand America, you must first understand baseball. There is some truth to that remark—some truth about baseball, to be sure, but also some truth about how American concepts and American problems are inseparable from their broader cultural context. For instance, I have found that non-Americans occasionally find it difficult to understand all the fuss over the "right to die" debate in America, and the vehemence with which it is sometimes argued. Why would anyone want to continue treating a patient in a persistent vegetative state with virtually no chance for recovery? Ah, well, I usually explain, you must also understand how the right to die is related to the right to life, and to the debate over abortion, and to American churches, and to the role of the church in small-town life; you must also

understand something about American hospitals and feminism and libertarianism and fundamentalism and natural rights and John Locke and Thomas Jefferson and so on and so on, ad infinitum. To understand America, I explain, you must first understand baseball.

Pluralism and Practical Action

The difficulty with moral concepts, of course, is that when we look at them in this way, as part of a society's form of life, they start to seem "merely" one sort of concept among many, as "only" relative to the way in which a people live. Hence relativism, hence the subjectivity of morals, and hence all the myriad debates in which moral philosophy has mired itself over the years. I believe that the constraints placed on morality by language and concepts prevent such a slide into relativism, but this is not the place to rehearse that debate. More important for our purposes is the relationship of moral pluralism to practical action. It is all very well to say that morality is embedded in a form of life, but how should we respond?

For one thing, it is important to realize that the bare fact of moral pluralism does not minimize the importance of moral conviction. Whatever else a moral judgment is, it is something we take seriously; it is no accident that we speak of moral *values*, with all the weight that word carries. And moral conviction need not be diminished by the recognition that others have moral convictions they take equally seriously. My recognition that others have differing moral beliefs about a given problem does not require me to sit back in respectful silence. One important mechanism for dealing with moral pluralism in the West is argument and rational persuasion. After all, communal living does require a certain amount of moral agreement.

Another more obvious but less often discussed consequence of recognizing pluralism is a redirection of one's intellectual energy. If moral concepts, and thus moral problems, are dependent on a culture's institutions, then clearly one important way to deal with those problems is to deal with the institutions. Cultural institutions are highly resistant to change, and it is not always clear what changes will solve problems and what changes will create them. But can anyone doubt that a great number of the problems in medical ethics are the result, for instance, of the way American doctors and medical students are trained? Or that many of these problems are fueled by the threat of malpractice lawsuits? Or that the abortion debate could ever be resolved without some broader changes in the circumstances that make abortion seem a necessary choice to so many women?

Hastings Center Report, July-August 1992

Yet if moral concepts are bound up with a society's way of life, then unless we expect all of the institutions, customs, and traditions of that society to be ordered and systematic, we should not expect moral concepts to meet the standards we would require of a systematic theory. Like other institutions, morality evolves in haphazard fashion, and moral disagreement inevitably emerges in response to broader societal changes. In fact, disagreement is so much a part of our notion of morality that we should reflect for a moment on what else we would lose if moral disagreement were to disappear. The result would bear little resemblance to what, at least in the West, we call morality. The concept of conscientious objection would vanish; we would have no moral reformers and no civil disobedience. We would lose the notion of one's moral ideals being self-chosen, of making up one's own mind about a matter of moral discretion. Also gone would be the idea of moral maturity, which would be replaced by conformity to the moral consensus. Moral reasoning would become like mathematical reasoning; all competent adults would agree which actions were right and wrong, and moral maturity would simply be a matter of acquiring the mental skills to reason correctly.

Moral disagreement will be with us as long as there is disagreement about what way of life is best for human beings. It is not at all obvious that this is a question that is answerable, even in principle.[12] There may be no best life, only better and worse lives. And if morality is tied to a form of life, then it is a mistake to think that we can eliminate moral differences without eliminating the differences in cultures, and in individuals, to which morality is tied. Though the biological characteristics humans share will mean that some lives, and some features of lives, are necessarily good or bad for human beings, there is no compelling reason, universally applicable, for adopting any one particular sort of life over all others —even if we had the choice, which we do not. For this reason, we should expect diversity in the sort of lives that people live, as well as the moral differences that inevitably follow.

References

1. See Grant Gillett, "Women and Children First," forthcoming in *Medicine and Moral Reasoning*, ed. B. Fulford, G. Gillett, and J. Soskice (Cambridge: Cambridge University Press); also his "Euthanasia, Letting Die and the Pause," *Journal of Medical Ethics* 14, no. 2 (1988): 61-67.

2. Nigel Barley, *Not a Hazardous Sport* (New York: Henry Holt, 1988), p. 205.

3. Joan Didion, "The White Album," in the *The White Album* (New York: Penguin, 1981), p. 11.

4. See, for example, Annette Baier, "Theory and Reflective Practices," in *Postures of the Mind* (Minneapolis: University of Minnesota Press, 1984), pp. 207-27; Robert L. Holmes, "The Limited Relevance of Analytical Ethics to the Problems of Bioethics," *Journal of Medicine and Philosophy* 15, no. 2 (1990): 143-59; and especially Stuart Hampshire, *Morality and Conflict* (London: Basil Blackwell, 1983).

5. Carl Elliott, "Everything Is What It Is," *Inquiry* 34 (1992): 525-38; Grant Gillett, *Reasonable Care* (Bristol: Bristol Press, 1989).

6. For instance, see Alasdair MacIntyre, *After Virtue* (Notre Dame, Ind.: University of Notre Dame Press, 1981); John Hardwig, "What About the Family?" *Hastings Center Report* 20, no. 2 (1990): 5-10; Marion Danis and Larry Churchill, "Autonomy and the Common Weal," *Hastings Center Report* 21, no. 1 (1991): 25-31; Steven H. Miles and Kathryn Montgomery Hunter, "The Case: A Story Lost and Found," Commentary and Overview. *Second Opinion* 15 (November 1990): 55-57.

7. See also the excellent criticism of MacIntyre's account of moral language in Paul Johnston, *Wittgenstein and Moral Philosophy* (London: Routledge, 1989), pp. 87-89.

8. Paul Auster, *New York Trilogy: City of Glass, Ghosts, the Locked Room* (New York: Viking Penguin, 1990).

9. For a more extended discussion of this broadly Wittgensteinian account of moral language, see Paul Johnston, *Wittgenstein and Moral Philosophy*; Grant Gillett, *Representation, Meaning and Thought* (Oxford: Oxford University Press, forthcoming) and Grant Gillett, "An Anti-Sceptical Fugue," *Philosophical Investigations* 13, no. 4 (1990): 304-21.

10. Clifford Geertz, *Local Knowledge* (New York: Basic Books 1983), pp. 62, 63.

11. Geertz, *Local Knowledge*, p. 64.

12. The best essay that I have read on this subject, and one I have drawn on here, is Stuart Hampshire's superb "Morality and Conflict," in *Morality and Conflict* (London: Basil Blackwell 1983).

[8]

CLINICAL ETHICS AS MEDICAL HERMENEUTICS

DAVID C. THOMASMA

*Professor and Director, Medical Humanities Program, Loyola University Chicago,
2160 South First Avenue, Maywood, IL 60153, U.S.A.*

ABSTRACT. There are several branches of ethics. Clinical ethics, the one closest to medical decisionmaking, can be seen as a branch of medicine itself. In this view, clinical ethics is a unitary hermeneutics. Its rule is a guideline for unifying other theories of ethics in conjunction with the clinical context. Put another way, clinical ethics interprets the clinical situation in light of a balance of other values that, while guiding the decisionmaking process, also contributes to the very weighting of those values. The case itself originates ideas, not only about which value ought to predominate in its resolution, but also provides the origin of clinical rules that can be used in other cases. These are interpretive rules. Some examples of these rules are presented as well.

Key words: clinical ethics, ethics, hermeneutics, interpretation, inductive reasoning, medical decision making, philosophy of medicine

1. INTRODUCTION

In the early days of medical ethics, it was not clear to practitioners of the discipline exactly which model of ethics was being employed. Often medical ethics was identified with professional ethics. For philosophers medical ethics was a branch of applied ethics, something pure philosophers looked down on for starters, since real philosophy was to be found in the major ethical theories themselves. Much of the philosophy of medicine in the 1970's dealt with the justification of medical ethics as an authentic region of concern for philosophy itself.[1]

Today the territory appears much clearer. There are a number of types of ethics about which discussion takes place. The important point is that in each, a differing kind of reasoning is appropriate. My thesis is that clinical ethics, one of these types, is actually a branch of medicine in which value-interpretation takes place. This, in turn, means that clinical ethics is a type of hermeneutics. Other types of ethical reasoning also might be called hermeneutical, but in an analogous way.

Theoretical Medicine **15**: 93–111, 1994.

94   DAVID C. THOMASMA

2. BRANCHES OF ETHICS

There are a number of types of ethics employed by thinkers when dealing
with medical issues. The types range from very abstract to very concrete,
deductive to inductive models of reasoning. With Glenn Graber, I have
examined these in detail elsewhere.[2] What follows is a necessarily brief
sketch that will establish the inductive nature of clinical medical ethics by
contrasting it with other models.

The most abstract and most deductive branch of ethics is that found in
philosophy of medicine itself. In this realm, philosophy of medicine contributes value-statements or general principles of interpretation, to medical
ethics. An example might be the development of the notion of primary of
the doctor-patient relationship for ethical resolution of cases.[3] Using this
value in medical ethics, one might argue that public policy and law should
encourage the decisional abilities of individuals with their physicians and
not try to mandate treatments. Similarly in clinical cases, one might
maintain that it is better to resolve ethical issues at the bedside than to
appeal to an ethics committee or other non-clinical entity for advice. If we
were to call this approach the "Rule of the Primacy of Relationships" we
might be able to call the application of such a rule to the realm of public
debate or clinical decisionmaking a kind of hermeneutics, since the rule
interprets the values that ought to predominate in such instances. This
would be stretching the idea of hermeneutics a bit far.

Another example of philosophy of medicine contributing a primary
value-principle to ethics is Engelhardt's argument that autonomy is the
necessary condition of possibility of ethics itself in his *The Foundations
of Bioethics*.[4] On this view, any violation of the principle of respect
for autonomy would, *ipso facto*, be a violation of ethics. It would represent an unethical act. In a way, this is hermeneutics "ahead of time," by
advance directive as it were, laying the groundwork for all subsequent
analyses.

A second, slightly more concrete instance of value-interpretation, is the
application of moral theory to a specific moral problem in medicine. This
is ethics applied to medicine. An example might be a utilitarian moral
thinker analyzing the problem of the use of fetal tissue transplants. In this
approach, an entire field of moral enquiry is applied to the analysis of a
large-scale medical ethics issue that has social and political, as well as
ethical, ramifications. Because of the reputed disjunction of such spheres
of moral enquiry, there is little chance of a thinker adopting one sphere
(traditionalist) engaging a person adopting another (e.g., existentialist).
MacIntyre argues this way in his Gifford Lectures.[5] If this be true, then

ETHICS AND HERMENEUTICS 95

the very choice to apply to an issue a special moral theory or mode of enquiry is itself a hermeneutical act, since it predisposes one ahead of time towards one set of ethical policy recommendations rather than another. In the instance just cited, a utilitarian would be much more likely than a traditionalist to approve of fetal tissue transplants on the grounds that such use is not illegal and can benefit a large number of people who are suffering. Once again, however, we would be stretching the notion of hermeneutics to speak of it at the juncture of choice of one's primary ethical system or the choice of which topics to address that might be amenable to the mode of analysis one adopts.

The third value-hermeneutical methodology is more properly what we would call medical ethics. It consists of the application of one or another principle to a medical ethics problem, without necessarily adopting the entire ethical theory that gave rise to and nurtured the principle. Thus, an eclectic medical ethicist might very well adopt the principle of respect for persons in analyzing a situation involving the consent of minors to a research protocol. This principle would function as one among many used to examine the issue, but the one that would predominate in the discussion. In this regard the ethicist might have pre-selected the principle because of its obvious applicability to the problems of assent to research when regarding minors, or the problems of surrogacy in the instances of parental consent. Nonetheless the act of pre-selection is again a kind of hermeneutical act, like pre-judgement of the text, that has caught the attention of hermeneutics scholars such as Gadamer.[6]

A fourth type of hermeneutics in medical judgement arises from clinical ethics. This is the one on which I intend to focus, so it merits a section of its own.

3. CLINICAL ETHICS AND HERMENEUTICS

Before proceeding further, it is now time to define hermeneutics. Hermeneutics is that act of interpretation across boundaries. It is also the discipline or study of that act, as it relates to epistemology, psychology, perceptual sciences, and other philosophical branches, such as metaphysics and theory of knowledge. I wish to focus on the act of interpretation itself. Note that I added to a standard definition to notion of interpreting across boundaries. If an assumption is made that interpretation can proceed without difficulty, whether that interpretation be of a text written in the past, a piece of music, even contemporary music, a work of art, or a person in the doctor-patient relationship, then the act of interpretation is usually not called a

96   DAVID C. THOMASMA

"hermeneutical" act, nor are the insights and methods of the discipline of hermeneutics summoned to clarify points in the interpretation. What makes interpretation hermeneutical is an historical problematic, that is, an intense realization of the historicity or conditionedness of any human action or human being. This intense realization is transcribed into a problem of a boundary or chasm between the interpreter and the interpreted. Both are bound up in the historical conditions of their existence. There is a boundary to be transcended, if possible, in the hermeneutical act.

At the risk of oversimplification, any interpretative act should be considered a hermeneutical one, given our awareness of historical conditions in which texts, music, art, and people themselves work out their own existence. With regard to the doctor-patient relationship, it is really astounding that any communication can take place. There is an imbalance of power in that relationship.[7] The level of suffering is entirely different for the one who actually suffers, the patient, compared to the one who must marshall corresponding feelings and responses of compassion. Then there is the gap of education about the disease, accident, and its remedies. In addition there may be a gap in class and income that might sometimes impede accurate understanding on the part of the patient and physician.

Bridging these and other gaps too numerous to mention, the physician and patient must understand each other, each other's roles, and the consequences of their relationship for healing and curing. Howard Brody has recently examined the implications of the doctor's healing power for both the doctor and the patient. His argument is that rather than diminishing the healing power of the physician, it ought to be employed by both parties in the relationship.[8] Seen in this light, the "working out" of the responsible use of power in the doctor-patient relationship is a hermeneutical branch of medicine itself. Insofar as the process of working out this power of healing involves ethics, then, clinical ethics is a branch of medicine itself, specifically it is the value-orientation of the act of clinical judgement that occurs between physician and patient.

I am reluctant to ascribe this act solely to the physician, since the judgement itself is formed from the dialogue and, indeed, the hermeneutics, that occurs between the parties rather than in the head of just one party, the doctor. My thesis is that clinical ethics is hermeneutical because it involves interpretation across all of the boundaries that naturally occur in an imbalanced relationship between physician and patient.[9]

4. MODEL OF CLINICAL ETHICS AS HERMENEUTICS

Since the beginning of modern clinical medical ethics, it has been no secret that the reasoning patterns of clinical judgement in medical care parallel of ethical judgement.[10,11] This realization is important for many reasons. For example, ethics education programs in medical schools have acquired a "clinical" focus of relevance and reality by stressing the similarity between medical and ethical decisionmaking.[12] Articles and books on the philosophy of medicine have sometimes underscored the relation of the ethic of medicine to clinical judgement.[13] More pointedly for our purpose, the nexus between clinical medicine and clinical ethics can help reveal structures of good decisionmaking in medicine that are not simple products of contractual models of the doctor-patient relationship. More is going on in that relationship than initially meets the eye.

My focus is on how the good emerges from medical and clinical judgement, and how the interaction of persons in context leads to that emergence. Put another way, the medical encounter in its context helps interpret the good through emergent values of doctors, other health providers, society, and patients. The case drives our thought, and compassion about the serious problems involved itself drives the case.

There is a powerful divinity-role played by modern medicine in its quest to overcome the exigencies of life and death. Counterbalancing this role is the standard account of rationalistic bioethics that deliberately removes particularity from the decisionmaking matrix. The purpose of this approach is to find some common ground among persons of varying belief-systems, in order to control biomedical technology's impact on personal autonomy, thus minimizing as far as possible the diversity of individuals and societies. Following a brief examination of this account, I will then discuss contextualism, as I call this approach. In particular I will offer some examples of clinical rules that function as hermeneutical interpretations of cases.

A responsible use of technological intervention with and for the sake of an individual patient requires not only rational analysis, but also a particular sensitivity to the particularities of the case and the emotional content of value commitments of the parties involved. The responsible use of power is a clinical ethics judgement in every case about the best balance of interventions and outcomes.

The most dramatic examples of taking such responsibility for the particularities of a case are culled from the problems of withholding and withdrawing care from the dying. But compassion is also required to assess properly the interventions to be given to the weak and debilitated elderly,

98   DAVID C. THOMASMA

to the demented, to individuals who wish to exercise their autonomy in
ways that are easily judged to be self-destructive, and to children, to
mention just a few of the challenges presented by modern medicine to
both physicians and patients alike.

4.1. *Casuistry*

I am very sympathetic to casuistry as the basic model for how the good
decision emerges in medicine. But more work must be done on the assumptions of casuistry. This becomes apparent when we begin to delve into the
ways in which medical judgement interprets experience by "mining" the
good. There is no time to explore all the ramifications of this kind of
question. We can only target two major problems with casuistry.

The most difficult assumption of casuistry is that it presupposes a unified
theory of human nature and social context by which one case can be
logically compared to another. This unified theory of human nature was
provided by the Natural Law Theory. But this theory, as it was employed
in the past, is now as discredited as is traditional casuistry. Toulmin and
Jonsen in their book, argue that casuistry arose as a method at just that
time in Western Civilization when the metaphysical superstructure of
Christianity began to collapse under the rise of the modern state, nationalism, and the age of reason.[14] They therefore make the case that casuistry
is eminently suitable for modern times, times of pluralism, times without
a moral consensus.[15] Yet it is difficult to ignore the need for some mode
of comparison by which one case is at the very least analogous to the other.
Otherwise we are lost in the same dilemma posed by Wittgenstein for which
the language games were a solution. Meaning is not wholly and completely
individual. It arises in a context beyond or encompassing the individual
case. The very basis for analogous cases is some perduring "something"
that crosses the boundaries of each case, each ethics-game as it were (to
continue the Wittgenstein analogy). Defenses of casuistry on this point by
Albert Jonsen and corresponding critiques by Tomlinson and Kopelman
have already appeared in these pages.[16,17,18]

There is a second, and related, problem. When casuistry began to be
discredited, it was done so by those who held that ethical theory was very
important. The method of ethical analysis changed from case-orientation
to deducing practical conclusions from principles. Reinstituting casuistry
as the model for both ethical and medical decisions neglects the importance
of ethical theory, and analogously, of the relationship of individuals within
the case and their values to the emergence of the good.

4.2. *Contextualism*

Just as Kant was awakened from his dogmatic slumbers by reading Hume, and by taking seriously the challenge to science that Hume's skepticism hurled, so too the deductive model of ethical reasoning has been hurled a challenge by casuistry (and postmodernism). It is closer to clinical judgement, it describes realistically (rather than ideally) how good decisions come about, and it is practical. Yet it neglects the importance of theory, and of the nexus of values that ethical theory seeks to protect.

Is there a middle ground between deducing the good decision from abstract and theoretical principles that ignore clinical realities, and educing the former entirely from the latter? Is there a middle ground between deduction and induction of the good?

A middle course between a generalist application of ethical theory and specialized case-by-case analysis is possible with a contextual grid for medical ethics.[19] It is only one example of work on contexts to which medical ethics must address itself. Neither axioms nor standard moral rules are sufficient (although they are necessary of course) to determine the validity of moral theory and ethical principles in resolving medical ethics problems. Additional rules, or guidelines for relating theory and practice, must be developed according to this approach. Among these rules is the context functioning as a formal adjustment to values in concrete circumstances. Earlier I emphasized the importance of consideration of the particularities of a case, including its context, for a properly compassionate analysis. This is also a concern of postmodernist ethics.

The root of the difficulty in medical ethics lies in a confrontation between an abstracting tendency in the long and rewarding history of ethics and the concrete, individual problems encountered by professionals. The latter must make quick decisions about very complex matters in order to benefit their patients. Contrariwise, ethical analysis must take careful note of numerous ethical theories, axioms, and other concerns in order to conduct a minimally decent conceptual and problematical analysis. This process takes time and, of necessity, becomes quite abstract. Health professionals and patients quickly lose interest in these abstractions and theoretical meanderings if they are not decisively and explicitly related to the realities of patient care. They must do ethics on the run.

Ethical principles appear abstract – or better, speculative – because they do not possess the same degree of social legitimacy as the values of everyday life. Moral abstractions frequently are seen by non-philosophers as empty of the normal ingredients of moral concerns people have in their day-to-day life. No doubt they can and do seep into that daily life, but the

100   DAVID C. THOMASMA

process of connecting theory to practice is a long and subtle one in most cases.[20] How often do we encounter physicians and patients who become impatient with "thinking" that has no practical consequence.

Thus, according to the contextualism theory, what is needed is a means by which to locate a moral problem and to exhibit the likely values and principles at issue within that locus. The context having been established by such a "grid," the discussion can proceed toward means for resolving the case by protecting the interests and values of those affected by it. But that is not all. The grid not only locates and focuses the moral discussion, it also hints at the cross-case commonalities that legitimize the very act of organizing similar cases, comparing them, and drawing conclusions about the new case.

There is a variability of contexts in the clinical resolution of cases that is noticeable to all who work in the medical setting. This variability does not describe so much the relativity of values and principles; rather, it describes how the weight they bring to bear on a case is partially determined by the medical specialty involved, the personal values of the patient, family, or social group, the personal and professional values of the health care professional involved, and the institutional setting in which the problem arises. Some principles and axioms will be given more weight than others in such a scheme, and one important component of the weighting will stem from the contexts. The good will arise out of the mix of these components.

Such a contextual grid is only one aspect, then, of what might be called context-variable moral rules. Other examples could be examined that do not fit the contextual grid pattern, but are moral rules which in other ways vary with the context. Further, the contextual grid I propose cannot encompass all of the variables in a case – but only the ones most likely to be affecting the emphasis of some values or principles over others. This is precisely where deductive models of ethical reasoning fall short.

An example follows: the rule of protection of autonomy is more likely to be given prominent focus in a primary care context than in a tertiary care one, wherein one's autonomy is virtually always depressed and hence concern for autonomy is diminished in favor of a goal of preservation of life and/or restoration of health.[21] Furthermore, the rule of protection of autonomy is more likely to be emphasized in cases in which there is no threat to others than in cases wherein the common good must be considered, sometimes to the detriment of personal autonomy. Finally, because the grid only *describes* most likely weights given to moral principles and rules in formulating an indicated course of action, one should not misconstrue the contextual grid as claiming that physicians in tertiary care settings do not care about protecting their patients' autonomy, or that public health officials stress social responsibility to the exclusion of individual well-being. All of these moral values bear upon a case. The grid only describes what values are most likely to take precedence over others.

The contextual grid theory rests on two distinctions. The first is the distinction between primary, secondary, and tertiary care settings, a standard distinction in medicine. This distinction forms one set of coordinates of the grid. Its importance for moral reasoning lies in the seriousness of the assault on personal wholeness brought about by the disease in question.[22] Thus, a patient's wishes are more likely to be sought and respected in a primary care setting than in an emergency room after a heart attack, where a paternalistic response may be, and often is, more appropriate. The second distinction or coordinate of the grid is that between the individual and the number of persons affected by the problem. The moral significance of this distinction is based on the increasing complexity of values the more different persons whose interests are affected by the outcome of the case enter our consideration, and our increased tendency to protect the commonweal the greater the number of affected persons. Recall again the purpose of the grid is to describe context-variable rules, i.e., which principles and axioms are likely to be given more weight than others in a given circumstance in formulating a moral policy or in developing an indicated course of action.

4.3. *Compassionate Analysis*

Advances have occurred in emphasizing the rights of patients not only to determine the treatments they desire and do not desire during the dying process, but also the development of the rights to choose treatments at any time during life, not just while dying. The efforts of patient advocacy groups in sponsoring and supporting legislation and court deliberations have been outstanding. The Living Will and Advance Directives, including the Durable Power of Attorney, now as recognized in the United States through the Patient Self-Determination Act implemented in December, 1991,[23] all point to eventual further clarification of these rights, for example, how they will have an impact on long-term care settings.[24] What is important to note is that the underlying motivation for the development of such instruments is the prevention of suffering, that is, to increase the role of compassion in decisions about life-prolonging technology.[25,26] It would make sense to extend these rights to even greater control over the dying process.

As noted earlier, medical technology gives us enormous power at all levels of life, but especially at the end of life. Yet concerns should not be

102   DAVID C. THOMASMA

confined to dispatching persons too early by injections, in active, direct euthanasia, while not meeting their physical and social needs. Another form of the "technofix" society is to prolong suffering in conditions of hopeless injury to life.[27] Daily life is full of interactions with "things" – non-human and fundamentally incomprehensible to most persons.[28] We sometimes get so used to technological processes that we behave as though they are substitutes for human and compassionate care. eating for many elderly and dying patients has been replaced by tubes; participating in the spiritual and material values of human life has been replaced by "merely surviving," as a being subjugated to the very products of human imagination.[29] The new experience that has replaced dignified suffering is artificially prolonged, opaque, depersonalized maintenance.[30]

Compassionate contextualism has the following features:

(a) Just as in aesthetics, one must know both the whole and the individual parts. Moral reasoning from both rationalistic and emotional openness means that the "big picture" is combined with the sophisticated understanding of the individual's plight, values, and possible outcomes. One is neither unduly swayed by reason or emotion, but by a balance between the two.

A good example might be a case in which a 14 year old child rejects a blood transfusion for religious reasons. She and her mother are recent converts to the Jehovah's Witnesses faith. She is the only surviving individual on an initial remission cancer protocol, but now suffers from pneumocystis carinii pneumonia. Her compromised immunological state with few white blood cells remaining means that, without a transfusion, she will die. She does not want to die, but she does want to be true to her fundamental religious principles. To complicate matters, her mother and she are converts based on the religion of her mother's third husband. She has changed religion with each marriage. The mother has a history of instability.

A clinical ethicist, unfamiliar with all the ramifications of the case, might argue on rational grounds that society grants power to pediatricians to protect the lives of such children. In some states, doctors have 48 hours during which they are to take over the case to protect the child while they seek a court order for custodial decisionmaking on behalf of the child. Yet a more complete understanding of the case includes an awareness of the girl's valiant fight against cancer, her maturity beyond her years, the strength of her own religious convictions, the bonds of love between the mother and child, and their sense of belonging to a religious community. All of these might be shattered in a decision to override her wishes and give her the transfusion. The latter may not be successful in any case.

ETHICS AND HERMENEUTICS 103

(b) The life of the patient has a certain "completeness" about it that transcends reason. It is discerned instinctively by the caregivers and surrogates. This "completeness" or wholeness of a life leads to decisions in some instances that might not otherwise be rationally defensible.

Consider the case of a nurse, daughter of a veterinarian and nurse, and eldest sister of three nurses. The youngest sister was driving a car, making a left turn, when the car was broadsided. The patient's head was broken from her spine at C2, and held on the body only by the muscle tissue of the neck. After stabilization it was determined that, although not brain-dead, significant damage had occurred to her brain. Even if she were to live, she would be in a permanent vegetative state and permanently paralyzed. Her parents, opening an ethics consult meeting with a prayer, tearfully expressed her view that she wanted to donate her organs. It became evident to everyone at the meeting, the hospital administrator, the neurologists, the chaplain, the nurses, and the ethicist, that her life would not acquire its divine completeness without donation of her organs. Her parents argued very successful, not only through reasonable statements, but also through their grief, that this and only this would give meaning to their daughter's commitment to care for others, and help them cope with her death. All of us agreed that she should have her organs taken prior to removing her from life-support systems.

This decision, important as it was, violated the law. The law requires that individuals be brain-dead before donation occurs. In her case, withdrawing life-support would contribute to the dying of the organs as well. The transplant team, a different group than that which met with the family during the ethics consult, refused to accept the decision on legal grounds, fearing they might be contributing to the death rather than taking the organs after a legal death had been proclaimed.

This case changed the way I think about organ donation, and led to a chapter I wrote arguing in favor of organ donation in a permanent vegetative state as well as when one is brain-dead.[31]

(c) The grounds for the decision are not ultimately made on the basis of current practice, although these principles are important, but on the basis of helping the person complete their life. In a spy novel by John Le Carré', *The Secret Pilgrim*, George Smiley says: "The purpose of *my* life was to end the time I lived in."[32] This statement gains particular poignancy when individuals combine reasons with compassion in dealing with issues at the end of life.

104   DAVID C. THOMASMA

5. CLINICAL ETHICS RULES

As argued so far, the context in which we work out resolutions of difficult cases assists, along with compassion for the individuals involved, in the clinical ethics reasoning necessary for such resolutions. I have called this doctrine "contextualism" because it emphasizes the importance of the particularities of cases in interpreting moral rules. In this environment, certain principles and rules for interpreting the relative weights of principles and values, are also emerging. Only a few examples will be offered regarding decision making for incompetent patients. A more complete analysis of my proposals regarding clinical ethics rules can be found elsewhere.[33]

5.1. *The Rule of Surrogate Decision Making*

By now it is well-recognized that by "incompetent" is meant an inability to execute decisions about one's care, whether the cause is senility, retardation, a stroke, mental illness, genetic disease, or any temporary or permanent incapacity. This statement is merely a negative elaboration on the common definition of a competence as a capacity for performance of a specific task. As Pellegrino defined it with respect to medical care, a "competent person possesses the capacity to make an explicit, reasoned, and intentional choice among alternatives."[34] This requires the capacity to receive information, perceive the relation of the information to one's own predicament, integrate it and calculate risks and benefits, make a choice among options, and convey or communicate that choice in some manner. Unless otherwise the case, one ought to assume that a person is competent. But incompetence can occur in any one of the categories Pellegrino mentioned, impairing that person's decision-making ability. It is for this reason that the wishes of patients and even their consent are sometimes not solicited nor honored in medicine.[35]

Closely related in outcome to the civil-rights-of-the-incompetent view is an argument that all incompetent patients must be treated the same as competent patients on grounds of fairness. When a patient has never been competent, one might try to appeal to an impartial committee, like an infant care review committee, to determine treatment decisions (in order to avoid subjective judgements). But the committee, seeking to avoid those judgements, and attempting to be fair to the patient, will often be forced to recommend treating the patient unless the issue of scarce resources rather than fairness governs the discussions. Evidence exists suggesting that committee decision-making is quite different than individual, and that an affirmative, interventionist course would most likely be chosen over a negative, withdrawing a course of treatment.[36]

In addition, the established set of criteria to which such a hospital ethics committee might appeal for withholding treatment from some incompetent patients fails to cover many situations. David Hilfiker noted in his article about a nursing home patient with pneumonia that, while there has been widespread discussion of principles involved in terminating treatment for comatose, dying patients, there has been much less about the incompetent and debilitated patient.[37] Responses only made it clearer that abstract thinking is difficult to apply at the bedside.[38,39,40]

5.2. *The Rule of Therapeutic Privilege*

Acting on behalf of incapacitated persons is quite difficult, especially if we are unsure of either their current wishes or unsure about their competence to express those wishes. If medicine's object is to protect or even restore autonomy and self-determination,[41] how can one protect this value while intervening in such a way that might disrupt that autonomy, neglect or ignore it, or even, destroy it permanently? Put another way, how can one maintain beneficence in face of uncertain benefit? The usual method is to calculate beneficence on the basis of the wishes of the patient, thus identifying what is best or the patient with his or her previously expressed wishes. However in dealing with incompetent patients, it is not always the case that one's best interests are served by a respect for prior wishes, or an effort to determine what someone would wish were that person now competent.

At this juncture an interpretent rule can be that of therapeutic assumption: The physician is justified in treating the disorder that renders the patient incompetent.[42] There is nothing essentially sacrosanct about respecting prior wishes of patient who were once competent. Because of the new situation that was perhaps not foreseen, these prior wishes themselves may now be suspect. Mooreim argues that respecting prior wishes for utilitarian reasons, given current and future economic pressures, may lead to rapid acceptance of a refusal of therapy (by prior wish). This may come to be the preferred social outcome.[44] If so, either one of two things must give. Either we will no longer seek the best interests of patients (but rather that of society), or we will sacrifice quality of care for inappropriately applied prior wishes.

106   DAVID C. THOMASMA

5.3. *The Rule of Medical Indications*

Veatch includes two other categories of patients: those who were never competent, and have no relatives or other agents to step into the guardian role. The third class is that of incompetent patients who do have guardians or family members able and willing to act as guardians. For Veatch both of these categories include patients who may once have been competent, but failed to make clear their wishes about the situations which eventually befell them. He argues that decisions can be made for such patients without appeal to subjective, substituted judgement criteria.

He confronts the fact that when patients have never expressed prior wishes, the principle of autonomy has no further merit. It makes no sense to try to respect a person's autonomy (read, "decision-making") when they have left no clues about what they would wish. Instead, and this is the danger in his position, one no longer aims at the best interests of the patient. Veatch holds these as now indeterminable. Instead, as he says, "the goal is not to serve the patient's best interests, but to honor his wishes out of respect for him."[45] But how can wishes not made be honored?

The willingness to abandon a search for the patient's best interests seems to lie in an identification of respecting persons with honoring their wishes, and in a repugnance for substituting one's own judgement about the quality of life for a missing capacity. This is an important, even necessary component to the whole notion of respect for persons. Consequently, there is much to admire in Veatch's position. But respecting wishes is a necessary but not a sufficient way to respect persons, especially in the absence of a decision-making capacity, precisely what is missing in never-competent patients. Keeping faith with such patients, then, requires some other kind of judgement.

There is a way to keep that faith, and not abandon it, as Veatch's reasoning has forced him to do. As noted, the flaw in that reasoning concentrates respect for persons on decision-making capacity. A better approach broadens our concerns to include medical indications, and the very nature of the assault on the body that led to the incapacity.

5.4. *The Vulnerability Principle*

In a previous work Edmund D. Pellegrino and I derived an axiom of vulnerability from the nature of medicine as a special kind of human activity.[46] We held that to attain the goal of the medical encounter – a right and good healing action for a particular patient – several axioms were necessary, the violation of any one of which imperil the goal. Observing the vulnerability principle was one of these necessary axioms.

The principle of vulnerability can be stated this way: In human relations generally, if there are inequities of power, knowledge, or material means, the obligation is upon the stronger to respect and protect the vulnerability of the other and not exploit the less-advantaged party. This is a principle of general ethics, applicable to all sorts of human relationships. It generates an obligation of altruism, i.e., taking others into account in our use of power, knowledge, or other possessions. This taking of vulnerability into account is a bilateral or multilateral affair when more than two persons are involved.[47,47,49]

5.5. *Rule Against Enthusiasms of Others*

For some, like C. Everett Koop, withholding treatment from incompetent patients is a violation of the patient's constitutional right to life. This is a vitalist position that few physicians would employ at the bedside.[50] The opposite view is expressed, for example, by Joseph Fletcher, an early, continuous, and strong proponent of a right to die. Fletcher says: "Death control . . . is a matter of human dignity. Without it persons become puppets. To perceive this is to grasp the error lurking in the notion that life, as such, is the highest good."[51]

Most persons are sympathetic with patients who must die a slow, lingering, painful death due to severe terminal illness. We can understand how, even when pain is controlled, the suffering that accompanies dying must also be addressed. For this reason a good argument can be made that doctors should assist in dying, in bringing about a good health, in the face of burgeoning medical technology.[52] For the most part this can be accomplished by what is called passive euthanasia, by withholding or even withdrawing medical technology at the patient's request. Sometimes this may be accomplished in the absence of an explicit request, as the Appleton Consensus suggests.[53] That technology was invented for the purpose of prolonging life. When it is used inappropriately, it unnecessarily prolongs the dying process. Withholding and withdrawing, then, are forms of taking responsibility for our technology.[54]

Keeping inappropriate technology out of the dying process at the request of the patient and family is a way of honoring the primacy of human life and human values over the mere brute existence of machines. Jonsen wonders just what exactly life support supports: "We talk about the maintenance of life; we don't often talk about the maintenance of personhood.

It interests me little," he says, "indeed, not at all, to be alive as an organism. In such a state I have no interests. It is enormously interesting for me to be a person . . . it is the perpetuation of my personhood that interests me; indeed, it is probably my major and perhaps my sole real interest."[55]

Does this honor include assisting at the suicide of elderly patients, as did Dr. Kevorkian did with his "death machine" at the request of Janet Adkins, or later, his assistance of nineteen others, many of whom suffered from chronic disorders rather than terminal ones? The heart of a massive public discussion ought to include the question about what sort of society we ought to be. Have we become so frighteningly fractured that people feel the need to dispatch themselves early in a chronic disease rather than trust others to care for them? Christine Cassell, M.D. is very worried that elderly persons, in light of the Cruzan decision, will want to commit suicide rather than subject themselves to possible violations of their values in nursing homes and hospitals after they become senile.[56] Evidence exists that there is a growing trend in elder suicide.[57] Will people increasingly feel threatened by high-technology hospitals where they are stripped of their values at the same time they are stripped of their clothing and put into the beds? Do we have to carry all sorts of lengthy legal documents on our person about our wishes regarding medical technology should we become ill or get in an accident? On a trip, we will be warned by relatives about our advance directives and living wills? "Don't leave home without them?"

5.6. *Two Rules for Protecting from Harm*

A clinical ethical principle is born of the first concern for the vulnerable. The greater the degree of incompetence, and the less the invasiveness of the procedure, the greater the quality of the preferences is required. Patients in persistent vegetative states or permanent comas or end-stage Alzheimer's disease or having suffered a severe stroke, are now all unable to speak for themselves. They have a high degree of incompetence. If the therapeutic plan turns on the question of withholding and withdrawing fluids and nutrition, these are considered less invasive procedures than using respirators and cardiopulmonary resuscitation. Withholding and withdrawing nutrition and hydration from such patients on the basis of their previous statements, according to this first ethical principle, can be done, but requires a very explicit, "clear and convincing" form of evidence. One form might be a living will or written advance directive. Informal discussion with relatives may be insufficient. Legal documentation is to be preferred.

On the other hand, all persons must be protected from another sort of harm. This is the harm brought to us courtesy of modern, high technology health care. For the most part we are able to control this technology by directing it to good human ends. Healing and curing patients are good examples. When highly technical means for curing individuals are employed, there is a danger that the means will begin to obscure the ends. This is especially true when the intervention has "frozen" persons in states that normally would have led to their deaths, just as modern medicine can freeze embryos on their way to their lives.

When individuals are in a permanent vegetative state or permanent coma they have been arrested from proceeding to their next adventure. We must take responsibility for the technology employed in keeping them alive in this state, far from the normal interactive, personal life they once enjoyed. They cannot be cured. They cannot be healed. Nancy Cruzan's family spoke of her in the past tense. There was a death in the family, but no burial. She was kept alive against her presumed wishes as conveyed by the family. Her life was in the hands of others. She and her family were controlled by the whims of others who fancied themselves as protectors of human life.

Arising from this additional concern to protect the vulnerable, then, is a second ethical principle. How may we protect incompetent patients from being at the mercy of others? How may we control the enthusiasms of the life-prolongers-at-all-costs? How should we properly direct our medical technology? This contrasting clinical ethics principle might be expressed as follows: The greater the permanent assault on the quality of personal, interactive human life, the less formal the quality of consent is required in order to withhold and withdraw medical treatment that might prolong life in such uncertain conditions, and the greater might be the reliance upon the patient's preferences as expressed informally to the family or as constructed by the family from the patient's value history.

6. CONCLUSION

These few clinical ethics rules follow directly from my thesis that clinical ethics can be compared to a hermeneutical judgement, an interpretation of a particular set of circumstances that define a case. From that judgement can be extrapolated "rules," which are actually interpretants (y) of situations (x). The context of the case permits us to apply some of these rules to it. This context, insofar as it suggests which rules to apply, also is a form of hermeneutics, as it guides us from the complex of the particularities of the case towards a more generalized form of resolution.

110   DAVID C. THOMASMA

REFERENCES

1. Engelhardt HT, Spicker S, eds. *Philosophy and Medicine*. Series for Dordrecht/Boston: Kluwer Academic Publishers, 1970 to the present.
2. Graber GC, Thomasma DC. *Theory and Practice in Medical Ethics*. New York: Continuum Publishing Co., 1989.
3. Pellegrino ED, Thomasma DC. *A Philosophical Basis of Medical Practice*. New York: Oxford University Press, 1981.
4. Engelhardt HT, Jr. *The Foundations of Bioethics*. New York: Oxford University Press, 1987.
5. MacIntyre, AC. *Three Rival Versions of Moral Enquiry: Encyclopedia, Geneaology, and Tradition*. Notre Dame, IN.: University of Notre Dame Press, 1990.
6. Gadamer HG. *Hermeneutics Versus Science?: Three German Views*. Notre Dame, IN.: University of Notre Dame Press, 1988. Also see Gadamer HG. *Gesammelte Werke*. Tübingen: Mohr, 1985–; *Truth and Method*. London: Sheed & Ward, 1975.
7. Brody H. *The Healer's Power*. New Haven: Yale University Press, 1992.
8. Ibid.
9. Pellegrino ED, Thomasma DC. *A Philosophical Basis of Medical Practice*. New York: Oxford University Press, 1981.
10. Fletcher J. Four indicators of humanhood: the enquiry matures. *Hast Ctr Rep* Dec. 1975;4:4–7.
11. Toulmin S. The tyranny of principles. *Hast Ctr Rep* Dec. 1981;11:31–39.
12. Pellegrino ED, McElhinney TK. *Teaching Ethics. Humanities, and Human Values in Medical Schools: A Ten-Year Overview*. Washington, D.C.: Society for Health and Human Values, Institute on Human Values in Medicine, 1982.
13. Pellegrino ED, Thomasma DC. *A Philosophical Basis of Medical Practice*. New York: Oxford University Press, 1981.
14. Jonsen A, Toulmin S. *The Abuse of Casuistry*. San Francisco, CA.: University of California Press, 1988.
15. McIntyre A. *After Virtue*. 2nd Edition. Notre Dame, IN.: University of Notre Dame Press, 1984.
16. Jonsen AR. Casuistry as methodology in clinical ethics. *Theor Med* 1992;12:295–308.
17. Tomlinson T. Casuistry in medical ethics: rehabilitated or repeat offender? *Theor Med* 1994;15(1):5–20.
18. Kopelman L. Case method and casuistry: the problem of bias. *Theor Med* 1994;15(1): 21–37.
19. Thomasma DC. The context as moral rule in medical ethics. *J. of Bioethics* 1984;5:63–79.
20. Graber GC, Thomasma DC. *Theory and Practice*.
21. Thomasma D. Beyond medical paternalism and patient autonomy: a model of physician's conscience for the doctor-patient relationship. *Ann Int Med* 1983;98:243–248.
22. Bergsma J, Thomasma, D. *Health Care: Its Psychosocial Dimensions*. Pittsburgh: Duquesne University Press, 1982.
23. PSDA well received in hospitals, despite early confusion. *Med Eth Advisor* March 1992;8:25–35.
24. Rouse F. Living wills in the long-term care setting. *J Long-Term Care Adm* Summer, 1988;17:14–19.
25. Mehling A. Living wills:preventing suffering or a deadly contract? *State Govern News* Dec 1988:14–15.
26. Mehling A, Neitlich S. Right-to-die backgrounder. *News from the Soc for the Right to Die* (newsletter) Jan. 1989:1–2.
27. Braithwaite S, Thomasma DC. New guidelines on foregoing life-sustaining treatment in incompetent patients: an anti-cruelty policy. *Ann Int Med* 1986;104:711–715.

ETHICS AND HERMENEUTICS   111

28. Giere R. Science and technology studies: prospects for an enlightened postmodern synthesis. *Science, Technology, & Human Values* 1993;18:102–111.
29. Illich I. *Medical Nemesis: The Expropriation of Health.* New York: Pantheon, 1976:106.
30. Ibid:154.
31. Thomasma DC. Making treatment decisions for permanently unconscious patients: the ethical perspective. In Monagle JF, Thomasma DC, eds. *Medical Ethics: A Guide for Health Professionals.* Rockville, MD.: Aspen Publishers, 1988:192–204.
32. Le Carré J. *The Secret Pilgrim.* New York: Alfred Knopf, 1991:12.
33. Thomasma DC. Ethical aspects of geriatric care. In Calkins E, Ford AB, Katz PR, eds. *Practice of Geriatrics.* Philadelphia/London: W.B. Saunders Co., 1992:136–143.
34. Pellegrino ED. Informal judgements of competence and incompetence. In Gardell Cutter MA, Shelp EE, eds. *Competency: A Study of Informal Competency Determination in Primary Care.* Dordrecht/Boston: Kluwer Academic Publishers, 1991:29–48.
35. Knight J. Judging competence: when the psychiatrist need, or need not, be involved. In *Competency, op. cit.*:3–28.
36. Williams P. Why IRBS falter in reviewing risks and benefits. *IRB* 1984;6:3.
37. Hilfiker D. Allowing the debilitated to die. *New Engl J Med* 1983;308:716–720.
38. Letters to editor, Allowing the debilitated to die. *New Engl J Med* 1983;308:862–863.
39. Hilfiker D. Response to letters to editor. *New Engl J Med* 1983;308:863.
40. Ibid.
41. Cassell E. The function of medicine. *Hast Ctr Rep* 1977:7:16–19.
42. Thomasma DC, Pellegrino ED. The role of the family and physicians in decisions for incompetent patients. *Theor Med* 1987;8:283.
43. Morreim EH. Competence: at the intersection of law, medicine, and philosophy. In *Competency*:93–126.
44. Abernathy V. Judgements about patient competence: cultural and economic antecedents. In *Competency*:211–226.
45. Veatch R. An ethical framework for terminal care decision: a new classification of patients. *J Am Ger Soc* 1984;32:667.
46. Pellegrino, Thomasma. *A Philosophical Basis.*
47. Goodin RE. *Protecting the Vulnerable: A Re-Analysis of Our Social Responsibilities.* Chicago: University of Chicago Press, 1985.
48. Veatch R. *The Foundations of Justice: Why the Retarded and the Rest of Us Have Claims to Equality.* New York: Oxford University Press, 1986.
49. Veatch RM. *A Theory of Medical Ethics.* New York: Basic Books, 1981.
50. Loewy E. Treatment decisions in the mentally impaired: limiting but not abandoning treatment. *New Engl J Med* 1987;317:1465–1469.
51. Fletcher JF. Four indicators of humanhood: the enquiry matures. *Hast Ctr Rep* 1974;4(6):4–7.
52. Cerne F. Mercy or murder? Physician's role in suicide spurs debate. *AHA News* July 2, 1990;26:1, 5.
53. Stanley JM, ed. The Appleton consensus: suggested international guidelines for decisions to forgo medical treatment. *J Danish Med Assoc (Ugeskr Laeger)* 1989; 151(11):700–706; reprinted in *J Med Eth* 1989;15:129–136.
54. Various Authors. The care of the dying: a symposium on the case of Betty Wright. *Law Med Health Care* 1989;17(3):205–268.
55. Jonsen A. What does life support support? In: Winslade W, ed. *Personal Choices and Public Commitments: Perspectives on the Humanities.* Galveston, TX.: Institute for the Medical Humanities, 1988:61–69. Quote:66–67.
56. Cassell C, Meier DE. Morals and moralism in the debate over euthanasia and assisted suicide. *New Engl J Med* 1990;323:750–752.
57. Conwell W, Rotenberg M, Caine ED. Completed suicide at age 50 and over. *J Am Ger Soc* 1990;38(6):640–644.

[9]

THE HYPERREALITY OF CLINICAL ETHICS:
A UNITARY THEORY AND HERMENEUTICS

HENK TEN HAVE

Katholieke Universiteit Nijmegen, Faculty of Medical Sciences, Department of Ethics, Philosophy and History of Medicine, P. O. Box 9101, 6500 HB Nijmegen, The Netherlands

ABSTRACT. Medical ethics nowadays is dominated by a conception of ethics as the application of moral theories and principles. This conception is criticized for its depreciation of the internal morality of medical practice and its narrow view of external morality. This view reflects both a lack of interest in the empirical realities of medicine and a neglect of the socio-cultural value-contexts of medical ethical issues, including the creative development of a broader philosophical framework for a practicable medical ethics. Several alternative approaches and conceptions have been proposed. The unified clinical ethics theory, developed by Graber and Thomasma, is an interesting attempt to synthesize these alternative approaches. It correctly identifies as the crucial problem the present disconnectedness of medical ethics from theoretical philosophy as well as the practice of medicine. In this paper, however, it is argued that the unitary theory should take more serious attention to the hermeneutic character of medicine as well as ethics. This implies that the unitary theory must in fact transform itself into an *interpretive* clinical ethics theory. The theoretical characteristics and practical consequences of an interpretive theory of medical ethics are discussed in the present paper.

Key words: clinical ethics, interpretive clinical ethics theory, unitary theory, hermeneutics, theory and practice in ethics, philosophy of medicine

1. INTRODUCTION

In *Amérique*, the French postmodern philosopher Jean Baudrillard, digesting his impressions of the New World, argues that America is neither dream nor reality; it is hyperreality, more realistic than reality itself.[1] Baudrillard derives this diagnosis from two symptoms:

(a) The New World is Utopia realized; it has accomplished what others in the Old World have only dreamt of. Everything is in existence because it has materialized immediately; it is not the result of a prior conceptualization. Words and ideas do not ontologically precede things and objects, but they present themselves as the world of actual, concrete experience. A way-of-thinking is made real through a way-of-life; everything in the world is factual and visible, thus unambiguous.

(b) At the same time, the empirical world is simulated reality; it is thoroughly artificial, a universe of perfect simulacra, and therefore more real than reality. Everything in the world is scenery, well-orchestrated simulation, like the smile of the dead person in his funeral home. The things we experience in the New World, are cinematographic but outside the cinema. People, cars, buildings, cities seem to emerge from the screen, materializing as the real world.

I will argue that the diagnosis of "hyperreality" also applies to clinical ethics as medical hermeneutics. This new conception of ethics is an interesting postmodern attempt to answer some recent criticisms of medical ethics. It focuses on what is considered the basic problem of contemporary medical ethics, *viz.* the discrepancy between theory and practice.[2] However, the characteristics of this new conception need analysis in order to clarify the type of answer it is inviting.

2. THE TRANSFORMATION OF MEDICAL ETHICS

The conception and role of medical ethics has been reshaped significantly over the last few decades. Traditionally, "medical ethics" used to refer to the *deontology* of the medical profession, to "codes of conduct which consist partly of ordinary moral rules, partly of rules of etiquette, and partly of rules of professional conduct."[3] In this sense medical ethics is essentially a set of problems that focus on the internal morality of medicine, *viz.*, the values, norms, and rules intrinsic to the actual practice of health care. Medicine is not considered a technical enterprise that can be morally evaluated from some exogenous standpoint. On the contrary, the professional practice of medicine presumes and implies a moral perspective; therefore, what is judged good medical practice is determined by the rules and standard procedures of the practice itself.

Since the 1960s, medical ethics has gone through various phases, gradually turning away from traditional deontology.[4] Initially, this development was induced by "internal" reasons: the biotechnological and scientific advances of medicine challenged the adequacy of the professional morality of medical practice. The next phase came about for "external" reasons. The unprecedented power of medicine generated problems not only for the individual patient and physician but for society as well. Consequently, the scope of medical ethics is considerably enlarged; there are new and more complex moral issues and new participants in an intensified set of moral debates. Medical ethics more and more is subsumed under a new category, *viz.*, *health care ethics* or *bioethics*. These new terms indicate that ethics deals not only with the problems arising in the physician-patient relationship, but also with the moral problems posed by other health care professionals, with the moral issues created by the health care system, and with the public policy implications of biomedical developments as a result of research.

Thus, the end-result of this gradual transformation of medical ethics was twofold:

First, it has produced a new profession of health care ethicists and bioethicists, possessing a specific body of knowledge and particular cognitive skills, specialized journals and societies, and newly-established centers and institutes.

Second, it has produced a socio-cultural movement of widespread public concern concerning medico-moral matters – particularly in those countries where advanced biomedical technology permeates public as well as private life.

There is today a growing awareness that the outcome of the aforesaid transformation process is unsatisfactory. The flourishing of medical ethics may have its benefits, but what are its costs? The professionalization and institutionalization of medical ethics received an enormous stimulus because both the adequacy and the relevance of medicine's internal morality were put into question. Ethicists have placed more and more emphasize on the crucial role of external morality: the principles, norms, and rules operative in society that are partly codified in the law. In their view, medicine and health care are nothing more than interesting domains in which general ethical theories, principles, and rules could be applied.

This shift from internal professional to external morality and the pre-dominant interpretation of medical ethics as "applied ethics" encouraged physicians to criticize present-day medical ethics for its lack of attention to the practical vicissitudes of health care, for its theoretical biases, and its conceptual alienation from clinical reality.[5,6] But it is also argued that the conceptual model grounding medical ethics is too limited and even reductive, when analyzed from the perspective of the tradition of philo-sophical ethics itself. Why should medical ethics be conceptualized as *applied* theory, rather than reflective practice?[7,8]

In addition, it is being suggested that there is a substantial discrepancy between the public's attention to moral questions and the actual impact of ethics on the routine practices of medicine, as well as the current direction of medicine's development. Moral issues tend to multiply everyday; but how successful are medical ethicists in addressing these novel issues? The media reflect a fascination with the myriad of moral problems in health care, but what will be the effect of these ethical debates on the decisions in everyday clinical medicine, on nursing practice, and on public health policies?

116   HENK TEN HAVE

3. THE DOMINANT CONCEPTION AND ITS CRITICISM

During the last thirty years, a new and unique view of medical ethics as a separate discipline disconnected from philosophy as well as medicine has emerged. But this disconnectedness is both its strength and its weakness. Only recently, after all, has the relationship between ethics and medicine reappeared as the subject of scholarly debate. The prevailing conception of medical ethics is continuously scrutinized and alternative conceptions developed.

The conception of medical ethics that serves as the mainstream of scholarly literature is that of applied ethics. This conception of medical ethics implies the following set of interdependent presuppositions:[9]

   (a) Ethics is application of ethical theory and ethical principles;

   (b) There is a body of ethical theories and principles waiting to be applied to a variety of practical, biomedical problems;

   (c) Professional ethicists have a special expertise in applying ethical theories and principles, whereas non-ethicists (e.g., physicians) supply problems for applied ethics;

   (d) Medical ethics is ordinary ethics applied to medicine. The context in which the problems arise is not peculiar in the sense of being characterized by intrinsic values which generate special problems. On the contrary, the medical context is seen as a practice-ground for a new profession of biomedical ethicists; and

   (e) The aim of medical ethics is to proffer practical recommendations and prescriptions, based on or deduced from ethical theories and principles.

This set of presuppositions makes clear why medical ethics is perceived as a specific discipline; it also defines the standards for the practice of medical ethics; ethics should perform three tasks: conceptual clarification, analyzing and structuring arguments weighing alternatives, and advising a preferable course of action.[10] The central contribution of medical ethics is therefore restricted. It does not necessarily result in judgments regarding what we should do. The ethicist provides the topography of arguments, and objectifies the options. The ethicist regards himself as a disinterested and neutral observer of medical practice, who is in the best position to weigh moral alternatives.

In recent years, the presuppositions underlying the conception of applied ethics have been critically questioned.

(a) The application of principles to cases has become paradigmatic of medical ethics. But, in fact, there is no consensus regarding the particular theoretical framework to guide the rational selection of principles to be

HYPERREALITY 117

applied. In ordinary practice, ethics is focused on mid-level principles –
such as respect for autonomy, beneficence, nonmaleficence, and justice.
These principles are then to be applied to dilemmas, cases, and problems
encountered in the practice of health care. From a specific principle, guidelines or recommendations can be derived in order to resolve various problematic situations. But there is no single rational criterion on the basis of
which to decide which principle is overriding; there is no definitive scheme
for ordering principles and for choosing between them. There are, of course,
a variety of moral theories, but in a pluralistic society no single moral
theory commands universal consensus. As long as the principles of applied
medical ethics are not integrated into some broader theoretical framework,
they tend to lead to conflicting judgments about particular actions and even
social policies. Even if one proceeds from some articulated moral theory
(e.g., consequentialism, contractarianism) one cannot evade the chaos of
conflicting moral judgments.[11]

The lack of agreement on which moral theory to apply on concrete
medical cases makes applied ethics counterproductive. Confronting physicians and medical students with a variety of conflicting but plausible
theories, applied medical ethics gives no moral guidance but produces the
conviction that whatever is done in problematic situations, some moral
theory will condone it, another will condemn it. Therefore, it is argued
that the belief in the primacy of applied ethics and the deductivist model
of applying general moral theories and intermediate principles have led to
an inadequate way of conceiving the relation of ethics to medicine.[12]

Because the dominant conception of medical ethics is too pragmatically
focused on application of principles, norms and rules, it is only loosely
embedded in philosophy, thereby lacking a more encompassing critical,
theoretical perspective on its own practical activities.

(b) The dominant conception has developed in a particular cultural
matrix. The fundamental ethos of applied medical ethics, its analytical
framework, methodology, and language, its concerns and emphases, and its
institutionalization have been shaped by beliefs, values, and modes of
thinking grounded in specific social and cultural traditions.

Nowadays, medical ethics itself has apparently become one of the most
powerful means to express and articulate these traditions. Comparing
medical ethics in China and the United States, Fox and Swazey remark:
"Using biology and medicine as a metaphorical language and a symbolic
medium, bioethics deals . . . with nothing less than beliefs, values, and
norms that are basic to our society, its cultural tradition, and its collective
conscience.[13] However, medical ethics only rarely attends to and reflects
upon the socio-cultural value system within and through which it operates.

Its usual assumption is that its principles, thoughts, and moral views are transcultural. H. T. Engelhardt, for example, distinguishes between two levels: that of secularized pluralistic society and that of the many particular moral communities with competing visions of the good life. Bioethics, in his opinion, should focus on the societal level, speaking across gulfs of moral discourse; it is a common neutral language, a secular moral grammar, guaranteeing a peaceable society. The most interesting task of ethics is on the first level: promoting and defending, in the context of health care, the general secular moral language of mutual respect.[14]

Critics agree that this is an important task; but it flows from a rather thin or minimalist conception of ethics.[15] Ethics is conceptualized as procedural; it is the regulation of social relations through peaceable negotiation. In order to speak the language of mutual respect, all other moral languages must be pacified.

But why should we abstain from our particular moral language in favor of a neutral common language? This question points to an important problem: how neutral is the common neutral language? Is Engelhardt's language itself not the specific moral language of a specific moral community? Is this language itself not the expression of a commitment to a certain "hypergood,"[16] in particular, that demands universal and equal respect and self-determining freedom – primal values in the liberal tradition? Such questions assume that the value of mutual respect and rights to privacy are not decontextualized standards but themselves expression of community-bound agreements.

Only recently there has been an increasing awareness that a critical examination of the value context is necessary for a better understanding of the strength and weakness of the currently dominant conception of medical ethics. R. Fox, for example, has shown how liberalism and individualism are very much characteristic of American bioethics. Focusing on autonomy and individual rights, other significant considerations (e.g., community and the common good, duties and responsibilities) are neglected, as are critical philosophical questions concerning attitudes toward medical progress and the role of health in communal life.[17]

Although within the philosophy of medicine in Europe the emphasis seems to be on the social aspects of medicine and the common good, rather than on the individual aspects and autonomy,[18] the dominating conception of medical ethics in, for example, the Netherlands seems in many respects not significantly different from that in the U.S.

(c) Another critique of the dominant conception of medical ethics is its inattention to the particularities of the practical setting. The theories and principles of applied ethics are necessarily abstract and therefore remote from the particular circumstances of a case, the concrete reality of clinical work, and the specific responsibilities of an individual person. By appealing to intermediate level principles, norms or rules, applied ethics may fail to realize the importance of the lived moral experience of health care professionals, as well as patients. The moral agent is taken to have an abstract existence. This point is critically elaborated by contemporary philosophers. Ethics, according to B. Williams, does not respect the concrete moral subject with his personal integrity. It requires that the subject give up his or her personal point of view and exchange it for an universal and impartial point of view. This is, Williams argues, an absurd requirement, because the moral subject is requested to give up what is constitutive for his or her personal identity and integrity.[19]

A similar issue is raised by Taylor in his recent work, in which morality and identity are considered two sides of the same coin.[20] To know who we are is to know to which moral sources we appeal. The community, the particular social space to which we belong, is the center of our moral experience. The use of ethical language depends on a shared form of life. This is in fact the old Wittgensteinian idea that all our understanding of language is a matter of picking up practices, being inducted into a particular form of life.

These criticisms imply that medical ethicists should be more appreciative of the actual experiences of practitioners and more attentive to the context in which doctors, patients, and others experience moral problems, e.g., the roles they occupy, the relationships in which they participate, the expectations they have. Doctor and patient are not a-historical, a-cultural, abstract rational beings; they are always members of communities, immersed in a tradition and participants in a culture.

Thus, the idea that a body of knowledge of normative theories and principles can be applied to medical practice, wrongly disregard the lived realities of health care. Moreover, it does not pay attention to the fact that moral concerns evolve within medical settings themselves and are a function of the social roles involved.

From these points of view two conclusions may be drawn:[21]

(a) morality is something we all participate in; medical ethics in particular is not the result of esoteric knowledge; anyone involved in the medical setting is *ipso facto* a moral participant and "expert" at least with regard to intuitive knowledge.

(b) the moral experience inherent in health care practices must be taken into account – more than the conformity of these practices with pre-existing ethical theories. From the perspective of applied medical ethics, abstracting from the reality of practices and appealing to moral principles and rules

120   HENK TEN HAVE

outside these practices, are necessary conditions to criticize health care
practices. The problem, however, is not only how such a standpoint external
to concrete practices is possible, but also whether appeals to external
morality are not vain without any knowledge of the morality internal to
the practices in question.[22]

4. ALTERNATIVE APPROACHES

From the various critiques, alternative approaches and conceptions of
medical ethics are nowadays being proposed and debated. None of these
developments is substantiated and accepted as the new medical ethics.
However, they all encourage a broader and deeper understanding of the
nature, scope, method,and applicability of ethics in the health care context.
Without offering a ready-made product, they heuristically point in the same
direction: *re-connecting medical ethics with both the more general perspectives of philosophy and the particularities of medical practices.*

In order to have a better understanding of the possibilities for such re-
connection, let me summarize the most promising new perspectives.

(a) In reaction to the perceived theoretical and methodological
weaknesses of applied ethics, new conceptions of medical ethics have
developed: phenomenological ethics,[23] hermeneutic ethics,[24] and narrative
ethics.[25] More traditional conceptions have been revitalized, notably the
new casuistry,[26] and the virtue approach.[27] In the Netherlands – as in many
other countries – these conceptions are well-known as philosophical and
moral perspectives. Nonetheless, as alternative approaches to medical
ethics, they are relatively unknown and unexamined. This unfamiliarity
could be the result of the recent professionalization of medical ethics. The
success of the dominating conception of applied ethics has more and more
segregated medical ethics from philosophy in general, hence underesti-
mating the need for a broader theoretical framework for practicing medical
ethics.

(b) A new perspective also emerges from the recent insights into the
relevancy of the social and cultural matrix in which medical ethics is
necessarily operating. For example, Callahan[28] argues that the ethical issues
in health care resource allocation and priorities in health policy should force
us to explore the goals and ideals of medicine as well as the meaning of
health in our way of life in modern society. What initially seem to be a set
of specific moral problems turns into a philosophical examination of the
place of health in human life and of the fundamental values of society.

However, research into the basic value systems relevant to medical

HYPERREALITY 121

ethical issues is relatively scarce. The data from sociological value research as well as the methodological experience of social scientists are unknown and virtually unused in the field of medical ethics.[29,30] The rigidly upheld partition between descriptive and normative ethics could explain the absence of empirical value studies in medical ethics. Only recently, however, has a more positive interaction between medical ethics and the social sciences evolved.[31]

(c) An interesting new conception of medical ethics is so-called "clinical ethics", popular (especially in the United States) but hardly practised in the Netherlands. It has emerged in response to the criticism that applied ethics is too far removed from the realities of medical practice. Clinical ethics has grown from an attempt to reorient medical ethics toward the daily health care setting.

The extent to which clinical ethics differs from the current conception of applied ethics can be summarized under four headings that characterize the basic ideas of clinical ethics:

4.1. *The Interdependence of Technical and Normative Dimensions of Medical Judgment*

This interdependence which is at the basis of clinical ethics, is repeatedly underlined by recent work in philosophy of medicine. It is argued that medicine is intrinsically a moral activity since it has a unique character as a healing relationship between physician and patient. Value judgments are pervasive in clinical decisions. The moral concerns are therefore inseparable from the technical concerns about the correct diagnosis and the most effective treatment: "medical reasoning involves ethical thinking."[32]

4.2. *Insider Perspective*

In formulating a clinical decision, the physician must take into account the ethical dimension. As a result of the special nature of the physician-patient relationship he or she is not a mere observer but an involved participant. This means that the realities of clinical decisionmaking are crucial for an understanding of the ethical dimensions. Clinical, ethical problems arising in the practice of surgery are not the same as those in pediatrics, obstetrics, or gynecology. They are not of the same nature "medically", but differ also with respect to the extent of risks and benefits. Specifically, the insider's perspective allows for the determination of whether risks are low in routine investigation, or substantial with questionable benefits. Clinicians are in the best position to identify moral issues in the context of the clinical situation. An insider perspective is needed to direct attention to the routine ethical questions in clinical encounters, but even more to develop empirical data relating to the process and outcome of clinical encounters: How do patients and physicians actually make decisions? What moral options are involved? What are the effects of personal and professional values in reaching decisions?

4.3. *Method of Induction*

Instead of a deductive method by which fundamental theories and principles are applied to practical moral dilemmas, an inductive methodology is being developed which begins with careful analysis of the empirical conditions. In this respect there is at the moment a renewed interest is classical casuistry.[33] In the casuistical method there are paradigm cases in which a particular moral maxim is clearly applicable. Analogies are then constructed regarding cases in which, due of different circumstances, another moral maxim appears less suitable. There is thus a range from more to less plausible arguments. The factual circumstances of a case are very relevant: they make different cases. The casuist's task is to determine the degree to which the relevant moral maxims fit the particular circumstances. Even more: which factors, personal preferences, and environmental conditions are relevant enough to be judged as moral facts?

In most cases the fit is not perfect; that means that the case is more or less convincing, probable, or arguable, but not certain. The casuistic approach corresponds largely to the *analogical* reasoning used in clinical decisionmaking. In diagnosis, therapy, and prognosis the clinician matches by analogy the case of a patient with other cases (i.e., those presented in textbooks) and classical descriptions or pathological theories. Like clinicians, the casuist aims not only at understanding a moral problem but at resolving it; she offers moral advice about the action which seems to be most appropriate in these particular circumstances. Unlike other ethicists, however, she organizes her ethical approach not around philosophical or moral principles but around clusters of factual circumstances relevant to medical decisions, such as patient preferences or medical indications.

4.4. *Ethics is an Inherent Reflective Function of Medicine Itself*

This is the logical consequence of the points just mentioned. When physicians consider ethics as an intrinsic feature of their craft, then ethical analysis of medical decisions cannot proceed from an externally imposed system, but is an inherent, "second-order function" of medicine ([2], p.

178). If a normative dimension is intrinsic to medical practice, then physicians have an obligation to reflect on the moral quandaries of medicine.

5. THE UNIFIED CLINICAL ETHICS THEORY

Overlooking the theatre of competitive approaches, one of the challenges to contemporary medical ethicists is to formulate a new conception and practice of medical ethics that can bridge the gap between the internal and external morality of medicine, as well as between medical empiricism and ethical normativism. It requires the development of a theoretical framework relevant to medical practice so that it may adequately take account of the norms and values inherent in the practice of medicine, but with sufficient critical distance so that it may provide a normative perspective on these practices. The crucial question therefore is: *How to develop a theoretical perspective on bioethics that reconnects bioethical concepts and practises with creative ideas and thoughts debated in philosophy in general as well as with the everyday realities of medical practise?*

Graber and Thomasma developed the unitary theory of clinical ethics out of a concern with the problematic relationship between theory and practice in medical ethics.[34] Having examined various models of theory-practice relation (for example, the model of applied ethics), they believe the new theory will avoid the weaknesses of these models and combine their strengths. The Unified Clinical Ethics Theory (UCET) therefore can incorporate elements of the virtue, deontological, and consequentialist theories of ethics. However, in the summary statement of UCET, given by the authors,[35] it is not obvious that it does indeed combine such theories. It is emphasizing the context of a case, the weighing of relevant values, and the role of interpreters but the normative justification for judging value *A* more important than *B* is that principle p′ takes precedence over p″.

At the same time, Graber and Thomasma consider UCET as a practical model of bioethical hermeneutics that combines both theory and practice. The hermeneutic aspect is repeatedly mentioned by the authors: all cases require interpretation; interpreters are involved in profound ways in analyzing the case and balancing its important features;[36] an essential part of making moral judgments is interpreting the fit between situation and principles.[37]

However, the pragmatic orientation of UCET has possibly prevented a further elaboration of this point of view, so that it is unclear how radical the hermeneutic perspective really is: is it methodological hermeneutics, paying adequate attention to the interpretive components of medical practice, or is it hermeneutic philosophy, trying to develop a theory of interpretation and to explain medicine as a hermeneutic science? If the last focus prevails, the crucial question for ethics as a practical enterprise is not so much to clarify action guides and make moral quandaries controllable but rather to make them communicable.

Because Graber and Thomasma have not further developed their hermeneutic philosophy, it may seem that hermeneutics has simply been incorporated as a tool into a hybridization of virtue, deontological and consequentialist theories. Even the name *"unitary* theory" suggests an harmonious combination of different approaches, whereas in fact the authors may have aimed at developing a more fundamental super-theory, absorbing specific ethical theories within a radical hermeneutic framework. If that is the real aim, the emphasis on virtues and principles as features of UCET wrongly suggests that their status can be reconciled with the role of interpretation. Interpreting seems necessary for knowing what virtues and principles apply in a specific situation. Hence, the importance of *interpreters* (not: interpretation) in UCET. The suggestion is that there are virtues and principles which are then analyzed and weighted by interpreters searching for guidelines in moral quandaries. However, from a hermeneutic perspective, virtues and principles are not independent of interpreters; they are not the precondition of interpretation but its result.

If clinical ethics should be considered as hermeneutics, as Graber and Thomasma advocate, then the implication is that the status and role of virtues and principles is of secondary importance in moral reasoning. What really is imperative is the development of an interpretive theory of medical ethics.

6. AN INTERPRETIVE CLINICAL ETHICS THEORY

A new interpretive theory of medical ethics can start with taking seriously the basic notions of the conception of clinical ethics. These notions imply that there are internal standards of professional practise. They also imply that this internal morality should be examined through reflective participation in health care practises. The first step towards a fusion of practise-internal and practise-external points of view is to re-orientate medical ethics on the moral principles, norms, and rules inherent in health care practises. Theoretically, the conception of clinical ethics invites such a re-orientation, arguing from a broader philosophical perspective on medicine and health care. But it is clear that for many of its practitioners "clinical ethics" in actual practise is not a notion denoting an alternative conception of medical ethics but rather a label specifying a particular field of application of ethical rules and principles. For them, clinical ethics simply means doing ethics in the clinical setting, without any necessity to change their conception and methods of applied ethics. Clinical ethics is then a special case of applied ethics. The initial impulse to re-orient ethics is neutralized; the dis-advantages of applied ethics can be overcome by introducing ethical discourse into the clinical world, and the same underlying values can be saved.

Thus, using the term "clinical ethics" does not necessarily imply that there is a new approach to medical ethics. At best it refers to the feeling that the common model of applied ethics needs amendment and revision. Clinical ethics itself is actually a borderline conception: it conveys new insights but it can easily be used to open up new contexts for the use of applied ethics without making these insights operational. In part, this is also the result of inadequate terminology: clinical ethics does indeed suggest only a new specific context, not a new conception of ethics adapted to all health care practices. However, what is important are the theoretical characteristics of clinical ethics as a radically different self-interpretation of ethics as well as its attentiveness and sensibility to medical realities. Graber and Thomasma demonstrate that it is possible to profit from its basic notions and its approach of medical practise, without reducing clinical ethics to applied ethics. UCET is an attempt to illuminate and explain the complicated interaction between the internal and external morality of health care practises. But in fact the implication of such attempt is very radical: complex bioethical problems must be understood within the broader framework of an interpretive, philosophical theory. Taken seriously, UCET is in fact ICET: *interpretive clinical ethics theory*. If in the end an ICET is needed, such theory should concentrate upon four characteristic parameters:[38,39]

6.1. *Experience*

As a particular branch of philosophy, ethics is proceeding from an empirical fund of knowledge, *in casu* moral experience. The moral dimension of the world is first and foremost experienced. Moral experience is our way of understanding ourselves and/in the world in moral terms.[40] Ethics is the interpretation and explanation of that primordial understanding. Before practising ethics we must already know, at least to some extent, what is morally desirable, obliged or right. Otherwise, we would not recognize what is appealing in a moral sense. But on the other hand, what we recognize in our experience is unclear and in need of elucidation and interpretation.

In short, we are approaching the moral dimension of the world from a set of prior understandings; they form the basis of our interest in what seems odd and strange to us, and what makes us reconstruct its meaning(s). We should, therefore, reflect upon our own moral experience as well as upon the moral sources and pre-understandings of our culture.

The starting-point of medical activity is the moral experience of the patient. The patient presents him- or herself to the physician as both puzzling and meaningful. The symptoms are deeply textured by his or her biographical situation, with his or her beliefs, values, habits and life-style. To ascertain what is wrong requires an interpretation, the more so since there is an initial distance between patient and physician. The meaning of the individual human being who is the patient requires interpretation for two reasons: (a) intrinsic strangeness; the experience of illness in this par-ticular patient is unique and unusual; (b) theoretical pre-understandings: the context in which the physician interprets the symptoms (e.g. the patho-logical models) is different from the context in which the interpretandum came into existence. It can reasonably be expected that moral experience differs according to the interpretive models used in various health care prac-tises and according to the specific complaints, illnesses and disabilities of the patients encountered in different health care settings. Different prac-tises should therefore be examined and compared.

6.2. *Attitudes and Emotions*

For ethics, the fundamental question is not so much 'What to do?' but rather 'How to live?' It is *praxis* not *poiesis* that is important.[41] The moral rele-vance of our actions should not be reduced to their effects; it is also deter-mined by an evaluation of what we do in executing our actions. This change of focus implies a re-orientation from activity to passivity, from acts to attitudes and emotions. Moral experience involves primarily feelings, for instance, of indignation, confusion or contentment; secondarily, these emotional responses can be made the object of moral thinking. A sharing of moral experience of patients and physicians, and of the emotions and attitudes involved, is therefore required during the execution of the research projects. Understanding and defining the morally relevant facts of a case do not involve the identification of relevant general principles and the deduction of a set of rules from which the correct response to the problem can be derived. The role of medical ethics is not so much explicate and apply ethical theories and principles but to interpret and evoke what is implied in moral experience. The notion "applied ethics" suggests wrongly that we already know which moral principles and rules to apply. However, rules and principles are in fact answers to what is evoked or appealed to in a particular case. First of all, we need to understand what the moral experience of vulnerability and appeal to assistance really means in this case. We need to discover why particular principles will motivate us in this case; why is there a particular ideal, rule or obligation? It requires close scrutiny of the medical situation in all its complexity.

6.3. *Community*

The interpretive reading of a patient's situation is not an individual doctor's affair. The medical prior understandings that orient the interpretation are the sediments of traditional cultural assumptions concerning the nature of the world and the body, and the results of a specific historical evolution of medical knowledge,particularly in the domain of a specific health care practise. Interpretation presupposes a universe of understanding. This is a consequence of the so-called hermeneutic circle; in order to interpret a text's meaning, the interpreter must be familiar with the vocabulary and grammar of the text and have some idea of what the text might mean. For man as a social being, understanding is always a community phenomenon: understanding in communication with others.The continuous effort to reach consensus through a dialogue with patients, colleagues and other health professionals, induces us to discover the particularities of our own prior understanding, and through that, to attain a more general level of understanding. Since the interpretation of moral experience takes place within the context of particular social practices, intimate knowledge of the historical, medical and scientific components of those practices is essential to the task of moral criticism. Ethics can not be practised without a high degree of engagement in medical work.

6.4. *Ambiguity*

Ethics should primarily aim at interpreting and understanding moral experience. But moral experience is complex and versatile. It implies that every interpretation is tentative; it opens up a possible perspective. Definitive and comprehensive interpretation is non-existent. A interpretive approach always has an ambiguous status: more than one meaning is admitted. That means that moral judgments and decisions which must be framed on the basis of understanding the thematic moral ordering of a person's life are fundamentally uncertain.

128   HENK TEN HAVE

7. THEORY AND PRACTICE

The "hyperreality" of clinical ethics as hermeneutics invites more empirical study of actual decision making processes. Like the empirical turn in contemporary philosophy of science, research projects should combine medical sociology and anthropology, philosophy and ethics to construct a more sophisticated view of moral experience in medicine and health care. During the daily clinical work at a hospital medical department significant ethical problems were encountered in 25 per cent of all patients;[42] although a variety of ethical problems were identified, it was not clear how and why problems were labelled as moral problems. A fine example of *in situ* research into the interpretation of moral experience is Bosk's study of the management of failure in a surgical service of a major American teaching hospital.[43] He investigated the set of background understandings, norms, and values that are invoked to categorize clinical events as errors.

By participant observation and interviews Bosk shows how the norms of clinical practice are constructed and learned during a surgical training program; surgeons are frequently using tactics of interpretation to make a distinction between inevitable blameless failures and unforgivable errors, and within the last category, between technical errors and moral errors. It appears that moral errors are considered more serious than technical ones. Bosk relates this unexpected finding to the nature of the doctor-patient relationship and to the conspicuousness of moral performance in surgery. He concluded that "postgraduate training of surgeons is above all things an ethical training."[44]

The examples suggest how theory and practice may be integrated into a clinical-ethical approach. With a combination of qualitative research methods (participant observation, case analysis, in depth interviews) we should analyse how moral problems occur in these practises, how they are defined, discussed, managed and resolved. Beginning with so-called "thick descriptions," the nature and role of the moral norms and rules inherent in specific practises can be described and understood. In a later phase analysis is concentrated upon the evolution and context of identified moral problems and dimensions. How can be explained that specific problems are now more common than in the past? How can be explained that some problems are defined as moral problems, and others not? How has the prevailing ethos of this community of health care practitioners been constituted?

But if medicine itself has to be considered as a hermeneutical enterprise, ethical analysis will be part of an interpretive theory of medicine. Working from an extensive knowledge of the theories and models in philosophy of medicine, and studying various sources (medical journals, presentations, autobiographies) changes in the self-interpretation of medicine must be described and explained. Research questions are, for example: How is medicine defined in various phases of its evolution and in different specialisms? What normative role is conceived for the physician-patient relationship? What kind of rationality is involved in medical decision-making? What concepts of disease, health, normality, and disability are in use in different settings? What kind of explanatory model is advocated? Which norms for professional conduct are advocated in the literature and in medical practice?

These questions should lead to developing a basic matrix identifying all fundamental characteristics of medicine's self-interpretation and relating them to each other in a coherent theoretical framework. Once a preliminary theoretical framework has been developed, empirical research data can be compared and evaluated, using this framework. To what extent is the internal morality that is functioning in various health care practices compatible with the philosophical self-understanding of those practices as reflected in the scholarly literature? How can the philosophical characterization of health care practices be amended, refined, differentiated in order to explain the actual contents, role, and effects of their internal morality?

Only then, we will observe how an interpretive clinical ethics theory has evolved into a reflective practice of clinical ethics.

Acknowledgement – This article developed from a conference organized by the Park Ridge Center for the Study of Health, Faith, and Ethics in December 1990 in Chicago. I am grateful to the Center and its staff for the opportunity to discuss the foundations of medical ethics. I would like to thank Professor Stuart F. Spicker for criticizing and improving the text of this article.

REFERENCES

1. Baudrillard J. *Amérique*. Paris: Grasset & Fasquelle, 1986.
2. Graber GC, Thomasma DC. *Theory and Practice in Medical Ethics*. New York: Continuum, 1989.
3. Downie RS. *Roles and Values. An Introduction of Social Ethics*. London: Methuen, 1974:1
4. Ten Have H, van der Arend A. Philosophy of medicine in the Netherlands. *Theor Med* 1985;6:1–42
5. Editorial. Medical ethics: should medicine turn the other cheek? *The Lancet* 1990:846–847.
6. Vandenbroucke JP. Medische ethiek en gezondheidsrecht: hinderpalen voor de verdere toename van kennis in de geneeskunde? *Ned Tijdschr Geneeskd* 1990;134:5–6.
7. Baier A. *Postures of the Mind. Essays on Mind and Morals*. London: Methuen, 1985.
8. Kass LR. Practicing ethics: where's the action? *Hast Ctr Rep* 1990;20:5–12.

130   HENK TEN HAVE

9. Ten Have H. *Een hippocratische erfenis: ethiek in de medische praktijk.* London: De Tijdstroom, 1990.
10. De Beaufort ID, Dupuis HM. *Handboek gezondheidsethiek.* Assen/Maastricht: Van Gorcum, 1988:19–20.
11. Brody B, ed. *Moral Theory and Moral Judgments in Medical Ethics.* Dordrecht: Kluwer Academic Publ., 1988.
12. Jonsen AR. Practice versus theory. *Hast Ctr Rep* 1990;20:32–34.
13. Fox RC, Swazey JP. Medical morality is not bioethics – Medical ethics in China and the United States. *Per Biol Med* 1984;27:337–360. Quote:360.
14. Engelhardt HT Jr. *The Foundations of Bioethics.* New York: Oxford University Press, 1986.
15. Callahan D. Minimalist ethics. On the pacification of morality. In Caplan AL, Callahan D, eds., *Ethics in Hard Times.* New York: Plenum Press, 1981:261–281.
16. Taylor C. *Sources of the Self. The Making of Modern Identity.* Cambridge: Cambridge University Press, 1989.
17. Fox RC. *The Sociology of Medicine. A Participant Observer's View.* Englewood Cliffs, NJ: Prentice-Hall, 1989.
18. Thomasma DC. The philosophy of medicine in Europe: challenges for the future. *Theor Med* 1985;6:115–123.
19. Williams B. Consequentialism and integrity. In Scheffler S, ed. *Consequentialism and Its Critics.* Oxford: Oxford University Press, 1988:20–50.
20. Taylor C. *Sources of the Self.*
21. Ten Have H, Kimsma GK. Changing conceptions of medical ethics. In Jensen UJ, Mooney G, eds., *Changing Values in Medical and Health Care Decision Making.* Chichester: John Wiley & Sons, 1990:33–51.
22. Jensen UJ. From good medical practice to best medical practice. *Int J Health Plan Mgt* 1989;4:167–180.
23. Zaner RM. *Ethics and the Clinical Encounter.* Englewood Cliffs, NJ: Prentice-Hall, 1988.
24. Carson RA. Interpretive bioethics: the way of discernment. *Theor Med* 1990;11:51–59.
25. Brody H. *Stories of Sickness.* New Haven/London: Yale University Press, 1987.
26. Jonsen AR, Toulmin S. *The Abuse of Casuistry.* Berkeley: The University of California Press, 1988.
27. Pellegrino ED, Thomasma DC. *For the Patient's Good: The Restoration of Beneficence in Health Care.* New York: Oxford University Press, 1988; *The Virtues in Medical Practice.* New York: Oxford University Press, 1993.
28. Callahan D. *What Kind of Life: The Limits of Medical Progress.* New York: Simon & Schuster, 1990.
29. Halman L, Heunks F, de Moor R, Zanders H. *Traditie, secularisatie en individualisering. Een studie naar de waarden van de Nederlanders in een Europese context.* Tilburg: University Press, 1987.
30. Inglehardt R. *Culture Shift in Advanced Industrial Society.* Princeton, NJ: Princeton University Press, 1990.
31. Weisz G, ed. *Social Science Prespectives on Medical Ethics.* Dordrecht/Boston/London: Kluwer Academic Publ., 1990.
32. Graber, Thomasma: 176.
33. Jonsen, Toulmin.
34. Graber, Thomasma.
35. Ibid: 194.
36. Ibid: 196.
37. Ibid: 201.
38. See note 9. Ten Have. *Een hippocratische erfenis.*

HYPERREALITY 131

39. See note 21. Ten Have., Kimsma.
40. Van Tongeren P. Ethiek en praktijk. *Filosofie & Praktijk* 1988;9:113–127.
41. Ibid.
42. Kollemorten I, *et al*. Ethical aspects of clinical decision-making. *J Med Eth* 1981;7:67–69.
43. Bosk CL. *Forgive and Remember: Managing Medical Failure*. Chicago: University of Chicago Press, 1979.
44. Ibid: 190.

[10]

HERMENEUTICAL CLINICAL ETHICS:
A COMMENTARY

STEPHEN L. DANIEL

*Director, Division of Education, American Academy of Neurology, 2221 University
Avenue, S.E., Suite 335, Minneapolis, MN 55414, U.S.A.*

ABSTRACT. Essays by Thomasma and ten Have recommend hermeneutical clinical ethics.
The use Thomasma makes of hermeneutics is not radical enough because it leaves out basic
interpretation of clinical practice and focuses narrowly on ethical principles and rules. Ten
Have, while failing to notice that the hyperreality of clinical ethics is a feature of all language,
rightly distinguishes four characteristic parameters of a thoroughgoing interpretive clinical
ethics: experience, attitudes and emotions, community, and ambiguity. Suggestions are made
for implementing hermeneutical ethics in clinical teaching.

Key words: Clinical ethics, hermeneutics, interpretation, ethics, philosophy of medicine,
medical decisionmaking, medical education

1. INTRODUCTION

Essays by Thomasma[1] and ten Have[2] contribute to the development of
clinical hermeneutics by focusing on ethical aspects of the clinical
encounter. Left out of discussion is the important role of interpretation in
the more scientific and technical aspects of clinical medicine, including
diagnosis and treatment. However, ethics does not lie at the periphery of
medicine. As Pellegrino and Thomasma remind us in their book *A
Philosophical Basis of Medical Practice*,[3] the end of medicine is a moral
one: the good of the person seeking help from the physician. Ethical considerations will therefore be an integral part of the approach to each and
every patient.

Of the two essays, ten Have's is more radical and consistent in its
espousal of a hermeneutical ethics in medicine. Thomasma views hermeneutics as a way to take account of various ethical theories in the
clinical context. I agree with ten Have that this is too weak a position.
If interpretation is the foundational act of clinical judgment, as I believe
it is,[4] it does not merely serve in an ancillary function to the conclusions derived from various ethical theories such as deontology and consequentialism.

134   STEPHEN L. DANIEL

2. CRITIQUE OF THOMASMA

Thomasma undercuts his argument that clinical ethics is hermeneutical when he devotes the final third of his essay to examples of various rules "for interpreting the relative weights of principles and values." While this exercise provides a useful critical review of current topics in the bio-ethical literature, it gives the reader little idea of how hermeneutics works. The closest we get to a hermeneutical approach is with the final two rules for "protecting the vulnerable from harm." The first, apparently reflecting the U.S. Supreme Court's reasoning in *Cruzan*,[5] uses the degree of incompetence as the weighting factor in determining the quality of patient preferences required for an ethical decision. Thus, for example (as in *Cruzan*), life-sustaining nutrition for a person in a persistent vegetative state may not be discontinued unless that person's preferences are stated in clear and convincing form. The second rule uses the level of permanent assault on the quality of "personal, interactive human life" as the criterion for relying on *less* formal indications of patient preference in making an ethical decision. This rule would also fit the *Cruzan* case, but with a different result than that reached by the Supreme Court. It all comes down to the language we use to describe a situation and the set of values, inherent in that language, that would lead us to the choice of one rule as opposed to another. This would be at the heart of a hermeneutical analysis, which focuses on the concrete particulars of language and experience. Thomasma's rules are removed from this process. Our expectation, considering the main thesis of the essay, would have been better met had we been led through interpretation of a case in which the issue of vulnerability arises. Then the "compassionate" part of Thomasma's contextualism could have been made evident in the care taken in interpretation to subordinate the interest of con-text (principle) to the interest of the text itself (the patient).

The conclusion of Thomasma's essay exhibits confusion about the interpretandum in clinical ethics. First "hermeneutical judgment" is equated with interpretation of "a particular set of circumstances that define a case." From this are extrapolated "rules" that are "interpretants of situations." These rules are then brought to "the case," whose "context" suggests which of them to apply. We appear to have been caught in a vicious circle – from case to rule to case again – unless it is the well-known "hermeneutical circle," i.e., rules, rather than being interpreted *by* cases, are part of the personal, professional, and cultural pre-understanding we bring to interpretation *of* cases. Hermeneutically, therefore, the case first mentioned could not be the same as the one mentioned later but must actually be a paradigm "case" based on the schematized circumstances shared by many

HERMENEUTICAL CLINICAL ETHICS 135

particular cases. For Thomasma, the "circumstances," "situation," or "contexts" are the middle terms allowing correspondence between general rules and particular cases. But it is far from clear that the circumstances of a case are generalizable. It would be more accurate to say that the language we use to describe one case may be analogous in meaning to the language we already have in our vocabulary from other cases. This explains why we would not expect a first-year medical student to gather from a set of rules the kind of ethical acumen gained by an experienced physician from encounters with her patients. The patient being the primary interpretandum, a ready recourse to rules betrays the wrestling with ambiguities demanded by an ethics of compassion. In the end, contrary to Thomasma, every ethical resolution of a clinical situation can be nothing but particular.

3. CRITIQUE OF TEN HAVE

I begin commentary on ten Have's essay with his notion that clinical ethics as hermeneutics is an example of "hyperreality." If I understand him, "hyperreality" refers to the modern phenomenon where words and ideas undeservedly become more real than the objects of our sense perception, which increasingly carry an aura of artificiality. I would agree that insofar as hermeneutics is a new language for the clinician, it risks being alien or irrelevant to the life of the clinic. But we should remember that Hermes, the mythical father of hermeneutics, is a trickster. In his Egyptian guise as Thoth he invented writing, which Plato has King Thamus in the *Phaedrus* denounce because it presents only a simulacrum of thinking which we mistake for the truth. Like writing, interpretation interrupts the dynamic flux of experience, introduces a rift or distance between matter (the object or event being interpreted) and spirit (its meaning for me). The spell of Hermes is that of the world as text or, what amounts to the same thing, the will-to-meaning. Following Derrida's idea of writing as paradigmatic for all language[6,7] we may regard every language or text as hyperreal. Hermeneutics is then the methodological attempt to penetrate through the textual veil of words to reveal their aspect as traces of spirit *in* matter, not above (*hyper*) matter.

I believe we can agree that the "matter" for clinical hermeneutics is a person's experience of bodily or psychic pain and/or suffering. It follows that the texts of suffering – bodily signs and stories of sickness[8] – will probably be more accessible to the skilled interpreter (e.g., literary critic, lawyer, or even laboratory scientist) than to the philosopher. One of ten

136 STEPHEN L. DANIEL

Have's objectives is understandably a defense of the value of philosophy
for clinical ethics. Yet his emphasis on a radical hermeneutics for medical
practice pushes us beyond the confines of philosophy to a more interdisciplinary conception of what we do when we make clinical decisions for
the good of the patient.

As ten Have correctly observes, a "unified clinical ethics theory" such
as that proposed by Thomasma makes a category mistake by introducing
hermeneutics as a supplement to various ethical theories rather than as the
broad framework for all theorizing in clinical medicine. He therefore wishes
to rename the approach he favors ICET: "*interpretive* clinical ethics theory."
This, however, still weights the discussion too much toward philosophical
theory (external morality) as opposed to clinical practice (internal morality),
a tension with which ten Have struggles throughout his essay. Should we
not rather speak simply of ICE: interpretive clinical ethics? This would
allow us to avoid the charge of a hyperreal "super-theory" which does not
necessarily give an accurate account of our ethical *praxis*, what we actually
do.

Ten Have identifies four "characteristic parameters" of interpretive
clinical ethics: experience, attitudes and emotions, community, and ambiguity. I believe these capture the most significant features of a hermeneutical approach to clinical ethics. I would further suggest that, with some
modifications, ten Have's order of arrangement reflects a natural progression of the levels of knowledge caregivers achieve in reaching clinical/
ethical decisions.

We start with "*in casu* experience," as ten Have calls it. However, it is
begging the question to describe it this early in the interpretive process as
"moral" experience, which ten Have equates with "understanding in moral
terms." I return to the question of the text. If it is the patient, as I have
already proposed, there is no reason to believe that he or she has an understanding of personal experience of disease in moral terms. If the text is
the experience of the caregiver, an element of bias may sway the interpretation away from the patient's values. In their manual of clinical ethics,
Jonsen, Siegler, and Winslade begin with medical indications as one of
the two weightiest ethical considerations in the physician-patient encounter.[9]
Medical indications bespeak the ideally objective and scientific interpretation of the patient's story/history, signs, and symptoms. They constitute
the logically prior literal sense of the text and, for the moment, bracket or
distance the interpretation from the question of subjective moral meaning
and value.

The second parameter in ten Have's schema is the focus on passive
attitudes and feelings, primarily in the patient but vicariously also in the

HERMENEUTICAL CLINICAL ETHICS 137

caregivers. If a clinical decision is to be ethical, it should arise out of perceived value. Consistent with an ethic of caring,[10,11] the cue to value is not a rational principle or maxim but something you hold passionately out of personal concern or anxiety for yourself or another. This explains why patient preference holds primacy among the ethical considerations in the manual mentioned above. Before a decision is made, the task of the clinician interpreter is through compassion to discern the patient's value as his (the patient's) affective reaction or spiritual understanding of the matter interpreted in "medical indications."

The third parameter recognizes community as the context for making clinical/ethical decisions. Here, finally, we enter the conflict of interpretations over various maxims, principles, professional codes, ethical theories, and paradigm cases making up the pre-understanding of a particular interpretive community composed of caregivers, patient, and significant others. This wisdom of the past may provide a ready and practical guide for decision if the community can reach consensus about the best interpretation. However, the novelty and complexity of a case may drive the interpreters into uncharted waters. Then the remaining guide for action will be a care which colors interpretation at every turn and ultimately respects the patient by letting her be, with or without "indicated" treatment.

Ambiguity fittingly constitutes the fourth and final characteristic parameter ten Have identifies for hermeneutical clinical ethics. In clinical medicine the comforting certainties of science never quite have the last say. Throughout the clinical process – because it involves persons and thus the life of spirit in matter – ambiguity keys us to several related aspects of interpretation: risk, chance, luck, and mystery. Common to these is the contingency of values or fragility of goodness for the patient and his or her interpreters.[12] It is a matter of luck for a patient to be in the hands of caregivers who happen to have the precise scientific knowledge and clinical experience to hold out the promise of successful treatment. Even with this, the outcome for the patient is never assured; and the mechanism of healing may never be fully known. There can be, however, a sense of ethical completeness about the clinical encounter if the caregivers bring compassion to the challenge of interpretation. This is risky business – allowing the heart to rule in reaching ethical decisions.

As ten Have concludes, there is a need for further study before hermeneutical clinical ethics can advance beyond the stage of hyperreality. This study may not be as scientific as he would like, but it must at least entail thick description of the "lived realities of health care." Projects in sociology, anthropology, and philosophy will enable medicine's self-interpretation by clarifying how the experience of various clinical spe-

138   STEPHEN L. DANIEL

cialists is mediated by language and social structures. The study, however, cannot be satisfied with description. It should recognize that a clinical-ethical decision may not only follow traditional principles and current accepted practice but also call them into question. If interpretive ethics is to be evolutionary, it should acknowledge that with each decision, and in the encounter of persons that provides the context for decision, spirit leaves a new trace in our experience of the world. I am skeptical of ten Have's rationalistic call for "a basic matrix identifying all fundamental characteristics of medicine's self-interpretation . . . in a coherent theoretical framework." Given the ambiguity and contingency of value, we probably need more projects like Robert Pirsig's in his semi-autobiographical fiction *Lila*, an extended case study in which personal suffering is interpreted and creatively assuaged through the perspective of a "Dynamic Quality" that preserves the tension between conflicting moral codes.[13]

4. CONCLUSION

The emphasis on interpretation in the essays by Thomasma and ten Have is salutary: it provides a ground for the discernment of spirit in the particularities of clinical experience and supports an ethic of caring in health care. The theory of hermeneutical clinical ethics will become a reflective practice if medical educators and clinicians can adopt several important operating ideas: (1) every clinical case is also ethical; (2) ethics is best learned through cases; and (3) accommodation between the value-free language of science and technology and the value-laden language of stories may be achieved through careful interpretation.

REFERENCES

1. Thomasma DC. Clinical ethics as medical hermeneutics. *Theor Med* 1994;15:93–111. This issue.
2. Ten Have HAMJ. The hyperreality of clinical ethics: a unitary theory and hermeneutics. *Theor Med* 1994;15:113–131. This issue.
3. Pellegrino ED, Thomasma DC. *A Philosophical Basis of Medical Practice*. New York and London: Oxford University Press, 1981.
4. Daniel SL. The patient as text: a model of clinical hermeneutics. *Theor Med* 1986;7:194–210.
5. *Cruzan v Director, Missouri Dept of Health*, 1990 US Lexis 3301 (US June 25, 1990).
6. Derrida J. *Of Grammatology*. Baltimore: Johns Hopkins University Press, 1976.
7. Derrida J. Plato's pharmacy. In his: *Dissemination*. Chicago: University of Chicago Press, 1981:61–171.
8. Brody H. *Stories of Sickness*. New Haven: Yale University Press, 1987.

HERMENEUTICAL CLINICAL ETHICS 139

9. Jonsen AR, Siegler M, Winslade WJ. *Clinical Ethics: A Practical Approach to Ethical Decisions in Clinical Medicine.* 2nd ed. New York: Macmillan Publishing Company, 1986.
10. Gilligan C. *In a Different Voice: Psychological Theory and Women's Development.* Cambridge: Harvard University Press, 1982.
11. Noddings N. *Caring: A Feminine Approach to Ethics and Moral Education.* Berkeley: University of California Press, 1984.
12. Nussbaum MC. *The Fragility of Goodness: Luck and Ethics in Greek Tragedy and Philosophy.* Cambridge: Cambridge University Press, 1986.
13. Pirsig RM. *Lila: An Inquiry into Morals.* New York: Bantam Books, 1991.

Part II
Applying the Methods

[11]

The Philosophical Review, Vol. XCVIII, No. 3 (July 1989)

ACTIONS, INTENTIONS, AND CONSEQUENCES: THE DOCTRINE OF DOING AND ALLOWING[1]

Warren S. Quinn

Sometimes we cannot benefit one person without harming, or failing to help, another; and where the cost to the other would be serious—where, for example, he would die—a substantial moral question is raised: would the benefit justify the harm? Some moralists would answer this question by balancing the good against the evil. But others deny that consequences are the only things of moral relevance. To them it also matters whether the harm comes from action, for example, from killing someone, or from inaction, for example, from not saving someone. They hold that for some good ends we might properly allow a certain evil to befall someone, even though we could not actively bring that evil about. Some people also see moral significance in the distinction between what we intend as a means or an end and what we merely foresee will result incidentally from our choice. They hold that in some situations we might properly bring about a certain evil if it were merely foreseen but not if it were intended.

Those who find these distinctions morally relevant think that a benefit sufficient to justify harmful choices of one sort may fail to justify choices no more harmful, but of the other sort.[2] In the case of the distinction between the intentional and the merely foreseen, this view is central to what is usually called the Doctrine of Double Effect (DDE). In the case of the distinction between action and inaction, the view has no common name, so for convenience we may call it the Doctrine of Doing and Allowing (DDA). (Because harm resulting from intentional inaction has, typically, been allowed to occur.) Absolutist forms of either doctrine would simply

---

[1]Thanks to Rogers Albritton, Tyler Burge, Philippa Foot, Matthew Hanser, Thomas Nagel, Michael Thomson, Derek Parfit, T. M. Scanlon, and to the editors of *The Philosophical Review* for valuable suggestions and criticisms.

[2]Harm here is meant to include any evil that can be the upshot of choice, for example, the loss of privacy, property, or control. But to keep matters simple, my examples will generally involve physical harm, and the harm in question will generally be death.

WARREN S. QUINN

rule out certain choices (for example, murder or torture) no matter what might be gained from them. Nonabsolutist forms would simply demand more offsetting benefit as a minimum justification for choices of one sort than for equally harmful choices of the other sort.

In this paper I shall examine the Doctrine of Doing and Allowing.[3] My aim is twofold: first, to find the formulation of the distinction that best fits our moral intuitions and second, to find a theoretical rationale for thinking the distinction, and the intuitions, morally significant. Both tasks are difficult, but the former will prove especially complex. What we find in the historical and contemporary literature on this topic is not a single clearly drawn distinction, but several rather different distinctions conforming roughly but not exactly to the distinction between what someone does and what he does not do. Special cases of inaction may be treated by an author as belonging, morally speaking, with the doings, and special cases of doing as belonging with the inactions. So in searching for the proper intuitive fit, we shall have to be alert to the possibility that the distinction between action and inaction (or between doing and allowing) is only a first approximation to the distinction we really want.

In evaluating various formulations of the doctrine I shall need special test cases. These will often involve improbable scenarios and repetitive structural elements. This is likely to try the reader's patience (he or she may begin to wonder, for example, whether we are discussing the morality of public transportation). But it may help to recall that such artificialities can hardly be avoided anywhere in philosophy.[4] As in science, the odd sharp focus of the test cases is perfectly compatible with the general importance of the ideas being tested. And the DDA is, I think, of the greatest general significance, both because it enters as a strand into many real moral issues and because it stands in apparent opposition to that most general of all moral theories, consequentialism.

Before beginning, I should emphasize that both the DDE and, especially, the DDA apply more directly to moral justification than to other forms of moral evaluation. It is therefore open to a de-

---

[3] I shall examine the DDE in a subsequent paper, "Actions, Intentions, and Consequences: The Doctrine of Double Effect."

[4] Think of Gettier cases, brain transplants, teletransporters, etc.

ACTIONS, INTENTIONS, AND CONSEQUENCES

fender of the DDA to admit that two *unjustified* choices that cause the same degree of harm are equally *bad*, even though one choice is to harm and the other not to save. I note this only because some writers have looked for such pairs in hope of refuting the doctrine.[5] Take the well-known example of an adult who deliberately lets a child cousin drown in order to inherit a family fortune.[6] The act seems so wicked that we understand the point of saying that it is no better than drowning the child. But if so, how can we hold that the difference between killing and letting die matters morally?

This objection seems to presuppose that if letting someone die is ever more acceptable, *ceteris paribus*, than killing someone, it must be because some intrinsic moral disvalue attaches to killing but not to letting die. And if so, this intrinsic difference must show up in all such cases.[7] But the doctrine may, and I shall argue should, be understood in a quite different way. The basic thing is not that killing is intrinsically worse than letting die, or more generally that harming is worse than failing to save from harm, but that these different choices run up against different kinds of rights—one of which is stronger than the other in the sense that it is less easily defeated. But its greater strength in this sense does not entail that its *violation* need be noticeably worse.

Such relations between rights are possible because moral blame for the violation of a right depends very much more on motive and

---

[5]For example, Michael Tooley in "Abortion and Infanticide," *Philosophy and Public Affairs* 2 (1972), p. 59.

[6]From James Rachels, "Active and Passive Euthanasia," *The New England Journal of Medicine* 292 (1975), p. 79.

[7]In "Harming, Not Aiding, and Positive Rights," *Philosophy and Public Affairs* 15 (1986), pp. 5–11, Frances Kamm rightly makes us distinguish between two ways in which killing might be intrinsically worse than letting die: a) killing might have some bad essential feature that cannot attach to letting die or b) killing might have some bad essential feature that, while not essential to letting die, can nevertheless be present in cases of letting die. If (b) is true then the moral equivalence of the two cases in which the child drowns would not establish a general moral equivalence between killing and letting die. For letting the child drown might be a special case in which letting die has the bad feature essential to killings but not to lettings die. And even apart from Kamm's point, the idea that intrinsically nonequivalent parts must always make an overall evaluative difference when embedded in identical contexts seems wrong. Consider aesthetics. There may certainly be important intrinsic aesthetic differences between two lampshades even though they create an equally bad overall impression when placed on a certain lamp.

WARREN S. QUINN

expected harm than on the degree to which the right is defeasible. Your right of privacy that the police not enter your home without permission, for example, is more easily defeated than your right that I, an ordinary citizen, not do so. But it seems morally no better, and perhaps even worse, for the police to violate this right than for me to. So there is nothing absurd in saying that the adult acts as badly when he lets the child drown as when he drowns the child, while insisting that there are contexts in which the child would retain the right not to be killed but not the right to be saved.

I.

The Doctrine of Doing and Allowing has been most notably defended in recent moral philosophy by Philippa Foot.[8] It will be convenient, therefore, to begin with two of the examples she uses to show the intuitive force of the doctrine.[9] In Rescue I, we can save either five people in danger of drowning at one place or a single person in danger of drowning somewhere else. We cannot save all six. In Rescue II, we can save the five only by driving over and thereby killing someone who (for an unspecified reason) is trapped on the road. If we do not undertake the rescue, the trapped person can later be freed. In Rescue I, we seem perfectly justified in proceeding to save the five even though we thereby fail to save the one. In Rescue II, however, it is far from obvious that we may proceed. The doctrine is meant to capture and explain pairs of cases like these in which consequential considerations are apparently held constant (for example, five lives versus one) but in which we are inclined to sharply divergent moral verdicts.

---

[8] In "The Problem of Abortion and the Doctrine of the Double Effect," in *Virtues and Vices and Other Essays* (Berkeley, Calif.: University of California Press, 1978), pp. 19–32, Foot argued that the distinction between doing and allowing could do all the work usually credited to the distinction between the intentional and the merely foreseen. In "Killing and Letting Die," Jay Garfield, ed., *Abortion: Moral and Legal Perspectives* (Amherst, Mass.: University of Massachusetts Press, 1984), pp. 178–185 and even later in "Morality, Action and Outcome," in Ted Honderich, ed., *Morality and Objectivity* (London, England: Routledge and Kegan Paul, 1985), pp. 23–38, she withdraws this claim, arguing instead that any intuitively adequate morality must assign an independent moral significance to the distinction between doing and allowing.

[9] From "Killing and Letting Die," p. 179.

ACTIONS, INTENTIONS, AND CONSEQUENCES

The first order of business is to get clearer on the crucial distinction that the doctrine invokes. In effect, the DDA discriminates between two kinds of agency in which harm comes to somebody. It discriminates *in favor of* one kind of agency (for example, letting someone drown in Rescue I) and it discriminates *against* the other kind (for example, running over someone in Rescue II).[10] That is, it makes these discriminations in the sense of allowing that the pursuit of certain goods can justify the first kind of harmful agency but not the second. I shall call the favored kind of agency *negative*, since on any plausible account it is usually a matter of what the agent does *not* do. For parallel reasons, I shall call the disfavored kind of agency *positive*. But, as indicated earlier, the distinction between positive and negative agency may or may not line up exactly with the ordinary distinction between doing and allowing or action and inaction. We may discover, as we consider various special circumstances, that certain actions function morally as allowings and certain inactions as doings. So let us begin by sifting various proposals for spelling out the nonmoral difference between the two kinds of agency.

One such proposal comes from some brief passages in the *Summa Theologiae* where Aquinas could be taken to suggest that the difference between the two forms of agency is one of voluntariness.[11] In harmful positive agency, the harm proceeds from the will of the agent while in harmful negative agency it does not.[12] St. Thomas seems to think that foreseeable harm that comes from action is automatically voluntary. But he thinks that foreseeable

---

[10]It seems clear than an agent's *not* doing something (for example, not saving someone from drowning) can be morally evaluated as justified, unjustified, right, or wrong, in precisely the sense in which these terms apply to actions. I shall therefore speak of assessing the justification or the rightness of someone's *agency* in some matter, meaning by this an evaluation of his knowingly acting or not acting.

[11]*Summa Theologiae XVII* (Cambridge, England: Blackfriars, 1970), 1a2ae Q. 6 article 3, pp. 15–16. The terms "positive agency" and "negative agency" are not, of course, St. Thomas's. This is the interpretation that he might give to them.

[12]In speaking of an inaction as harmful or as producing harm (or in speaking of harm as coming from it) I am not begging the question against Aquinas. For I mean these expressions only in the weak sense of connecting the inaction with a harmful upshot, and not in any sense that would imply that the harm was voluntary.

WARREN S. QUINN

harm coming from inaction is voluntary only when the agent could and *should* have acted to prevent it. Positive agency would therefore include all foreseeably harmful actions and those foreseeably harmful inactions that could and should have been avoided. And negative agency would include the foreseeably harmful inactions that could not or need not have been avoided.

But what kind of "should" (or "need") is this? If we take it to be moral, the doctrine becomes circular.[13] Inactions falling under positive agency are harder to justify than inactions falling under negative agency. Why? Because by definition the latter need not have been avoided while the former, if possible, should have been.

We could, however, avoid the circularity by taking the "should" to be premoral, reflecting social and legal conventions that assign various tasks to different persons. And we might think that these conventions play a central role in an important premoral, but morally relevant, notion of causality.[14] The helmsman's job is to steer the ship, and this is why we say that it foundered *because* of his careless inaction. The loss of the ship would thus be like the death in Rescue II, which happens because of what we do. And both cases would contrast with the death in Rescue I, which we do not, in the relevant sense, bring about. Voluntariness would thus be seen as a distinctive kind of causal relation linking agency and its harmful upshots in the cases of action and conventionally proscribed inaction (positive agency), but not in the case of conventionally permitted inaction (negative agency). So formulated, the doctrine would not only be clear but would have an obvious rationale. Harmful negative agency is easier to justify because in such cases the harm cannot, in the relevant causal sense, be laid at the agent's door.

I have two objections to this proposal. First, there is little reason to treat most instances of the neglect of conventional duty as posi-

---

[13]It may be, of course, that Aquinas's account of the voluntary is not meant as part of the theory of justification and is therefore not directed to the distinction between positive and negative agency. It might instead be part of the theory of praiseworthiness and blameworthiness, which presupposes an independent account of what can and cannot be justified. If so, there could be no charge of circularity. For harmful inaction clearly does deserve blame only if it could and should, morally speaking, have been avoided.

[14]I am indebted here to Michael Thompson, who thinks that something like this is suggested in the work of Elizabeth Anscombe.

ACTIONS, INTENTIONS, AND CONSEQUENCES

tive agency. We can usually explain in other ways just why morality takes these tasks so seriously. If human communities are to thrive, people will have to perform their social roles. That is why, in a variant of Rescue I, the private lifeguard of the lone individual might not be morally permitted to go off to save the five, even though a mere bystander would be. To explain this difference, we would not also need to suppose that the private lifeguard and bystander stand in different causal relations to the person's death. There is, moreover, room to think that the special duty of the private lifeguard should be put aside, especially if his employer is a pampered rich man, and the five are too poor to afford personal attendants. But this kind of circumstance would have no justificatory force where death was the upshot of clearly positive agency. In Rescue II, for example, it would not matter that the man trapped on the road was rich and spoiled while the five were poor and worthy.

My second objection is more general. The type of proposal we are examining relationalizes the special moral opprobrium attaching to positive agency by reference to its special causal properties. Since negative agency is not, in the intended sense, the cause of its unfortunate upshots, the moral barriers against it are lower. But this leaves the doctrine open to a serious criticism. For there are other conceptions of causality according to which we are in (the original) Rescue I every bit as much a cause of death as in Rescue II. What matters, according to these conceptions, is whether a nonoccurrence necessary for a given effect was, relative to a certain standard background, surprising or noteworthy. In this sense, we may say that a building burns down because its sprinklers failed to work, even though their failure was traceable to the diversion of water to another more important fire. That the diversion was quite proper is nothing against the claim that the failure of the sprinklers helped cause the loss of the building. And something similar holds for Rescue I. The fact that we did not save the one because we quite properly saved the others would not show that his death was not in part due to our choice.

So even if there is a causal notion that corresponds to Aquinas's idea of the voluntary, it is in competition with other causal notions that may seem better to capture what is empirically important in scientific and ordinary explanation. And it is arguable that the defense of the doctrine should not depend on a causal conception

WARREN S. QUINN

that we would otherwise do without. If the doctrine is sound it ought to remain plausible on an independently plausible theory of causation. In any case, this is what I shall assume here. So I shall grant opponents of the doctrine that the permissible inactions we are considering, no less than the impermissible actions, are partial causes of their harmful upshots. This will force me to try to make sense of the doctrine on other grounds.

But this still leaves the task of stating the nonmoral content of the distinction between harmful positive and harmful negative agency. Perhaps the difference should, after all, be put in the most simple and straightforward way, as the difference between action that produces harm and inaction that produces harm. If we think of action along the lines proposed by Elizabeth Anscombe and taken up by Donald Davidson—a conception whose basic outline I propose to adopt—individual actions are concrete particulars that may be variously described.[15] To say that John hit Bill yesterday is to say that there was a hitting, done by John to Bill, that occurred yesterday. To say that John did not hit Bill, on the other hand, is to say that there was no such hitting. Taking things this way, the distinction between harmful positive agency and harmful negative agency would be the distinction between harm occurring because of what the agent does (because of the existence of one of his actions) and harm occurring because of what the agent did not do but might have done (because of the noninstantiation of some kind of action that he might have performed).[16]

Surprisingly, most moral philosophers who write on these matters reject this way of drawing the distinction. Jonathan Bennett, a severe critic of the DDA, dismisses Davidson's conception of

---

[15]G. M. A. Anscombe, *Intention* (second edition) (Oxford, England: Blackwell, 1963), especially sec. 26, pp. 45–47. See also Donald Davidson, *Essays on Actions and Events* (Oxford, England: Clarendon Press, 1980). See there "The Logical Form of Action Sentences," pp. 105–122; "Criticism, Comment and Defence," pp. 122–144, esp. pp. 135–137; and "The Individuation of Events," pp. 163–180.

[16]What I see as right in the Anscombe-Davidson view is the suggested metaphysics—the claim that action is a matter of the presence of something and inaction a matter of its absence. And I think that our intuitions about whether something is an action or inaction as we think about it morally are metaphysically relevant. So I am not greatly worried that someone pursuing the Anscombe-Davidson line might discover criteria of action and inaction that would radically conflict with our judgments in moral thought.

ACTIONS, INTENTIONS, AND CONSEQUENCES

action without argument.[17] Most likely he minds its failure to provide a clear criterion for distinguishing action from inaction in all cases, one that would tell us, for example, whether observing a boycott (by not buying grapes) or snubbing someone (by not acknowledging his greeting) consists in doing something by way of inaction or simply in deliberately not doing something. Bennett is reluctant to assign moral work to any distinction that leaves some cases unclear, especially where there is no theoretically compelling reductionistic theory for the clear cases. But I am disinclined to adopt such a standard. Almost no familiar distinction that applies to real objects is clear in all cases, and theoretical reducibility is a virtue only where things really are reducible. In any case, the imposition of such a standard would shut down moral theory at once, dependent as it is on the as yet unreduced and potentially vague distinctions between what is and is not a person, a promise, an informed consent, etc.

But Bennett is not simply negative. He proposes an ingenious and, for limited applications, clearly drawn distinction between positive and negative *facts* about agency as a respectable way of formulating the doctrine.[18] (Not of course to save it, but to expose it.) Roughly speaking, an event is brought about by someone's positive instrumentality, as Bennett calls it, when the event is explained by a relatively strong fact about the agent's behavior—for example, that he moved in one of a limited number of ways. Negative instrumentality, on the other hand, explains by reference to relatively weak facts about behavior—for example, that the agent moved in any one of a vast number of ways.

The trouble is that this distinction gets certain cases intuitively wrong. Bennett imagines a situation in which if Henry does nothing, just stays where he is, dust will settle and close a tiny electric circuit which will cause something bad—for example, an explosion that will kill Bill.[19] If Henry does nothing, he is by Bennett's criterion positively instrumental in Bill's death. (For only one

---

[17]"Morality and Consequences," *The Tanner Lectures on Human Values* II (Salt Lake City, Utah: University of Utah Press, 1981), pp. 54–55.

[18]Bennett, pp. 55–69.

[19]Bennett, pp. 66–68. If Henry's body were *activating* the device—if he were depressing a trigger or conducting a current—we might see his agency as positive despite his motionlessness. But Bennett doesn't assign any such role to Henry's body.

WARREN S. QUINN

of Henry's physical actions, staying still, will cause the death, while indefinitely many will prevent the death.) But suppose Henry could save five only by staying where he is—suppose he is holding a net into which five are falling. Surely he might then properly refuse to move even though it means not saving Bill. For his agency in Bill's death would in that case seem negative, much like that in Rescue I.

Bennett also misses the opposite case. Suppose the device will go off only if Henry makes some move or other. In that case his instrumentality in the death would, for Bennett, be negative. But those who would rule out Rescue II would surely not allow Henry to go to the rescue of five if that meant setting off the device. For his agency in the death of Bill would in that case seem positive.[20] Bennett's distinction, however admirable in other ways, is not the one we seem to want. Perhaps this is already clear when we reflect that, according to him, the instrumentality of someone who intentionally moves his body (in, for example, following the command "Move in some way or other—any way you like!") is negative.

Philippa Foot also rejects the idea that the distinction between positive and negative agency is that between action and inaction.[21] She claims that it would not make any interesting moral difference if respirators (presumably sustaining patients who would otherwise die) had to be turned on again each day. Active turning off and passive not turning on would be morally the same. To be relevant to the present issues, her idea must be that this would not make a difference even in cases where some great good could come about

---

[20]That Bill's death would in this case be a side-effect of the rescue does not distinguish it from Rescue II. For in neither case is the death of the one intended. It might be objected that here but not in Rescue II the killing would not be *part* of the rescue. But if Henry's movement sets off the explosion (for example, by triggering a fuse sensitive to movement) then Henry's killing Bill does seem part of the rescue, at least in the sense that he kills Bill by the very movements that form part of the rescue attempt. Of course there could be circumstances in which Henry's movement would not so much set off the explosion as allow it to be set off. Suppose, for example, Henry's remaining where he is prevents dust from settling upon and thereby triggering an explosive device below him. In such a case, I agree that he might go off to save the five. For although he will be active in Bill's death, his agency will involve taking his body from where it would save Bill to where he can make use of it to save the five, a special circumstance that I shall discuss later.

[21]"Morality, Action and Outcome," p. 24.

ACTIONS, INTENTIONS, AND CONSEQUENCES

only if a particular respirator were not running. Let us see whether this is right. Suppose there are temporary electrical problems in a hospital such that the five respirators in Ward B can be kept going only if the one in Ward A is off. On Foot's view it should not matter whether a hospital attendant keeps the five going by shutting down the one or, in case it is the kind that needs to be restarted, by simply not restarting it.

It would be very odd to think that if the single respirator were already off, the attendant would be required to restart it even if that meant shutting down the five in Ward B. So Foot's idea must imply that if the single respirator were running, the attendant could just as properly shut it down to keep the others running. Now while there seems something more objectionable about shutting the respirator down, I think that all things considered it might be permitted. One reason is that we could perhaps see it as a matter of the hospital's allocating something that belongs to it, a special kind of circumstance that we shall consider later. But suppose the hospital is an unusual one in which each patient must provide his own equipment and private nursing care. Suppose further that you are an outsider who happens for some reason to be the only person on the scene when the electrical problem arises. In this case, it seems to matter whether you keep the respirators in Ward B going by not restarting the one in Ward A (it being of the type that needs restarting and the private nurse having failed to show up that day) or whether you actually shut it down. The first case seems rather like Rescue I and the second uncomfortably like Rescue II.

Foot goes on to offer what she takes to be a different and better interpretation of the distinction. She thinks what matters is not the difference between action and inaction but the difference between two relations an agent can have to a sequence of events that leads to harm. It is one thing to *initiate* such a sequence or to *keep it going*, but quite another to *allow it to complete itself* when it is already in train.[22] Agency of the first two kinds is positive, while agency that merely allows is negative. One problem with this account arises when we try to explain the difference between allowing a sequence to complete itself and keeping it going when it would otherwise

---

[22]Ibid., p. 24, including footnote 2 on p. 37.

WARREN S. QUINN

have stopped. We might have thought that the former was a matter of doing nothing to stop it and the latter was a matter of doing something to continue it. But that would seem to take us back to the rejected distinction between action and inaction.

Another problem concerns forms of help and support which do not seem to consist in keeping already existing dangerous sequences at bay. Suppose I have always fired up my aged neighbor's furnace before it runs out of fuel. I haven't promised to do it, but I have always done it and intend to continue. Now suppose that an emergency arises involving five other equally close and needy friends who live far away, and that I can save them only by going off immediately and letting my neighbor freeze. This seems to be more like Rescue I than Rescue II, but it doesn't appear to be a case in which I merely allow an already existing fatal sequence to finish my neighbor off. For he was not already freezing or even, in some familiar sense, in danger of freezing before the emergency arose. Or if we think he was in danger, that danger was partly constituted by what I might fail to do. We might simply stipulate, of course, that any fatal sequence that appears to arise from a *failure* to help someone is really the continuation of a preexisting sequence. But then we seem to be falling back on the notion of inaction as fundamental.

II.

I am therefore inclined to reject Bennett's and Foot's positive suggestions, despite their obvious attractions. May we then return to the simple and straightforward way of drawing the distinction, as between harm that comes from action and harm that comes from inaction? I think not. Cases involving the harmful *action of objects or forces* over which we have certain powers of control seem to demand a more complex treatment. Consider, for example, the following variant of Rescue II (call it Rescue III). We are off by special train to save five who are in imminent danger of death. Every second counts. You have just taken over from the driver, who has left the locomotive to attend to something. Since the train is on automatic control you need do nothing to keep it going. But you can stop it by putting on the brakes. You suddenly see someone trapped ahead on the track. Unless you act he will be killed. But if you do stop, and then free the man, the rescue mission will be aborted. So you let the train continue.

ACTIONS, INTENTIONS, AND CONSEQUENCES

In this case it seems to me that you make the wrong choice. You must stop the train. It might seem at first that this is because you occupy, if only temporarily, the role of driver and have therefore assumed a driver's special responsibility to drive the train safely. But, upon reflection, it would not make much moral difference whether you were actually driving the train or merely had access to its brake. Nor would it much matter whether you were in the train or had happened upon a trackside braking device.[23] The important thing from the standpoint of your agency is that you *can* stop the train and thereby prevent it from killing the one.

But this is not the only thing that matters, as can be seen in a different kind of case. Suppose, in a variant of Rescue I (Rescue IV), you are on a train on which there has just been an explosion. You can stop the train, but that is a complicated business that would take time. So you set it on automatic forward and rush back to the five badly wounded passengers. While attending to them, you learn that a man is trapped far ahead on the track. You must decide whether to return to the cabin to save him or stay with the passengers and save them.

May you stay? I think you may.[24] We would be more tolerant of

---

[23]Suppose that you and a friend are off, by car, on a rescue mission that unexpectedly turns into Rescue II. You are sitting in the passenger seat, and your friend is driving. For some reason he hasn't noticed the trapped person, but you have. If you do nothing, your friend will inadvertently run over and kill the man. Can you really think that the end of rescuing the five would *not* justify your friend the driver in deliberately killing the man, but *would* justify you in keeping silent (or in not pulling up the hand brake)? I find this implausible. And it seems equally implausible to suppose that your obligation to yell or pull the brake comes from your having, temporarily, assumed the role of driver. What matters is that the mission has become illicit precisely because, as you can see, it requires that someone be killed. So it has also become illicit to try to *further* the mission, whether by deliberate action or omission.

[24]At least if you are not the driver or his designated replacement—that is, someone charged with a special moral responsibility to see to it that the train kills no one. If you have that responsibility but lack a special duty toward the injured people (you are not also their doctor), then there would be something extra on the moral balance in favor of stopping. But we should not build this complication into our account of the difference between positive and negative agency. For the force of this extra factor seems independent of facts about agency. It does not seem to derive from any supposition that, if you stay with the passengers, you will really be taking the train forward or will somehow be party to the fatal action of the train itself.

WARREN S. QUINN

inaction here than in Rescue III. And this is because of your intentions. In Rescue III you intend an action of the train that in fact causes the man's death, its passing over the spot where he is trapped.[25] Not, of course, because he is trapped there. But because the train must pass that spot if the five are to be saved. In Rescue IV, however, things are different. In that case you intend no action of the train that leads to the man's death. The purposes for which you act would be just as well served if the train's brakes were accidentally to apply themselves.

In Rescue III, but not in Rescue IV, the train kills the man *because* of your intention that it continue forward. This implicates you, I believe, in the fatal action of the train itself. If you had no control, but merely wished that the rescue would continue—or if, as in Rescue IV, you had control but no such wish—you would not be party to the action of the train. But the combination of control and intention in Rescue III makes for a certain kind of complicity. Your choice to let the train continue forward is strategic and deliberate. Since you clearly *would* have it continue for the sake of the five, there is a sense in which, by deliberately not stopping it, you *do* have it continue. For these reasons your agency counts as positive.

The surprise in this is that we must bring the distinction between what is intended and merely foreseen into the DDA. But the two doctrines do not therefore merge. As I shall try to show in another paper, the DDE depends on something different—on whether or not a victim is *himself* an intentional object, someone whose manipulation or elimination will be useful. But the victim is not in that way involved in the special kind of positive agency we find in Rescue III. What is intended there is not something for him—that he be affected in a certain way—but some action of an object that (foreseeably but quite unintentionally) leads to his death.

---

[25]In Rescue III you intend an action of the train that immediately kills the man. But it would make no difference if, in a variant of the case, you did not intend that the train pass over the spot where the man was trapped, but merely intended that it pass over some nearer part of the track (where that would foreseeably lead to its passing over the fatal spot). Nor would it matter, in a further variant of the case, if the intended action of the train would lead to the man's being killed by some immediate cause other than the train. All that is essential is that you intend some action of the train that you can foresee will cause the man's death.

ACTIONS, INTENTIONS, AND CONSEQUENCES

To the idea of positive agency by action, we must therefore add positive agency by this special kind of inaction. But this is, I think, the only complication we need to build into the doctrine itself. (Other more minor qualifications will be discussed in the next section.) We may now construct the doctrine in stages, starting with some definitions. An agent's *most direct contribution* to a harmful upshot of his agency is the contribution that most directly explains the harm. And one contribution explains harm more directly than another if the explanatory value of the second is exhausted in the way it explains the first.

In the absence of special circumstances involving the actions of objects, an agent's contributions to various effects in the world are those of his voluntary actions and inactions that help produce the effects. So in ordinary cases, his most direct contribution to any effect is the action or inaction that most directly explains the effect. In Rescue I, for example, our most direct contribution to the death of the one is our failure to save him. Our going off to save the five contributes less directly. For it explains the death precisely by explaining the failure to save.[26] In Rescue II, on the other hand, our most direct contribution to the death of the man trapped on the road is our act of running him over.

In special circumstances, that is, where harm comes from an active object or force, an agent may by inaction contribute the harmful action of the object itself. This, as we have seen, happens just in case the object harms because the agent deliberately fails to control it and he fails to control it because he wants some action of the object that in fact leads to the harm. Having defined this much, the rest is straightforward. Harmful positive agency is that in which an agent's most direct contribution to the harm is an action, whether his own or that of some object. Harmful negative agency

---

[26]We fail to rescue the one *because* we rescue the five instead. But notice that this account implies, in the previously mentioned puzzle cases of boycotting and snubbing (cases where we are unsure whether there is a genuine action by way of an inaction or merely a deliberate inaction), that the agent's most direct contribution to the upshot is an inaction. Grape sales decline because we don't buy grapes, and we don't buy them *because* we are boycotting. Happily, this means that we do not have to decide whether boycotting is a genuine action in order to determine the boycotter's agency in the intended upshot. It will turn out on either hypothesis to be negative.

WARREN S. QUINN

is that in which the most direct contribution is an inaction, a failure
to prevent the harm.

III.

We should now look briefly at certain kinds of cases in which
common-sense morality seems to qualify the doctrine as I have just
described it, permitting us to harm or even kill someone in order
to help others. I am not thinking here of the avoidance of great
catastrophes. The doctrine, as already indicated, need not be absolutist. And even in its nonabsolutist form, it cannot contain everything of moral relevance. Special rights to do that which produces
harm and special duties to prevent harm must also be factored in.
In this way the doctrine has the force of one important *prima facie*
principle among others. Rights of competition, to give a familiar
example, legitimate certain kinds of harmful positive agency—
such as the shrewd but honest competition in which you take away
another person's customers. The right to punish is another familiar example. On the other side, special duties to aid may arise
from jobs, contracts, natural relations, or from the fact that
someone's present predicament was of your making.[27] These special duties explain why some instances of negative agency seem no
easier to justify than active harmings.

These familiar rights and duties do not require that the doctrine
be qualified. They merely oppose it in particular cases. But other
situations seem either to require special amendments to my definitions of positive and negative agency or to show that in certain
situations the doctrine lacks its usual *prima facie* force. Qualifications of the first sort sometimes seem required where harm arises
from the active *withdrawal* of aid. In one kind of case you actively
abort a project of rescuing or helping that, knowing what you now
know, it would have been wrong to undertake. For example, you
stop the train in Rescue III, and the five therefore die. In another
kind of case, you remove something from where it would help
fewer to where it would help more, for example, a raft that is pres-

---

[27]If you have advertently or inadvertently poisoned someone who can
yet be saved by an antidote that you actually have, then you seem to be in
no moral position to go to the rescue of five others rather than staying to
save him.

ACTIONS, INTENTIONS, AND CONSEQUENCES

ently within the reach of one drowning victim but that could be moved to the vicinity of several other victims.[28] The object might be your body. You might, for example, cushion the fall of one baby if you stay where you are, but cushion the fall of several others if you move. In all these cases harm comes to someone because you decide to act rather than to do nothing. But because your action is a certain kind of withdrawing of aid, it naturally enough seems to count as negative agency.

In other cases, harmful positive agency seems to lack some of the *prima facie* opprobrium that usually attaches to it. Sometimes this is because the harm would have been avoided but for some blameable fault of the person harmed. Suppose, for example, that the person in Rescue II who blocks the road had been repeatedly warned not to stray where he might interfere with important rescue efforts. If so, we might feel somewhat more justified in proceeding with the rescue (although never, I think, as justified as we feel in Rescue I). People must, after all, accept some responsibility for the predicaments they stupidly and wrongly bring upon themselves.[29]

In a quite different kind of case, someone may have a special liability to be harmed by a physical or psychological interaction that is generally innocuous and, therefore, of no general moral significance. He might have a rare disease that makes any kind of physical contact very harmful to him. Or he might become dangerously hysterical if we yell in his presence. In such cases we might feel that we could try to save other people from some se-

---

[28]It seems important in this kind of case that those who are saved by your action have just as much right to the raft as the one who suffers. Removing it from the reach of its owner would, for example, be very questionable. It also seems important that the person from whom the raft is taken is not already using the raft to save himself. It is one thing to remove it from his reach and quite another to push him off it.

[29]The responsibility of others also comes in when we know that an action will occasion aggression by a third party—for example, if I know that Jones will murder you if I rescue five of his enemies who are drowning. If it seems that I may proceed with the rescue in this case it is because we shall, quite sensibly, attribute the blame for your death to Jones and not to me. In this kind of situation it is important that the action I undertake is morally pressing. Had Jones threatened to murder you in case I mowed my lawn, my ignoring the threat might well seem a kind of active provocation.

Medical Ethics

WARREN S. QUINN

rious danger even if it would mean brushing up against him or yelling. For, unlike standard instances of harmful positive agency, the attempt would not seem to count as an aggression against the victim; since he does not suffer because of any *general or typical* liability to harm. And this seems sensible. Morality must to some degree reflect the standard human condition. In particular, it must be capable of defining a class of presumptively innocent actions.[30]

Another qualification concerns large public and private projects, like the building of skyscrapers, highways, and dams. We are clearly permitted to help initiate such projects even though we know that in their course some deaths or injuries are practically inevitable. For one thing, the harm is usually remote from what we do. And, more important, the actual harm will generally have been preventable, and its occurrence will be much more directly traceable to the wrongful agency of persons more immediately concerned. It is of course essential that we do not in any way intend the harm that may occur, and take reasonable precautions to prevent it.

In the celebrated Trolley Problem, we seem to find yet another exception to the doctrine's strictures against harmful positive agency.[31] In this case a runaway trolley threatens five who are trapped on the track where it is now moving. If the driver does nothing the five will die. But he can switch to a side-track where only one person is trapped. Most people think the driver may switch tracks. But switching is positive agency while doing nothing

---

[30]But this qualification does not apply to special liabilities created by *external* features of a situation. If driving by Smith's house would set off an explosive device that would blow him up, then driving by, even when it would be necessary to rescue five others, would count as an aggression rather than a failure to help. And this also makes sense. For there seems to be no way in which we can define the class of presumptively innocent actions by prescinding from unusual external circumstances. Removing a ladder is not presumptively innocent when someone is high up on it. And driving down a public road is not presumptively innocent when someone is trapped on it. But entering someone's field of vision (where that sets off no devices, etc.) seems quite different, even where the person will, because of a rare mental illness, be harmed by it.

[31]I believe the case was introduced by Foot in "The Problem of Abortion and the Doctrine of the Double Effect," p. 270. See also Judith Jarvis Thomson, "The Trolley Problem," in *Rights, Restitution, and Risk: Essays in*

ACTIONS, INTENTIONS, AND CONSEQUENCES

appears to be negative agency. So the case looks like a counterexample.

But if we look again, we can see that the driver's passive option, letting the train continue on the main track, is really a form of positive agency. This is because the only possibly acceptable reasons for him not to switch would be to prevent the death of the man on the side-track or to keep clean hands. But the clean-hands motive begs the question; it presupposes that the doctrine does not also speak against not switching. So in deciding the status of his possible inaction we must put this motive aside. This leaves the aim of preventing the death of the man on the side-track. But if the driver fails to switch for this reason, it is because he intends that the train continue in a way that will save the man. But then he intends that the train continue forward past the switch, and this leads to the death of the five. So, by my earlier definitions, his choice is really between two different positive options—one passive and one active.[32] And that is why he may pick the alternative that does less harm. Properly understood, Trolley Cases are no exception to the doctrine.

IV.

Perhaps we have found the basic form of the doctrine and the natural qualifications that, when combined with other plausible moral principles, accurately map our moral intuitions. But someone will surely object that intuitiveness and correctness are different things and that intuitions about particular kinds of cases may reflect nothing more than conditioning or prejudice. What we need, therefore, is a more philosophical defense of the doctrine, a rationale that can be called upon to support the intuitions.

Moral Theory (Cambridge, Mass.: Harvard University Press, 1986), pp. 94–116. And Jonathan Glover discusses a fascinating real-life trolley case in *Causing Death and Saving Lives* (Harmondsworth, England: Penguin Books, 1977), pp. 102–103. During World War II British intelligence apparently had the power to deceive the German command about the accuracy of rocket attacks on London. Had they chosen to do so—and they did not—they could have redirected the rockets to less densely populated areas outside the city.

[32]This solution to the trolley problem works equally well for versions in which the choice belongs to someone who happens upon a trackside switch.

WARREN S. QUINN

Foot locates a kind of rationale in the distinction, borrowed from the law but applied to morality, between negative and positive rights. Negative rights are claim rights against harmful intervention, interference, assault, aggression, etc. and might therefore naturally seem to proscribe harmful positive agency, whether by action of the agent himself or by action of some object to which, by strategic inaction, he lends a hand. Positive rights, on the other hand, are claim rights to aid or support, and would therefore seem to proscribe harmful negative agency. Foot's idea seems to be that general negative rights are, *ceteris paribus*, harder to override than general positive rights.[33] And while this seems intuitively correct, it is not obvious why it should be so.

The thesis that negative rights are harder to override immediately implies that negative rights take precedence over positive rights. And it is the thesis of precedence that matters most to us, since it applies directly to circumstances, such as the ones we have been considering, in which the two kinds of rights compete with each other—situations in which the positive rights of one person or group can be honored just in case the negative rights of another person or group are infringed. In Rescue II, for example, the positive rights of the five to be saved from death compete in this way with the negative right of the trapped person not to be killed.

The weakest thesis of precedence would hold that in such oppositions the negative rights prevail just in case the goods they protect (the goods that would be lost if they were overridden) are at least as great as the goods protected by the positive rights (the goods that would be lost if they were overridden). The goods in question are life, health, freedom from injury, pleasure *de facto* liberty, etc.—goods that do not include or presuppose the moral good of respect for any of the rights in conflict.[34] All other things being equal, the weakest thesis of precedence would forbid us to

---

[33]See "The Problem of Abortion and the Doctrine of the Double Effect," p. 27. Foot does not actually speak of "general" positive and negative rights. But I think that is what she means. For natural or contractually acquired "special" positive rights may sometimes bind as strongly as general negative rights. We saw, for example, that a private lifeguard in Rescue I might not be permitted to leave to save the five.

[34]In presenting versions of the precedence thesis, I am supposing (*contra* John Taurek in "Should the Numbers Count?" *Philosophy and Public Affairs* 6 (1977)) that the numbers do count—for example, that saving two

ACTIONS, INTENTIONS, AND CONSEQUENCES

kill one person to save another, but would permit us to kill one in order to save two.

A very strong thesis of precedence, on the other hand, would rule out any infringement of certain very important negative rights (for example the right not to be killed or the right not to be tortured) no matter what positive rights were in competition with them. This would still allow positive rights protecting more important goods to prevail over negative rights protecting less important goods—would permit us, for example, to knock one person down in order to save another from serious injury. But it would not permit us, for example, to kill or torture one to save any number of others even from death or torture.

A perhaps more plausible intermediate thesis would hold that no negative rights are absolute, but would accord to the most important ones considerably more force than they have on the weakest thesis. Such a view might well accommodate the ordinary thought that while someone may not be killed to save five, he might be killed to stave off the kinds of disasters that consequentialists dream up. It might go on to state some kind of criterion for when negative rights must give way; or it might, in Aristotelian fashion, leave the matter to moral perception.[35]

If, on the other hand, negative rights do not take precedence over positive rights then either the reverse is true or neither takes precedence over the other. If positive rights actually take precedence, then we might, as seems absurd, kill two to save one. Suppose one person is drowning and two are trapped on the road. A morality that permitted us to run over and kill the two in order to save the one seems not only odious but incoherent. For once we have decided to kill the two, we have placed them in at least as much danger as the one was in originally. And that would presumably activate their positive rights to be saved from their predica-

---

lives generally does twice as much good as saving one. I am also supposing that goods of different kinds (for example, preservation of life and relief from suffering) can be compared and at least roughly summed up, and that in cases of conflicting rights we can make at least a rough comparison of the overall good protected by the rights on each side of the conflict.

[35]Or it might include a criterion that itself requires intuition to apply—by claiming, for example, that a negative right may be justifiably infringed just in case it would be contemptible of its possessor to insist on it. That is the kind of criterion that I find attractive.

WARREN S. QUINN

ment—rights that would collectively outweigh the positive rights of the one who is drowning.

If there is going to be precedence, it clearly has to be precedence of negative rights. But this leaves open the possibility that neither kind of right takes precedence over the other, that is, that in the competitions we are considering the rights protecting the greater balance of good should, *ceteris paribus*, prevail. In such a moral system the person trapped on the road in Rescue II could not with moral authority object to our running over and killing him. For we shall be saving five others each of whom values his life just as much as he values his. This moral system is perfectly coherent. But it has unappealing aspects.

In such a morality the person trapped on the road has a moral say about whether his body may be destroyed only if what he stands to lose is greater than what others stand to gain. But then surely he has no real say at all. For, in cases where his loss would be greater than the gain to others, the fact that he could not be killed would be sufficiently explained not by his authority in the matter but simply by the balance of overall costs. And if this is how it is in general—if we may rightly injure or kill him whenever others stand to gain more than he stands to lose—then surely his body (one might say his person) is not in any interesting moral sense *his*. It seems rather to belong to the human community, to be dealt with according to its best overall interests.

If it is morally his, then we go wrong if, against his will, we destroy or injure it simply on the ground that his loss will be less than the gains of others. The same is true of his mind. If we may rightly lobotomize or brainwash him whenever others will gain more than he will lose, then his mind seems to belong not to him but to the community. There is an obvious parallel here with his different, and much less important, relation to his property. An object does not belong to him if he may have and use it, and others may not take it from him, only as long as his keeping it would be better for him than his losing it would be for them.[36] Whether we are speaking of ownership or more fundamental forms of possession, something is, morally speaking, his only if his say over what may be

---

[36]And something similar holds for damage. You don't own something if others may damage it whenever that is best for all concerned.

ACTIONS, INTENTIONS, AND CONSEQUENCES

done to it (and thereby to him) can override the greater needs of others.[37]

A person is constituted by his body and mind. They are parts or aspects of him. For that very reason, it is fitting that he have primary say over what may be done to them—not because such an arrangement best promotes overall human welfare, but because any arrangement that denied him that say would be a grave indignity. In giving him this authority, morality recognizes his existence as an individual with ends of his own—an independent *being*.[38] Since that is what he is, he deserves this recognition. Were morality to withhold it, were it to allow us to kill or injure him whenever that would be collectively best, it would picture him not as a being in his own right but as a cell in the collective whole.[39]

This last point can be illustrated not by thinking of bodies or minds but of lives. The moral sense in which your mind or body is yours seems to be the same as that in which your life is yours. And if your life is yours then there must be decisions concerning it that are yours to make—decisions protected by negative rights. One such matter is the choice of work or vocation. We think there is something morally amiss when people are forced to be farmers or

---

[37]Reference to the specific moral relation that I have in mind (in saying that someone's body and mind are his and not the community's) is made most naturally by a particular moral use of the possessive pronoun. This makes repeated reference awkward, and tempts me to talk in ways that are potentially misleading. I have spoken of a person's mind as belonging to him and have drawn an analogy with property. But both moves are dangerous. The intended sense of "belong" derives from the special use of the possessive. And the analogy with property is, as indicated, inexact. Both relations ground rights of say in what is to be done, but a person's mind or body are definitely not property—not even his property.

[38]I mean here to invoke the ordinary sense of "being," in which human persons, gods, angels, and probably the higher animals—but not plants, cells, rocks, computers, etc.—count as beings.

[39]It would make no difference, I think, if the overall good of the whole were thought to be a mere sum of the good of its parts—that is, if the whole were regarded as a mere colony without a morally significant higher-order function of its own. To deny the precedence of negative rights would still be to limit a person's moral protections precisely by this test: whether or not granting the protections would best serve the collective good. It would be to suppose that he may rightly be killed or injured if the cost to him does not outweigh the sum of the benefits to others. And this seems to me a clear enough way in which he would be regarded, morally, as a cell in the collective whole.

WARREN S. QUINN

flute players just because the balance of social needs tips in that direction. Barring great emergencies, we think people's lives must be theirs to lead. Not because that makes things go best in some independent sense but because the alternative seems to obliterate them as individuals. This obliteration, and not social inefficiency, is one of the things that strikes us as appalling in totalitarian social projects—for example, in the Great Cultural Revolution.

None of this, of course, denies the legitimate force of positive rights. They too are essential to the status we want as persons who matter, and they must be satisfied when it is morally possible to do so. But negative rights, for the reasons I have been giving, define the terms of moral possibility. Their precedence is essential to the moral fact of our lives, minds, and bodies really being ours.

But it might be objected that the weakest thesis of precedence would give us some degree of moral independence, and at the same time would let us do the maximum good, honoring as many positive rights as possible. On that thesis, it would not be proper to kill one person to save another who is equally happy and useful— it would not be proper, say, to flip a coin. But it could be right to kill one to save two or even five to save six. Why then adopt a stronger thesis? The answer, I think, depends on how important the relevant forms of legitimate control are to us—the extent to which we wish to belong, in the sense under discussion, to our-selves.[40] And this might depend on the aspect of ourselves in question.

We feel, I believe, most strongly about assaults on our minds. Here most of us are far from minimalists about the precedence of negative rights. The idea that against our will we could justifiably be brainwashed or lobotomized in order to help others cuts deeply against our sense of who and what we are. Here it seems the sense of our own rightful say leads almost to absolutism. We feel less strongly about our persons (at least those parts that do not directly affect our minds) and labor. But even here we wish, I think, to have a kind of defensive say that goes far beyond the weakest

---

[40]I am not claiming that any person or persons have actually designed morality with an eye to giving themselves the degree of say they find fit-ting. But I do think that light can be shed on the (timeless) content of morality by considering the importance to us of what would be realized or unrealized in the design of various moral systems.

310

ACTIONS, INTENTIONS, AND CONSEQUENCES

thesis of precedence. A system that gave you some authority over what might be done to you but allowed us to kill or injure you whenever that would even slightly maximize the overall good would seem a form of tokenism.

It must be said that something like the precedence of negative rights can be accepted by a certain kind of consequentialist—one who thinks that a person's having an effective say over what is done to him (but not over what is done to others) is, in itself, a kind of good that can be added to the more familiar goods of life or happiness.[41] This kind of consequentialism would grant each of us a kind of special authority against interference. But it is unclear that it would thereby give us the moral image of ourselves we think fitting. For it locates the ultimate ground of proper deference to a person's will in the fact that such deference maximizes the general balance of good. In such a system, it is not so much his right to have his way that really matters as the general goodness of letting him have his way.

A consequentialist might reply that anything other than a consequentially grounded system of rights leads to absurdities, and that in praising the virtues of a rights-based morality I can be saying no more than that there is value in the social influence of such a system—that it is good if people's rights are respected and bad if they are violated. But circumstances can arise in which respecting someone's negative rights will lead to an abuse of the negative rights of others. And in at least this kind of case it would be incoherent, the consequentialist will insist, to suppose that negative rights can override their positive counterparts.[42] Suppose B and C will be murdered unless we murder A. A has a negative right against our murdering him, and B and C have positive rights that we help prevent their being murdered. If the ground of the system of rights lies in the value of respect for (or at least nonvio-

---

[41]Amartya Sen makes room for what he calls goal rights in "Rights and Agency," *Philosophy and Public Affairs* 11 (1982), pp. 3–39.

[42]Samuel Scheffler develops such an argument in *The Rejection of Consequentialism* (Oxford, England: Clarendon Press of Oxford University Press, 1982), pp. 80–114. Sen, in "Rights and Agency," Section VI and VII, tries to make room within a consequentialist framework for kinds of agent-relativity that would undermine the argument. But I find these agent-relative features poorly motivated as elements of a possible consequentialism.

WARREN S. QUINN

lation of) rights, then surely the positive rights of B and C must prevail. For only by murdering A can we maximize the value that the entire system aims at.

But this objection misses the mark. The value that lies at the heart of my argument—the appropriateness of morality's recognizing us as independent beings—is in the first instance a virtue of the moral design *itself*. The fittingness of this recognition is not a goal of action, and therefore not something that we could be tempted to serve by violating or infringing anybody's rights. It is also true, of course, that we think it good if people actually respect each other's rights. But this value depends on the goodness of the moral design that assigns these rights. It is not that we think it fitting to ascribe rights because we think it a good thing that rights be respected. Rather we think respect for rights a good thing precisely because we think people actually have them—and, if my account is correct, that they have them because it is fitting that they should. So there is no way in which the basic rationale of a system of rights rules it out that a person might have a right not to be harmed even when harming him would prevent many others from being harmed in similar ways.

The rationale that I have proposed is anticonsequentialist not only in its assignment of priority to negative rights, but also, and more fundamentally, in its conception of the basic social function of morality. For consequentialism, it seems fair to say, the chief point of morality is to make things go better overall—to increase average or total welfare within the human community. But on the view presented here, an equally basic and urgent moral task is to define our proper powers and immunities with respect to one another, to specify the mutual authority and respect that are the basic terms of voluntary human association. The doctrine we have been discussing addresses this task directly. And this is why it is far more than a casuistical curiosity. Whether we ultimately agree with it or not, we should recognize that, in giving each person substantial authority over what can rightly be done to him, the doctrine conveys an important and attractive idea of what it is to be a citizen rather than a subject in the moral world.

University of California, Los Angeles

[12]

The Philosophical Review, Vol. 101, No. 2 (April 1992)

DISCUSSION

Quinn on Doing and Allowing

John Martin Fischer
Mark Ravizza

1.

In "Actions, Intentions, and Consequences: The Doctrine of Doing and Allowing," Warren Quinn undertakes a discussion of the Doctrine of Doing and Allowing (DDA).[1] He aims to find the formulation of the distinction between doing and allowing that best fits our intuitions, and a theoretical rationale for thinking the distinction morally significant.

Quinn sets out the distinction between doing and allowing by considering two Rescue cases. In Rescue I, you can save either five people who are in danger of drowning in one location or a single person who is in danger of drowning somewhere else, but you cannot save all six. In Rescue II, you can save five people who are drowning, but to do so you must drive over and thereby kill someone who is trapped on the road (this person could otherwise be freed later). Quinn maintains that you are perfectly justified in saving the five in Rescue I, but that it is far from obvious that you are justified in saving the five in Rescue II. The DDA must account for these intuitions. In particular, DDA must discriminate against one kind of agency—which Quinn calls "positive agency"—and in favor of another kind of agency—which he calls "negative agency." Quinn warns that the distinction between positive and negative agency may not line up exactly with the traditional distinction between action and omission (or even that between doing and allowing). It is nevertheless intended to be continuous with and to capture the idea behind the traditional distinction between doing and allowing.

Quinn defines an agent's *most direct contribution* to a harmful consequence of his agency as the contribution that most directly ex-

---

[1] *Philosophical Review* 98 (1989): 287–312.

FISCHER AND RAVIZZA

plains the harm. For example, in Rescue I our most direct contribution to the death of the one is our failure to save him; our saving the five explains the death of the one less directly. In contrast, in Rescue II our running over the one most directly explains his death. Employing this definition, Quinn defines harmful *positive* agency as agency in which the agent's most direct contribution to the harm is an action of his own or that of some object controlled by him.[2] Harmful *negative* agency is agency in which the agent's most direct contribution to the harm is an inaction, or a failure to prevent the harm. Thus, allowing the single individual to drown in Rescue I is an example of negative agency, whereas driving over the single individual in Rescue II is an example of positive agency.

Quinn suggests that this explication captures the idea behind the distinction between doing and allowing—or that it is at least closely related. Further, he claims that the DDA (so understood) can effectively sort through various puzzling cases, including Rescues I, II, III, and IV. In Rescue III, you are travelling on a train to rescue five who are in imminent danger of death. The driver has left you in charge of the train, and you can stop it by pulling on the brakes. You suddenly see someone trapped ahead on the track, and unless you act he will be killed. But if you do stop the train and free the man, the rescue mission will be aborted. In Rescue IV, you are on a train on which there has just been an explosion. Since stopping the train is a complicated business that would take time, you set the train on automatic forward and rush back to the five badly wounded passengers. While attending to them, you learn that a man is trapped far ahead on the track. You must decide whether to return to the cabin to save him or stay with the passengers and save them. Quinn believes that you must stop the train in Rescue III, but that you may stay with the five passengers in Rescue IV. And he claims that the DDA, as he interprets it, implies these results.

Quinn also claims that the DDA provides a solution to the Trolley Problem.[3] Quinn applies the DDA to a trolley case in which a

---

[2] We have stated the doctrine as we believe Quinn intends it. His formulation is, "Harmful positive agency is that in which an agent's most direct contribution to the harm is an action, whether his own or that of some object" (301).

[3] Quinn first simply applies the DDA to "trolley cases" (304); but in note 32 (305) Quinn claims that he has provided a "solution to the Trolley

QUINN ON DOING AND ALLOWING

driver of a trolley must choose between letting the trolley run over
five persons who are trapped on the track ahead, and shunting the
trolley onto a different track on which there is only one person.
Initially it might seem that the Trolley Problem presents a counterexample to DDA. This is because intuitively it seems permissible
for the driver to shunt the trolley, but DDA would appear not to
yield this result (since switching appears to be positive agency,
whereas doing nothing seems to be negative agency). To avoid this
result, Quinn argues that the driver's choice is really between two
different *positive* options, and thus the driver may act in a way
which produces less harm. Failing to switch the trolley is argued to
be a form of positive agency, because by not switching the trolley
the driver intends that it continue forward, and ultimately this
leads to the deaths of the five. Since the driver's most direct contribution to the deaths of the five can be traced to the action of an
object which he controls (i.e., the trolley that he intends to continue
forward), letting the trolley continue on its present course is a form
of positive agency.

Finally, Quinn suggests a rationale for the DDA. He points out
that negative rights protect agents from harmful positive agency,
while positive rights protect agents from harmful negative agency.
But negative rights are in general more stringent than positive
rights, because they guard the authority of an individual to make
decisions about the things most important to him—his mind, body,
and life. Thus, it is alleged to be reasonable that the proscription of
harmful positive agency should be stronger than the proscription
of harmful negative agency.

2.

We wish to take issue with all four claims developed above: that
Quinn's explication of the distinction between doing and allowing

---

Problem." The Trolley Problem was first articulated in Philippa Foot,
"The Problem of Abortion and the Doctrine of the Double Effect," reprinted in *Virtues and Vices and Other Essays* (Berkeley: University of California Press, 1978), 19–32; and further developed in Judith Jarvis Thomson, "Killing, Letting Die, and the Trolley Problem" and "The Trolley
Problem," reprinted in *Rights, Restitution, and Risk: Essays in Moral Theory*,
ed. W. Parent (Cambridge: Harvard University Press, 1986), 78–116.

renders it continuous with the standard conception of the distinction, that the DDA (so explicated) sorts through the four Rescue cases successfully, that it provides a solution to the Trolley Problem, and that its rationale can be given by reference to the relative stringency of negative rights (in the way suggested by Quinn). We shall argue that the four claims face related difficulties. First, we shall show how the notion of positive agency in Quinn is much broader than the ordinary notion. Further, we shall show how this leads to difficulties with both the Trolley Problem and the Rescue cases. Finally, we point out that the alleged rationale for the distinction is inapplicable insofar as the distinction departs radically from the ordinary distinction between positive and negative agency.

2.1

Consider again Quinn's claim about the version of the trolley case he discusses. In this case, the trolley driver must decide what to do: if he does nothing, the trolley will run over five, but if he shunts the train to the right (thereby saving the five), the trolley will run over one. Quinn claims that this is a choice between two types of positive agency. As pointed out above, failure to switch the trolley is alleged to be positive agency, because by not switching the trolley the driver intends that it continue forward, and ultimately this leads to the deaths of the five. (This is positive agency insofar as the driver's most direct contribution to the death of the five is the action of an object which he controls—the trolley.) Further, Quinn claims that exactly the same analysis applies to the version of the trolley case in which the choice belongs to a bystander (rather than the driver).[1] (In this case a bystander could shunt the train onto the right spur, thus saving five but causing the death of one.) That is, in the bystander version, if the bystander were to refrain from shunting the trolley, this would also count as positive agency. Finally, presumably Quinn would have to say the same thing about a third version of the trolley case, in which there is one person on the main track and five on the side track. How could switching the positions of the potential victims in this way make a difference to

---

[1]Quinn, 305 n. 32.

QUINN ON DOING AND ALLOWING

whether the bystander's refraining from switching would count as positive or negative agency?

But now it is evident that Quinn is committed to an extremely implausible view—a view which is radically discrepant with the ordinary conception of positive agency. He is committed to the claim that if a bystander in the third case were to refrain from switching the trolley and the trolley were to run over the one person, this would count as *positive* agency. But surely this is a paradigmatic case of "allowing." It is thus unreasonable to suppose that Quinn has given us a perspicuous explication of our inchoate concept of positive agency; Quinn's notion of positive agency is considerably broader than the ordinary notion.

2.2

It is precisely this feature of Quinn's proposal that renders it incapable of solving the Trolley Problem. The Trolley Problem, as developed by Philippa Foot and Judith Thomson, involves various pairs of hypothetical cases. The problem is to develop a satisfactory principle which distinguishes the members of the various case pairs. It will be useful here simply to focus on one such pair.

Let us call the first case Bystander. It is the second version of the trolley case developed above. That is, a bystander can either shunt the trolley to the right, thereby saving the five but causing the death of one, or he can refrain from shunting the trolley, which would result in the deaths of the five. Judith Thomson thinks that it is plausible that one may shunt the trolley to the right in Bystander, thereby saving the five.

Consider now Fat Man.[5] A person is standing on a bridge watching a trolley hurtling down the track toward five innocent persons. The brakes have failed, and the only way in which the person can stop the train is to impede its progress by throwing a heavy object in its path. A fat man is standing on the bridge next to the person, and the person could push him over the railing and onto the track below. If he does so, the fat man will die, but the five will be saved. (One can imagine that the person would not actually need to push the fat man to get him to topple; perhaps he is peering over the

---

[5]Judith Jarvis Thomson, in Parent, 83–84.

FISCHER AND RAVIZZA

handrailing, watching the lamentable scenario below, and the person can simply wobble the handrailing, thus causing him to topple.) Thomson thinks that it is *impermissible* to save the five in this case; indeed, she says, "Everybody to whom I have put this case says it would not be [permissible to kill the fat man]."[6]

Now we can state (one version of) the Trolley Problem as follows. In virtue of what is it permissible to save the five in Bystander but not in Fat Man? The challenge is to produce a principle that distinguishes these cases and that generalizes suitably. It is simply a *presupposition* of the Trolley Problem that it is permissible to save the five in Bystander but not in Fat Man. A *solution* to this problem (which is what Quinn has allegedly offered us) would present a suitable method of differentiating the cases. (In contrast, a *dissolution* of the problem might provide reason to question the presupposition.)[7]

But consider now Fat Man. Quinn's version of the DDA is supposed to imply that it is impermissible in this case to save the five. But it seems that by exactly the sort of reasoning that led Quinn to say that refraining from switching the trolley in Bystander would (on his approach) be positive agency, we should conclude that refraining from pushing the fat man would (on Quinn's approach) count as positive agency. And of course it would follow that it would be permissible in Fat Man (as in Bystander) to save the five. By reasoning parallel to that employed by Quinn in Bystander, we have it that in refraining from pushing the fat man, one intends that the trolley continue forward. But then one's most direct contribution to the deaths of the five is the action of an object (the trolley) over which one has control. Thus, Quinn has *not* provided a solution to the Trolley Problem. And the difficulty here stems from the same source identified above—an overly broad account of positive agency.

---

[6]Thomson, in Parent, 109.

[7]For preliminary work toward a dissolution of the problem, see John Martin Fischer, "Tooley and the Trolley," *Philosophical Studies* 62 (1991): 93–100; "Thoughts on the Trolley Problem," in *Ethics: Problems and Principles*, ed. John Martin Fischer and Mark Ravizza (Fort Worth, Tex.: Harcourt Brace Jovanovich, 1991), 308–17; "The Trolley and the Sorites," *Yale Journal of Law and the Humanities* 4 (1992): 105–26; and Fischer and Ravizza, "Thomson and the Trolley" (manuscript).

QUINN ON DOING AND ALLOWING

2.3

Exactly the same sort of difficulty plagues Quinn's discussion of the Rescue cases. It is supposed to follow from Quinn's DDA that it is impermissible to save the five in Rescue III (in which you are at the controls of the train and must run over one to save the five), whereas it is permissible to save the five in Rescue IV (in which you have rushed back to save five wounded passengers and the train is on automatic pilot). But we do not see how Quinn's account has this result.

Consider Rescue IV. Why exactly shouldn't one reason as follows? If you refrain from rushing back to the controls of the train, you intend that it continue forward. This leads to the death of the one. Thus, your most direct contribution to the death of the one can be traced to the action of an object (the train) over which you have control. Your behavior in saving the five would then seem to count as positive agency, and the putative difference between Rescue III and Rescue IV would disappear.

Quinn might attempt to defend his DDA as follows. He might say that there is a principled way of distinguishing between Bystander, on the one hand, and such cases as Fat Man and Rescue IV, on the other. That is, Quinn might say that in Fat Man and Rescue IV the agent would *not* have the relevant intentions about the train, insofar as intentions don't "transfer" in the way required by our argument. So, for example, whereas the person in Fat Man would have the intention to refrain from pushing the fat man, this does not imply that he has any intention *about the trolley*. Similarly, whereas you would have the intention to attend to the five in Rescue IV, this does not imply that you have any intention about the train. In contrast, in Bystander your intention would be not to shunt the trolley, which implies an intention that it continue forward: the original intention is about the trolley, and thus no *transfer* of intentions from one object to another is required.

Note, however, that the claim that intentions *never* transfer from one object to another is too strong. Consider a case similar to Bystander, Bystander*. In Bystander* a train is coming down the track. If you do nothing it will continue along, thus activating a mechanism that both causes it to slow down (and ultimately stop) and causes *another* train (ahead on the track) to start up and ultimately run over the five. Presumably, Bystander and Bystander*

FISCHER AND RAVIZZA

are morally equivalent; specifically, if it would be permissible for the bystander to shunt the trolley in Bystander it would also be permissible for the bystander to shunt the trolley in Bystander*. But if intentions never transfer from one object to another, then Quinn must distinguish the two cases. This is because (on the supposition that intentions never transfer) Quinn must consider the bystander's refraining from shunting the train in Bystander* to be *negative* agency. Thus, on the supposition in question, Quinn must say that whereas it is permissible to shunt in Bystander, it is impermissible to shunt in Bystander*—an evidently implausible result.

What is necessary, then, in order to defend Quinn's DDA is some sort of "restricted transfer" of intentions. That is, whereas intentions must be transferred in a case such as Bystander*, they cannot be transferred in such cases as Fat Man and Rescue IV. Can some sort of restricted notion of transfer of intentions be developed that implies these results (congenial to Quinn's purposes)?

We do not see how to formulate a perfectly general restricted transfer principle. But it might be worthwhile to consider the following constraint on the transfer of intentions within a limited domain of cases. Consider the class of cases in which there is "already" a causal sequence in motion that threatens to result in some harm. The following specifies the *only* condition in which transfer of intentions is permissible: One can transfer intentions across any of the elements in the causal chain that are necessary to the chain's resulting in the harm.

This restricted notion of transfer of intentions appears to imply the results required by Quinn. In Bystander*, if the bystander refrains from shunting the train, he would have an intention about the newly activated train: the intention to refrain from shunting the first train implies an intention about the second train. Thus, as in Bystander, one has a choice between two forms of positive agency. Further, the restricted transfer principle seems to block the transfer of intentions in such cases as Fat Man and Rescue IV. Take, for example, Fat Man. One might have an intention about the fat man—to save his life. Given the restriction on transfer of intentions, this does *not* imply an intention about the train, insofar as the fat man is in the relevant sense causally isolated from the train. A similar point applies to Rescue IV. Whereas one can have an intention about the five, this need not imply an intention about

QUINN ON DOING AND ALLOWING

the train, insofar as the five are in the relevant sense causally isolated from the train. So if one attends to the five, one's most direct contribution to the death of the one would be *negative* agency.

But we do not think that this restricted transfer principle is acceptable. To see this, imagine that the situation is as in Rescue IV except for the following changes. When you run back to attend to the five, you see that they all have broken necks and are lying on the throttle of the train in such a way as to keep it going. The only way to stop the train is to move all of them, but this will kill them. Call this case Rescue V. In Rescue V the five wounded individuals lying on the throttle are necessary parts of a causal chain that threatens some harm—the death of the one on the track ahead. In refraining from moving the five, one would have an intention about the five—to save their lives. Given the situation, this implies an intention about their lying on the throttle—that they continue to do so. And an intention that the wounded individuals continue to lie on the throttle implies an intention about the train—that it continue forward. The restricted transfer principle cannot block this transfer of intentions; indeed, it explicitly licenses it. If this is correct, then Quinn must assimilate Rescue V to Rescue III and distinguish it from Rescue IV. But it is highly implausible to suppose that Rescue IV and Rescue V are morally different in such a way that it would be permissible to save the five in Rescue IV but not in Rescue V.

To summarize: Quinn himself does not discuss the issue of transfer of intentions. We have pointed out that if intentions are allowed to transfer in intuitively plausible ways, then Quinn's explication of DDA is unacceptable: the account of positive agency is too broad. Further, we have argued that Quinn can adopt neither a blanket proscription on transfer nor a certain restricted notion of transfer. We cannot think of any other plausible restriction on transfer of intentions that would render Quinn's DDA acceptable.

2.4

In this paper we have pointed out that Quinn's explication of the distinction between positive and negative agency—apart from any restriction on transfer of intention, which is not discussed by Quinn—renders his notion of positive agency excessively broad. We have argued that this leads to difficulties in the Trolley Problem and Rescue cases. Finally, we note that the disparity between

FISCHER AND RAVIZZA

the ordinary notion of positive agency and Quinn's notion renders his alleged rationale for the DDA inapplicable.

On the ordinary notions of positive and negative agency, positive agency tends to result in violations of *negative rights*, which are supposed (by some) to be more stringent than positive rights. But on Quinn's account, positive agency departs significantly from the ordinary notion, and thus there is no reason to think that on his account positive agency will tend to result in violations of negative rights. Indeed, think again about the situation described above in which a bystander simply refrains from shunting a train that then runs over one person; Quinn must deem this positive agency. Compare it with Rescue II, in which the only way of saving the five involves killing the one. It is unilluminating to claim that the bystander in the above trolley case violates a negative right of the one, whereas you simply fail to secure a positive right of the one in Rescue II. Note that the individuals' interests and the nature of the individuals' potential losses in both cases (the relevant version of Bystander and Rescue II) are precisely the same. Insofar as Quinn's notion of positive agency departs radically from the ordinary notion, the correlation between positive agency and negative rights is attenuated, and Quinn's rationale for DDA disappears.[8]

University of California, Riverside

---

[8]We have benefited from support from the Center for Ideas and Society, University of California, Riverside.

[13]

ACTIVE AND PASSIVE EUTHANASIA

JAMES RACHELS

Abstract The traditional distinction between active and passive euthanasia requires critical analysis. The conventional doctrine is that there is such an important moral difference between the two that, although the latter is sometimes permissible, the former is always forbidden. This doctrine may be challenged for several reasons. First of all, active euthanasia is in many cases more humane than passive euthanasia. Secondly, the conventional doctrine leads to decisions concerning life and death on irrelevant grounds. Thirdly, the doctrine rests on a distinction between killing and letting die that itself has no moral importance. Fourthly, the most common arguments in favor of the doctrine are invalid. I therefore suggest that the American Medical Association policy statement that endorses this doctrine is unsound. (N Engl J Med 292:78-80, 1975)

THE distinction between active and passive euthanasia is thought to be crucial for medical ethics. The idea is that it is permissible, at least in some cases, to withhold treatment and allow a patient to die, but it is never permissible to take any direct action designed to kill the patient. This doctrine seems to be accepted by most doctors, and it is endorsed in a statement adopted by the House of Delegates of the American Medical Association on December 4, 1973:

> The intentional termination of the life of one human being by another — mercy killing — is contrary to that for which the medical profession stands and is contrary to the policy of the American Medical Association.
>
> The cessation of the employment of extraordinary means to prolong the life of the body when there is irrefutable evidence that biological death is imminent is the decision of the patient and/or his immediate family. The advice and judgment of the physician should be freely available to the patient and/or his immediate family.

However, a strong case can be made against this doctrine. In what follows I will set out some of the relevant arguments, and urge doctors to reconsider their views on this matter.

To begin with a familiar type of situation, a patient who is dying of incurable cancer of the throat is in terrible pain, which can no longer be satisfactorily alleviated. He is certain to die within a few days, even if present treatment is continued, but he does not want to go on living for those days since the pain is unbearable. So he asks the doctor for an end to it, and his family joins in the request.

Suppose the doctor agrees to withhold treatment, as the conventional doctrine says he may. The justification for his doing so is that the patient is in terrible agony, and since he is going to die anyway, it would be wrong to prolong his suffering needlessly. But now notice this. If one simply withholds treatment, it may take the patient longer to die, and so he may suffer more than he would if more direct action were taken and a lethal injection given. This fact provides strong reason for thinking that, once the initial decision not to prolong his agony has been made, active euthanasia is actually preferable to passive euthanasia, rather than the reverse. To say otherwise is to endorse the option that leads to more suffering rather than less, and is contrary to the humanitarian impulse that prompts the decision not to prolong his life in the first place.

Part of my point is that the process of being "allowed to die" can be relatively slow and painful, whereas being given a lethal injection is relatively quick and painless. Let me give a different sort of example. In the United States about one in 600 babies is born with Down's syndrome. Most of these babies are otherwise healthy — that is, with only the usual pediatric care, they will proceed to an otherwise normal infancy. Some, however, are born with congenital defects such as intestinal obstructions that require operations if they are to live. Sometimes, the parents and the doctor will decide not to operate, and let the infant die. Anthony Shaw describes what happens then:

> ...When surgery is denied [the doctor] must try to keep the infant from suffering while natural forces sap the baby's life away. As a surgeon whose natural inclination is to use the scalpel to fight off death, standing by and watching a salvageable baby die is the most emotionally exhausting experience I know. It is easy at a conference, in a theoretical discussion, to decide that such infants should be allowed to die. It is altogether different to stand by in the nursery and watch as dehydration and infection wither a tiny being over hours and days. This is a terrible ordeal for me and the hospital staff — much more so than for the parents who never set foot in the nursery.*

I can understand why some people are opposed to all euthanasia, and insist that such infants must be allowed to live. I think I can also understand why other people favor destroying these babies quickly and painlessly. But why

---

Address reprint requests to Mr. Rachels at the Department of Philosophy, University of Miami, P.O. Box 8054, Miami, FL 33124.

*Shaw A: 'Doctor, Do We Have a Choice?' The New York Times Magazine, January 30, 1972, p 54

should anyone favor letting "dehydration and infection wither a tiny being over hours and days?" The doctrine that says that a baby may be allowed to dehydrate and wither, but may not be given an injection that would end its life without suffering, seems so patently cruel as to require no further refutation. The strong language is not intended to offend, but only to put the point in the clearest possible way.

My second argument is that the conventional doctrine leads to decisions concerning life and death made on irrelevant grounds.

Consider again the case of the infants with Down's syndrome who need operations for congenital defects unrelated to the syndrome to live. Sometimes, there is no operation, and the baby dies, but when there is no such defect, the baby lives on. Now, an operation such as that to remove an intestinal obstruction is not prohibitively difficult. The reason why such operations are not performed in these cases is, clearly, that the child has Down's syndrome and the parents and doctor judge that because of that fact it is better for the child to die.

But notice that this situation is absurd, no matter what view one takes of the lives and potentials of such babies. If the life of such an infant is worth preserving, what does it matter if it needs a simple operation? Or, if one thinks it better that such a baby should not live on, what difference does it make that it happens to have an unobstructed intestinal tract? In either case, the matter of life and death is being decided on irrelevant grounds. It is the Down's syndrome, and not the intestines, that is the issue. The matter should be decided, if at all, on that basis, and not be allowed to depend on the essentially irrelevant question of whether the intestinal tract is blocked.

What makes this situation possible, of course, is the idea that when there is an intestinal blockage, one can "let the baby die," but when there is no such defect there is nothing that can be done, for one must not "kill" it. The fact that this idea leads to such results as deciding life or death on irrelevant grounds is another good reason why the doctrine should be rejected.

One reason why so many people think that there is an important moral difference between active and passive euthanasia is that they think killing someone is morally worse than letting someone die. But is it? Is killing, in itself, worse than letting die? To investigate this issue, two cases may be considered that are exactly alike except that one involves killing whereas the other involves letting someone die. Then, it can be asked whether this difference makes any difference to the moral assessments. It is important that the cases be exactly alike, except for this one difference, since otherwise one cannot be confident that it is this difference and not some other that accounts for any variation in the assessments of the two cases. So, let us consider this pair of cases:

In the first, Smith stands to gain a large inheritance if anything should happen to his six-year-old cousin. One evening while the child is taking his bath, Smith sneaks into the bathroom and drowns the child, and then arranges things so that it will look like an accident.

In the second, Jones also stands to gain if anything should happen to his six-year-old cousin. Like Smith, Jones sneaks in planning to drown the child in his bath. However, just as he enters the bathroom Jones sees the child slip and hit his head, and fall face down in the water. Jones is delighted; he stands by, ready to push the child's head back under if it is necessary, but it is not necessary. With only a little thrashing about, the child drowns all by himself, "accidentally," as Jones watches and does nothing.

Now Smith killed the child, whereas Jones "merely" let the child die. That is the only difference between them. Did either man behave better, from a moral point of view? If the difference between killing and letting die were in itself a morally important matter, one should say that Jones's behavior was less reprehensible than Smith's. But does one really want to say that? I think not. In the first place, both men acted from the same motive, personal gain, and both had exactly the same end in view when they acted. It may be inferred from Smith's conduct that he is a bad man, although that judgment may be withdrawn or modified if certain further facts are learned about him — for example, that he is mentally deranged. But would not the very same thing be inferred about Jones from his conduct? And would not the same further considerations also be relevant to any modification of this judgment? Moreover, suppose Jones pleaded, in his own defense, "After all, I didn't do anything except just stand there and watch the child drown. I didn't kill him; I only let him die." Again, if letting die were in itself less bad than killing, this defense should have at least some weight. But it does not. Such a "defense" can only be regarded as a grotesque perversion of moral reasoning. Morally speaking, it is no defense at all.

Now, it may be pointed out, quite properly, that the cases of euthanasia with which doctors are concerned are not like this at all. They do not involve personal gain or the destruction of normal healthy children. Doctors are concerned only with cases in which the patient's life is of no further use to him, or in which the patient's life has become or will soon become a terrible burden. However, the point is the same in these cases: the bare difference between killing and letting die does not, in itself, make a moral difference. If a doctor lets a patient die, for humane reasons, he is in the same moral position as if he had given the patient a lethal injection for humane reasons. If his decision was wrong — if, for example, the patient's illness was in fact curable — the decision would be equally regrettable no matter which method was used to carry it out. And if the doctor's decision was the right one, the method used is not in itself important.

The AMA policy statement isolates the crucial issue very well; the crucial issue is "the intentional termination of the life of one human being by another." But after identifying this issue, and forbidding "mercy killing," the statement goes on to deny that the cessation of treatment is the intentional termination of a life. This is where the mistake comes in, for what is the cessation of treatment, in these circumstances, if it is not "the intentional termination of the life of one human being by another?" Of course it is exactly that, and if it were not, there would be no point to it.

Many people will find this judgment hard to accept. One reason, I think, is that it is very easy to conflate the question of whether killing is, in itself, worse than letting die, with the very different question of whether most actual cases of killing are more reprehensible than most actual cases of letting die. Most actual cases of killing are clearly terrible (think, for example, of all the murders reported in the newspapers), and one hears of such cases every day. On the other hand, one hardly ever hears of a case of letting die, except for the actions of doctors who are motivated by humanitarian reasons. So one learns to think of killing in a much worse light than of letting die. But this does not mean that there is something about killing that makes it in itself worse than letting die, for it is not the bare difference between killing and letting die that makes the difference in these cases. Rather, the other factors — the murderer's motive of personal gain, for example, contrasted with the doctor's humanitarian motivation — account for different reactions to the different cases.

I have argued that killing is not in itself any worse than letting die; if my contention is right, it follows that active euthanasia is not any worse than passive euthanasia. What arguments can be given on the other side? The most common, I believe, is the following:

"The important difference between active and passive euthanasia is that, in passive euthanasia, the doctor does not do anything to bring about the patient's death. The doctor does nothing, and the patient dies of whatever ills already afflict him. In active euthanasia, however, the doctor does something to bring about the patient's death: he kills him. The doctor who gives the patient with cancer a lethal injection has himself caused his patient's death; whereas if he merely ceases treatment, the cancer is the cause of the death."

A number of points need to be made here. The first is that it is not exactly correct to say that in passive euthanasia the doctor does nothing, for he does do one thing that is very important: he lets the patient die. "Letting someone die" is certainly different, in some respects, from other types of action — mainly in that it is a kind of action that one may perform by way of not performing certain other actions. For example, one may let a patient die by way of not giving medication, just as one may insult someone by way of not shaking his hand. But for any purpose of moral assessment, it is a type of action nonetheless. The decision to let a patient die is subject to moral appraisal in the same way that a decision to kill him would be subject to moral appraisal: it may be assessed as wise or un-

wise, compassionate or sadistic, right or wrong. If a doctor deliberately let a patient die who was suffering from a routinely curable illness, the doctor would certainly be to blame for what he had done, just as he would be to blame if he had needlessly killed the patient. Charges against him would then be appropriate. If so, it would be no defense at all for him to insist that he didn't "do anything." He would have done something very serious indeed, for he let his patient die.

Fixing the cause of death may be very important from a legal point of view, for it may determine whether criminal charges are brought against the doctor. But I do not think that this notion can be used to show a moral difference between active and passive euthanasia. The reason why it is considered bad to be the cause of someone's death is that death is regarded as a great evil — and so it is. However, if it has been decided that euthanasia — even passive euthanasia — is desirable in a given case, it has also been decided that in this instance death is no greater an evil than the patient's continued existence. And if this is true, the usual reason for not wanting to be the cause of someone's death simply does not apply.

Finally, doctors may think that all of this is only of academic interest — the sort of thing that philosophers may worry about but that has no practical bearing on their own work. After all, doctors must be concerned about the legal consequences of what they do, and active euthanasia is clearly forbidden by the law. But even so, doctors should also be concerned with the fact that the law is forcing upon them a moral doctrine that may well be indefensible, and has a considerable effect on their practices. Of course, most doctors are not now in the position of being coerced in this matter, for they do not regard themselves as merely going along with what the law requires. Rather, in statements such as the AMA policy statement that I have quoted, they are endorsing this doctrine as a central point of medical ethics. In that statement, active euthanasia is condemned not merely as illegal but as "contrary to that for which the medical profession stands," whereas passive euthanasia is approved. However, the preceding considerations suggest that there is really no moral difference between the two, considered in themselves (there may be important moral differences in some cases in their *consequences,* but, as I pointed out, these differences may make active euthanasia, and not passive euthanasia, the morally preferable option). So, whereas doctors may have to discriminate between active and passive euthanasia to satisfy the law, they should not do any more than that. In particular, they should not give the distinction any added authority and weight by writing it into official statements of medical ethics.

[14]

Journal of medical ethics, 1988, **14,** 115-117

Editorial

Euthanasia, withholding life-prolonging treatment, and moral differences between killing and letting die

Raanan Gillon   *Imperial College and King's College, London University*

Several papers in this issue relate to the questions of – or as some would have it, the question of – (a) when and why to forego life-prolonging treatment and (b) whether intentional killing of patients who want to die can ever be justified, let alone legalised. Arguments about these questions have also been rehearsed recently in the British Medical Association's (BMA) report on euthanasia (1), in the Hastings Center's Report on foregoing treatment (2), and at a valuable international conference held at Lawrence University in Appleton, Wisconsin, in which doctors and ethicists from ten countries, mostly in Europe and America, sought areas of agreement on these matters (3).

As Gavin Fairbairn points out in this issue of the journal (4), what is morally true of acts causing death is equally true of omissions causing death, *'other things being equal'*. The qualification is vital, for 'other things' often are not equal, yet discussion in contemporary medical ethics seems increasingly to ignore this fact and move to the unqualified claim that killings are necessarily morally equivalent to lettings die. Were *that* true then medical decisions to forego life-prolonging treatment resulting in an earlier death than would have occurred had treatment been given would necessarily be morally equivalent to decisions to kill resulting in the same reduction of life-span.

In analysing these issues it is thus important to distinguish between two quite different claims. The first is that there is a necessary moral *equivalence* between killing and letting die. The second is that there is a necessary moral *difference* between killing and letting die. Both claims are false but it is only the second to which contemporary philosophers have addressed themselves, demonstrating unequivocally that there is no necessary moral difference between killing and letting die. The famous example offered by James Rachels (5) in which one villain drowns his young cousin in order to inherit while another, intending to do the same is spared the effort because his cousin falls in his bath, hits his head and drowns 'naturally', is one of many that show there can be no *necessary* moral difference between killing and letting die. This is an important conclusion to hammer home to those who simplistically assume that just because a death results from an omission to do something it is morally preferable to a death that results from doing

something; who assume, for example, that a death that results from not connecting a patient to a respirator is necessarily morally preferable to a death that results from disconnecting a patient from a respirator.

However, from the conclusion that there is no necessary moral difference between killing and letting die it simply does not follow that they are necessarily morally equivalent; all that follows is that there are cases where letting die is morally equivalent to killing (and of course vice versa). Plenty of counterexamples are available to demonstrate that it would be equally absurd to claim that killing is necessarily morally equivalent to letting die – as Philippa Foot pointed out so long ago, sending poisoned food to starving people in the underdeveloped world is clearly worse than allowing them to die of starvation by not sending them food (6). If a doctor kills his patient in order to get away for the weekend or because he wants to free a bed for the next 'take' that is clearly wrong; yet not resuscitating the same patient because he or she is in persistent vegetative state or because he or she has refused resuscitation may well be morally required. It is probably safe to assert that there are *no* arguments in the philosophical literature that explicitly set out to show that killing is necessarily morally equivalent to letting die, *tout court*, let alone that succeed in doing so. (Papers purporting to falsify this claim will be welcomed – though not without astonishment!). But of course it is true that where there are no morally relevant differences (ie 'other things being equal') *then* killing and letting die are morally equivalent: that is an analytic truth, true by virtue of the language used, but it is not an enlightening truth and on the contrary tends to be a very misleading one.

Medicine, law and everyday morality distinguish clearly between a strong universal though *prima facie* prohibition on killing and a very much more equivocal attitude to letting die. The assumption underlying this general approach seems to be that all of us owe a strong *prima facie* duty to all others not to kill each other but that we may or may not, depending on the circumstances and the relationships involved, owe a duty to each other to preserve each other's lives. Expressed in rights language the assumption may be put thus: all of us have a strong *prima facie* right against all others that they must not kill us: we may or may not

116   *Editorial: Euthanasia, withholding life-prolonging treatment, and moral differences between killing and letting die*

have rights against others that they prolong our lives, depending on who those others are, our relationships with them, and the particular circumstances.

Are there any moral justifications that underpin this common tendency to distinguish morally between killing and letting die or is it mere unsupported intuition and custom? Since the desire to undermine the distinction is most often manifested by consequentialist philosophers it may be best to start with consequentialist justifications for maintaining it.

The first is that so long as most killings continue to be perceived by most people as being far worse than most lettings die (at present an indisputable empirical fact), it is from a consequentialist point of view important – case for case – to concentrate on prevention of killings more than on prevention of allowings to die, whether or not people are right in their perception of such an important difference between the two. For given such perceptions, the prevention of a killing will produce more benefit than the prevention of a letting die.

Secondly, it is probably true to say that more resources are usually necessary for the prevention of a letting die than for the prevention of a killing (ie keeping people alive when they would otherwise die is likely to require more resources, especially in the medical context, than stopping people killing others typically requires). So once again from a consequentialist point of view it would seem likely to maximise welfare and thus be better if we continued to differentiate morally between killing and letting die and concentrated on preventing the former by maintaining a powerful *prima facie* moral prohibition on killing.

The third consequentialist justification for distinguishing morally between killings and lettings die is that in the large majority of cases killing people harms them in comparison with letting them go on living. Conversely while this is also often true about not trying to keep people alive, there are very many cases (especially and increasingly so in the medical context) in which letting people die harms them less than keeping them alive – and trying to keep them alive – would harm them. So while a general injunction against killing people can easily be seen to conduce to maximising welfare (it is a further question to be considered below whether the injunction should extend to voluntary euthanasia) it seems highly unlikely that an equivalent general injunction to keep people alive wherever possible would also maximise welfare.

A fourth, and in medicine particularly important, moral difference between the moral injunctions against killing and against letting die rests on the moral assumption that people's autonomy ought to be respected, in so far as such respect is compatible with respect for the autonomy of all affected. This principle is supportable from both consequentialist and deontological moral perspectives. Now it might be thought that respect for autonomy is neutral between

killing and letting die, but this is surely not the case, for while a doctor who imposes life-prolonging treatment on a patient who competently rejects it is clearly failing to respect the patient's autonomy, a doctor who refuses a patient's request to be killed does *not* infringe the patient's autonomy (except in very rare cases where the patient is unable to kill himself). Autonomy is after all by definition *self*-rule and the patient's ability (and indeed in Britain legal right) to kill himself is not, except in the rare cases indicated, infringed by the doctor's refusal. On the contrary, in cases where the doctor has a moral objection to killing it would infringe the *doctor's* autonomy if he were required to kill the patient, albeit at the patient's competent request.

Equally the doctor *would* infringe the patient's autonomy by imposing treatment, including life-prolonging treatment, against the patient's will. This last argument can be expressed even more strongly in rights language in a way that should be persuasive to anyone who believes that people have a right not to be confined in hospitals, given medicines, operated on or subjected to any other form of medical treatment, against their will (assuming that danger to others is not involved and assuming that they are sufficiently in their right mind not to be properly regarded as mentally incompetent to make autonomous decisions).

Seen from the perspective of medical ethics – with its central concern to benefit patients medically with minimal harm (or without undue burden) in the context of respect for the patients' autonomy and the need to act justly – there seems little doubt that doctors must not do things to patients against the patients' will. Doctors *offer* their services, they don't and should not impose them, even to prolong life (given the standard provisos alluded to above). Thus the withholding of life-prolonging medical treatment when the competent patient refuses it is not only morally permissible but morally required, a conclusion shared by the BMA, the Hastings Center Report and the Appleton international consensus.

Voluntary euthanasia – the deliberate ending of life in the context of severe and incurable disease at the competent request of the patient – continues to be rejected by most 'official' medical ethics pronouncements, including that of the BMA, with the exception of official Dutch medical ethics and *de facto* Dutch law, for both of which it is acceptable provided it is carried out according to guidelines agreed between the Dutch medical and legal authorities. Here the deliberations of the Appleton international conference are instructive, for the consensus accepted that requests for voluntary euthanasia might, where incurable disease and suffering were involved, be morally justified. However all the participants, including the Dutch (two of whom movingly described the intolerable circumstances of patients for whom they had administered euthanasia under the terms of the Dutch guidelines) agreed that it was safer for statutes against intentional homicide to remain in force.

The Dutch believed nonetheless that there should be a mechanism such as their own whereby doctors in strictly specified circumstances should not be prosecuted – somewhat as, to give a less weighty analogy, offered by Jean Davies in this issue of the journal (7), members of the emergency services are not prosecuted for jumping red lights in the course of attending emergency calls, though the law against doing so remains. This, however, was to go too far for most of the other participants at Appleton, for whom the importance of the general prohibition of killing people outweighed the benefits of permitting doctors to do so, even in those cases where requests for such voluntary euthanasia were morally justifiable – and where to accede to them better fitted the description 'helping to die' rather than 'killing', to use the distinction proposed by Jean Davies (7).

Much of the opposition to voluntary euthanasia turns on slippery-slope worries. The Dutch have instituted a social experiment which in the coming years should give some indication of how justified or how exaggerated such worries are. Meanwhile spurious philosophical claims or suggestions that when doctors forego life-prolonging treatment their omissions are necessarily morally equivalent to killing their patients must be rejected: in particular such ideas should not be allowed to bolster nonsensical notions that somehow doctors fall into the same moral camp as murderers unless they do all they possibly can to prolong their patients' lives, regardless of their patients' wishes, regardless of the burdens on the patients, regardless of the costs and opportunity costs to others, regardless of the quality of life prolonged and regardless of the probabilities of achieving such prolongation. Such a result would indeed be a disastrous misinterpretation of the now uncontentious claim that there is no *necessary* moral difference between killing and letting die.

References and notes

(1) *Euthanasia – Report of a British Medical Association working party*. London: British Medical Association, 1988.

(2) *Guidelines on the termination of life-sustaining treatment and the care of the dying – a report by the Hastings Center*. Briarcliff Manor, NY. The Hastings Center, 1987.

(3) *An international consensus statement on foregoing life-prolonging treatment* (in press). Correspondence in advance of publication to Professor J Stanley, Edward F Mielke, Professor of Ethics in Medicine Science and Society, Lawrence Univeristy, Appleton, Wisconsin 54912, USA.

(4) Fairbairn G J. Kuhse, Singer and slippery slopes. *Journal of medical ethics* 1988; 14: 132–134.

(5) Rachels J. Active and passive euthanasia. *New England journal of medicine* 1975; 292: 78–80 (and variously reprinted).

(6) Foot P. The problem of abortion and the doctrine of the double effect. *Oxford review* 1967; 5: 5–15 (and variously reprinted).

(7) Davies J. Raping and making love are different concepts: so are killing and voluntary euthanasia. *Journal of medical ethics* 1988; 14: 148–149.

[15]

VITAL DISTINCTIONS, MORTAL QUESTIONS

DANIEL CALLAHAN

DEBATING EUTHANASIA & HEALTH-CARE COSTS

he euthanasia issue is entering a new phase, one likely to be complicated and painful. Though California voters recently defeated an initiative to put a euthanasia referendum on the ballot, public opinion surveys, here and abroad, indicate growing support for active euthanasia and assisted suicide. The de facto legalization of euthanasia in Holland does not necessarily signal the beginning of a larger trend, but its occurrence is a significant break with a long-standing prohibition in Western societies.

This already difficult set of issues is almost certain to be further complicated by the growing need to ration health-care resources. The decision of the Oregon legislature in 1987 to deny organ transplants under its Medicaid program, and to spend the money instead on prenatal care, will not remain an isolated event. Less dramatically but more pervasively, the failure to control medical costs has stimulated a national effort to reduce unnecessary and wasteful treatments. Medical care of the dying or the critically ill—long believed to be a frequent source of doubtful expenditures—has emerged as a place to curtail heavy medical costs.

The conflation of the allocation and euthanasia issues is becoming increasingly evident. On one side are those who argue, with apocalyptic dread, that economic excuses and rigid cost-benefit analysis will now be deployed to carry out what is otherwise unthinkable: to rid our society of the retarded, the handicapped, and the burdensome elderly. David Andrusko, an editor of the *National Right to Life News*, has called this trend a ''juggernaut of death.'' On the other side are those who argue that it is precisely the denial of a right to die that grievously exacerbates our financial plight. Patients need more power, they say, including the right to active euthanasia and assisted suicide and the means to curb the physicians' appetite for aggressive medicine regardless of a patient's prospects. As William S. Kilbourne, Jr., put it in the *Euthanasia Review*, ''not all the torture dealt out by all of the totalitarian

governments in the world causes as much pain as overtreatment of the terminally ill.''

These new developments raise two questions. Does the long-standing Western tradition that rejects active euthanasia and assisted suicide have the intellectual resources to withstand the growing pressures to legitimate them? Does that same tradition also have the resources to cope with the allocation issue, and to do so in a way that respects human life and dignity? I think that it is rich enough to encompass both problems simultaneously, but that at some crucial points it needs further work and elaboration. The tradition must strengthen the arguments against active euthanasia and, at the same time, develop morally justifiable criteria for limiting life-sustaining health care at the societal level by defining the circumstances when such limitation is necessary or sensible.

> **1** Does the long-standing Western tradition that rejects active euthanasia and assisted suicide have the intellectual resources to withstand the growing pressures to legitimate them?

What is behind the change in public opinion on euthanasia? A great deal of the emerging debate is coming to turn on not simply what is, or may be, happening, but also on what it means and how it should be interpreted. Let me venture an interpretation.

CHANGING ATTITUDES Since the 1970s, death has been an institutional event, with over 80 percent of deaths occurring in hospitals. Even those dying in nursing homes are likely, in an acute crisis, to be taken to a hospital. Hospitals themselves have become different institutions, more than ever oriented to intensive care. Once in hospitals, patients are faced with a strong bias toward aggressive technological care. They will be treated by doctors nervous about malpractice suits, but in any case trained to save life unless there is a powerful presumption against it and, most

DANIEL CALLÀHAN, *a former editor of* Commonweal, *is the director of The Hastings Center. He is author of* Setting Limits: Medical Goals in an Aging Society (Simon and Schuster).

important, increasingly ingenious in the extension of life against great odds. When a patient dies in a'hospital it is almost always now the result of some conscious decision, the result of a medical power able to give almost every patient at least a few more hours or days. Patients are as a rule more quickly put on respirators than was the case twenty years ago, and they are much more likely to be fed artificially should their critical illness render them incapable of or uninterested in eating.

Beyond the hospital setting there have been other important general trends. The broadest and most encompassing is the increase in chronic illness, particularly that ensuing upon acute episodes of life-saving interventions. More of those episodes are followed by a long decline toward death, often marked by sporadic acute recurrences where the patient is brought through once again. An increase in the time between the determination of a terminal illness, or fatal disease, and death is still another important change, now reaching three years in the case of cancer deaths. An extended life with a chronic illness, and an extended dying, are growing consequences of improved medical care. As Arthur Barsky, M.D., has noted in his new book, *Worried Sick: Our Troubled Quest for Wellness* (Little, Brown, 1988), "while more effective medical care enables us to live longer, the *proportion* of life spent in ill health has actually *increased*." It is these "failures of success" that account for the rising incidence of some late-onset diseases, such as Alzheimer's.

General public awareness of these shifts is an important reason, I am convinced, for the rise of interest in active euthanasia. Public opinion surveys have indicated a sharp shift in that direction. Comparative Louis Harris surveys show that 53 percent of respondents in 1973 opposed active euthanasia (with 37 percent favorable), while by 1985, 61 percent were favorable, with only 36 percent opposed. These changes closely parallel changes in medical practice, especially the shift to deaths in institutional settings. It is plausible to think that the public has become more fearful of an extended or painful death, and wants active euthanasia to regain mastery over medical attitudes and technologies it believes can no longer be controlled.

There is an alternative interpretation. In this view, our culture is now disposed to take the value of life less seriously than it once did. The greatest danger is not that patients will be overtreated or their lives too long extended, but that socially burdensome patients will be targeted for elimination, sacrificial victims on the altar of cost-benefit analysis. I have no doubt that the seeds of such a possibility are present—one can find some indication of just about any trend one likes in this area—but there is as yet no good *evidence* that it is strong or widespread. A reported increase in mortality rates in some places as a result of the diagnostic related groups (DRG) cost-containment strategy under Medicare is, however, the kind of evidence that should be followed. Its meaning is not yet clear.

In any event, the fear of a shift to active euthanasia, a fear made more credible by the polls, has been the stimulus behind prolife resistance to almost all proposed legal changes. Living will legislation, for instance, is looked upon as the leading wedge of a value system whose acceptance will lead first to legitimating active euthanasia, and then to killing the weak and powerless. While there is now said to be less total resistance to policy change among prolife groups, and some actual recent initiatives, their political power has intimidated politicians. Within medicine, a fear of indictment in some places for termination of treatment and a more generalized anxiety about malpractice suits (however overblown in actuality) has created a climate of uneasiness. For most physicians, the course of least resistance is simply to treat, and the more aggressive their treatment, the safer they feel. Here is where things come full circle: an awareness of that physician-nervousness serves all the more to increase patient anxiety. It begins to seem that only acceptance of a policy of active euthanasia will prevent the possibility of overtreatment.

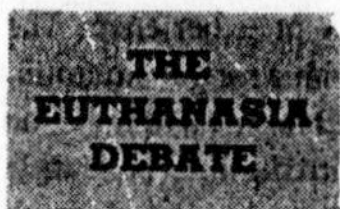

While the euthanasia movement has deep historical roots, going back to Greek and Roman times, it has had a special force in the West for a number of decades (and in England since the nineteenth century). Its primary argument has always been a relatively simple one: a dying person (or one whose life has become intolerably burdensome) has the right to have his or her life ended by another if that is necessary to avoid suffering. The popular phrase "mercy killing" refers to the killing of one person by another as an act of kindness, not as an act of malice or self-interest on the part of the one who does the killing (or assists in a suicide). The moral foundation of this claimed right is that our body is our own, and that our life should be subject to our self-determination. We have, then, a right to end our own life; and if we cannot accomplish that on our own, another person has the right to end it for us, as an act of compassion. These arguments gain weight from the reality that contemporary medicine can and does draw out our dying, or our suffering lives, beyond all decent limits. That we could, by providing more choice to patients, also reduce unnecessary and unwanted costs is still another important consideration; individual and social good could be jointly served.

The persuasiveness of these arguments seems to be growing for many. Can they effectively be resisted—as I think they must be? The most common objection to active euthanasia is based on the abuses it could engender. Even if one grants a right to have one's life ended, how could it safely be enacted into law? How could even a carefully drawn law avoid possible outright coercion of dying patients, or more likely their subtle manipulation? There are many reasons why the death of one person can be of advantage to another. In a society less than pleased to care for those who are costly or burdensome, the social pressures in that direction would be all the stronger.

Beyond that plausible possibility is the further danger of a move to involuntary euthanasia. If there are some lives "not worth living"—and not just the lives of the terminally ill but of others whose quality of life is low—why not, then, for their sake as well as that of society, simply end those lives? The right to die could become a duty to die. The likelihood that society will ride this slippery slope, from voluntary to involuntary, *may* increase once the principle of direct killing has been introduced. Reasons of both expediency and mercy will have been used to make that introduction acceptable.

To all of these long-standing objections, I would add another. Precisely because of the growing need for health-care rationing, there is all the more reason to avoid the possible abuses of active euthanasia. The attraction of using it as a way of assisting cost-containment efforts would increase the risks of abuse all the more. The cleaner the separation between rationing and euthanasia, the better.

Nonetheless, more work is needed to develop the reasons for opposition to active euthanasia, reasons that do not depend too heavily on possible abuses. Those of us who use such arguments against euthanasia should realize that, for all of their intuitive plausibility, they rest upon a calculus of probabilities that has little grounding in history or experience. The often-invoked Nazi analogy has limited value for our situation. The Nazis did not start with voluntary euthanasia and move on to involuntary euthanasia; they started with the latter, and their rationale for involuntary euthanasia had nothing to do with either self-determination or the avoidance of medical over-treatment. These slippery slope arguments are, then, not fully adequate.

A traditional religious position has supplied the missing argument: self-determination does not extend to a right to take our own life; God alone has the right to take innocent life. For many, that belief remains the ground for resistance. But it will have limited force in the secular domain. We need a more philosophical argument, not dependent on religious premises, that might have a comparable force, and that would apply even if one granted that patients have a right to take their own lives (now legal in most states). If such a right is conceded, does it follow that another may be given the right to kill such patients? I do not think so.

John Stuart Mill, in his classic work, *On Liberty*, argued that the one exception to our right to do with our person as we will is the right to sell ourselves into slavery. "By selling himself for a slave," he wrote, "[a person] abdicates his liberty; he foregoes any future use of it beyond the single act . . . The principle of freedom cannot require that he should

be free not to be free. It is not freedom to be allowed to alienate his freedom."

There is a parallel here: to cede to another the right to kill us is to give that person the power to remove our freedom once and for all. The reason even voluntary slavery is wrong is not simply that we ought not, in the name of mercy or freedom, be able to alienate our freedom so fundamentally, but also that no other person should be given so total and decisive a power over our life. That is the most basic threat to, or violation of, the right of self-determination that can be imagined. However strong the motive to do so, that fundamental right cannot be set aside without contradicting its very nature. If I am by right master of my fate, I cannot transfer my right of mastery to another, nor can any other person receive it from me.

To ask another to be the agent of my death, moreover, would cease to be simply an expression of my isolated autonomy. It would create a profound relationship between that other person and myself, transcending our individual acts. From the side of the person who killed me his would be an irrevocable act, one that becomes his act as much as mine. From my side, I would be recruiting an accomplice, asking him to take into his hands a decisive power over me, one that could not be recalled once he had acted. I see no moral basis for so ultimate a transfer of the power of life and death. It is more than the principle of self-determination historically has, or morally should, encompass.

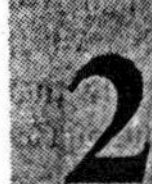

The euthanasia and allocation debates are easily likely to mutually confuse, even pollute each other. To avoid that, it is necessary to be clear about the difference between directly killing a known patient and making an allocation decision whose effect will be to allow many to die who might otherwise be saved. How can it be morally plausible to condemn the one but allow the other? In the first section, I have tried to sketch, all too briefly, why I think that the traditional prohibition of direct killing has been correct: active euthanasia runs the risk of corruption and wrongly extends to another the right to control our bodies.

But of late, the strongest challenge to the tradition has been a denial that there is a meaningful distinction to be made between killing and allowing to die, between an act of commission and one of omission. While this challenge comes most strongly from those favoring the legalization of active euthanasia, it seems to draw at least implicit or inadvertent support from some prolife groups as well. Supporters of euthanasia argue that if there is no serious distinction to be drawn between killing and allowing to die, then our present acceptance of allowing to die ought to be extended to active killing, when such killing would be more merciful. Prolife groups may

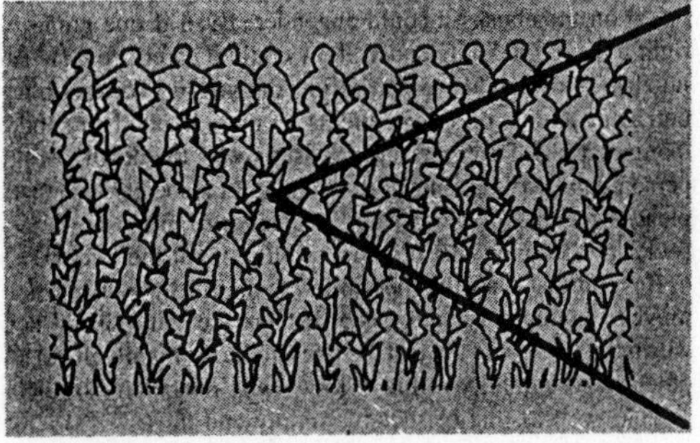

acknowledge a strictly logical distinction between the two, but argue that "allowing to die" is a slogan that has come to be used as a legitimizing rationale to end the lives of those who are burdensome or judged to have lives not worth living. This simultaneous challenge from the liberals and the conservatives promises maximum confusion, making it that much harder to discuss carefully the euthanasia issue and all but impossible to consider coherently the allocation problem.

MAINTAINING THE DISTINCTION My contention is that, properly understood, the distinction between killing and allowing to die is still perfectly valid for use, both in the euthanasia debate and in the allocation discussion. The distinction rests on the commonplace observation that lives can come to an end as the result of (a) the direct action of another who becomes the cause of death (as in shooting a person), or as the result of (b) impersonal forces where no human agent has acted (death by lightning or by disease).

The purpose of the distinction is to separate those deaths directly caused by human action, and those caused by nonhuman events. It is, as a distinction, meant to say something about human beings and their relationship to the world. It attempts to articulate the difference between those actions for which human beings can rightly be held responsible and those of which they are innocent. At the heart of the issue is a distinction between physical causality—the realm of impersonal events—and moral culpability—the realm of human responsibility.

Little imagination is required to see how the distinction between killing and allowing to die can be challenged. The standard objection encompasses two points. The first is that people can die equally by our omissions as well as our commissions: we can refrain from saving them when it is possible to do so and they will be just as dead as if we shot them. Our decision itself, and not necessarily how we effectuate that decision, is the reason for their death. That fact establishes the basis of the second point: if we *intend* a person's death, it can be brought about as well by acts we omit as by those we commit; the crucial moral point is not how the person dies, but our intention. We can, then, be responsible for the death of another by intending that they die and we accomplish that end by standing aside and allowing them to die.

Despite these criticisms—resting upon ambiguities that can readily be acknowledged—the distinction between killing and allowing to die remains valid. It has not only a logical validity but, no less important, a social validity whose place must be as central in moral judgments about allocation as in individual patient decisions. As a way of elucidating the distinction, I propose that it is best understood as expressing three different, though overlapping, perspectives on nature and human action: metaphysical, moral, and medical.

Metaphysical The first and most fundamental premise of the distinction between killing and allowing to die is that there is a sharp difference between the self and the external world.

Unlike the childish fantasy that the world is nothing more than a projection of the self, or the neurotic person's fear that he or she is responsible for everything that goes wrong, the distinction is meant to uphold a simple notion: there is a world external to the self that has its own, and independent, causal dynamism. A conflation of killing and allowing to die mistakenly assumes that the self has become master of everything within and outside of the self. It is as if the conceit that modern humans might ultimately control nature has been internalized: that, if the self might be able to influence nature by its actions, then the self and nature must be one.

But, of course, that is a fantasy. The fact that we can intervene in nature, and cure or control many diseases, does not erase the difference between the self and the external world. It is as "out there" as ever, even if more under our sway. But that sway, however great, is always limited. We can cure disease, but not always the chronic illness that follows the cure. We can forestall death with modern medicine, but death always wins because of the body's inherent limitations, stubbornly beyond final human control. We can distinguish between an aging body and a diseased body, but in the end they always become one and the same body. To attempt to deny the distinction between killing and allowing to die is, then, mistakenly to impute more power to human action than it actually has and to accept the conceit that nature has now fallen wholly within the realm of human control.

Moral At the center of the distinction between killing and allowing to die is the difference between physical causality and moral culpability. On the one hand, to bring the life of another to an end by an injection is to directly kill the other—our action is the physical cause of death. On the other hand, to allow someone to die from a disease we cannot cure (and that we did not cause) is to permit the *disease* to act as the cause of death. The notion of physical causality in both cases rests on the metaphysical distinction between human agency and the action of external nature. The ambiguity arises precisely because we can be morally culpable of killing someone (unless we have a moral right to do so, as in self-defense) and no less culpable for allowing someone to die (if we have both the possibility and the obligation of keeping that person alive). Thus there are cases where, morally speaking, it makes no difference whether we killed or allowed to die; we are equally responsible morally. In those cases, the lines of physical causality and moral culpability happen to cross. Yet the fact that they can cross *in some cases* in no way shows that they are always, or even usually, one and the same. We can usually dissect the difference in all but the most obscure cases. We should not, then, use the ambiguity of such cases to do away altogether with the distinction between killing and allowing to die. Ambiguity may obscure, but it does not erase the line between the two.

There is one group of ambiguous cases that is especially troublesome. Even if we grant the ordinary validity of the distinction between killing and allowing to die, what about those cases that combine (a) an illness that renders a patient unable to carry out an ordinary biological function (to eat or breathe unassisted, for example), and (b) our decision to turn off a respirator or remove an artificial feeding tube? On the level of physical causality, have we killed the patient or allowed the person to die? In one sense, it is our action that shortens the person's life, and yet in another sense it is the underlying disease that brings that life to an end. I believe it reasonable to say that, since this person's life was being sustained by artificial means (respirator or tube), and that was necessary because of the presence of an incapacitating disease, the disease is the ultimate reality behind the death. Were it not for the disease, there would be no need for artificial sustenance in the first place and no moral issue at all. To lose sight of the paramount reality of the disease is to lose sight of the difference between ourselves and the outer world. Our action may hasten, but does not finally cause, this death.

I quickly add, and underscore, a moral point: the person who, without good moral reason, turns off a respirator or pulls a feeding tube, can be morally culpable if there is no good reason to do so. (To cease treatment may or may not be morally acceptable.) The moral question is whether we are obliged to continue treating a life that is being artificially sustained.

There is an analogous issue of importance. Physicians frequently feel morally more responsible for stopping the use of a life-saving device than for not using it in the first place. While the psychology behind that feeling is understandable, there is no significant moral difference between withholding and withdrawing treatment. The point of this now almost universal denial is precisely that an intervention into the disease process does not erase the underlying disease. To accept the fact that a disease cannot be controlled, though an effort was made to do so, is as morally acceptable as deciding in advance that it cannot be successfully controlled.

Medical The main social purpose of the distinction between killing and allowing to die has been that of protecting the historical role of the physician as one who tries to cure or comfort patients rather than kill them. Physicians have been given special knowledge about the body, knowledge that can be used to kill or to cure. They are also given great privileges in making use of that knowledge. It is thus all the more important that their social role and power be, and be seen to be, a limited

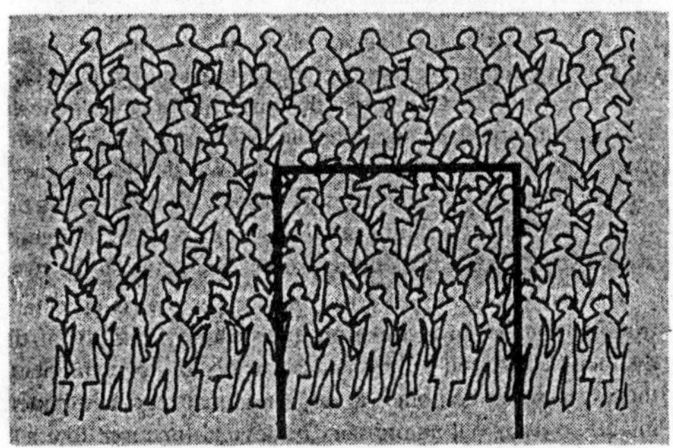

power. That power may be used only to cure or comfort, never to kill. Otherwise, it would open the way for powerful misuse and, no less important, represent an intrinsic violation of what it has traditionally meant to be a physician.

Yet if it is possible for physicians to misuse their knowledge and power in order to kill people directly, are they therefore required to use that same knowledge always to keep people alive, always to resist a disease that can kill the patient? The traditional answer has been: not necessarily. For the physician's ultimate obligation is to the welfare of the patient, and excessive treatment can be as detrimental to that welfare as inadequate treatment. Put another way, the obligation to resist the lethal power of disease is limited—it ceases when the patient is unwilling to have it resisted, or when the resistance no longer serves the patient's welfare. Behind this moral premise is the recognition that disease (of some kind) ultimately triumphs, and that death is both inevitable and not always the greatest human evil. To demand of physicians that they always struggle against disease, as if it were always in their power to conquer it, would be to fall into the same metaphysical trap mentioned above: that of assuming that no distinction can be drawn between natural and human agency.

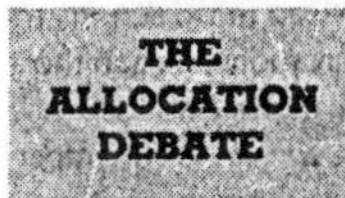

If the implications of doing away with the distinction between killing and allowing to die are momentous for the euthanasia debate and the treatment of individual patients, they are equally grave in their implications for the allocation debate. It is hard, in fact, to see how we can have a reasonable allocation debate without making the distinction central to that debate. Without it, we face a number of stark alternatives. If we cannot morally distinguish between killing and allowing to die, then every allocation decision can be construed as directly killing those who lose out in the process. A refusal to provide life-saving coverage under an entitlement program will be seen as a means of active *involuntary* euthanasia. To allocate money, say, to education rather than to health care could be seen as a decision to kill people for the sake of education (more specifically, to kill the sick to help children).

Given that understanding, health needs would ordinarily trump all other social claims (unless they could be justified also on health grounds); any other choice would be seen as direct killing. I do not invoke here a hypothetical worry. Even now, those who have tried to limit health allocations have been accused by some of using financial arguments as a covert way of ridding society of people unwanted on other grounds, or simply thought too burdensomely expensive to be worth support. Others have been no less quick to complain: for a society to deny health resources to the needy, or to want to limit an entitlement program, is a murderous course, a selfish way to keep for oneself resources that would save the lives of others.

I believe that way of thinking, whether from right or left, is misleading and harmful. To deny the distinction between killing and allowing to die, and then to use that denial as a way of circumventing a necessary debate or decision about allocations, only adds a social error to a metaphysical one. To say this is not to deny that allocation decisions have important life-and-death implications, or that some allocation decisions could be used to mask abominable moral attitudes or practices; or that, in practice, some allocation decisions can be wrong or unfair. I am only trying to say that issues of this kind must be decided on their merits and not dealt with by ignoring or confusing the distinction between killing and allowing to die. That helps nothing.

How, then, can we make difficult allocation decisions in ways that avoid any suggestion that they are being used as a way of wrongly killing people? Or of making them in ways that properly allow us to let disease shorten, or end, life? This problem is all the more complicated for affluent nations. For nations that have nothing, there are only "lifeboat" choices, that is, giving only to one because there is not enough for both. For affluent countries the decision is more complex. We could in this country always spend more on health care. But when would it become unreasonable to do so?

It is not easy to find a moral foothold for making such judgments. They must certainly meet some reasonable tests of justice and fairness, both substantively and procedurally. They ought also to reflect some coherent vision of a good society. I will not take up those important questions here. Instead, I want to focus on the problem of finding the limits of our obligations to others. The Catholic tradition, ordinarily thought to be quite conservative on these matters, has long accepted in principle that the imposition of a grave burden on others is a justifiable reason for a person to choose to forgo life-saving care. An important implication of this principle—though rarely drawn—is that neither society nor families have an obligation to take on excessively heavy financial burdens to save the life of another. We can be asked to do our duty toward one another; we cannot be required to act heroically, or severely to jeopardize the welfare of others for whom we may also be responsible.

This principle, though well established, has been little analyzed, perhaps partly because until recently in most developed countries it has usually been possible for families or society to bear the financial burdens, however heavy. The needed resources were available. In practice, moreover, it has been a principle that few would be likely to invoke, particularly within the family; though theoretically justifiable, it could

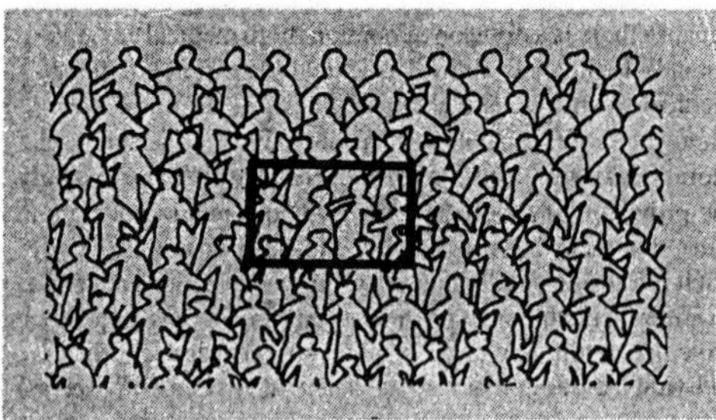

look selfish, and in application could evoke feelings of great doubt and guilt.

There is another problem about the use of this principle. It is inherently communitarian. It recognizes that the common good of families, or society, can and should on occasion take precedence over individual welfare. That is the kind of principle that Americans at least have been reluctant to embrace. To suggest that individuals may not have an unlimited claim on the assistance of their families or neighbors, or that the latter in turn may have only limited obligations to one another, is a disturbing thought. It has ordinarily been evaded by calls to remove excessive burdens from families and to lay them on the state. Only now, when the resources of the state are being stretched and demands upon it seem to be reaching an intolerable limit, can the principle be considered more openly and directly.

Yet how are we to do so in a responsible, fair, and humane way? We might best approach the problem in stages, working first to minimize financial burdens by voluntary methods and then gradually using more stringent methods.

Voluntary methods of choosing treatment   Some 25-30 percent of Medicare costs, for instance, are incurred by 5 percent or so of its beneficiaries in their last year of life. Almost everyone can think of friends or family members who seem to have received unnecessary treatment in their dying. A long-standing assumption of many is that greater patient choice, particularly in terminal illness, would significantly reduce costs. Yet there is no actual evidence that greater choice would reduce costs. In the Medicare case, the available evidence suggests that behind the high costs lies the difficulty of making a prognosis that death is imminent. Moreover, no one has shown that the costs, though high, are unreasonable or unjust.

There is an even greater difficulty in relying upon voluntary methods to do a decisive job in lowering costs. As the history of the debate over "death with dignity" and allowing to die has shown, it has been exceedingly hard in practice to make termination decisions. Even when there is general agreement that excessive and unwanted care should not be given, disagreements among physicians and family members, uncertainty of prognosis, and fear of legal or moral liability, have made individual decisions troublesome. "Living will" and durable power-of-attorney statutes are certainly desirable for individual welfare, and may be of some economic help. So is ready access to hospice services and facilities. But there is little in the history of such legislation to date to indicate that it can overcome the reluctance of contemporary medicine to declare that anyone is, in fact, dying, and to give up the hope for therapeutic success that is its driving impetus and the greatest source of constantly escalating costs.

Screening for access to treatment   A number of experiments and policies have been established in recent years both to evaluate better the efficacy of various treatments and to limit, by preliminary screening, access to therapies that are expensive and unlikely to be helpful to some patients. Second opinions prior to surgery, strict criteria of efficacy for admission to intensive-care units, and development of standards for the use of various diagnostic procedures and treatment therapies, are among the techniques being used. Efforts to evaluate the efficacy of various therapies, while widely commended as a goal, have been pursued only fitfully, especially with respect to the development of standards for the termination of a particular treatment. None of these evaluation, prognosis, and screening methods will be of much economic benefit unless their use becomes mandatory. The increased use of preliminary screening will also have to be matched by methods designed to stop those treatments already underway which are ineffective for a significant prolongation of life.

Useless and financially burdensome treatment A striking feature of efforts to increase patient choice and to use scientific methods of evaluation and screening, is that they build upon widely accepted values. The appeal to a combination of freedom and science is a powerful one. Their use to promote efficiency and economic savings only enhances their attractiveness. The same cannot be said for taking the next step: that of possibly refusing to continue what some, but not all, would consider useless treatment, and the use of "excessive financial burden" as a reason to deny treatment that might be efficacious. These work directly against the grain. It would seem to many an outrageous denial of freedom to refuse the choice of a treatment when, at least in the eyes of some, that treatment is perfectly valid. It would seem an offense against justice to deny someone a treatment judged medically and scientifically valid on the grounds of its costs, either to a family or to a society.

But these are just the kinds of decisions we may have to make. Let me stalk them by moving through a sequence. When the death of the whole brain was proposed in the late 1960s as the standard for declaring a person dead, there was great resistance. Physicians argued that it should be left to them to make a choice between the traditional definition—spontaneous cessation of heart and lung activity—and the newer definition of brain death. That argument eventually lost. Today brain death is the accepted medical and legal standard. Once a patient has been declared dead by that standard, medical treatment must be stopped; to continue would be to treat a dead body, by definition "useless" treatment. This standard applies even if, in the eyes of his or her family, a patient is by their lights not dead.

Let us take another step. What about the continued treatment of patients in a permanent vegetative state (PVS)? (PVS is commonly defined as that condition in which higher brain [neocortical] functions have been lost, but the brain stem remains alive.) Should that treatment be considered "useless"? Patients have lived on in this state for years—ten years in the instance of Karen Ann Quinlan and thirty-seven years in another famous case—and there may be ten thousand such patients in the United States today. Recently, various court decisions have upheld the validity of terminating treatment,

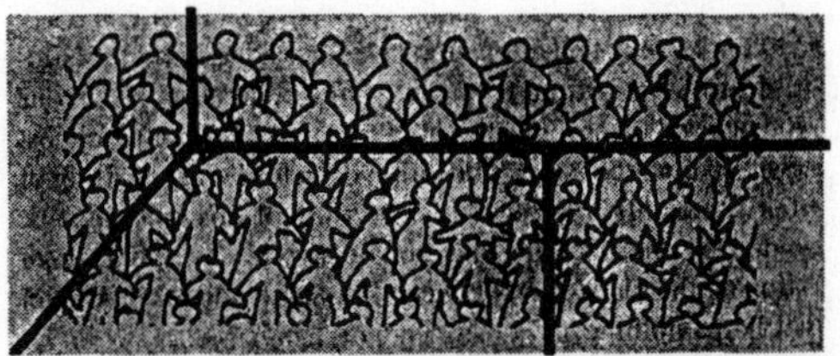

including artificially provided food and water. But there are many who think that this is nothing more than a form of direct killing, equivalent to active euthanasia. There is just enough scientific uncertainty about diagnosing PVS (or making definite judgments about the state of consciousness of those in that condition) to give these opponents a small degree of medical credibility. Proponents of continued care, moreover, argue that it is a moral, not a medical judgment, to say that a life of permanent unconsciousness is not a life suitable for sustenance. The moral judgment, they claim, should recognize that no one has the right to judge that the life of another is meaningless.

How might one respond to that view? It is not the task of medicine to decide whose life is worth living; that is indeed a moral issue. But it is the task of those who provide care to make prudent judgments concerning treatment that provides no known medical benefits, and, based on present medical knowledge, to determine when someone has lost the capacity for meaningful personal life—at least to the extent that such life requires some minimal level of intact higher brain activity. These judgments may be wrong, but they are not patently irresponsible or indifferent to human life. They are no more and no less than what they claim to be: prudent judgments based on available knowledge.

Those who make such judgments can reasonably conclude that continued treatment of a PVS patient is "useless" and economically indefensible. A family would certainly be justified in claiming that any financial burden imposed upon it was excessive (for the cost of any useless treatment would be excessive); and the society could well claim that it had no obligation to provide expensively useless treatment (Medicaid has most commonly paid the costs of PVS victims).

There has obviously been a great societal reluctance to follow through on such logic. PVS is an ambiguous category because there is a division of opinion, both medical and moral, about whether sustaining patients by artificial feeding is medical treatment, and about whether it is useful or useless. There are those who believe there are neither medical nor solid moral reasons to stop treatment of those in PVS, particularly the provision of food and water (which some do not want to call "treatment" in any case). Theirs may be a minority voice, but it is a strong one. For another, those who believe continued treatment (including food and water) of PVS is unjustified have been willing to support only court decisions pertinent to individual cases in that respect. There have been no concerted efforts to have Medicaid or Medicare deny payment for care of

PVS, or to have private insurance carriers do so. It is hard to see how a debate on that reimbursement issue can be forestalled much longer.

Let us take a step to the next category, even more troubling, that of possibly denying the provision of expensive medical treatment that is undeniably efficacious. The most difficult case would be one in which the expensive available treatment is effective and where the prognosis for a full and extended life span is high. This is now the case with kidney, heart, and liver transplants. Since the cost of such transplants is totally beyond the economic capacity of the average family, there has rarely been discussion about families' obligations to take on those costs. Instead, they have resorted either to government support or to public appeals.

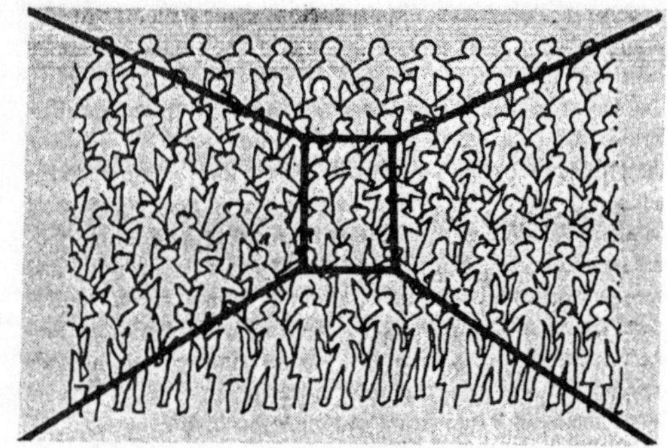

SOME BOUNDARY STANDARDS

Must we, however, judge that, in an otherwise affluent society, a government decision to refuse to support organ transplantations would be morally unjustifiable? Or to refuse other forms of expensive, efficacious treatment as well? Can a government claim that the provision of some forms of treatment constitutes a grave and excessive burden—which is, in effect, what the state of Oregon has done? No clear answer can be given to a question of this kind, in part because much depends upon particular circumstances. But it is possible, I believe, to fashion some general standards for assessing those circumstances. I will call them boundary standards.

The first such standard is that government cannot automatically be required to pay the costs of whatever new treatments result from scientific advance. Government cannot be held hostage to medical progress, which in the nature of the case is constantly devising new, and often more expensive, treatments and cures. This is an obvious point, but, in practice, it is widely assumed that, once a treatment has proved efficacious, government is obliged to pay for it; such has been the history of organ transplantation, as it moved from the experimental to proven therapy. The automatic presumption in favor of reimbursement for whatever treatment has been shown efficacious now must give way to one that is more neutral, that is, one subject to other considerations than progress and proven efficacy.

A second standard is that government cannot be obliged to meet every individual medical need, however valid that need. In an earlier time when medicine was comparatively less effective, there was a relatively uniform range of medical costs. Individual costs of care varied, but only within a relatively narrow range. Medical progress has not only raised the costs of care in general, it has also widened the range of costs. As more can be done to save the lives of individuals, and to save the lives of those afflicted with relatively uncommon conditions or syndromes, the range of spending possibilities broadens. Cases with costs of $500,000 to $1 million become more common; and whole categories, such as neonatal care, increase the discrepancies within individual medical subspecialties. To ask government, in the wake of these develop-

ments, to provide individual care regardless of the cost, is to ask too much. That is another way of urging the government to sign blank checks, the amount of which is to be determined by unchecked medical progress as it constantly redefines and expands the concept of "need."

A third standard is that government has the obligation to encompass the full range of human needs, not simply health needs, and to address the entire range of conditions and programs that together make up a coherent society. That is a way of saying that a government would be imprudent, if not irresponsible, to give over a disproportionate share of its resources to meet health-care needs, even if some of those needs are matters of life and death for individuals. Societies need education for their children, police and fire protection, national defense, roads and transportation systems, jobs and economic infrastructures, social welfare programs, and so on. It is a long list.

We can ask what is a proportionate share for each of those categories, and as a society we will argue about that. But there is no reason to exempt the health-care sector from that debate. Government would be well justified, I believe, to say that it cannot allow health claims always to override other social claims, to allow expensive individual health needs to overcome public interest needs (organ transplants over schools), or to allow issues of life and death always to trump issues of social amenities (hospitals over parks).

I offer here no formula for making those hard allocation decisions. But I do want to suggest that, just as we would consider it neurotic and hypochondriacal for an individual to give over an excessive portion of his or her psychic energy and economic resources to the preservation of health, the same is possible for a society. We need to scale down the priority routinely given to health-care needs, and to stand firm in the face of the inevitable medical progress that promises to deliver some benefit, even life itself, to some individuals if only we will collectively pay for it. We need to develop a strong capacity to say no to some of these possibilities. We need to combine an ability to determine limits with sensitive and open public debate about just what it is that makes for a good society, and what is the proper and sensible place to be given to the pursuit of health and the avoidance of death.   □

[16]

Utilitarianism and Respect
for Human Life

T. L. S. SPRIGGE
Edinburgh University

I

Bentham and Mill and probably most utilitarians (though Sidgwick is in part an exception) have a good deal in common with Hobbes and Spinoza as moral thinkers. For they share a commitment to deriving ethics from the actual and normal motivations of human beings as creatures of the natural world rather than, like Kant and many religious moralists, from some transcendent realm to the requirements of which natural man has a duty to submit without expecting any help therefrom in the satisfaction of his natural inclinations. In the present context I shall call all such thinkers ethical naturalists, though I do not mean this expression in any very precise technical sense, only to indicate a commitment to somehow deriving morality from natural fact.

The derivation of ethics from actual and normal motivations for our ethical naturalists has two aspects. First they believe that the reasons a moralist may propose to us for being moral must exhibit morality as somehow satisfying what we are inevitably after in life anyway; reasons of other sorts can have no psychological hold on us and it would be somehow absurd if it were otherwise. Secondly they believe that the respect for other individuals which morality imposes consists in a concern with their natural satisfactions. Doubtless all these thinkers had difficulties in producing a moral theory which satisfied these two requirements. In the case of Bentham and Mill these derive from the problem of reconciling the concern for a person's own happiness which figures in the first requirement and that for others which figures in the second, and Hobbes and Spinoza face problems which are not so different. None the less there is no doubt that they all sought somehow to satisfy these requirements.

However, the two groups of thinkers differ, in ways which are sometimes important, on what those basic motivations of human beings are from which ethics must somehow be derived in this double sense. For Hobbes and Spinoza the basic motivation is the desire to survive. The quest for pleasurable experience is decidedly secondary to this, and of significance only or mainly as a mark of the organism's success in its basic survival drive. (Or at least that is the implication of

2   *T. L. S. Sprigge*

their viewpoint taken in the initially most natural way, though it is arguable that Spinoza's conception of survival incorporated the idea of survival in a maximally fulfilled form.) With the utilitarians, in contrast, it is the minimization of unpleasant and maximization of pleasant experience which is the basic, indeed the only, ultimate goal. So much is true of Bentham without doubt. Mill's position may need some qualification to allow for his doctrine of quality but the upshot, so far as there is a definite one, will be something not very different, such as the best life as a whole, taking quality and quantity into account, considered from a purely hedonic point of view.

The precise way in which the two groups move from their psychological views to their ethical conclusions is rather different though perhaps equally problematic. But they all hold that each person's own most basic drive, whether to survive or to be happy, can become the reason for cooperating with others in forms of life supposedly calculated to maximize satisfaction of such drives for all.

It is aguable (1) that Hobbes and Spinoza are more realistic in their psychology but that (2) we would be more reasonable beings if our psychology were more of the kind specified by the utilitarians. So far as (1) goes, when one considers the struggle to survive people put up under appalling conditions without much apparent reason for expecting any great happiness in the future, it does seem that most people are more concerned with survival than happiness. And this seems intelligible in evolutionary terms. Those organisms disposed to put up the best fight for life are those most likely to survive and breed. There is something a bit unrealistic in saying that humans typically struggle to live because they judge that pleasure will outweigh pain in the future, and that therefore its maximization for oneself requires one's survival. Yet there is something very compelling in the claim that ultimately nothing is good or bad in any intrinsic way except experiences which feel worth while or bad in the actual having of them. Personally I believe that this is the only rational view and that it is more than simply some personal stance, since to think of anything as good or bad is precisely to think of it as having qualities of which the only conceivable actual species are species of pleasure and pain.[1] But to reach that reasonable view is to go somewhat beyond simply living on the basis of one's unreflective drives. Doubtless both groups oversimplify the nature of basic human drives, but Hobbes and Spinoza seem right, as against the utilitarians, as to what is ordinarily most basic in actual behaviour while the latter may have a better conception of the kinds of motives which will come to weigh most when people become more reflective.

---

[1] I have argued for this at length in T. L. S. Sprigge, *The Rational Foundations of Ethics*, London, 1987, chs. v–vii.

Utilitarianism and Respect for Human Life 3

Its failure to take proper account of the normal human concern with sheer survival blunts the claim of utilitarianism to be rooted in what people typically most aim for. It also provides part of the explanation of the clash which many people feel between utilitarianism and many ordinary moral beliefs on the whole issue of respect for human life.[2] For much ordinary moral thought regards cessation, or at any rate premature cessation, (perhaps vaguely conceived as cessation before the organism has tired of life and no longer has the basic drive to survive) as either the worst, or at any rate very nearly the worst, thing that can happen to it from its own point of view, while a hedonistic ethic certainly does not imply this (thus the Epicureans were particularly insistent that death is not an evil). For such ordinary moral thought rests on a concern to respect all equally coupled with the belief that survival is the primary good and cessation the primary evil for each, while the utilitarian's corresponding concern to respect all equally takes the form of the belief that the suffering or joy of any one matters as much as that of any other but that survival as such, and other than as a means to a predominantly pleasant life, has no value.

So it might seem that if one is to have a naturalistic ethic close to ordinary motivations a Spinozistic or Hobbesian one must either replace or be combined with a utilitarian one, for even if pure utilitarianism is somehow more rational, it has less of that appeal to the natural man which is a main recommendation of a naturalistic ethic. For the natural man, it seems, typically wants to go on living even when his hedonic prospects are not bright.

That may explain some of the apparent tension between utilitarianism and ordinary moral thought on matters of life and death. For utilitarianism cannot altogether endorse the view that cessation is the worst or nearly the worst of evils for each individual. Rather it must align itself with the long line of philosophers, from Epicurus on, who have argued that it is only through misconception that we can think of the state of being dead as itself an evil. And it is surely true that, discounting any supposed troubles in store in an after life and taking death as complete personal cessation, it can only be through confusion that we think of it as something bad for anyone. Even if the fear of death is too deeply rooted genetically to be avoided we can see on reflection that the genuine evil of someone's death must be cashed in terms of sorrow caused to others and the loss of such happiness as he himself might have enjoyed in future.[3]

[2] I am grateful to Dr. Vinit Haksar for discussion of these matters and for helpful comments on a first draft of this paper, and to him and Mr. George Morice for bibliographical help.

[3] Thomas Nagel has argued tentatively against the tradition that death is not an evil (*Mortal Questions*, Cambridge, 1971, ch. i). See also Steven Luper-Fox, 'Annihilation', *Philosophical Quarterly*, xxxvii (1987), 233–52. However, the old arguments, as given most eloquently by Lucretius, seem to me unassailable.

4   *T. L. S. Sprigge*

Let us now consider how great the tension with ordinary thought[4] which follows from utilitarianism's necessarily purely hedonistic conception of the evil of death really is and whether its implications are so far from the views on killing which most ordinary people will ever manage to accept that it must relinquish any claim to provide a criterion of right and wrong continuous with ordinary human feeling. Those who reject it for that reason doubtless often think that they are rejecting an excessively naturalistic ethic, but from a perspective like that of Hobbes or Spinoza it may be concluded rather that it is not sufficiently so.

II

Do the sheerly hedonic concerns of utilitarianism (taken in combination with relevant facts about human life) imply a condemnation of killing so much weaker than that which most people will continue to feel, however reflective they become, as to destroy any supposed basis utilitarianism can find in an appeal to our natural goals when reflectively scrutinized?

I have been presenting the issue entirely in terms of hedonistic utilitarianism and this is often thought in a worse position in this connection than preference utilitarianism. For the latter can be taken as holding that killing is wrong because it prevents certain purposes being carried out. However, I shall concentrate on hedonistic utilitarianism because, contrary to prevailing opinion, it seems to me far more rational than preference utilitarianism.[5]

My concern is not with the general issue between consequentialist ethical systems and deontological or agent-relative ones but with the charge that specifically hedonistic utilitarianism can only muster so superficial a condemnation of killing that only the most eccentric can take it seriously once this is grasped. This charge can be made in the interests of a non-hedonistic consequentialism (such as one for which premature death is a non-hedonic evil) or of a deontological ethic for which certain acts of killing are proscribed without consideration of their consequences. Thus I shall have nothing to say as to which alternative ethic would be preferable for one who rejected hedonistic utilitarianism on this or some related ground.[6]

---

[4] See R. G. Henson, 'Utilitarianism and the Wrongness of Killing', *Philosophical Review*, lxxx (1971), 320–37, for a good example of the claim that utilitarianism cannot deal acceptably with the wrongness of killing. See also Philip E. Devine, 'Homicide Revisited', *Philosophy*, lv (1980), 329–47.

[5] For my reasons see T. L. S. Sprigge, 'Utilitarianism', *An Encyclopaedia of Philosophy*, ed. G. H. R. Parkinson, London, 1988, pp. 590–612, especially pp. 606–8, and less fully Sprigge, *The Rational Foundations*, pp. 23–5.

[6] The bearing of the opposition between consequentialism and deontological ethics on the matter of killing crops up several times in the collection (including its introduction) *Consequentialism and its Critics*, ed. Samuel Scheffler, Oxford, 1988.

Utilitarianism and Respect for Human Life 5

Some disapprove of utilitarianism for even raising questions as to why killing humans, with some special exceptions, is wrong. But if utilitarianism has a reply to moral scepticism, and the right reply, that is (as I see it) a strength not a weakness. For it is not always the most contemptible people who have moments of extreme moral scepticism when they wonder whether perhaps everything is, after all, permitted, and it is one part of a sensible moral philosophy to have something to say to people in such a state, by reminding them of the concrete facts, attention to which will dispel this mood. Utilitarianism has always presented itself as the rationale of much of the ordinary moral convictions of most people in (what it conceives to be) a decent civilization as well as the goad to seeing that there are among these convictions some which are better transcended. Those philosophers who insist on the terrible results of utilitarian thinking do little justice to the strengthening of moral decency which a rational grounding for one's better feelings can give.

I am not attempting a full utilitarian treatment of such controversial matters as abortion, capital punishment, and war, but only with countering the common suggestion that utilitarianism runs foul of views about killing almost universal in a society like ours. That suggestion arises because for utilitarianism the main evil is the causing of pain (that is, any kind of suffering), while the condemnation of killing by ordinary morality seems to rest on treating premature death, especially violent death, as an evil greater than that of the suffering it involves either for the victim or those emotionally or practically affected by it. Thus killing someone is typically thought much worse than producing the same amount of pain in other ways (and to an extent which can hardly be met by putting it down to the prevention of the pleasures the victim might have enjoyed if he had lived).

I am speaking of the killing of humans. I shall not consider issues about the killing of animals here, and shall speak as though utilitarianism were concerned solely with the effects of conduct on human sentience. This would be historically and morally wrong if it were done for any purpose other than the present one of simplification.

To counter the charge that utilitarianism can only offer views on killing which no one not besotted with theory is likely to endorse I shall argue for just one main point: (1) There is little reason to think that utilitarianism has implications in this area which would be widely shocking to most people in our community. I should also like to argue, what can only be implied in this article, that: (2) In the debates common in our society about various different sorts of killing (abortion, capital punishment, war, rebellion and terrorism etc) most of the various positions advocated can be brought under the wing of utilitarianism. That may, indeed, discredit utilitarianism conceived as a simple de-

6   *T. L. S. Sprigge*

cision method for the quick resolution of all difficult questions. But if it is conceived rather (as is more sensible and equally true to its traditions) as a constructive clarification of what needs to be decided, it is only to be expected that it will not bring instant solutions but will only aid in a much more gradual movement towards a consensus.

It is not only those hostile to utilitarianism, but also some whose turn of mind is on the whole of a utilitarian sort, who are induced by this clash to see some inadequacy in a purely utilitarian approach to the requirement of respect for human life. Thus Jonathan Glover, in perhaps the fullest recent philosophical treatment of the ethics of killing, has qualified a commitment to what is for the most part a purely utilitarian approach, by supplementing this with a principle of autonomy which allows him to conclude: 'Except in the most extreme circumstances, it is directly wrong to kill someone who wants to go on living, even if there is reason to think this desire is not in his own interests.'[7] And many others have objected to the lack of respect for the individual's autonomy implied by a purely utilitarian ethic.[8]

It is doubtless true that pure utilitarianism does not ascribe that degree of importance to autonomy which many moral philosophers think an adequate moral theory should. But it can show a good deal of concern with it, and to me it seems plain that placing a higher value upon it than hedonistic utilitarianism can do is pretty pointless, (and I doubt if Mill really meant to do so either in *Utilitarianism* or even in *On Liberty*).

Obviously autonomy of various sorts is often a great hedonic good, or at least its absence a great hedonic evil. For it is a fact that people do not like 'to be pushed around'. And that gives a very good reason for not pushing them around, *ceteris paribus*. Most of the time we want to work out our own destiny for ourselves, though the extent to which this is so differs from person to person, and from culture to culture. But should we think invasions of autonomy are bad for reasons other than that they lower the quality of life?

One problem for those who place such a high value on autonomy is

[7] Jonathan Glover, *Causing Death and Saving Lives*, Harmondsworth, 1977, p. 83. As Vinit Haksar has shown there is some unclarity as to whether Glover thinks of autonomy as a good to be pursued in conjunction with welfare or whether respect for the autonomy of those one is immediately dealing with is a constraint upon the promotion of good. See Vinit Haksar, *Equality, Liberty and Perfectionism*, Oxford, 1979, pp. 134–5. On the whole he seems to mean the second.

[8] Lawrence Haworth ('Autonomy and Utility', *Ethics*, xcv (1984), 5–19) has claimed that utilitarianism must give a special place to autonomy. I do not find his argument, based on the claim that only autonomous pleasures can be regarded as pertaining to a person's real good, very convincing. I grant that some pleasures forced on us in a somewhat extrinsic way may not be deeply satisfying, but surely any utilitarian worth his salt will think a deeply satisfying pleasure good whatever the explanation of how it first became a pleasure. Education, for example, should promote the capacity for fresh kinds of pleasures, not only those which would have been such anyway. Cf. Devine, 335.

Utilitarianism and Respect for Human Life 7

that there may be people who would rather not be too autonomous, and would rather rely on others to tell them what to do. Do we respect their autonomy by leaving them dependent beings, or by 'forcing them to be free'? In its own way it is a curious form of paternalism which insists that being the lord and master of one's fate is a supreme good for us all whether we will be the happier thereby or not. Why should people have more autonomy than they want, or more than they can be happy with? Why insist that being the lord and master of one's fate is a supreme good for us all whether we will be the happier thereby or not? It may be said that autonomy is not the kind of thing that could be forced on people. But if our autonomy can be decreased by external pressures then presumably it can also be increased, and the latter may be as open to the charge of paternalism as the former. It may be, for example, that there are forms of autonomy, such as a strong commitment to thinking out everything for oneself, which make it more difficult to stand up under stress.[9] To say that it still brings more benefits than harm may be true, but needs to be shown.

Most people (I surmise) in the Western world disapprove of the Indian system of arranged marriages. But suppose it is actually a rather positive ingredient of a social system so far as happy lives go, should we think it ought to be destroyed simply in the interests of autonomy? I do not say it is a positive thing, hedonically, but should we be right to condemn the system if it could be shown that it makes for more happiness than the alternative life patterns likely to replace it? Or should we refuse to consider the possibility that the best system would be a compromise between completely arranged and completely autonomous marriages?

I am far from denying either the instrumental or intrinsic value of autonomy in practical life, understood in such straightforward ways as 'the ability and willingness to undertake for oneself the ordinary tasks of daily life',[10] or as possession of a critical intellect, which does not adopt opinions on the mere say-so of authority. But I am denying it an intrinsic value other than its own felt satisfactoriness and an extrinsic value other than its facilitation of felicific conduct.

A more serious criticism of utilitarianism than its supposed disrespect for autonomy, and more relevant to its possible inadequately negative view of killing, is its apparent failure to do justice to the value pertaining to particular individuals. However, this disrespect can be exaggerated. It is a common criticism that utilitarianism simply sees individual persons as receptacles for pleasure and pain, and that it matters little which receptacle is used so long as the collection of

---

[9] Cf. John Benson, 'Who is the autonomous man?', *Philosophy*, lviii (1983), 5–17.
[10] Benson, 8.

8   *T. L. S. Sprigge*

receptacles as a whole contains as much pleasure and as little pain as possible.

So far as that is taken as suggesting that the utilitarian, in his anxiety to remove suffering, only cares about the terrible time some individual is having, or may end up having if we do not act, as an addition to the total sum of human suffering, the criticism is rather silly. The utilitarian realizes that suffering is (at least at the level of ordinary description which a deeper metaphysical account—say in terms of streams of consciousness—may clarify but not reject in essential content) a state of persons, and what motivates him is the desire that persons should not be in that state. When Bentham wished to see vexation reduced by an improved legal system, or the misery of prisoners reduced by prison reform, he was upset at the thought of real people suffering, not at some impersonal load of pain. Utilitarian opposition to torture is simply the decent human response of being shocked that people should be made to undergo such things. Such statements as that 'it is of the essence of utilitarianism to view people not as ends in themselves but as a means to the production of happiness'[11] are somewhat grotesque. For utilitarianism each person is an end in himself if that means, what I presume most people effectively take it to mean, that what matters to him is an instance of the one kind of thing which does matter in itself. Its concern with happiness and unhappiness is not with something to which a human life is a means but with that which mainly constitutes it.

Where there seems some justification to the criticism, however, is that classical utilitarianism may seem to suggest the idea that people are replaceable. Thus utilitarians tend to support abortion of one child in order to have another later, where it is clear that the aborted child would have had some very serious impediment to an ordinarily decent life. In contrast, some believers in the right to life will argue that that very child had the right to the best life that could have been offered it, and should not have had its life terminated so that a child with better chances of happiness could be produced instead.[12]

The idea that human beings are replaceable does sound unattractive and a society in which we thought of each other as suitably killed in order that another should have existence instead would not be a good one in which to live. But there seems a difference between thinking of someone as replaceable once he is there as a figure in the world, making his own peculiar contribution to the human race, and thinking of a being who, represents only a rather general possibility of such a figure as replaceable.

Suppose a man in reciprocated love with another's wife, and that (for

[11] Devine, 334.
[12] See, for example, Haksar, pp. 130–39.

Utilitarianism and Respect for Human Life 9

whatever reasons) divorce or separation is impossible without the husband's consent, which is unobtainable. Might not such a couple in some cases be able to argue thus? If we kill the husband we can live together and have children who will bring more happiness into the world than ever this husband does (whom we may imagine to be gloomy and unpopular, though not a monster). And would not the utilitarian have to say that such a killing, *ceteris paribus*, would be right? It would be no good saying that the husband would then lose the chance of some future happiness, which it is likely would outweigh the gloom he brings to existence. For even if this were so, the happy children who will not be born unless he is extinguished, will surely outweigh that good.

One can say, of course, that all these things are uncertain, and that it is safer to assume that most people's lives are worth living and that there can never be certainty that the appropriate children will even be born. But that hardly seems sufficient to meet the objection that utilitarianism cannot deal properly with the wrongness of killing. The utilitarian must either show why our normal sentiments which would condemn such a deed point the right way, or support views which will be felt appalling by most.

One of the fullest discussions of these matters from a utilitarian or nearly utilitarian standpoint is certainly Glover's and he does not escape this sort of charge. True, as we have seen, he is not strictly a utilitarian. Rather his position on killing is based on an approach of 'respecting people's autonomy and on the nature of their lives'.[13] Thus he holds that the only direct reasons which make killing wrong are three: (1) that it is wrong, other things being equal, to reduce the amount of worthwhile life; (2) that it is wrong, other things being equal, not to respect a person's autonomy; (3) that it is wrong, other things being equal, to cause pain. In addition, we have: (4) various so-called side effects, such as effects on the family, or an increase of general feelings of insecurity in society.

If we set aside (2) for the reasons given, we are left with a utilitarian position which seems to invite the charge that for utilitarianism each individual is simply a vessel for filling up with as much happiness as possible and well replaced by any more capacious vessel if there has to be a choice. For if the main reason I have for not killing someone is simply that doing so will reduce the amount of worthwhile life, then it will appear right for the couple in love to kill the woman's husband in the circumstances described. And much of Glover's actual detailed discussions suggest that he does tend to think of people as replaceable, even if not to the extent that critics may say he is logically committed.

The utilitarian must surely somehow recognize a special badness in

<hr>

[13] Glover. p. 136.

the premature cessation of each particular person which cannot be equated with a mere numerical decrease in the amount of worthwhile life. Otherwise he must draw not only such unpalatable conclusions as we have indicated but also ridiculous ones such as that killing and failing to conceive as many children as one can (provided they have the prospect of a life more worthwhile than not) are on a par.

We are here in sight of two famous dilemmas for the utilitarian. (1) Is it average or total happiness that matters? The answer gives us average or total utilitarianism. (2) Does the morality of an action turn mainly, or even only, on its effects on the happiness or unhappiness of those who do exist or will exist anyway? Or does it turn equally on the happiness or unhappiness it promotes or prevents merely by promoting or preventing the very coming into existence of certain possible people? The first alternative may be called personal utilitarianism (since it emphasizes the concern due to nameable individuals), the second impersonal utilitarianism (since its concern is with the quality of sentient life generally). There are many intermediate stances which can be taken towards both dilemmas but their general tendency is usually more in one direction than the other.

To me it seems that a totalistic and impersonal utilitarianism is more reasonable than any of the alternative answers to these dilemmas of which I know. Any such position will have some surprising implications but none so bizarre as those associated with average utilitarianism, with its implication that there is a good reason for killing off all those who lower the hedonic average. And its difficulties sometimes seem greater than they are through its not being realized that the total happiness in question is not that of any one generation, but of all future sentient life—though here we are simplifying by considering only human experience—which can be affected by our actions. This greatly reduces any value to be attached to building up the total of human happiness in the near future by breeding a larger population where this would reduce the average in ways which are likely to continue into the indefinite future either in terms of exhaustion of resources or by breeding a psychologically sick generation whose deficiencies will affect future generations for the worse.

The faults of the more obvious sort of totalistic and impersonal utilitarianism are not put right by any kind of average and/or personal utilitarianism, but by a rejection of the unduly arithmetical terms in which these dilemmas are posed in the first place. For one can be a utilitarian in the sense of holding that the basic positive factors in favour of action must be pleasures gained and pains prevented without thinking that the weighting of pleasures and pains when grouped together can ever be a matter of sheer arithmetic. That was the strength of Mill's much criticized appeal to quality. No amount of

Utilitarianism and Respect for Human Life 11

headaches of a mild kind for a moment or so for everyone can equal horrible torture for one.[14] Nor can genuinely fulfilling ecstasy be neatly balanced against an eternity of the pleasures of mild drowsiness. But I do not accept that recognition of that is recognition of the failure of the main utilitarian insight.

The alternative view which I support is that what matters, in terms of final rational evaluation, is the effect upon the hedonic worthwhileness of sentient life as a whole, or upon such a whole of sentient life as includes all the action's foreseeable effects on sentience. What contributes to the hedonic worthwhileness of a whole of sentient life is a mix of quantity, however precisely that is understood, and quality, which cannot (so far as I can see) be reduced to rule. The kind of imaginational exercise suggested by C. I. Lewis and Hare according to which one imagines one's way into the lives of all those affected and asks which one would choose, if one was somehow to live through them all, seems about as good as any.[15] I have tried to give my own rather similar view in *The Rational Foundations of Ethics* (Chapter 7). This is a totalistic and impersonal position which tries to take some account of quality. It can claim to be hedonic so far as everything which counts towards the goodness or badness of such a whole situation is cashable hedonically even if the totting up cannot be reduced to arithmetic.

People sometimes object to utilitarianism of this type on the ground that it lets individuals and their individual claims just drop out of the picture. Now certainly a main ethical problem is the adjudication of personal claims and certainly most of us will not easily be brought to cooperate willingly in arrangements in which we think our own claims will be slighted. But that does not preclude our being brought to see that our claims should only be satisfied so far as that produces the best upshot on the whole for sentient life or even our finding within our personal drive to happiness ground for joining in a scheme in which the principle of final arbitration is conceived in this way. However, I am not concerned here with the justification of utilitarianism but with its implications and their supposed unacceptableness to ordinary moral feeling. So in what follows I shall assume that some sort of total and impersonal, but not strictly arithmetical, utilitarianism represents the final truth and ask whether it implies attitudes to killing which most reflective people are likely to continue to find unacceptable.

Doubtless it does if taken in conjunction with some very thin view of what makes humans happy or unhappy. But I see no reason for associating it with such a view. For on any reasonable view of human

[14] A straight statement of this kind of objection is made by T. Goodrich in 'The Morality of Killing', *Philosophy*, xliv (1969), 134ff. For a good reply see S. Talmage, 'Utilitarianism and the Morality of Killing', *Philosophy*, xlvii (1972), 47, 55–63.

[15] See R. M. Hare, *Moral Thinking*, Oxford, 1981, ch. 7, and C. I. Lewis, *An Analysis of Knowledge and Valuation*, La Salle, 1946, pp. 546ff.

life there are various different whole styles of life which can be compared for the general felt worthwhileness they possess in the living of them. These lives incorporate sentiments, rules, tastes, habits of a great variety and they cannot be simply atomised so that any bit can be dropped without this affecting the form in which the rest can survive. And utilitarian thinking of an adequate sort will bid us live much of our life in the style which is best from our point of view and in our society without continually appealing to the ultimate principle of utility on the basis of which it can be recommended. Moreover, even when we do thus reflect, the preservation or improvement of such a style will be one of the main things to be considered.

This sounds a bit like rule utilitarianism. However, it is not like any form thereof which is a genuine alternative to act utilitarianism. For the suggestion is, first, that in reflecting on our actions from a utilitarian point of view we must always remember as a main consideration the way in which it will affect the style of life of ourselves and our fellows, and, secondly, that we will do best, so far as the promotion of happiness goes, to live the relevant style of life without such reflection for much of the time.

This leads us to a question highly relevant to all matters about killing: Is the ideal utilitarian society one in which everyone is a utilitarian? Should the utilitarian regard it as one of the tasks of those who can influence social developments to encourage utilitarian styles of thinking at the expense of others?

Before answering this it must be noted firmly that it would be an absurdity if the main content of a utilitarian ethic consisted in precepts regarding the way in which good utilitarians would behave in the company of good utilitarians. For most people are not presently inclined to act in predominantly utilitarian ways and there is no likelihood of this changing in the foreseeable future. (Bentham himself was aware how mistaken it could be to attempt promulgation everywhere of a single utilitarian norm both in legislation and morality.)[16] And even those who may officially hold views of a utilitarian character are not going to be actuated by utilitarian thinking all the time. For in the first place much of their behaviour will be determined by concern with their own welfare and of those close to them rather than with the greatest happiness of the greatest number, and secondly even when they are living by ideals which are less egoistic than this, their ideals will not in practice normally simply be those derivable from a utilitarian calculation.

But is it even desirable that we should all be utilitarians all the time?

---

[16] Consider in this connection 'Essay on the Influence of Time and Place in Matters of Legislation', *The Works of Jeremy Bentham*, ed. John Bowring, 11 vols., Edinburgh, 1843, i. 169–94 (also in *Traités de législation civile et pénale*, ed. P. É. L. Dumont, 1802, iii. 325–95).

Utilitarianism and Respect for Human Life   13

Suppose someone is training to win a race. Are they doing so because they think their winning will be for the greatest happiness of the greatest number? Hardly. Nor would it be easy to persuade them to step back and ask themselves if it is so, and withdraw if it seems not to be. (It is only in cases with special political implications that the idea of raising such a question would occur.) It is doubtful if they are even doing it because they judge it to be for their own greatest overall happiness. They will be very happy if they win but they are not doing it in order to get that happiness. (This, the most usual of objections to psychological hedonism, seems right, though it may still be, as I think, that past hedonic reinforcement, positive and negative, is the essential determinant of all goals which are more than the end states of instinctive actions.) At least much of the time they are simply hooked on the end of winning.

Now consider preparations for a wedding. The best man is working out what he must do with the ring, the bride's father is thinking out his role, the happy couple are practising the tone of voice in which to make their responses, and so forth. Are they seeking to do what they think will best promote the happiness of all affected, or even their own? Their aims are more direct—to do the right thing. But what if they step back and consider the ultimate point of what they are up to? Perhaps the father thinks that he wants to give his daughter a wedding she will look back on with pleasure. And perhaps the daughter is concerned to give her parents the kind of wedding they want. None of this, however, makes much sense unless there is someone who directly wants the wedding to satisfy certain criteria of a successful occasion, not because that makes them happy, but just because that is a direct goal of theirs.

Thus people have many goals which do not consist in happiness for themselves or for others. Nor is this something that the utilitarian would wish to change. In his reflective utilitarian moments he will want life to be lived in a maximally satisfying way, but he will realize that this requires that people want to achieve things and contemplate things of certain sorts, not because they contribute to the maximization of general, or even their own, happiness, but simply because they find them good. In other words the good utilitarian life requires that certain sorts of activities, achievements, and objects of contemplation be liked for their own sakes and that various things attract or repel us without their attraction or repulsiveness taking the form of a utilitarian judgement as to their usefulness or harmfulness. And even looked at from the reflective utilitarian point of view, the enjoyment of each of these is good in itself and not merely good as a means to the swelling of an aggregate.

Having, or regarding as good, many emotional attitudes whose propositional content is not directly utilitarian does not require any

14   *T. L. S. Sprigge*

sort of bad faith on the part of a utilitarian or a schizoid personality. One can step back and see the sexual instinct as necessary for human life without wanting to have sexual feelings replaced by judgements about their utility, or regarding the way things present themselves to sexual feeling as in contest with the content of utilitarian opinions.

In much the same way utilitarianism can quite consistently stress the importance for human life of various moral attitudes whose propositional expression does not take the form of utilitarian judgements. These can be valuable either because having them is itself an enrichment of human life or because they are useful in a less immediate way. And the same may be true of various feelings which, without being themselves moral judgements, pass naturally into moral judgements. Just as it would be absurd to think that utilitarianism implies that a love of music is to be superseded by a rational judgement as to the contribution of music to the sum of human happiness, so is it a mistake, only less absurd because more understandable, to hold that utilitarianism should aim to purge us of everything which could be called a moral attitude except endorsement of the principle of utility. And closely associated with certain desirable moral attitudes are certain attitudes to our fellows. Utilitarians should not forget the importance that attaches to our thought about our own and each other's character and conduct both as an influence on our own and as a direct satisfaction or dissatisfaction.

It is useful in this connection to draw a contrast between rational utilitarian judgements at the level of critical reflection and judgements which belong to the give and take of ordinary life. R. M. Hare has elaborated an account of a contrast between reflective and intuitive moral thinking which is in many respects similar to that I wish to make.[17] But whereas for Hare judgements of the second kind typically turn on rules of thumb for dealing with questions quickly in ordinary life, I would stress the direct value of the feelings, which we may call moral sentiments, which they express, as enrichments of human life, comparable to the enrichment given it by music, (so that Hare's archangel who lacked them would be inferior in the richness of his life to one who possessed them).

Thus a utilitarian might take a broadly anti-abortion stand on the ground that a society which permits it readily will be poor in certain moral and quasi-moral sentiments of respect for human life, and in certain forms of personal relationship, which are direct sources of happiness as well as important social controls. Of course, there will be utilitarian argument on the other side; my point is that a utilitarian interpretation can clarify the issue for reasonable people on both sides.

---

[17] Hare, *Moral Thinking*, especially chs. 2 and 3.

Utilitarianism and Respect for Human Life   15

Some of the harshness of Jonathan Glover's determinedly utilitarian (apart from the qualification concerning autonomy) discussions of the morality of various kinds of killing arises from his not seeming to do adequate justice to the value, both intrinsic and extrinsic, of a variety of feelings about our fellows and about protecting their lives which are not themselves utilitarian in content. Much more stress needs to be put on the way in which a special sentiment of disapproval for certain acts is bound up more or less intrinsically with ways of feeling towards our fellows which are among the chief goods of human life. And even when the main reason why these feelings are desirable lies simply in their steering us away from actions which Glover is only prepared to call bad in virtue of their side effects, it may be that we will not be the sort of people which it is for the best that we should be if we do not feel that there is something rather more intrinsically undesirable about such action.

From the point of view of ultimate critical utilitarian reflection a large part of what makes killing another human wrong in all those ordinary circumstances in which it counts as murder lies in an elaborate complex of human goods which depend on each of us regarding it as taboo, and on the particular damage to such goods which stem from each individual murder. But it gives a very misleading impression to express this as the view that murder is wrong not in itself but only in its side effects, as Glover tends to do (or rather thinks he would have to if he could not invoke respect for autonomy as a booster to pure utilitarianism).[18] For at that level the very distinction between side effects and direct effects is somewhat arbitrary. Thus if a utilitarian argues that infanticide (and, some might add, too ready resort to abortion) is wrong on account of its psychological effects on those who arrange and do the deed, and thin end of the wedge effects, (which would put any children at risk who prove a nuisance to their guardians with a vast subsequent coarsening of human relations) he may be as completely against it as anyone can be against anything. It would sound misleadingly tepid to say that he only condemns it for its side effects. Anyway, it is none too clear what is meant by asking whether an act (or type of act) is bad in itself or for its side effects, since effects can be pushed one way or the other by mere redescription.[19]

Moreover, the moral sentiments which a utilitarian may hold it desirable for us to have (not simply as means to an end but as part of the utilitarian end of a happy form of human life) towards the killing of a baby, and which we express in terms of moral outrage, may be as

---

[18] Glover, pp. 126ff. seems to me misleading in this way in a manner not sufficiently offset by the explanation on p. 40.

[19] This is, after all, the brunt of Glover's case against the commissions/omissions distinction.

16   *T. L. S. Sprigge*

direct a response as that of liking or disliking certain musical sounds. And the same goes for many other forms of killing. That they seem directly wrong to us, in ways which are not based upon a utilitarian calculation, may be a great utilitarian good.

It seems sufficiently evident that people will be happier in a society in which these sentiments are widespread and that therefore the preservation of those various attitudes which one can sum up as respect for human life should be given very high importance.

The reasons why people are liable to be happier in such a society are many. They consist both in effects relatively external to those sentiments and ones intimately involved with their very nature. We are each of us safer in a society with a strong sense of human solidarity which includes respect for human life, and are so particularly in respect of that wish to survive for as long as possible which a contract theorist like Hobbes saw as the main motive for making the contract. But also we enjoy being respected by others and have fuller and deeper relations with others on account of our mutual trust and respect. The case for abiding by and promoting a pattern of life which is happier in the living of it than likely alternatives is at least as good as is the case for spending resources on education in the good things of culture and supporting and engaging in the arts.

It may be said that no one has collected evidence for the claim that this kind of caring society is a happier one than a more callous one. Perhaps not. And if somehow I were convinced that some way of life of a more callous kind was hedonistically much better for the community as a whole, and that our community could become such a community without passing through intervening phases which would outweigh the increase in value, perhaps I would then think that it might be proper to attempt to move society in that direction. But the mere fact that we might be happier if we were different sorts of being would not be sufficient reason for weakening our dedication to ideals which are essential for our happiness as we are.

And in any case, there is plenty of evidence at the level of common sense psychology for the belief that a caring society is the hedonically better off, and that we should be very careful in pulling it apart by trying to weaken our revulsion against killing, but should aim rather at strengthening it. I even suggest that that gives some justification to the special concern shown to save nameable people at risk of death in an accident in spite of allowing a few 'statistical' deaths to be inevitable on the roads.[20]

There is a tendency to think that resting fundamental moral principles on empirical facts (such as our usually very strong wish to

----

[20] Compare Glover, pp. 210–16.

Utilitarianism and Respect for Human Life 17

survive as long as possible) somehow renders them superficial. Its tendency to encourage such thought is one objection to excessive use of quite fanciful examples in moral philosophy. But it is a great mistake for empiricists, at least, to think in this way, for according to empiricism it is precisely empirical facts, of any pervasiveness, which are real facts about the world in contrast to the more stipulative nature of necessary truth. A rationalist may think otherwise, but then rationalists have tended to think that these facts are necessary truths (though truths about nature, not about a transcendent realm) rather than empirical. Either way resting moral principles upon fundamental facts about human beings does not make them somehow superficial. So if the wrongness of killing depends upon facts about human psychology it does not therefore cease to be a fundamental moral principle. It may be objected that for the utilitarian it certainly contrasts with the principle of utility, which, however much utilitarians may try to wriggle out of the fact, has *a priori* status. Even if this is so, (as is debatable) it remains true that moral principles derivable from it 'only' in conjunction with very basic facts about human nature are not being thereby treated as somehow of less than fundamental importance.

All this is not to deny that a sensible utilitarianism may have to challenge some widely held moral views.

It has been pointed out that common moral feeling regards it as worse seriously to hurt an animal than to kill it, but worse to kill than seriously to hurt a human being. Utilitarianism may seem bound to challenge this distinction by assimilating the status of humans to animals in this respect. And that may be a ground of objection to utilitarianism for some people.

How would a Hobbesian or Spinozist view this matter? Would they perhaps assimilate the cases by moving rather to the second attitude for animals as well as humans? After all animals have as direct an inclination to struggle for survival as do humans.

The historical Spinoza (and I presume Hobbes) thought that we had no duties to animals, essentially because they could not co-operate with us in promoting the good life and were not involved in any implied contract with us. But someone sharing the psychological views of these two thinkers but who based ethics upon a universalizability principle might be led to this. For they might see ethics as resting upon a recognition of the equivalence of the will to live in all beings. This was roughly the position of Schopenhauer and Schweitzer.

But let us return to utilitarianism. Suppose (to use for once the kind of fanciful example I basically dislike) a Nazi type extermination of large groups of people with suffering kept minimal with the aid of extraordinarily powerful tranquillisers on all concerned or affected. Would the regime responsible be worse or better than one which

18   *T. L. S. Sprigge*

tortured its enemies in atrocious ways without killing them? The
utilitarian might be inclined to think the latter the worse, while
perhaps most people would respond more negatively to the former. I
believe my own fairly spontaneous reaction is that of the utilitarian.
The torture of people in some countries today seems worse to me than
any readiness to execute supposed enemies of the state quickly. But it
remains the case that one who has feelings whose pervasiveness is
essential for the happiness of society would feel horror at the thought
of a society in which one group of humans is ready to annihilate
another, however painlessly. He could also recognize reflectively that
such a society would have deprived itself of the chief elements of
human well being—quite apart from the fact that in reality such
alleged painlessness would certainly be a myth.

My defence of the capacity of utilitarianism to give a reasonable
account of the wrongness of killing has concerned mainly the problems
supposedly springing from a purely hedonistic conception of what is
good or bad in itself and its consequent inability to see that 'continued
human life is of value as such, independently of any judgement
concerning its worthwhileness'.[21] But the drift of some arguments
concerning the homicidal implications of utilitarianism is to show
rather that it is its consequentialism, hedonistic or otherwise, which
has these appalling implications. For even if utilitarianism can show
that, though death is not the evil men tend to think it, still the killing
of one's fellows is, that does not yield the kind of agent relative
condemnation of killing entrenched (with many qualifications) in
ordinary morality. Thus it has been suggested ironically that a group
of utilitarians plotted the assassination of President Kennedy in a
reasonable expectation that this might lead to legislation in the US
against the private possession of fire arms and thus save many lives.
Even though that was not the result, it was perhaps genuinely probable
that it would be, in which case the act was objectively right from a
utilitarian perspective (and right in intention in any case).[22]

But I suggest that the worry produced in most people at the idea of
so-called utilitarians acting thus springs from a good idea of the
terrible quality of life which would be bound up with and consequent
upon such behaviour. This is just the same old problem as that of the
punishment of the innocent man in the interests of the greatest good. It
is evident that the world will get worse if people break down the barrier
of sentiment they have against certain types of action. Are there,
indeed, any known cases where someone acting in any such manner to
bring about a surplus of good has succeeded in doing so? If so, they

[21] Devine, 332.
[22] Don Locke, 'Why the Utilitarians shot President Kennedy', *Analysis*, xxxvi (1975–6),
153–5.

Utilitarianism and Respect for Human Life 19

must be so rare as to be a bad basis for prediction. The utilitarian has every reason to insist on the truth that personal callousness spreads. If I hear of terrorists who have killed their friends to stir up feeling against enemies who will be thought to have done it, I am shocked, having a well founded sense that they are moving even further from the type of life which can possibly promote good than I might previously have thought.

It will scarcely be profitable to pursue further some of the far fetched tales which some philosophers tell in order to discredit utilitarianism. Their main point is clear enough, namely that there is a general feeling that killing people, except under very specific conditions, is very wrong, and wrong in a way which cannot be adequately cashed in terms of suffering before the killing by the victim, his loss of opportunities for happiness later, and the sadness of the bereaved. Thus even if someone has every reason to believe the life of another wretched, and that there will be more relief than sorrow at his death, it is still considered wrong to kill him. I have rejected Glover's attempt to explain this by an appeal to a special principle of respect for individual autonomy not cashable in hedonic terms. Must I then hold that in the last resort such killing would be right, at least if done in secret, so that no damaging precedent is set etc. etc.?

I answer that a readiness to kill someone without his consent (possibly some quite extraordinary circumstances excepted) must express an attitude of such negativeness to another that it is for the good of us all that we should, so far as possible, never feel it towards our fellows.[23] That it expresses such a negative feeling follows from various facts. First, there is the fact that aggression finds its psychological consummation or fulfilment in killing someone; secondly, that one can only wish to be responsible for someone's departure from the world if one thinks him quite unloveable; and thirdly, that people by and large do not want to die so that making someone die by force is necessarily to take up a hostile stance towards him. So if we hear of someone ready to kill we deplore his having such a feeling.

It would be strange and regrettable if there was not some tendency to respond with a related dismay even to cases of requested mercy killing. Too eager a response to such a request suggests absence of an important sentiment against killing and a failure to appreciate the value of the individuality of others, a failure in love, to put it more strongly. That there are some cases where the loving act precisely is to kill seems, however, hard to deny.

But my purpose here is not to decide just what killing is justified from a utilitarian point of view, and how that squares with any

[23] Cf. R. E. Ewin, 'What is wrong with killing people?', *Philosophical Quarterly*, xxii (1972), 139.

20   *T. L. S. Sprigge*

particular species of common morality. I have only sought to show that utilitarianism does not have a particularly light hearted attitude to killing, even though it does not include the desirability of each person's survival for as long as possible in the ultimate rationale of moral judgement which it professes to provide.

III

To sum up:

From a utilitarian point of view what matters is how conduct affects the sum of sentient life, and I have simplified here by confining attention to human life. Conduct is right or wrong in virtue of whether it makes life as a whole a better or a worse affair in hedonic terms, though this cannot be made a matter of sheer arithmetic. But this whole of life includes the felt goodness and badness of styles of feeling bound up with certain ways of relating to others (a point perhaps better made by Spinoza than Bentham).

One of the main conditions of human life being worthwhile is that each individual should belong to a community in which there is mutual respect and does not have to participate in communities in which he is not respected. Perhaps in the past this goal could be realized if respect for others was confined to members of one's own community, where this meant something less than the human race. For there was no need to participate in a larger community, except in very limited ways, or in warfare, and a reduced form of respect to aliens encountered then was perhaps compatible with a reasonable life. But that is not practicable in the modern world and humans can only avoid participation in a community where they are not respected to the extent that humans in general respect each other.

This respect implies that (possibly subject to some very special exceptions) relations between people will not reach a point of such aggression that they are ready to kill each other. That requires that there are sentiments about killing which cannot be reduced to judgements about what will best promote the sum of human happiness.

But each one of us who has these sentiments can see it as a utilitarian good that so far as possible we should all continue to have them and this extraordinarily important good can only be promoted if we all keep these sentiments alive in ourselves.

Granted we have these sentiments we will not want to kill, and it would make us very unhappy if in some moment of passion we did so. That is an additional, if not the main reason for avoiding killing if it ever becomes a temptation.

The idea of killing one person with the intention of replacing him with happier others proposes an end which will make us miserable,

Utilitarianism and Respect for Human Life 21

granted we are the sorts of people that it is for our own and the general happiness that we should be.

To the extent that our attitudes are of this desirable sort we will have some appreciation of the special quality of feeling contributed to the totality by each particular individual we know (and realization that there is some such special contribution made by individuals we do not know). Thus we will no more want to see one individual's special contribution to the total cut short earlier than need be than we would want to destroy works of art. Human happiness requires a taste for particular sorts of good, and each human individual is a particular good.

This may seem starry eyed, for are not some people hardly contributors to human good at all, or at least such that their contribution to the worsening of human life far outweighs this? Well, perhaps that is, after all, true in some cases, but we are going to have much happier relations with each other if our normal expectation is that every one has something special to offer. Only in very striking cases (such as some horrible tyrant) does it become appropriate to decide that the bad far outweighs the good. And if in such cases utilitarianism supports tyrannicide that will hardly be held against it by many reflective people.

But would not people who might replace a person we kill equally offer their own distinctive contribution to the good of sentient life? Doubtless so, but it does not augur much of a taste for what is good if one prefers what is completely unknown to what is a going concern. It would be foolish to tear down the buildings of a fine old city on the ground simply that something better is likely to be put in its place.

These considerations offer a rational justification of the general condemnation of such killing as is universally stigmatized as murder. They also suggest an approach, which cannot be developed further here, to controversial questions about killing which will be utilitarian in character while respectful of moral sentiments which utilitarianism is wrongly thought bound to treat lightly. Thus when the more obvious felicific calculations of the desirability of abortions under certain circumstances, or the use of aborted embryos and foetuses for experimental or other medical purposes, have been considered, great weight must still be given to the emotional congruence of whatever policy we support with attitudes to fellow humans which it is a great utilitarian good that we should have.[24]

[24] It seems clear enough that countenancing infanticide of children merely on grounds of parental convenience would not be thus congruent, so that the kind of utilitarian case for infanticide viewed with alarm by critics of utilitarianism (see, for example, Haksar, p. 132) does not seem to me one which would be made by someone whose serious concern was with the advancement of human happiness. The case of quite grossly abnormal children is more problematic, but however he decides it the utilitarian will not be obviously at loggerheads with some settled consensus of normal moral feeling.

[17]

ALLEN BUCHANAN

Advance Directives and the Personal Identity Problem

I. THE VALUE OF ADVANCE DIRECTIVES

Recent years have seen a marked increase in the use of and enthusiasm for advance directives for medical care. Perhaps the most familiar type of advance directive is the living will, a document whereby a person when competent issues more or less specific instructions as to which forms of care or treatment she wishes to have or not to have under certain circumstances, when she is no longer competent to decide. The other main type of advance directive, usually called a durable power of attorney, is the designation of a proxy, a trusted individual or committee of individuals who are to make decisions for a person after she becomes incompetent. It is possible to combine the two: a person may designate a proxy but also lay down instructions that place limits on the proxy's discretion to decide.

What is the value of advance directives—or, more precisely, what values are they supposed to serve? Either of two answers is usually given. First, advance directives are said to protect us from unwanted, virtually futile medical interventions that at best may prolong a miserable or meaningless existence. Second, some contend that advance directives are valuable because they allow self-determination, which is said to be valuable for its own sake. These answers, though correct as far as they go, are seriously incomplete. Indeed, they give a foreshortened picture not only of the value of advance directives, but also of the moral life.

In addition to protecting its author from unproductive bodily invasions and allowing her to exercise self-determination, an advance directive can allow her to relieve emotional and financial burdens that would otherwise fall on others. By issuing an appropriate advance directive one can *do good*

I am grateful to Dan W. Brock, Joel Feinberg, Deborah Mathieu, and Daniel I. Wikler for helpful comments on an earlier version of this article.

to others.[1] Viewing advance directives in this broader way can be liberating. Instead of being seen simply as devices for protecting the patient or for exercising autonomy for its own sake, they might in addition become vehicles for *new forms of altruism*, new ways of exercising the virtue of charity. For example, instead of specifying that if one comes to be in a persistent vegetative state all means of life support are to be withdrawn, a person with a strong sense of social obligation might instead request to be sustained in such a condition until his organs and other transplantable tissues are needed to save or enhance the lives of others. For several reasons, then, advance directives are of great potential value. Nevertheless, serious objections can be raised against their use, as we shall see.

II. The Moral Authority of Advance Directives

Those who have shown unreserved enthusiasm for the use of advance directives have perhaps made the following assumption: if, as the courts and most bioethicists now agree, the competent individual has a virtually unlimited right to refuse treatment, even life-sustaining treatment, then the same choice ought to be respected when a competent individual makes it concerning a future decision situation through the use of an advance directive.

I have argued elsewhere that this assumption is dubious because it overlooks several morally significant asymmetries between the contemporaneous choice of a competent individual and the issuance of an advance directive to cover future decisions.[2] For example, even if at the time

1. For a person who takes a direct interest in the well-being of others who will be affected by what is done to her after she becomes incompetent, an advance directive can make a significant contribution to its author's own good in two ways. First, the issuance of an advance directive can contribute to its author's well-being *while she remains competent* by reducing her anxiety about the distress her loved ones would experience in making difficult decisions without her guidance, and by assuring her that they will not be subject to crushing and wasted financial costs. Second, there is a sense in which our interests can survive us. I have an interest in how my family will fare after my death, and that interest survives me in the sense that whether or not it is satisfied will depend upon events that occur after I am gone. An advance directive can help me ensure that my "surviving interests" are satisfied. To the extent that one's well-being, or at least the goodness or success of one's life, depends on how one's interests in general fare—including one's surviving interests—an advance directive can make an important contribution to it.

2. Allen Buchanan, with Dan W. Brock and Michael G. Gilfix, *Surrogate Decision-Making for Elderly Individuals Who Are Incompetent or of Questionable Competence*, report prepared for the Office of Technology Assessment, U.S. Congress, 1986, chap. 3. See also Allen

279 *Advance Directives and
the Personal Identity Problem*

an advance directive was issued an individual was well informed about the options available should she develop a particular disease or be in a certain condition, therapeutic options and hence prognosis may change between the time the directive was issued and the time at which it is to be implemented. A second morally relevant difference is that the assumption that a competent person is the best judge of her own interests is weakened in the case of a choice about future contingencies under conditions in which those interests have changed in radical and unforeseen ways.

A third and equally significant asymmetry is that important informal safeguards that tend to restrain imprudent or unreasonable contemporaneous choices are not likely to be present, or if present, to be as effective, in the case of an advance directive. If a competent patient refuses life-sustaining treatment, those responsible for her care can and often do urge the patient to reconsider her choice, and in some cases this can prevent a precipitous and disastrous decision. This safeguard, if it occurs at all, is unlikely to come into play as forcefully during the process of drawing up an advance directive. For when the decision to forgo life-sustaining treatment is a remote and abstract possibility it is less likely to elicit the same protective responses that are provoked in family members and health care professionals when they are actually confronted with a human being who they believe can lead a meaningful life but who chooses to die.

Once these three asymmetries are appreciated, it should be clear that even if the competent patient has a virtually unlimited right to refuse life-sustaining treatment, it does not immediately follow that a refusal of life-support ought always to be respected if it is expressed in an advance directive. After more complex argumentation, however, we might well conclude that in spite of these asymmetries the law ought to regard valid advance directives as having the same force as a competent patient's contemporaneous choice. For we might be persuaded that attempts to limit the authority of advance directives would in practice lead to their being ignored by paternalistic physicians or families, thus robbing them of their value. The well-documented persistence of unjustified paternalistic behavior by physicians indicates that this is a significant danger.[3]

Buchanan and Dan W. Brock, "Deciding for Others," *Milbank Quarterly* 64, supp. 2, in press.

3. Allen Buchanan, "Medical Paternalism," in *Paternalism*, ed. Rolf E. Sartorious (Minneapolis: University of Minnesota Press, 1983), pp. 61–81; Buchanan, Brock, and Gilfix, *Surrogate Decision-Making for Elderly Individuals*, chap. 3; Charles W. Lidz et al., *Informed Consent* (London: Guilford Press, 1984), esp. pp. 8–9.

III. Loss of Personal Identity

There is, however, a much more profound and potentially grave threat to the moral authority of advance directives which remains even if we conclude that, all things considered, the asymmetries cited above do not provide sufficient grounds for limiting that authority. This is the objection that the very process that renders the individual incompetent and brings the advance directive into play can—and indeed often does—destroy the conditions necessary for her personal identity and thereby undercut entirely the moral authority of the directive.

This challenge rests upon the assumption that whatever the correct theory of personal identity turns out to be, it will include the claim that psychological continuity is (at least) a *necessary condition* for personal identity. In what follows I will accept this assumption for the sake of argument. Though I believe it can be adequately defended, I shall not attempt to do so here. I think it is also fair to say that this view about personal identity is already so widely held and well supported in the philosophical literature that the threat it appears to pose to advance directives ought to be taken seriously.[4]

The notion of psychological continuity, of course, is inherently vague, since the continuity between mental states (including memories, affective states, and dispositions) admits of degrees. Thus the question arises: just how "close" must various types of interconnections among such states and dispositions be to support an ascription of psychological continuity?

Nevertheless, the fact that there is a twilight does not show that we cannot distinguish between noon and midnight. There are some cases in which human beings suffer permanent neurological damage so severe that psychological continuity is utterly destroyed—cases in which there is no psychological continuity regardless of how low we set the standard of continuity necessary for the preservation of personal identity. This is so because some neurological damage causes the permanent extinction of all psychological properties and states, while stopping just short of the point at which (according to the whole-brain or brain death criterion) the individual ceases to live.[5] An individual who is in a "persistent vegetative

---

4. For an influential recent discussion of the psychological continuity view see Derek Parfit, *Reasons and Persons* (New York: Oxford University Press, 1986), pp. 204–9. See also H. P. Grice, "Personal Identity," in *Personal Identity*, ed. John Perry (Los Angeles and Berkeley: University of California Press, 1975), pp. 73–95.

5. For a detailed explanation of the whole-brain death criterion, according to which death occurs when there is a permanent cessation of all functioning throughout the brain (includ-

281

*Advance Directives and
the Personal Identity Problem*

state," an irreversible deep coma, fits this description, as do infants born with no cerebral cortex (anencephalics). In such cases the being has no psychological states or properties, only "vegetative," that is, autonomic, ones. For present purposes, such cases are wholly unproblematic, because on the conception of personal identity we are investigating, which I shall call the psychological continuity view, such patients have without question suffered a loss of personal identity. Difficulties arise, however, when irreversible neurological damage falls short of permanent unconsciousness but is nonetheless so severe as to call into question the persistence of enough psychological continuity to preserve personal identity.

The most troubling sort of case might seem to be the following: advanced Alzheimer's dementia has resulted in such extensive, permanent neurological damage that the patient's memory has been destroyed, his cognitive processes have been virtually obliterated, and all that remains is basic perceptual awareness. Unlike the persistently vegetative patient, the profoundly demented Alzheimer's patient can see and hear or at least has visual and auditory sensations (though this is not to say that he can distinguish conceptually and label appropriately what he sees and hears). In addition, the patient in question (again, unlike the permanently unconscious patient) is capable of pain and even of physical pleasure, though of fleeting and rudimentary sorts.[6]

Such cases have seemed to some to rob advance directives of their moral authority.[7] Their argument may be reconstructed as follows:

(i) One person's advance directive has no moral authority to determine what is to happen to *another person.*

(ii) In some cases of severe and permanent neurological damage, for example, that due to advanced Alzheimer's dementia, psychological continuity is so disrupted that the person who issued the advance directive no longer exists.[8]

---

ing lower and higher brain centers), see *Defining Death,* Report of the President's Commission for the Study of Ethical Problems in Medicine and Biomedical and Behavioral Research (Washington, D.C.: U.S. Government Printing Office, 1981).

6. Office of Technology Assessment, U.S. Congress, *Losing a Million Minds: Confronting the Tragedy of Alzheimer's Disease and Other Dementias* (Washington, D.C.: U.S. Government Printing Office, 1987), pp. 68–83. This chapter also contains a bibliography on Alzheimer's disease.

7. Rebecca Dresser, "Life, Death, and Incompetent Patients: Conceptual Infirmities and Hidden Values in the Law," *Arizona Law Review* 28, no. 3 (1986): 379–81.

8. Premise (ii) in the slavery argument is *not* offered as a claim about which individuals

Therefore

(iii) In such cases the advance directive has no moral authority to determine what is to happen to the individual who remains after neurological damage has destroyed the person who issued the advance directive.

Let us call this the slavery argument, since it portrays advance directives, not as vehicles for self-determination, but as sinister devices to subjugate other persons.

The slavery argument, however, is invalid—conclusion (iii) does not follow from the conjunction of premises (i) and (ii). To make it valid, another premise must be added:

(ii′) The individual who remains after neurological damage has destroyed the person who issued the advance directive is a (different) *person*.

Although the addition of premise (ii′) renders the argument valid, it also makes it vulnerable to the charge that it is unsound, because the truth of premise (ii′) can be challenged.

The key to appreciating the force of this challenge is to understand what sort of judgment we are making when we judge that the psychological continuity necessary for personal identity no longer exists. Psychological continuity, as we have already noted, admits of degrees, just as the decision-making capacities that constitute competence are a matter of degree.[9] Further, just as *where* we set the threshold for competence is a matter of choice, not a decision uniquely determined by the facts of the case, so also a choice must be made as to what degree of psychological continuity we will regard as necessary for personal identity and how much diminution of psychological continuity we will regard as the destruction of the person. As with the threshold of decision-making capacity for compe-

____

the law presently considers to be persons. Instead, the argument is intended to express a severe limitation on the *moral* authority of advance directives, a limitation which the law, if it is to be morally sensitive, *ought* to recognize.

9. *Making Health Care Decisions*, Report of the President's Commission for the Study of Ethical Problems in Medicine and Biomedical and Behavioral Research (Washington, D.C.: U.S. Government Printing Office, 1982), pp. 55–62. For a more detailed analysis of competence, see Buchanan, Brock, and Gilfix, *Surrogate Decision-Making for Elderly Individuals*, chap. 2.

283   *Advance Directives and*
                                           the Personal Identity Problem

tence, however, our choice of a degree of psychological continuity necessary for preservation of the person (or a degree of psychological discontinuity sufficient for the loss of personal identity) need not be *arbitrary*. There may be sufficient reasons for setting the threshold at one level rather than another, just as there are sufficient reasons for setting the threshold of decision-making capacities required for competence at one level rather than another.[10]

IV. How Much Psychological Continuity Is Enough?

It must be emphasized that the psychological continuity view does not itself answer the question "Just how much psychological continuity is necessary for the preservation of personal identity?" If the degree of psychological continuity necessary for preservation of personal identity is set rather *low* or, conversely, if the degree of diminution of psychological continuity compatible with the preservation of personal identity is set rather *high*, then *there will be very few if any real-world cases in which we would be justified in concluding that neurological damage has destroyed one person but left a living, different person*. For reasons that will soon become clear, a conception which sets the level of psychological continuity necessary for personal identity rather low may be called a *conservative* criterion of personal identity.

The crucial point is this: if we adopt a conservative (low threshold) criterion of psychological continuity, then those cases in which we can confidently conclude that the person, Jones, has ceased to exist (because neurological damage has so severely diminished psychological continuity) will be cases in which neurological damage is so catastrophic that we would be equally confident in concluding that the living being who remains is *not a person at all* and hence, *a fortiori*, not a *different* person, Jones II.

Although there is dispute about precisely which properties are jointly necessary and sufficient for personhood, there is considerable consensus in the philosophical literature as to what at least some of the necessary

---

10. In particular, it can be argued that, other things being equal, the greater the risk and the more complex the information that a reasonable person would want to take into account in making a given decision, the higher the level of decision-making capacities the individual should have in order to be considered competent to make the decision. See Buchanan, Brock, and Gilfix, *Surrogate Decision-Making for Elderly Individuals*, chap. 2.

conditions are.[11] The following cognitive capacities are among the strongest candidates for necessary conditions:

(a) the ability to be conscious of oneself as existing over time—as having a past and a future, as well as a present;

(b) the ability to appreciate reasons for or against acting; being (sometimes) able to inhibit impulses or inclinations when one judges that it would be better not to act on them;

(c) the ability to engage in purposive sequences of actions.

If any of these three, or anything even roughly similar to any of them, is at least a necessary condition of being a person, then it appears that the profoundly demented patient described above is not a person. It must be emphasized, however, that lack of personhood does not imply lack of moral status altogether. The very fact that a being can experience pleasure and pain may itself impose significant limitations on how we may act toward it.

It might be objected that this reasoning is flawed by an equivocation on 'person', because that term, as it occurs in debates about personal identity, embodies a *metaphysical* concept of persons, while the term 'person' is used in a *moral* sense when it is said that features (a)–(c) are necessary conditions for being a person. Thus even though the living being that remains after neurological damage produces a drastic diminution of psychological continuity may not be a person in the moral sense, it does not follow that that being is not a person in the metaphysical sense, and hence that he is not a different person from the person who issued the advance directive. And if he is a different person, then the advance directive of another person has no moral authority concerning how he is to be treated.

There are two difficulties with this objection. The first is that it rests on the very dubious assumption that a metaphysical and a moral sense of 'person', or a metaphysical and a moral concept of persons, can be neatly distinguished. The fact that philosophers typically appeal to our intuitions about responsibilities and commitments—that is, to basic *moral* concepts—in order to support their metaphysical theses about the criterion of identity for persons casts serious doubt on this assumption. Second, and more important, unless the concept of a person implicated in the psycho-

11. Joel Feinberg, "The Problem of Personhood," in *Contemporary Issues in Bioethics*, ed. Tom L. Beauchamp and LeRoy Walters, 2d ed. (Belmont, Calif.: Wadsworth, 1982), pp. 108–16, and Mary Ann Warren, "On the Moral and Legal Status of Abortion," in ibid., pp. 25–60.

                                    *Advance Directives and
                                          the Personal Identity Problem*

logical continuity view is in some sense the concept of *moral* personality, it is difficult to see why showing that psychological continuity has not been so severely diminished as to result in a loss of personal identity would establish that an advance directive still has moral authority. In other words, if the concept of a person implicated in the psychological continuity view is a purely metaphysical, nonmoral concept, then it is hard to understand why certain marks on paper made by a person in *this* (metaphysical) sense should *ever* be thought to create obligations or confer authority, since obligations can be created and authority conferred only by persons in the moral sense.

Indeed, it is not surprising that it is difficult, if not impossible, to distinguish a purely metaphysical, nonmoral sense of 'person', at least if we are looking for a criterion of personal identity that articulates or builds upon our ordinary, pretheoretical concept of personal identity. For surely our ordinary judgments typically, if not exclusively, are motivated by moral concerns—in particular, the ascription of responsibility, the recognition of rights and obligations, and the acknowledgment of commitments.

I suggested earlier that if the degree of psychological continuity necessary for the preservation of personal identity is set rather low, the cases in which we should be most confident in declaring that neurological damage has destroyed personal identity (without causing death) will *not* be cases in which we would judge that one person (Jones) is replaced by another person (Jones II). Instead, they will be cases like that of the profoundly and permanently demented individual with Alzheimer's dementia, where neurological damage has destroyed a person, and all that survives is a terminally ill nonperson with what we may call radically truncated interests. If this is so, then we will not be faced with a choice between implementing a formerly existing person's advance directive and protecting the rights and interests of another person who will be harmed, indeed destroyed, if the first person's advance directive is implemented. Instead, our task will be that of deciding whether following a formerly existing person's instructions is compatible with discharging whatever obligations we may have toward a living being whose existence will probably be brief no matter what we do and whose mental capacities are much less sophisticated than those of a small child or of a nonhuman animal such as a dog, and who virtually always suffers debilitating and painful physical ailments as well.[12] Should

12. Office of Technology Assessment, *Losing a Million Minds*, pp. 77–78.

we follow the advance directive and terminate support for the surviving individual, or should we ignore the advance directive (now that its author has ceased to exist) and attend only to the interests of the surviving individual?

The nature of the surviving being's interests provides an answer to this question. These consist solely in the interest in avoiding pain and the interest in having whatever fleeting, fragmentary, and unanticipated experiences of simple physical pleasure his or her damaged nervous system still allows. The crucial point is that our obligations to such a being are at best quite limited because of the radically truncated character of its interests. In the case of those "primitive" species of nonhuman animals who have such radically truncated interests, it is hardly controversial to conclude that our obligation is simply the negative one of not inflicting suffering (or that at most we are obligated to give them pleasure if we can do so at little cost to ourselves and without compromising the interests of other beings with more robust interests).[13]

It is tempting to believe that in such a case there is no moral conflict at all—no question of weighing the authority of the advance directive against the interests of the surviving being. For if the person who issued the advance directive no longer exists, then it would appear that her advance directive would be wholly irrelevant to the question of how we may treat this other individual. According to this line of thought, there is no conflict because the advance directive becomes *inapplicable*—null and void—with the extinction of its author. The advance directive exerts no moral pull whatsoever; all that is morally relevant is whatever moral status accrues to the (radically truncated) interests of the surviving individual.

This conclusion, however, will not stand scrutiny. A person who issues an advance directive may do so not only to exercise control over what happens to her*self* after she becomes incompetent, but also to protect certain interests she has in what happens to her body after she, the particular person who she is, no longer exists.

---

13. The fact that a profoundly and permanently demented Alzheimer's patient is a *human being* with radically truncated interests certainly makes a difference to most of us, psychologically speaking. Our greater sense of identification with members of our own species, unbolstered by any arguments of principle, may even be sufficient to justify behaving differently toward human beings with truncated interests simply because they are human beings, if we *choose* to do so. But none of this shows that we have robust, positive *obligations* toward them.

287   *Advance Directives and*
                        the Personal Identity Problem

Persons often have interests that survive them. Most persons, for example, have an interest in the well-being, both financial and personal, of their loved ones, and many have an interest in how their mortal remains are treated. These are "surviving interests" in the sense that whether they are satisfied or thwarted depends upon events that occur or do not occur after the person no longer exists.

Suppose that you have issued an advance directive including the instruction that if you become permanently and profoundly demented—that is, if you are "succeeded" by a terminally ill nonperson with truncated interests—all life-support efforts are to be withdrawn. Presumably you have a legitimate interest in what happens to your living remains under these circumstances, just as you have a legitimate interest in what happens to your body after you are pronounced dead. Your advance directive is a tool for protecting that interest.

Your interest in not having your remains sustained by life-support systems may be based on your notion of personal dignity or fittingness, or it may be based on your commitment to avoiding what you believe to be unjustifiable burdens on your family or on society. Part of what makes advance directives so attractive to many people is that they can serve as a device for securing such surviving interests.

Just as the interest in the treatment of one's corpse is a legitimate interest of persons, so is one's interest in what happens to one's living remains. We would be justified in thwarting the latter interest only if satisfying it required the thwarting of other, morally weightier interests. In the type of case under discussion, however, following an advance directive will not thwart morally weighty interests. Instead, it will only result in the earlier death of a severely physically debilitated, suffering, terminally ill being who possesses only radically truncated interests.

So the advance directive is applicable and does override whatever extremely limited obligations we may have to sustain the life of the surviving individual in such cases. The legitimate interest one has in determining what happens to one's living remains makes the advance directive applicable, even though the person who authored it no longer exists. And in the absence of countervailing weighty moral interests that would speak in favor of sustaining those living remains, we should acknowledge the legitimacy of the person's interest by following the advance directive.

The preceding argument establishes that *if* the degree of psychological continuity necessary for the preservation of personal identity is set very low, then three conclusions follow. First, adoption of the psychological continuity view of personal identity does *not* undercut the moral authority of advance directives because the slavery argument is invalid or, if modified to achieve validity, unsound. Even if the person who issued the advance directive no longer exists, it does not follow that following the advance directive is inflicting one person's will upon *another person*. Second, if the being that remains after neurological damage undercuts personal identity is not a person but a being with radically truncated interests, our obligations toward that being are quite limited. Following an advance directive to achieve a painless termination of life support for a being with such radically truncated interests need not involve the violation of any obligations toward that being. Third, whether neurological damage that results in the diminution of psychological continuity presents us with a choice between following one person's advance directive and preserving another person's life will depend upon the degree of psychological continuity required for the preservation of personal identity. If it is set quite low, such choices will only rarely, if ever, be necessary.

This is an important result. For if faced with such a choice we would have to disregard the advance directive. To do otherwise would be to give one person a wholly illegitimate, nonconsensual power of life and death over another person. So if the threshold for psychological continuity were set so high that loss of personal identity was a frequent occurrence, then the authority of advance directives would be frequently undercut. If the threshold is set low, however, the mere possibility of loss of personal identity will not threaten the legitimacy of advance directives. However, nothing said so far supports the further claim that the degree of psychological continuity *ought* to be set so low.

V. ATTEMPTS TO RAISE THE THRESHOLD

Indeed, some proponents of the psychological continuity view have adduced hypothetical examples calculated to convince us that we do or should set the threshold rather high—or, conversely, that we do or should regard some disruptions of psychological continuity far less drastic than those wrought by advanced Alzheimer's dementia as constituting a loss of personal identity.[14] The two examples that follow have been used to sup-

14. Donald Regan, "Paternalism, Freedom, Identity, and Commitment," in *Paternalism*, ed. Sartorious, pp. 113–38.

 *Advance Directives and
the Personal Identity Problem*

port the high threshold (that is, radical as opposed to conservative) view in the following fashion. First, those who offer them surmise that most thoughtful and morally discerning people would respond to the cases in a certain way. Then they suggest that the explanation, or at least the best explanation, of these moral responses, or at least the best way to render them principled and consistent, is to acknowledge a concept of personal identity that sets the threshold of psychological continuity necessary for persistence of personal identity quite high.

The first case is that of a young nineteenth-century Russian nobleman who is, he sincerely professes, committed to socialist ideals. Since he knows that later in life he will inherit vast wealth and may be tempted to abandon his socialist ideals, he extracts a promise from his young wife. If, after he inherits the fortune, he attempts to renege on his commitments to redistributing it to the poor (freeing his serfs, and so on), she is to prevent him from doing so. Those who employ this example first conclude that we think it proper for the woman to resist her middle-aged husband's attempts to keep the wealth for himself or that at the very least we recognize that she faces a serious conflict of moral obligations.[15] This first conclusion seems unexceptionable. However, those who employ the example go on to contend that this moral assessment presupposes or at least is best explained by the judgment that we regard the young nobleman and the middle-aged husband as *different persons*.

This latter conclusion, however, is as unconvincing as it is gratuitous. To understand the wife's predicament we need only recognize that the obligations a person acquires through a promise made to another can sometimes conflict with other obligations she has toward *him*, and that a person may find it advisable to use a promise extracted from another to prevent *himself* in the future from abandoning his current commitments.

This is not to say that the wife would or should choose to honor the promissory obligation at the price of other values or obligations. She might, for example, conclude that her youthful husband had been deluded, brainwashed by leftist friends, and that his commitment had been formed under duress or at a time when he lacked competence to make it. (Similarly, we might conclude that a particular advance directive for medical treatment was invalid because issued under duress and hence fails to confer authority or create obligations.) If, on the other hand, the wife be-

15. Derek Parfit, "Later Selves and Moral Principles," in *Philosophy and Personal Relations*, ed. A. Montefiore (London: Routledge and Kegan Paul, 1973).

lieved that her youthful husband's commitment to socialist ideals and his decision to ask her to make the promise were ones he was competent to make and were substantially voluntary, then she might conclude, with justification, that she should resist his current pleas. Clearly, one obvious condition for being released from a promise does not apply here: the wife cannot justify not acting on the promise on the grounds that the promisee failed to foresee the current situation and would not have wished the promise to be carried out in it. His whole point in asking her to make the promise, rather, is that he did foresee that he would be tempted to abandon his ideals.

Moreover, if we were to take literally the proposal that the man who extracted the promise no longer exists, we would get a dissolution, not an explanation, of the wife's serious *moral* conflict. For now her current husband is simply making the outrageous and immoral claim that he is entitled to her former husband's property. Though the "widow" may, for prudential reasons or out of love for her second husband, *prefer* to misuse the money her first husband entrusted to her, she can view this as a conflict of *moral obligations* only if she is either confused or self-deceiving. In sum, the first example does nothing to support the claim that the threshold of psychological continuity either is or should be set so high as to wreak havoc with the moral authority of advance directives.

The second example is no more persuasive. It concerns an elderly saintly man who is for good reason awarded the Nobel Peace Prize. After the prize is awarded it comes to light that some sixty years earlier a very young man—who not only bore the same name as the Nobel laureate, but also had a body and brain identical with those of the laureate—ferociously attacked and injured a policeman in a brawl.[16] Purveyors of this example contend that it supports their claim that we do or at least should conclude that the young rowdy and the saintly laureate are different persons, that the links of psychological continuity stretching from the former to the latter are sufficiently tenuous as to fall short of the appropriate degree of continuity necessary for the persistence of a single person.

This conclusion, as in the Russian nobleman case, is supposed to provide an explanation, or the best explanation, of our moral responses to the case. Presumably the relevant moral response would be an unwillingness to punish the saintly elderly laureate for the crime of the rowdy youth. But

16. Parfit, *Reasons and Persons*, p. 326.

it should be obvious that there is another way of explaining this response that is at least equally plausible as an explanation and that does not require us to embrace the radical conclusion that the young man and the laureate are different persons.

We may, instead, conclude that *mercy*—which presupposes guilt and hence the preservation of identity—is appropriate in this case, for several reasons. First, in this case punishment would not serve at least two of the goals that are usually thought to justify it: it could neither *reform* the person on whom it would be inflicted (since he has already not only reformed himself, but become saintly), nor *deter* or *prevent* him from committing further crimes (since he is not now the sort of person who will ever commit any crime). Second, to the extent that we think of the criminal as having incurred through his crime a "debt to society," we may decide not to punish him because we believe that through the extraordinary efforts that earned him the Nobel Peace Prize the laureate has more than discharged that debt.

It might be objected that even if his debt to *society* has been discharged, the crime the young man committed wronged a *particular person*, the policeman, and that *this* debt has neither been paid to nor forgiven by that individual. To show mercy would be to fail to appreciate the nature of the criminal act—the fact that it was the wronging of a particular person. Consequently, the objection goes, we cannot explain the judgment that the laureate should not be punished by saying that it is an appropriate exercise of mercy. Instead, we can explain our judgment that he should not be punished—or at least justify it—only on the assumption that the laureate and the youth are different persons.

This objection contains a grain of truth, but it is nonetheless spurious. All it establishes is that showing mercy by not punishing the laureate is one thing, while deciding not to require him to render compensation for his wrong to the policeman is another. If, as seems appropriate, we view the offense as both a public and a private wrong, *we* may show mercy for the former, while acknowledging that it is up to the *victim* whether to forgive the latter.

Suppose the policeman has remained seriously incapacitated and wracked with pain since the injury. To the extent that we feel that the laureate owes him compensation, this belief *supports* the conclusion that the youth and the laureate are the same person. And, as we have seen, our feeling that the laureate should not be punished does *not* presuppose that he and the youth are not one and the same person. So it seems that the second example, like the first, fails to provide solid support for the conclusion that we do or should set the threshold of psychological continuity necessary for the preservation of personal identity quite high. Therefore, neither of these examples supports the claim that there will be a significant number of cases in which neurological damage is severe enough to undercut the moral authority of an advance directive by destroying its author while leaving in his place another *person*.

It might also be argued that a healthy and reasonable conservatism weighs heavily in favor of setting the threshold of psychological continuity required for the persistence of personal identity rather low. Some of our most important social practices and institutions—those dealing with contracts, promises, civil and criminal liability, and the assignment of moral praise and blame—apparently presuppose a view of personal identity according to which a person can survive quite radical psychological changes and hence a high degree of psychological *discontinuity*. If this is so, then given the value of these practices and institutions, we would have to have extraordinarily weighty reasons for giving up the view of personal identity upon which they are founded. But as we have seen, examples like those of the Nobel laureate and the Russian nobleman do not supply such reasons, since our responses to them can be explained quite well without assuming loss of personal identity. Nor, it should be recalled, does adoption of the psychological continuity view itself commit us to setting the threshold lower (or higher) than our social practices and institutions presuppose. That view is simply neutral as to what degree of psychological continuity is required for the persistence of the person. It appears, then, that since the value of preserving some of our most basic institutions and practices speaks in favor of setting the threshold of psychological continuity necessary for personal identity low, and there is nothing of comparable weight on the other side of the balance, we clearly ought to set (or rather leave) the threshold low.

The issue may not be quite so clear-cut as this, however. Consider what would occur if a much higher threshold of psychological continuity were *consistently* employed so that our expectations would adapt to it. Ponder, in particular, how such a change would affect the practice of issuing advance directives and more generally our practices of caring for incompetents.

If people knew that the degree of psychological continuity considered

*Advance Directives and
the Personal Identity Problem*

necessary for the preservation of personal identity was rather high and if they were confident that there were reliable methods for ascertaining when such a degree of continuity had been lost, they would take this into account. I would know, for example, that after I became incompetent I might suffer sufficient neurological damage so that others would judge that *I* no longer existed, but without the damage (at least for a time) being so catastrophic that what remained was not a person at all. I would know that if this occurred, I would be declared dead and my will would be read. The declaration of my death would have definite and predictable social, moral, and legal implications: my family would no longer be responsible (morally or legally) for the care of the different person who remained after I ceased to exist. Nor, presumably, would they have any special standing in decisions concerning the treatment or nontreatment of that person.

What I am suggesting is that it is a mistake simply to assume that a significant raising of the threshold of psychological continuity necessary for the preservation of personal identity would be incompatible with some of our most valuable social practices and institutions. It is also a mistake to assume that such a shift would undermine the practice of issuing advance directives. Instead, what might occur would be a revision of those institutions and practices and a narrowing of the scope of the authority of advance directives. There would be no conflict between honoring one person's advance directive and preserving the life of the different person who succeeded him because the authority of the advance directive would be understood by all concerned to begin with the onset of incompetence and to terminate with the loss of personal identity.

Nevertheless, it is worth contemplating what the cost—both moral and financial—of such a shift would be. There would, of course, be *transition costs*. Greater or lesser degrees of confusion, lack of coordination, and anxiety might result, depending upon how the new conception of personal identity—along with the new legal definition of the death of a person it requires—is implemented. But even after the transition had been achieved there would be major social, legal, and moral problems to deal with. The new system would result in the "births" of large numbers of "new persons" who would as it were spring full-blown into the world and who would not, strictly speaking, be the sons, daughters, husbands, wives, or friends of anyone. Such "new persons" would have no financial assets (or debts), nor would any individual or family be legally responsible for them. Of course, it might be possible to restructure our practices concerning family responsibility to include "quasi obligations" of family members to the "successor persons" of their deceased loved ones. Indeed we might fashion legal obligations of a limited sort and impute them to the "predecessor person" himself. The price of setting the threshold for psychological continuity high is that doing so enormously complicates and magnifies the problem of intergenerational justice.

The strangeness and complexities of the arrangements needed to cope with the new problem of intergenerational justice—and the potential for conflicts of obligations they generate—numb the mind. I sketch them here only to emphasize that those who have advocated adopting a view of personal identity that significantly raises the threshold of psychological continuity necessary for the preservation of the person simply have not thought through the disturbing implications of their proposal. Even worse, as I have already argued, they have given us no good reasons for undertaking the radical revision of our practices, institutions, and ways of thinking of ourselves and our relationships with one another that taking their proposal seriously would require.

VI. A Compromise Position

I have argued that even if the psychological continuity view is accepted, it does not follow that we should recognize a high threshold of psychological continuity as necessary for personal identity. And from this it follows that we have no reason to fear that the moral authority of advance directives will dissolve with or soon after the onset of incompetence, thus rendering them useless.

Even if I am correct in this, however, there is another thesis, held by Derek Parfit, the most prominent proponent of the psychological continuity view, which remains unscathed by my criticisms thus far. This is the claim that since psychological continuity is a matter of degree, we should acknowledge in our morality and social practices and institutions the implications of the fact that personal identity is not an all-or-nothing affair, but rather a matter of degree. In other words, the moral and social significance we attach to personal identity should reflect the fact that being the same person is not an either/or proposition, but a matter of more or less.

According to Parfit, not only philosophers but also ordinary people have tended to assume that personal identity is or depends upon some deeper, metaphysical fact. This, he believes, is a mistake. Psychological continuity

295   *Advance Directives and*
                                the Personal Identity Problem

is all there is to personal identity. There is no deeper (or other) fact of the matter. And the importance we attach to personal identity should reflect the fact that there is no deeper fact.

I propose to understand this latter thesis as follows. In real-life situations, the judgment that A is the same person as B typically has moral implications. Once we see that personal identity depends on psychological continuity (and not on any further or deeper fact) we should acknowledge that the character and force of the judgment that A is the same person as B *vary* with the degree of psychological continuity between the psychological states (or psychological properties) of A and those of B. For example, we ordinarily think that if A, the man we now see before us, is the same person as B, the cold-blooded killer who assassinated the president a year ago, then A is culpable for that killing. But, Parfit suggests, if personal identity depends upon psychological continuity, then the lesser the degree of psychological continuity, the lesser the culpability.

The application of this general thesis to the case of advance directives is straightforward. The greater the degree of psychological continuity between A, the competent person who issued the advance directive, and B, the (incompetent) individual whose body (and brain) are spatiotemporally continuous with A's, the greater the moral authority of the advance directive, that is, the more *weight* A's wishes, as expressed in the advance directive, should be accorded in determining what is to be done to or for B.

If taken at face value, this proposal does not represent a mere revision, even a radical revision, of our conception of personal identity. Rather, it is a proposal to do away with personal identity judgments as we ordinarily understand them and to replace them with judgments about differing degrees of psychological continuity and the differing moral weights that correspond to them. Once we accept the psychological continuity view, the thesis that psychological continuity is necessary for personal identity, along with the seemingly unexceptionable claim that psychological continuity is a matter of degree, the replacement of "all-or-nothing" moral judgments (A is responsible or he is not, A's wishes should be dispositive or they should not count at all) with varying moral weight judgments may seem inescapable.

But this is not so. There are powerful pragmatic reasons for maintaining a social consensus according to which degrees of psychological continuity which meet or exceed a particular threshold are sufficient for an *unqualified* judgment of personal identity, a judgment which carries with it *max-*

imal moral force. And this is so even if the moral weights corresponding to degrees of psychological continuity below the threshold may vary, diminishing as the degree of psychological continuity decreases. Similarly, being a competent adult depends on a complex of skills and capacities, and the possession of these skills and capacities is always a matter of degree. Nevertheless, there may be decisive pragmatic reasons for recognizing a certain threshold of the relevant skills and capacities as necessary for maturity and for ascribing, in an *all-or-nothing* fashion, a distinctive social and legal status to persons whose skills and capacities fail to meet that threshold. So from the claim that the psychological continuity upon which personal identity depends is a matter of degree, it does *not* follow that personal identity judgments should be replaced by judgments about varying degrees of psychological continuity and corresponding moral judgments concerning the varying weights of rights and obligations.

What sorts of pragmatic considerations might count in favor of the social recognition of a threshold of psychological continuity that might be used to make "all-or-nothing" personal identity judgments? First of all, any other approach faces daunting epistemic obstacles. Attempts to make numerous fine-grained judgments about degrees of psychological continuity would require far richer data than we ordinarily have or could acquire, even with great cost and effort. The various moral weights to be assigned to interests, rights, or obligations on the basis of these judgments of psychological continuity would be correspondingly ill founded and unreliable. Second, even if these epistemic difficulties could be surmounted, tailoring the ascriptions of rights and responsibilities to reflect such fine-grained distinctions would require institutions whose constituent rules would be so complex as to preclude most if not all people from mastering them well enough to achieve a stable framework for legitimate expectations and the efficient social coordination that depends upon such a framework.

Again, an analogy may help. Being designated a mature person (or competent adult), as opposed to a minor, carries with it a fairly clear-cut bundle of legal rights and social privileges and responsibilities. Of course, it is theoretically possible to fragment this bundle, by distinguishing different rights and obligations (or giving the same rights and obligations different weights) and mapping them onto varying degrees of the several skills and capacities which together constitute maturity. But here, as in the case of attaching different moral weights to rights, obligations, or interests in

*Advance Directives and
the Personal Identity Problem*

such a way that the weights correspond to different degrees of psychological continuity, greater sensitivity may come at a prohibitive price—costly information gathering that results nonetheless in inaccurate judgments and inefficiently complex institutions.

One of the attractions of a system that designates thresholds as markers for ascriptions of status (such as that of competent adult) and assigns bundles of rights (and obligations) indiscriminately to all who enjoy the status in question is that it facilitates coordination by sharply limiting the number and sensitivity of judgments upon which people must agree if their expectations are to be sufficiently congruent. It has long been noted that the social recognition of rights minimizes the need for complex consequentialist reasoning (and the potential for disagreement, error, and lack of coordination which such reasoning carries with it). Indeed, the appeal to rights typically avoids consequentialist reasoning by declaring consequences to be irrelevant. Similarly the use of a threshold of psychological continuity in the making of personal identity judgments not only reduces the number of estimates of degrees of psychological continuity, it also simplifies the ascription of rights and obligations by bundling them together and avoids the problem of recognizing different weights for rights and obligations corresponding to different degrees of psychological continuity.

If, as I am suggesting, a strong pragmatic case can be made for singling out a threshold of psychological continuity for personal identity judgments, there is nevertheless a way in which the (alleged) fact that personal identity is *really* a matter of degree could still be accommodated. We might attach full moral force to the rights and obligations that we ascribe to those who clearly meet or exceed the socially recognized threshold, while attaching diminishing moral significance to those obligations and rights (or to the interests that the rights serve) as we move "downward" from the threshold.

In the case of advance directives, this would amount to the following procedure. So long as the degree of psychological continuity which we take to be necessary for the preservation of personal identity is present, the advance directive has full moral authority. (Recall, however, my earlier argument that this "full authority" may *not* be as robust as the authority of the competent patient's contemporaneous decision.) As we move "downward" from this threshold, through lessening degrees of psychological continuity, the moral authority or force of the advance directive diminishes correspondingly. In other words, for cases that fall *below* the threshold—and only for those—the weaker the degree of psychological continuity, the more readily the advance directive may be overridden by competing moral considerations, including our concern for the well-being of the incompetent individual. Presumably a point is eventually reached at which the degree of psychological continuity between the author of the advance directive and the incompetent individual is so small that the advance directive of the former has no authority at all over the latter, at least if the incompetent individual can be said to have interests of any morally significant sort.

Thus even where diminution of psychological continuity is great enough to lead us to conclude that the incompetent individual is not the person who issued the advance directive, we might nevertheless conclude that there is enough psychological continuity to give the wishes expressed in the advance directive *some weight* in our decision concerning the treatment of the incompetent individual. This would amount to recognizing as morally significant the especially intimate relationship between these individuals while at the same time acknowledging that they are distinct individuals.

The virtue of the compromise view is that it acknowledges both the value of our current institutions and practices, which to a large extent do treat personal identity as an all-or-nothing affair, *and* the implications of the view that personal identity depends upon something, namely, psychological continuity, which admits of degrees.

That such a strategy is coherent is again made clear by the analogy used earlier. We can (1) admit that maturity (being a competent adult) depends upon skills and capacities that admit of degrees (and that there is no "deeper fact" about maturity), (2) single out a threshold level of these skills and capacities as necessary for maturity, (3) ascribe a bundle of moral rights and obligations only to those who meet or exceed the threshold level, and (4) ascribe successively more restricted (less weighty, more easily overridden) rights and obligations to those who fall further and further below the threshold. Thus nascent obligations and rights (or morally considerable interests) would ripen as the individual moves toward the threshold of maturity.

VII. CONCLUSIONS

The results of our investigation of the claim that a proper understanding of personal identity poses a serious challenge to the authority of advance

*Advance Directives and
the Personal Identity Problem*

directives can now be summarized. The thesis that psychological continuity is at least a necessary condition for personal identity is plausible and widely held. Yet on any reasonable interpretation of this thesis it is undeniable that there can be and indeed are some cases in which neurological damage results in loss of personal identity without being so complete as to result in death, as defined by the widely accepted whole-brain death criterion. Since those who are permanently unconscious have no *psychological* states or properties, there has been loss of personal identity in these cases, no matter how high or low we set the degree of psychological continuity necessary for the preservation of personal identity. Such cases pose no radical challenge to the moral authority of advance directives, however, because they are not cases in which following one (formerly existing) person's advance directive will end another, different person's life, since the permanently unconscious are not persons at all.

Nor do cases of profound and permanent dementia pose such a challenge, for in these cases neurological damage, though it falls short of permanent unconsciousness, destroys at least some of the necessary conditions for personhood. Here, too, as in the case of the permanently unconscious being, we are not faced with a choice between respecting the wishes of one (formerly existing) person and protecting the interests or rights of another person. There is this important difference, however: the profoundly demented individual, though not a person, is by virtue of her capacity for pleasure and pain a being with morally considerable interests. For this reason a genuine conflict may arise—between implementing the advance directive and acting in morally appropriate ways toward the profoundly demented individual. Such a conflict, however, is neither so fundamental nor so intractable as a conflict between the rights of two persons. One reason for this is that the profoundly and permanently demented Alzheimer's patient is not like a happy and otherwise normal individual who has simply lost some of his cognitive functions. On the contrary, the advanced Alzheimer's patient not only has radically truncated interests, but also has a very limited life expectancy and typically suffers a number of serious and often painful physical ailments as well. Our obligations toward such beings are to minimize their pain and to provide comfort, not to prolong their lives by costly medical interventions.

The psychological continuity view of personal identity does not itself provide an answer to the question: Where should we set the threshold for psychological continuity—what degree of psychological continuity is necessary for the preservation of personal identity? If the threshold is set high, then we will be forced to conclude that there will be many cases in which neurological damage destroys the person who issued an advance directive but leaves in his place a different person, over whose fate the advance directive can have no authority. If it is set low, the cases in which we are confident that loss of personal identity has occurred will be those in which what remains is not a person and, *a fortiori*, not a different person.

Some philosophers have adduced hypothetical examples to support the conclusion that we ought to set the threshold very high. These examples do not succeed, however, because our moral responses to them can be explained just as well (or better) by alternative hypotheses that do not presuppose loss of personal identity.

Setting the threshold high might not be incompatible with the existence of some of our most valued social practices and institutions—those involving commitment and responsibility—nor even with a coherent practice of implementing advance directives. For such institutions, as well as the practice of advance directives, may be flexible enough to adapt to a new conception of personal identity. However, the moral and social costs of the restructuring of our practices and institutions which such a shift in the threshold would mandate would be very high, and as yet we have no good reasons to incur them. Thus the fact that neurological damage can destroy the psychological continuity necessary for personal identity does not, as some have argued, undermine the moral authority or value of advance directives as a basic tool for dealing with problems of decision making for those who are incompetent.

A quite different implication of the psychological continuity view is that the very attempt to locate a threshold of psychological continuity (whether high or low) reveals a failure to understand that personal identity judgments, understood as all-or-nothing claims, ought to be replaced with judgments concerning degrees of psychological continuity, along with corresponding judgments concerning the moral weight of rights, obligations, or interests—including the moral weight to be accorded to interests expressed in advance directives. We have seen, however, that the thesis that the psychological continuity upon which personal identity depends admits of degrees does *not* entail that we should abandon the use of all-or-nothing personal identity judgments, any more than the fact that maturity depends upon skills and capacities that are a matter of degree entails that it is a mistake to designate as mature only those who possess the skills and capacities in question to a certain degree. There is nothing incoherent about designating a certain degree of psychological continuity as neces-

*Advance Directives and
the Personal Identity Problem*

sary for the persistence of personal identity *and* recognizing that psychological continuity is a matter of degree *and* admitting that psychological continuity is all there is to personal identity.

Nor is there any inconsistency in combining the threshold approach with social practices and institutions that recognize the diminishing moral authority of an advance directive as the degree of psychological continuity decreases below the threshold. Moreover, I have indicated why such a way of thinking about personal identity—which I have labeled the compromise position—may be advisable. It allows us to preserve the core of some of our most valuable practices and institutions, those which presuppose the use of all-or-nothing personal identity judgments, while acknowledging that personal identity is simply a matter of psychological continuity and does not depend on some deeper, metaphysical fact. This compromise approach allows us to make a significant place for advance directives among our social institutions and practices without presupposing a dubious metaphysical theory of personal identity. For cases in which justified all-or-nothing personal identity judgments can be made, valid advance directives have their full moral force. For cases in which psychological continuity has diminished to points below the threshold that grounds all-or-nothing personal identity judgments, the moral force of advance directives is correspondingly weakened and may disappear altogether.

This is not to say, however, that advance directives are never morally problematic. Perhaps the most troubling case for according an advance directive absolute authority would *not* be one in which we think that there has been a loss of personal identity. Instead, it might be of the following sort. An apparently valid advance directive specifies that no life-sustaining treatments, including antibiotics, are to be used on the individual if she suffers loss of cognitive function. The patient does suffer a serious loss of cognitive function due to a discrete neurological injury, such as a stroke. She is now a mentally handicapped person, but clearly a person—and indeed the same person—nonetheless. Moreover, the patient is otherwise healthy, is apparently quite happy, and wants to live. Then she develops a life-threatening pneumonia. Following the advance directive will result in the easily avoidable death of a happy and reasonably healthy, though mentally handicapped, person. Suppose also that she is judged not to be competent to rescind the advance directive. There is clearly a sense in which a decision to ignore her advance directive would interfere with her earlier autonomous choice.

Cases like this challenge the depth of our commitment to individual autonomy and with it the assumption that the moral authority of advance directives may never be limited on paternalistic grounds. I am not convinced that it is possible to provide a conclusive argument to show that paternalism is never in principle justified in any such case. My aim here, however, is not to evaluate paternalistic challenges to advance directives but rather to evaluate a more fundamental objection rooted in the problem of personal identity.

It is important to emphasize, however, that the combination of factors that makes cases such as this so disturbing will probably be quite rare. And it is worth repeating that the challenge such cases pose to the authority of advance directives does not rest on the assumption that there has been a loss of personal identity.[17] The fact that neurological damage can result in loss of personal identity without death is not, I have argued, a serious challenge to the moral authority of advance directives.

17. For a more comprehensive treatment of advance directives see Allen Buchanan and Dan W. Brock, *Deciding for Others: The Ethics of Surrogate Decision-Making* (Cambridge: Cambridge University Press, forthcoming).

[18]

Journal of medical ethics, 1988, **14**, 173-1.

Philosophy, medicine and its technologies

Brenda Almond   *University of Hull*

Author's abstract

*There is a need to bring ethics and medical practice closer
together, despite the risk and problems this may involve.
Deontological ethics may promote* sanctity *of life*
considerations against the quality *of life considerations
favoured by consequentialists or utilitarians; while talk of*
respect *for life and the* value *of life may point to more
qualified ethical positions.*

*This paper argues for a respect-for-life position,
dismissing a utilitarian cost-benefit outlook as too
simplistic; but an unqualified fixed principles approach is
also ruled out, both because of its unacceptable
consequences in individual cases and also because of its
reliance on the slippery slope argument which, it is argued,
is logically and psychologically deficient.*

*The case of genetic engineering provides an example in
which the notion of respect may operate, but in which
broad general principles also apply. A cautious
conservatism towards accepted principles is recommended
in the development of medical technologies.*

Developments in medical technology over the last two
decades as well as changes in the law have created a
much livelier interest in medical ethics than prevailed
in days when death was indisputable and un-
postponable, and life, once established in the womb,
could only be suppressed at the cost of drastic danger to
the pregnant woman. The current situation is one in
which humans, to cite a much-used phrase, have an
opportunity, if they wish to take it, to 'play God'. Life
may be created in the laboratory test-tube. The nature
of that life can be altered by gene-splicing. Those who
reach a point of death through the deterioration of a
vital organ may have their lives prolonged by organ
transplantation; those unable to eat and unable to
breathe may be intravenously fed and artificially
respirated; and when death is inevitable, the process of
dying may be indefinitely prolonged. Possibly the
balance of power between humans and nature is about
to be restored by AIDS: an infectious virus illness of
long latency and inevitable fatality which is beyond the
reach of medical control or cure. This too, has already

Key words

Medical technology; philosophy and medicine.

produced legal and ethical dilemmas, though these are
of a different order from the dilemmas that arise from
medical advance.

Ever since the development of the first atomic
weapons, and the doubts about their use expressed by
the scientists who produced them, people have been
aware that scientific advance divorced from ethical
sensitivity is a Frankenstein capable of destroying its
creators. In a different metaphor, it is Adam and Eve in
the Garden of Eden choosing to eat of the tree of
knowledge and neglecting to eat of the tree of Good and
Evil. But philosophy in recent decades has itself posed
a barrier to any linking of science and morality in the
shape of the fact-value distinction. Empiricist
philosophy itself – the philosophy in which scientific
advance is grounded – has firmly separated theory
from practice: considerations about the nature of
morality from decisions about what to do. Only
recently, with the challenge to fundamental
presuppositions of empiricism from logic (Quine,
Putnam) and from philosophy of science (Kuhn,
Feyerabend, Lakatos) has it become possible for moral
philosophy to shake itself free of the restraints imposed
on it by Hume, and pursued in the present century by
both logical positivists and linguistic philosophers.

This transformation of philosophy has, as it
happens, coincided with the perceived need of medical
science to find an acceptable ethical framework for
difficult practical decisions. Faced with new
developments in intensive care, in cardiac
resuscitation, organ transfer and the new techniques of
reproduction, some philosophers have duly rushed in,
as the philosopher David Lamb has put it, where
neurologists or other medical professionals rightly fear
to tread (1). It seems even, in some cases, that they
have failed to apply the imaginative exercise of seeing
that, unlike the debates of the philosophy classroom,
the ethical arguments that win the day in medicine
have serious and significant consequences in the lives
of ordinary people. They may themselves, personally,
for example, find ultimately that their dying is
agonisingly prolonged as a result of arguments they
have successfully urged about the definition of death,
or the moral and legal constraints that should be placed
on physicians. On the other hand, of course, they may
have their life cut short because arguments in the other

174 *Philosophy, medicine and its technologies*

direction have won the day. Or, to change the example: because some ethical theorists have won a political argument centred on civil liberties in relation to the issue of testing for HIV infection, certain other individuals may be exposed to infection and die prematurely of AIDS, who would *not* have died had policies based on stressing responsibility for others won the day.

So, however they choose to use it, philosophers do have a new freedom; applied philosophy is accepted *within* philosophy and made welcome in many practical areas outside it. The skills that moral philosophers have to offer are their familiar weapons of argument and counter-argument, but the situations in which they must deploy these weapons are wholly novel: they are situations in which bad arguments can actually kill, or at least add needlessly to the sum of human suffering. There is a need for caution, then, and due consideration – for testing an argument in hypothetical application to one's own case, and for asking the question, previously considered inappropriate in philosophical discussion: 'Is what I propose to say likely to be useful or helpful to those currently confronting this problem personally?' It need hardly be said that such a question would retrospectively eliminate many of the articles that have been published on the subject of abortion.

Despite these caveats, however, the need to bring ethics and medical or scientific practice closer together overrides the risks involved. As a recent group of commentators on this issue has written: 'Almost every action within the medical setting either explicitly or implicitly contains two judgements, one ethical and one scientific, and there is constant interplay between what is technically possible and what is morally desirable' (2). There is clearly, then, a need for what the moral theologian Ian Ramsey called a 'human and not a tyrannical technology' (3) – a need, in other words, to attempt to marry or harmonise scientific expertise and moral sensitivity.

It is worth remarking, too, that today's discussions take place in the shadow of a single appalling precedent: that period just before and during World War II when certain medical professionals abandoned normal ethical sanctions and operated briefly, albeit under enormous pressures, in separation from the traditional and proper concerns of medicine. It is right to recall that brief phase of Nazi medicine as a counter to the arguments of those who might today wish to press ahead in various areas without restraint in the name of scientific progress.

But given that a need is acknowledged, there is less agreement about what should be the starting-point for the project of linking morality and medical science. Should that starting-point be ethical theory or medical practice? Is it, in other words, better to start by setting out broad ethical positions before going on to draw detailed practical conclusions? Or is it preferable to start from the standpoint of the particular: a problem-oriented or case-by-case approach? In deciding between these alternatives, practical considerations may reasonably be allowed to play some part. When, for example, the goal is to initiate professionals-in-training into a concern for the moral aspects of their work, it is probably enough simply to ask which method is more *effective*, or is found more acceptable by those involved. And it may well be that the case-by-case approach – arriving at principles from the detail of particular instances – is right for these situations. But for forming a wider overview of the situation – for seeing things on a macro rather than a micro scale, as is necessary for legal or political decision-making, it may be that it is necessary to set out broad principles first and to move on from them to particular conclusions.

Again, where what is at issue is doctor-patient interaction, consideration of particular cases may be appropriate, but where a whole area of scientific research, such as, for example, genetic engineering, is in question, keeping one's eye on the detail may be a way of failing to see the wood for the trees.

In the end, however, it is likely that, provided the reasoning is sound, both these methods of approach will ultimately lead to the same destination. Ethical theory must complete itself in the realm of the particular; while close attention to the moral aspects of particular cases should in the end bring an understanding of certain broad ethical positions. Either way, the road to be travelled is likely to be via some broad but specifically *medically-oriented* principles such as those proposed, for example, by Gillon: autonomy; beneficence; non-maleficence, and justice ('fair adjudication between competing claims') (4).

For present purposes a combination of these methods may be most appropriate: starting with a specific example and seeing what broad considerations it involves. We might consider for this purpose an actual case cited by a consultant in Scotland: the sterilisation without her knowledge or consent of a young married woman whose first child had just been stillborn (personal communication). The case as described seems to flout most principles: the woman's right to make her own decisions; her right to information; the consultant's duty to respect these rights; the woman's loss of the child-bearing capacity, and so on. But when the consultant added further factual information: that delivery of the child had revealed an advanced stage of cancer and an urgent need to proceed to a treatment which necessarily resulted in sterility, it becomes clear that another principle was operating – most would say rightly in this case: a consideration of the practical consequences, together with a presumption in favour of producing the best or happiest outcome possible in the circumstances, irrespective of rigorist or legalistic considerations.

What this case reveals, then, is the central conflict to be found in very many instances and cases, between the autonomy principle and the principle of beneficence – between respect for patients' preferences or rights and consideration of their *interests*. While this is characteristic of the ethical dilemmas that arise in the clinical setting, the area of medico-scientific research gives rise to another range of moral considerations. Both kinds of problem are involved, however, in situations which involve patients themselves in experimental procedures. In these overlap cases, there is, for ethics committees in hospitals, not only the problem of balancing the patient's autonomy against the patient's best interest. There may also be a need to balance the interests of current patients against those of future unknown patients – or to trade the good of many for the comfort or risk of a few. In these cases, the patient's autonomy and the need for informed consent may be set against the welfare of future patients – the greatest good of the greatest number – which may only be achievable by involving present individuals in experimental procedures, either as subjects or controls.

There are areas of research, however, which may pose ethical dilemmas without directly involving patients, and so without raising the issue of autonomy: such areas, for example, as genetic engineering and, in particular, the manipulation of human genetic material. A different way, then, of formulating the ethical issues may be needed to produce principles of the level of generality that is required to set these issues, too, in an appropriate moral context.

The term 'deontological' is commonly used to characterise the views of those who favour strict adherence to rules or principles above practical utility. But in medicine, it seems to be distinctive of a deontological approach that it stresses one basic moral intuition in particular: that of the *sanctity* of life (5). It is characteristic of a consequentialist position, on the other hand, which bases decisions on outcomes – an approach contrasted with the first as 'teleological' – that it regards *quality* of life considerations as decisive (6). And those who might wish to avoid philosophical absolutes of any kind but are nevertheless disturbed by the extent to which humans are prepared to manipulate nature or human materials, and to exploit it/them without limit for ends they deem to be desirable, may speak of a *respect* for life requirement (7). There may also be a presumption in favour of the *value* of life which equates with none of these, but is used to express the view, which sounds truistic but which is in fact a non sequitur – that life is worth living and should therefore be preserved at all costs (7).

The mention of costs here reminds us that there is another dimension to these ethical and medical arguments: the economic and the political. The standpoint of those who introduce cost-benefit considerations tends to be utilitarian or outcome-oriented. It usually involves appeal to quality-of-life considerations, and does not see the *value* of life as absolute or uncomputable.

For people who stand on the consequentialist side of the ethical debate the case-by-case approach to ethical judgement may be favoured not simply for methodological reasons, but for deeper and more ideological reasons. They may wish to make the claim that all judgements are essentially individual and particular. And, despite the claims of some rule-utilitarians to the contrary, it would seem to be an essential aspect of the utilitarian position that consequences should be calculated in particular settings. They are relevant to an occasion and an instance. This applies even where following a broad rule is advocated for the majority of cases. Utilitarians who deny this have in fact unwittingly lined up with deontologists.

This emphasis on particular cases brings utilitarians close to the views of those who favour the kind of situation ethic advocated by some religious thinkers (8). Religion, on the whole, however, may be expected to be found in alignment with the approach to medical ethics that stresses the importance of principles. It is an extremely important force within medicine, first because there are a number of key areas where religious absolutism conflicts (a) with what some patients want, as well as with what has been conceded to them by law, such as, for example, abortion – and (b) with what some medical professionals would wish to offer but are not allowed to by law, such as the early termination of suffering by euthanasia in cases where death is inevitable. On the whole, religion operates as a conservative influence in medicine, since the pronouncements of the main religions on most subjects were formulated *before* the technological advances that have given rise to so many current dilemmas.

This is not, however, to decry a principled approach, far from it. On the contrary, some further considerations will be advanced here – and one argument in particular will be discussed – which might incline the uncommitted or undecided towards a principled approach in the modified 'respect for life' sense, and away from an uncritical acceptance of the notion that maximising welfare – doing the best for everyone in a particular situation – is the right way to proceed. These considerations will have special force when it comes to issues which are not directly part of the clinical person-to-person encounter, but relate to matters of the moral limits to scientific advance, as in the case of genetic engineering, and the growing number of possibilities of interfering with what human beings are in the habit of calling 'the natural'.

The first of these considerations concerns what the Greeks called *hubris* – an arrogance which takes the form of humans placing themselves on a level with the gods. Perhaps it was this sort of *hubris* that was referred to in the introduction to a medical ethics textbook which stated 'With the help of biological and behavioural sciences, human beings are seizing control over human nature and human destiny' (9).

The feeling that there is such a moral lapse, despite the fact that we appear to have no word for it in the English language, is expressed by contemporary commentators in such claims as that human life – and perhaps life in all its forms – is intrinsically deserving of respect. David Lamb has used this notion of respect-worthiness to suggest that human material, such as embryos, or parts of the bodies of the dead, may be deserving of a modified degree of respect, as compared with actual human beings who receive full respect (10).

It may also be expressed in terms of feelings of outrage at certain developments. Mary Warnock advances this kind of consideration in discussing embryo research, speaking of 'barriers which should not be passed' and 'things which, regardless of consequences *should not be done*' (11). She cites Dr Robert Edwards as having argued that if the results of IVF research are beneficial (a) to the infertile or (b) to researchers into genetic disease and others with a legitimate interest, it must be right. Against this, Warnock insists 'No one's morality consists of nothing but a calculation of benefits and harms' (11).

These reservations are not, however, universally shared. For example, Diana Brahams, writing in the *New Law Journal*, speaks of the need to convert such wholly negative and destructive events as abortion into something of positive value. She would, it seems, advocate harvesting of parts from anencephalic neonates, from aborted fetuses, and from fetuses deliberately conceived for this purpose, where this might help another family-member. (She does not discuss the case of a pregnancy entered into for this purpose as a commercial venture.)

In pressing her case, Brahams uses another philosophical category rather than the one usually introduced, declaring that there is 'no *logical* objection to the use of fetal organs for transplantation' (12). This appeal to logic when ethics seems a doubtful ally is a striking new development in terms of the relation between philosophy and medicine. It is necessary to remember, however, that logic, being the science of tautologies, has nothing to say on *either* side of these or any other substantive issues.

Beyond these considerations, however, lies a yet wider context, in which the basic assumptions of Western medicine and science are challenged, either by the introduction of an Eastern or philosophically holistic perspective, or by, for example, a feminist analysis of the broad structures which shape the ethical setting for particular medical dilemmas.

One commentator has summed up the questions involved here in the following terms: 'What images of health, disease, normalcy, womanhood, sexuality, etc undergird the present delivery of health care and development of new biomedical technologies?' (13). She also asks: 'Should the new technologies be developed in the absence of basic nutritional, health and medical care in Third World countries?' (13).

These broader perspectives throw into sharp relief the extent to which a stress on autonomy and the rights of patients is part of a much wider liberal political perspective, based on a belief in freedom and self-determination. This is of course in itself an ethical stance, and one which would not necessarily command the support of people brought up within different traditions, with different expectations and desires. This constitutes a reminder that ethics, culture – of which the practice of medicine is a part – and, again, religion, are a closely-woven cloth.

For all these reasons, then, the piecemeal approach of utilitarianism, with its simplistic practical assumptions, needs to be treated with cautious suspicion, or, at least, care. An unqualified principle-based approach, however, is equally suspect. This may best be demonstrated by consideration of one argument which plays a uniquely important role in principled approaches: the metaphor of the slippery slope.

This argument tends to make its appearance when a single paradigm case is used to break a general principle, taboo or restriction. For example, the case of a child born without limbs, hearing, sight or brain-function may be cited as justifying euthanasia for defective new-born babies. Defenders of the slippery slope argument then suggest that this constitutes the thin end of the wedge (or first foot on a slope) the end result of which is that cases bearing less and less resemblance to the paradigm lose the protection of the moral taboo. So, for instance, it may be that a child with a mild form of Down's Syndrome will not be kept alive, or that an adult paraplegic, who nevertheless wants to live, will have his or her life prematurely terminated.

The slippery slope argument take two forms: one a logical argument, the other a comment on human psychology. Its effectiveness varies according to which form is in question. It is scarcely valid as a logical argument, as an examination of its basic form shows: a certain principle, the argument suggests, entails a certain action towards which we may be sympathetic (letting a grossly handicapped infant die, for example). It also might *seem* to entail another action we do *not* approve of (killing a moderately handicapped infant, perhaps). The advocate of the slippery slope argument then reasons: since the second action is wrong, the principle must be wrong. And since the principle is wrong, the first action must be wrong, too. Set out like this, it is clear that the slippery slope argument involves a double fallacy: other considerations could make the second action wrong; and even if a principle is wrong, not all actions compatible with it are necessarily wrong.

As a psychological argument, however, the slippery slope argument is more effective. Humans may be more disposed to take larger steps as a result of practice in taking smaller steps. A little bit of killing may lead to a hardened moral sensitivity which permits in the end of a great deal of killing.

But most commentators seem agreed that psychologically a stand may be taken at any point on the 'slope' of some particular medical issue that is judged appropriate in the light of current knowledge and medical expertise. And unless this flexibility is permitted, anomalies arise and harsh consequences may follow.

For example, *anomalously,* abortion of an anencephalic fetus may be legally and morally permissible (because it is not potentially capable of meaningful life outside the womb – hence not to be regarded in law as *viable*) but once born, it must be treated for its brief existence as a life. And, *harshly,* in Ireland, for example, such a fetus must be carried to term (12).

So the slippery slope argument is ineffective in establishing that principles should never under any circumstances be violated. As commentators on Kant's rigoristic presentation of moral principles have seldom failed to point out, principles may be of greater or lesser degree of generality, and their exact formulation can make all the difference to their acceptability.

Formulations of an ethical position in terms of the concept of respect for life, then, may seem preferable to those put forward in terms of fixed principle, as permitting the degree of flexibility that is in fact needed here.

It is this concept, too, that seems most relevant to ethical discussion surrounding such issues as the new technology of reproduction, genetic engineering and the use to which human tissue and organs may be put. To take the issue of genetic engineering as an example, it may be denied that important ethical issues *are* involved here, on the grounds that what is being achieved by genetic engineering, is simply a more sophisticated version of what generations of rose-growers, dog-breeders and farmers have tried to achieve in more traditional ways. And indeed, where what is at issue is the production of frost-free varieties of wheat or heavy-cropping apple-trees, it may be hard to see that ethical issues do arise. And certain other problems – the creation through gene-splicing of pests, viruses or microbes – while they *do* give rise to problems, may be perceived first as *practical* problems, rather than as moral ones. Inevitably, though, they *become* moral problems if they can harm or endanger *people*. It may be said that if there is no *intention* to harm, even if the results are catastrophic, then the scientists responsible have done nothing morally wrong, unless they have also been careless. However, in a situation where the consequences of the release of a new organism are irreversible and essentially unpredictable, it could be argued that this constitutes morally blameworthy irresponsibility. As far as public policy is concerned, some countries have banned experimental releases of this kind of organism; some impose no controls at all, and others require reporting and the seeking of official sanction for individual releases. Because of the uncertainties, it would seem that the moral requirement of concern to prevent avoidable harm would justify the latter as the *minimum* position.

However, the view that only the prevention of harm is involved here becomes less convincing once one moves away from the area of plants and micro-organisms and considers the creation of animal hybrids; or the creation of anencephalic clones for

spare-part surgery – or of a race of giants, or of a low-intelligence slave class. Even on such subjects, however, ethical opinion is divided. Jonathan Glover argues that the genetic alteration of human-kind is not morally objectionable, providing only *willing* parents donate their genetic material (14).

But R M Hare has reportedly argued that the possibility of genetic misfits – Chernobyl-type disasters in the genetic area – means that it would be wrong to experiment with human material. D H M Brooks, on the other hand, argues that there could be no moral objection to the creation of a happier society by the development of a race of willing slaves endowed with appropriate emotions (15).

On the whole, however, it seems right that interference with human genetic material should come under a special taboo – one which might also cover treatment of dead human tissue. While organ removal is widely regarded as ethically acceptable – in the case of kidneys, its endorsement is almost a moral requirement – there will be limits most people would acknowledge. (Would anyone be prepared to see human tissue made into high-protein food for calves, for example?). So it seems that a moral sensitivity does in fact operate in these areas which is neither deontology – expressible in terms of principles – nor teleology – a matter of undesirable consequences. Is this in its negative form what Warnock expressed as 'outrage'; in its positive form what others have expressed as 'respect'?

I should like to suggest that it is not precisely this, but rather something capable of a more rational formulation. What these issues involve is competing views of human nature: what humans are; what they may become; and how they may best find their fulfilment. Another way to put this is to say that, common to many ethical and religious theorists is a certain conception of human flourishing. In practice, an understanding of human nature in its various historical and cultural settings, as well as of human beings as biological organisms, suggests an ethical framework in which this flourishing is most likely to be achieved. As J S Mill put it, in the last chapter of *Utilitarianism* (16), this may after all involve adherence to certain principles of broad generality – the principle of justice, for example – that human beings have come to value over millenia. So, while repudiating a narrowly principle-based approach in human affairs we are no doubt right to be as the moral theologian Ian Ramsey put it, 'cautiously conservative towards the principles we already hold' (17).

These are not only principles for life, but also for death and dying. And indeed, in death and suffering, religion and medicine find a common focus. In expressing reservations, in feeling instinctively that it would be right to hold back, or at least to move only with caution in areas of technological advance that may affect human nature itself, we may be rightly holding on to what we know, and wisely hesitating about the plunge into the unknown. For, as David Lamb has pointed out, the issues are not insignificant. On the contrary, in his words: 'At stake is the *idea* of the humanness of our human life and the meaning of our embodiment, our sexual being, and our relations to our ancestors and descendants' (7).

Thirty years ago, a leading spokesman of the Christian religion was prepared to defend human manipulation of nature in strong terms. In 1958 Ian Ramsey wrote: 'The only sense in which the "unnatural" is wrong is that according to which "natural" is the perfection of creation towards which we aspire; and the knowledge whereby we are enabled to control the actual and mould it after the image of the ideal comes to us by the grace of God working through the devotion of human investigators. If it enables us to deflect the course of gametes into channels through which they will contribute to the making of a better civilisation than would result from their being left alone, it is showing us the way to use actual "nature" for the creation of the ideally "natural" ' (18). He added that interference with nature may not be a *failure* of reverence, but rather that *refusing* to interfere might itself be a kind of irreverence – ignoring, as he put it, God's guidance to doctors and technologists.

But thirty years have passed since then and thirty years have seen many changes which could not have been contemplated when Ramsey was reflecting on these themes. I do not think that, writing today, anyone with ethical sensitivity could pronounce so firmly in favour of unqualified further advance in medicine and its technologies. The ethical test to apply in all such developments is that these should not merely perpetuate the life of a biological organism unwilling to accept its necessary mortality, but that they should harmonise, too, with a higher notion of human existence – human existence which at its best, acknowledges its own transitoriness. This principle operates not merely to suggest self-restraint in the development of medical technologies but also to govern practice in the person-to-person encounters of clinical medical practice.

Brenda Almond is Director of the Social Values Research Centre, University of Hull.

References

(1) Lamb D. The death of reason in intensive care. *Times higher educational supplement* 1988 Mar 25; 17.

(2) Moros D A *et al*. Thinking critically in medicine and its ethics: relating applied science and applied ethics. *Journal of applied philosophy* 1987; 4: 229

(3) Ramsey I. Inaugural address to BMA. *British medical journal* 1972; 279: 214

(4) Gillon R. *Philosophical medical ethics*. Chichester: John Wiley and Sons, 1985.

(5) This position, espoused for example by E Anscombe, is set out clearly in Glover J. *Causing death and saving lives*. Harmondsworth: Penguin, 1977.

(6) The utilitarian approach is exemplified in Singer P, Kuhse H. *Should the baby live?* Oxford University Press, 1985.

(7) Lamb D. *The slippery slope*. Beckenham: Croom Helm, 1988.

(8) See, for example Fletcher J. *Moral problems in medicine*. Princeton NJ: Princeton University Press, 1954.

(9) Lammers S E, Verhey A. *On moral medicine*. Grand Rapids, Michigan: Williams B Berdmans Publishing company, 1987: preface: ix.

(10) See reference (8): chapter 9.

(11) Warnock M. Do human cells have rights? *Bioethics* 1987; 1: 1 – 14.

(12) Brahams D. Transplantation, the fetus and the law. *New law journal*. 1988; 137: 91 – 93.

(13) Lebacqz K. Bio-ethics: some challenges from a liberation perspective. See reference (9): 64 – 69.

(14) Glover J. *What sort of people should there be?* Harmondsworth: Penguin, 1984.

(15) Brooks D H M. Dogs and slaves: genetics, exploitation and morality. *Proceedings of the Aristotelian Society* 1987 – 88; LXXXVIII: 31 – 64

(16) Mill J S. *Utilitarianism*. London: Dent, 1954.

(17) Ramsey I. *Christian ethics and contemporary philosophy*. London: SCM Press, 1966.

(18) Ramsey I. See reference (17) and quoted in *Journal of medical ethics* 1987; 13: 190.

[19]

The Philosophical Quarterly Vol. 33 No. 132

Vol. 33 No. 132   July 1983

IN VITRO FERTILIZATION:
THE ETHICAL ISSUES

By John Harris

Human beings who appear to be attempting to play God attract the sort of hostility usually reserved for Gods who forget themselves so far as to aspire to do likewise. And just as "acts of God" are synonymous with disaster, so acts of scientists can appear disastrously divine. The spectre of Dr. Frankenstein, the representative "mad scientist", is standardly invoked as a dire warning of what to expect when researchers tamper with the ultimate constituents of what matters. However grotesque, there is a certain appropriateness to its invocation in the context of the discussion and speculation surrounding recent work on so-called "test-tube" babies.

The storm of interest and protest that this work has attracted and continues to attract[1] is, as is often the case, not on account of what is being done but for fear of what the work demonstrates can or might be done. The work in question,[2] initially undertaken to remedy infertility, involves the fertilization of human eggs "*in vitro*" and the growing of the resulting embryos in the laboratory for subsequent transplantation into mothers who have experienced difficulties in conceiving by more economical means. However, two of the leading people in this field, Dr. R. G. Edwards and Mr. Patrick Steptoe, whose work generated the first successful test-tube baby, have pointed the way clearly to new and controversial uses of their work[3] and others have been quick to follow. These controversial possibilities have led the British Medical Association first to condemn such work and to forbid their members to assist, then almost immediately to withdraw the ban and finally to set up an ethical sub-committee to report on the rights and wrongs of all such work. The moral

---

[1] See for example: *The Guardian*, 1st October 1982 and 8th October 1982, *The Observer*, 3rd October 1982, *The Sunday Times*, 3rd October 1982 and *The London Standard*, 27th September, 1982.

[2] That of R. G. Edwards and Patrick Steptoe. See particularly *Human Conception* In Vitro Edwards and Purdy ed. (London, 1981).

[3] loc. cit.

218   JOHN HARRIS

concern of the Government has also been stirred so far as to establish its own
ethical committee, the Warnock Committee, to make a similar report.

For all its innocent beginnings (and maybe endings too) the work of
Edwards and Steptoe and others has opened up possibilities and perhaps even
more important, public discussion of possibilities,[4] that have hitherto figured,
if at all, only in the dreams and discussions of moral philosophers. I shall start
in Section I by reviewing what is now being done by researchers in the field of
in vitro fertilization and indicate what such researchers believe will or may
become possible in the relatively foreseeable future. Section II will explore the
moral status of the embryo with a view to establishing the permissability of
killing such a being *in vitro* or *in vivo*. Section III will examine the question of
whether or not experiments on embryos raise different moral issues and
require different justification from those involved in deciding whether embryos may be killed or aborted. Finally, in Section IV we will consider whether
the possibilities opened up by *in vitro* fertilization constitute a slope so slippery
that we dare not step onto it.

                                       I

WHAT'S HAPPENING NOW

At the moment eggs can be removed from a woman and fertilised in a dish
on the laboratory shelf. These embryos can then be implanted in a woman so
that she can grow them and give birth to the resulting baby in the normal way.
About fifty such children have been born to women treated by Edwards and
Steptoe. If the embryos are not implanted they can continue to grow *in vitro* (at
the moment they have been so grown for up to nine days). They can then be
"flattened"[5] for examination, simply thrown away like most aborted embryos,
used for experiments and or for therapy (more of which anon), or they may be
frozen for future use.[6]

The Spare Embryo

Most eggs obtained for fertilization are provided by women who wish to
have a child and the embryos are re-implanted in the donor mother. So called
"spare" embryos are produced when, usually as a result of fertility hormones
being used, women produce multiple eggs which are all fertilised but of which
only one (or perhaps two) are re-implanted because of the added risks
attached to the prospect of multiple births. The remaining embryos are thus
"spare". Of course other spare embryos could and have been produced
deliberately and not as the bonus by-product of a fertility clinic. Indeed many

        [4] See *The Guardian*, 25th October 1982.
        [5] See Report in *The Guardian*, 8th October 1982.
        [6] This is the practice in Australia: See Edwards and Purdy, op. cit.

IN VITRO FERTILIZATION 219

such embryos were produced by Dr. Edwards and other workers in order to test and develop fertilization techniques.[7]

Permutations

We should note for the record a number of possibilities that arise. The eventual "host" mother may not be the donor of the egg cell and the donor of the sperm may or may not be known to the donor of either the egg cell or to the eventual host mother. So the possibilities are that because of conceptual problems (though of course not necessarily so):

(1) A woman may donate her own oocyte or egg cell to be fertilised either by her husband or partner or by some other donor spermatozoa, for re-implantation into herself.

(2) A woman may donate an oocyte for fertilization in any of the above ways for implantation in another woman either so that woman can have "her own" child (perhaps fertilised by her husband or partner) or so that the original donor can (for whatever reasons)[8] avoid pregnancy but still have "her own" baby.

Where a woman accepts a donor oocyte with the intention of giving birth to and bringing up the child as "her own" we might call this "prenatal adoption",[9] where the intention is that the resulting child be returned to the donor of the oocyte (or perhaps of the sperm) it might be called "uterine leasing" or "postnatal parenthood". And of course the baby might go to some "stranger".

Freezing

We have almost run ahead of ourselves, but not by very much. The question of whether or not it is dangerous to the embryo to freeze and thaw it is not yet finally resolved, and this is important if the above possibilities are to be realised as we shall see. There have been decades of work on freezing and thawing mammalian embryos and other living tissue and very high success rates are now normal. Indeed, it is standard practice to freeze and "bank" some strains of experimental mice. So that while the prognosis of success with human embryos is very good indeed the problem remains that, as Clifford Grobstein has said, "Ninety per cent success rates . . . may be acceptable for laboratory and domestic animals. In humans it is the ten per cent failure rate that is of concern – particularly if these are partial failures, not detectable until after birth or even later in life".[10]

---

[7] *The Observer*, 3rd October 1982.

[8] She may have a condition that makes birth dangerous.

[9] Edwards and Purdy, p. 360.

[10] Clifford Grobstein: "Coming to terms with test-tube babies", *New Scientist*, 7th October 1982.

But the prognosis for freezing is so good that in Australia for example it is regarded as morally acceptable to freeze spare embryos precisely because, since it may be possible to thaw them later and implant them, this does not amount to killing them.[11]

We should note also that one of the possibilities adumbrated above, that of donor embryos for "host" mothers, could be achieved "most effectively" with frozen-thawed embryos because these can be held until the uterus of the recipient is in the most receptive stage of the "cycle".[12] Although such donations are of course possible without resort to freezing.

Finally, freezing generates one further permutation, that of:

> (3) *Post Mortem* conception and birth, since frozen egg and sperm may be thawed and brought together after the death of either or both of the donors and frozen-thawed embryos may be implanted after the death of the donors.

IMMEDIATE AND PROXIMATE POSSIBILITIES

Firstly and of course the main use of *in vitro* fertilization techniques is in the treatment of infertility. It is estimated that there are for example 2½ million infertile couples in the United States, seventy five per cent of whom could be helped by the techniques now developed.[13] But although *in vitro* fertilization techniques were developed primarily to treat infertility many other uses immediately suggest themselves.

Suppose that a young woman were to have eggs removed from her ovaries and fertilised by her husband (or anyone). She could then freeze and store these for implantation whenever career permitted or fancy took and with a supply of embryos in the bank a couple or either one of them could be sterilised without losing the capacity to have children. These may seem frivolous uses to some but they have important effects. For example, since we know that the incidence of Down's syndrome increases sharply in the last decade of fecundity (between 35 and 45) a mother wishing to give birth during these years could *conceive* much earlier when the chances of avoiding Down's syndrome are much higher. But better still, the chances are that it will be possible to check whether the embryo had Down's or other genetic disorders before freezing and implantation and so virtually abolish this risk. Indeed as R. G. Edwards has noted:

> Identifying embryos with genetic abnormalities would offer an alternative to amniocentesis during the second trimester of pregnancy, and the "abortion *in vitro*" of a defective preimplantation embryo, still free-living, minute and undifferentiated, would be infinitely

[11] Edwards and Purdy, p. 361.
[12] Grobstein, *op. cit.*, page 16.
[13] *The Guardian*, 25th October 1982. About one in ten women are infertile.

IN VITRO FERTILIZATION 221

> preferable to abortion *in vivo* at twenty weeks of pregnancy or there-
> abouts as the results of amniocentesis are obtained. It would also be
> less traumatic for parents and doctor to type several embryos and
> replace or store those that are normal rather than having the threat of
> a mid-term abortion looming over each successive pregnancy.[14]

Further, there are good prospects[15] of sexing embryos which will make it possible for parents to choose to implant "boys" or "girls" in order of preference or in preferential order. It will also be possible to implant only those embryos of the preferred sex. This may have more "respectably medical" uses in that embryos can be screened for sex-linked disorders.

Cell and Tissue Banks

R. G. Edwards was able to report recently[16] that "it is now possible to contemplate the use of "tailor-made" embryonic tissue grown *in vitro* for grafting into adults". The special advantages of this possibility are that "Grafts of embryonic tissue may offer a wider scope than those taken from neonates or adults, because tissue could be obtained from organs which do not regenerate in adults, and the risks of graft rejection can possibly be eliminated".[17] Edwards goes on to list a number of specific possibilities that arise.

Foetal tissue can be used to replace bone marrow in patients that have for example been exposed to radiation and foetal liver cells injected into the placenta can prevent the expression of inherited anaemia. It may be also that tissue grafted from neonates may be used to "restore immune deficiencies in old people"[18] and a "practical approach to controlling immunological ageing may involve a combination of dietary manipulation, chemical therapy and cell grafting . . . Other recent reports have indicated that pancreatic cells may be used to repair diabetes and cultured skin cells grafted to repair lesions . . . Human amniotic epithelial cells . . . could be useful in repairing inherited enzyme defects in recipient children and adults".[19]

Further Edwards reports that there are indications that foetal brain tissue might be capable of repairing neural defects in adults and "there are reports that kidney cells may be transplanted into the human brain in order to cure illnesses such as Parkinson's disease".[20] "Myocardial tissue . . . should be obtainable from embryos growing *in vitro* without great difficulty,"[21] and might be used by cardiologists for repair of the major vessels of the heart.

Finally, there are various indications that the ultimate and most intractable problems of tissue and cell grafting and of transplantation procedures may be

---

[14] Edwards and Purdy, p. 373.

[15] op. cit., p. 372 ff. [16] op. cit., p. 380. [17] Ibid.

[18] Ibid. [19] op. cit., p. 381. [20] Ibid.

[21] Ibid. The pancreas may also be transplanted from the foetus at 20 weeks and may be used eventually to cure diabetes.

222   JOHN HARRIS

solved by methods of *in vitro* embryology. Edward notes a number of methods
for completely avoiding rejection by "tailoring embryos to suit a particular
recipient"[22] and lists two strong advantages in using foetal tissue. The first is
that "foetal tissue . . . might not be rejected by incompatible donors as strongly
as adult tissue" and the second that "Tissues compatible with an adult host
might also be obtained through cloning" or by otherwise genetically tailoring
matched or compatible tissue.[23]

We have for the moment looked sufficiently far into the future and we must
now return to our starting point and ask what arguments there are against the
continuation of such work and the realization of these possibilities?

> There is only one argument for doing something; the rest are argu-
> ments for doing nothing.[24]

Cornford's jibe at academics in 1908 is particularly apposite in considering
the case against *in vitro* fertilization. The arguments for doing nothing or
rather for doing nothing of the sort fall into two broad categories. There are
the arguments which are all variants of the "slippery slope", the lower reaches
of which we have just been examining. The other arguments all turn either on
the issue of whether it is morally permissible to kill the embryo, or on whether
it is morally permissible to use it or parts of it for our own purposes. We will
examine both groups of arguments, attempting the slippery slope last.

                                        II

THE MORAL STATUS OF THE EMBRYO
The two questions to which we require answers before we can decide what
an appropriate response might be to the possibilities we have been considering
are: when does life begin? and when does life begin to matter morally? It is
often thought that the answer to the second question is the same as that to the
first but as we shall see this cannot be the case.

When Does Life Begin?
To many it has seemed that conception is the obvious answer to the
question when does life begin. Over any rival candidates it seems to have the
decided edge that it is an identifiable event from which point the egg begins
the continuous process that leads to maturity. But of course the egg is alive
well before conception and indeed it undergoes a process of development and
maturation without which conception is impossible. The sperm too is alive and
wriggling. Life is a continuous process that proceeds uninterrupted from
generation to generation continuously (or at least sporadically) evolving. It is

---

[22] op. cit., p. 382.   [23] Ibid.
[24] F. M. Cornford, *The Microcosmosgraphia Academica* (Cambridge, 1908).

IN VITRO FERTILIZATION 223

not then life that begins at conception. But if not life, is it not at least the new *individual* that begins at conception?

A number of "things" may begin at conception. Fertilization can result not in an embryo but in a tumour which can threaten the mother's life. This tumour, called a hydatidiform mole, would not presumably be invested with all the rights and protections that many believe spring fully armed into existence at fertilization.

Even when fertilization is, so to speak, on the right tracks, it does not result in an individual of any kind. The fertilised egg becomes a cell mass which eventually divides into two major components: the embryoblast and the trophoblast. "The embryoblast becomes the foetus and the trophoblast becomes the extraembryonic membranes, the placenta and the umbilical cord. The trophoblastic derivatives are alive, are human, and have the same genetic composition as the foetus and are discarded at birth".[25]

A further complication is that the fertilised egg cannot be considered a new individual because it may well become two individuals. The fertilised egg may split to form twins and this can happen as late as two weeks after fertilization.

Life then is a continuum and the emergence of the individual occurs gradually. At this point it is commonly argued that if life does not begin at conception and if it cannot be said that a new individual human being begins there, at least the potential for a new human being is then present complete with its full genetic makeup in all its uniqueness and individuality. And since the fertilised egg is potentially a human being we must invest it with the same rights and protections as actual human beings.

The Potentiality Argument

There are two sorts of difficulty with the potentiality argument which are jointly and severally fatal to it. The first is that the fact that something will become x (even inevitably, which is not the case with the fertilised egg), is not a good reason for treating it now as if it had become x. We will all, inevitably, die but that is, I suppose, an inadequate reason for treating us now as if we were dead.

The second difficulty is that it is not only the fertilised egg that is potentially a new human being. The unfertilised egg and the sperm are just as potentially new human beings. To say that the fertilised egg is a potential human being is just to say that if certain things happen to it (like implantation) and certain other things do not (like spontaneous abortion) it will eventually become a human being. But precisely the same is true of the egg or sperm. If certain things happen to the egg (like meeting a sperm) and certain things happen to the sperm (like meeting an egg) and certain other things do not (like meeting a

[25] H. W. Jones, Jnr., "The Ethics of *In Vitro* Fertilization – 1981" in Edwards and Purdy, p. 353. See also Grobstein (1982).

224   JOHN HARRIS

contraceptive) then they will eventually become a new human being. So if we are somehow morally required to actualise all human potential then we are all in for a highly exhausting time.

All that can safely be said of the fertilised egg is that it is live human tissue. Life itself does not begin at fertilization, nor does human life, they both continue. What we need is not an account of when life begins but of when life begins to matter morally and why it matters morally. The question must be what should lead us to accept the embryo or the foetus or the neonate or the child or anything at all as having that range of qualities that makes for personhood? In virtue of what are we morally required to accept something as a person and consequently morally required to refrain from treating it in ways we may not treat people?

The Concept of the Person

The concept of the person is a topic for a book or at least a paper of its own. I cannot here hope to develop such a concept.[26] I think, though, that sufficient can be said to show whether or not there is good reason to think that the embryo, foetus or neonate are persons, and so see what protections we are morally obliged to afford them, not in virtue of their potential but in virtue of what they are.

It is important to remember that what we need to identify are those features, whatever they are, which both incline us and entitle us to value ourselves and one another and which licence our belief that we are more valuable (and not just to ourselves) than animals, fish or plants. In other words we are looking for the basis of our belief that it is morally right to choose to save the life of a person rather than a dog where both cannot be saved and that this choice is not merely a form of species prejudice, arbitrary but understandable. So the features we are looking for, although they will be possessed by normal mature adult human beings will not simply catalogue the differences between such beings and animals.

A concept of self will not simply be a means of self-justification. For example, the question of whether or not there are people on other planets is a real one. If there are, we need not expect them to look or sound or smell like us. They may not be organic at all and perhaps reproduce by mechanical construction rather than genetic reproduction. But if we are able to answer the question in the affirmative we will be distinguishing people on other worlds from animals, machines or plants on those worlds. We will be deciding

---

[26] See my *Violence and Responsibility* (London, 1980) Chapter 1, and also my "The Political Status of Children" in *Contemporary Political Philosophy*, ed. Keith Graham (Cambridge, 1982). A similar view is taken by, *inter alia*, P. Singer *Practical Ethics* (Cambridge, 1982) and M. Tooley in "Decisions to Terminate Life and the Concept of the Person" in *Ethical Issues Relating to Life and Death*, ed. J. Ladd (Oxford, 1979).

whether the appropriate response to them is to have them for dinner in one sense, or in the other. And if these people are technologically very much our superiors, we may hope to persuade them for the same reasons that we are people, not just like them maybe, but *enough* like them. But in what respect?

Each of us will have our own reasons for valuing our own lives and each of us is able to appreciate that the same is true of others, that they too value their own lives. What we have in common is our *capacity* to value our own lives and those of others however different our *reasons* for so doing may be or may seem to be. These features tell us both how to recognise other beings as people and also tell us why it is wrong to kill such creatures against their will. They are people because they are capable of valuing life and it is wrong to kill them because they do value life.

The wrongness of killing another person is on this view chiefly the wrongness of permanently depriving her of whatever it is that makes it possible for her to value her own life. So that, although each person may find different and unique value in their own life each is equally wronged by being deprived of a life, the continuation of which they value. We can thus see what is wrong with ending such a life without in any sense sharing the values that make it worthwhile. If we discover persons on other worlds we may recognise them as persons and appreciate the wrongness of killing them without in any way understanding "what makes them tick" or what they could possibly value, so long as it is clear that they are capable of valuing their existence.[27]

Persons – A Definition

A person will thus be any individual capable of valuing its own life. Such a being will, at the very least, be able to conceive of itself as an independent centre of consciousness, existing over time with a future that it is capable of envisaging and wishing to experience.

To take the concept of the person further than this is a task for another occasion. We have, however, come far enough to draw two conclusions. The first is that we require an account of the moral difference between persons on the one hand, and animals, fish, plants and perhaps robots on the other. Such a concept will tell us how in principle we might recognise people when we encounter them. If the concept of the person that I have sketched above is unacceptable, some other such concept that will do the same job is still required. Our second conclusion is that on the concept of the person I have outlined neither eggs, nor sperm, nor embryos nor yet neonates will possess

---

[27] On this conception of the person neither suicide, aiding suicide nor voluntary euthansia will be wrong, for individuals, by wishing to die show either that they do not value life or that they value death more. To frustrate the wish to die will thus be as bad as to frustrate the wish to live. We must of course be sure that if we kill people in accordance with their wish to die that *all aspects* of that act are in accord with their wishes.

226 JOHN HARRIS

the requisite degree (or indeed any degree) of self-consciousness required. But these beings are unlikely to qualify on any other account of what it is to be a person. This is because neither their state of consciousness or any other capacities they possess are relevantly distinguishable from those of many animals.

We can conclude that even if the concept of the person just outlined is rejected, no such concept will be able relevantly to distinguish the moral status of the embryo from that of many animals without the aid of the fatally flawed potentiality argument, and so the prospect of concluding that the embryo shares the rights and protections of normal adult human beings is vanishingly small.

It will also be a consequence of the arguments developed here that since neonates and very young children are not capable of wishing to live, it will be no more wrong to kill them, side-effects apart,[28] than to kill other creatures of comparable capacities like dogs and sheep. The side-effects in the case of neonates and young children are likely to be importantly different than is the case with embryos and since we are here concerned principally with *in vitro* embryology we will be content simply to note this for the record.

Abortion

We should also note before moving on that anyone or any society that permits either abortion or methods of "contraception" which prevent implantation of the fertilised egg, takes the view that the embryo is of less value than the mature human being. It cannot be morally worse to end the life of an embryo *in vitro* than it is to do so *in vivo*. Nor can it be morally worse to fertilise an egg *in vitro* knowing that you will not allow the fertilised egg to be implanted or carried to term than it is to fertilise *in vivo* with the same attitude to implantation or the prospect of birth. The motives of science are not more obviously corrupt or more frivolous than the motives of sex, so that even without accepting or even considering arguments about the moral status of the embryo, a society or an individual that has concluded that I.U.D.'s and some contraceptive pills are permissible forms of birth control, or that abortion is permissible, either freely or where the disutility of continuing a pregnancy can be demonstrated, must conclude that *in vitro* fertilisation and the non-implantation of "spare" embryos is also permissible on the same terms. That is, either with the same freedom permitted to the use of I.U.D.'s and other methods of contraception that prevent implantation, or with the same freedom that abortions are standardly performed.[29]

---

[28] Of course, one side-effect will be that if their parents wish them to live, *they* can be wronged by killing their embryo.

[29] Around 150,000 abortions are performed in the United Kingdom each year (149,746 in 1979): *Office of Population Census – Abortion Statistics* (1979), AB No. 6., H.M.S.O.

IN VITRO FERTILIZATION 227

By far the most significant of the new moral dilemmas posed by *in vitro* fertilization techniques are the questions of experiments on and use of tissue from embryos and the problem of whether such techniques leave us bootless on a slippery slope.

III

EXPERIMENTS ON EMBRYOS

Our investigations into the moral status of the embryo (and I use 'embryo' indiscriminately for all stages of development from zygote or blastocyst through to the end of the third trimester of pregnancy) have indicated that the embryo is not a person and that it is not morally wrong to end the life of such a being. Are there any reasons why we should not use the embryo for experimental purposes, for observation or indeed for the provision of tissue or organs in any of the ways described in Section I?

Pain and Suffering

Certainly it does not follow from our conclusion that there is nothing morally wrong with killing an embryo, or that there is nothing morally wrong with doing other things to or with it. For example, we may hold that it is wrong to inflict pain on creatures whom it is permissible to kill and that if they are to be killed we must do so as painlessly as possible. This is, I suppose, the attitude of most people to the killing of animals for food and other human purposes. Where pain is inflicted on such creatures (and where it isn't for the creatures' own good, as in most surgical operations) we demand, or we ought to demand, that the gains for humanity are of an importance to warrant the cruelty and suffering involved.

If, as seems likely, the embryo is not capable of feeling pain in the first few weeks of life (probably up to eighteen weeks) because it lacks a sufficiently established nervous system, this reason for not interfering with it cannot apply and it will not for similar reasons where adequate anaesthesia is used. We should also note and be concerned that many abortions are carried out after eighteen weeks and are performed in circumstances that are careless of the pain that might be inflicted on the embryo.

So, although the gratuitous infliction of pain gives us one reason to object to experiments on the embryo, it is an objection that can very easily be met.

Consent

To many people the idea of experiments on living human embryos is deeply disturbing, as is the prospect of using tissue or organs from such beings to save the lives of human persons or to repair disabling defects. But the idea and the wide-spread practice of using tissue and organs from live adults seems to be

228   JOHN HARRIS

far from disturbing. Skin grafts, cornea, kidney and bone-marrow transplants from children and adults to one another are not uncommon, nor of course is the use of cadaver organs and tissue. In each case however the crucial difference seems to be the ability to give and the actual giving of consent.

With live adults and children the wrongness of performing operations upon them and of taking away even "spare" parts against their will is straightforwardly related to the wrongness of killing them against their will and consent will remain effectively the *sine qua non* of such operations.[30] However, with cadaver transplants the situation is far from straightforwardly similar. The current practice is to require consent either from the potential donor while alive, perhaps in the form of a will or kidney donor card or suchlike, or to obtain consent from the next-of-kin after death. And by and large people seem to want the obtaining of such consents to be mandatory. Now of course, all things being equal, it is always a good idea not to ignore people's wishes and sensibilities over such matters. However, all things are decidedly not equal.

The necessity of obtaining consent for cadaver transplants costs many hundreds of lives each year in this country alone. Where there is no kidney donor card, for example, the necessity to find next-of-kin and find them in any condition to entertain the question of transplants from their nearest and dearest means that many potential donor organs are lost. Other vagaries of consent can have more disastrous consequences. Following a BBC Panorama programme in 1981 on the subject of transplants thousands of potential donors tore up their cards and the consequent short-fall of donors meant that many hundreds went without the transplants they desperately needed, either to stay alive or to improve the quality of their lives.

Transplantation Orders

The dead person cannot be wronged or harmed by the transplant of their organs "against their will" for they have no will – they are not there to be harmed. Is the squeamishness, sentimentality or ignorance of relatives of the dead a sufficiently important value to warrant protection at the cost of hundreds of lives annually?[31] The State has the power to order a *post mortem* examination regardless of the wishes of the deceased or his or her relatives and often does so order when there is nothing so important as the saving of a life to be gained by so doing. If the State can order *post mortem* examination of the dead on the slightest of pretexts, where for example there is the vaguest of suspicions as to the cause of death, how much more important and useful it

---

[30] There may, of course, be occasions when even the killing of the innocent (perhaps in war?) is morally permissible, even without their consent.

[31] There is an estimated shortfall of 1000 kidney transplants alone. Of course if transplantation orders were to be instituted there would have to be complete confidence in the criteria for brain death and that no life support systems would be prematurely switched off.

IN VITRO FERTILIZATION   229

would be to be able to order *post mortem* transplantation! If the ability to use cadaver organs for transplants were automatic there is no doubt that many hundreds, perhaps even many thousands of lives could be saved annually at the same "social cost" that we already (willingly?) pay for judicial certainty as to the cause of death.

If we return now to the issue of experiments with and transplants from the embryo we find related problems and issues. Unlike the articulate child or adult, the embryo cannot give or withhold consent, and this is not just a contingent difficulty about the development of speech, it reflects the fact that the embryo has no self-consciousness at all. If we are justified in killing or aborting the embryo, and do just this, its life will be lost and its death is a useless waste, not of life primarily, though living cells and tissue die, but of life-saving potential. If we can use it to save and ameliorate the lives of persons in being, would it not be both wasteful and morally wrong not to do so?

There are two sorts of problems here which turn on the question of whether the embryo can be said to be moribund or not and on the issue of whose consent is required.

Condemned to Death?

> How about the foetus which is not growing satisfactorily or which is cleaving abnormally? Do we regard this embryo as having condemned itself to death . . .? Is it not time that we started regarding these early embryos as collections of cells, and not as foetuses? Those that are not replaced in the mother are condemned to death, just as sperm that is spilt on the floor is condemned to death.[32]

These remarks of Patrick Steptoe strangely echo those of John Locke:

> Indeed having by his own fault forfeited his own life by some act that deserves death, he to whom he has forfeited it may, when he has him in his power delay to take it and make use of him for his own service; and he does him no injury by it. For whenever he finds the hardship of his slavery outweight the value of his life it is in his power by resisting the will of his master, to draw on himself the death he desires.[33]

Although Locke was referring to slavery the principle to which they are both appealing is the same, that death is wasteful and that when you are justified in ending a life you may also be justified in forbearing to take that life and making use of it instead. Of course, the issue of slavery is much more complex and for Locke the morality of the decision is in part determined by its being preferable to the slave, given a justified alternative of death.

[32] Edwards and Purdy, p. 364.
[33] John Locke, *Second Treatise on Government*, (Oxford, 1966), Chapter IV, p. 14.

 JOHN HARRIS

But Steptoe is surely right to suggest that if the embryo is moribund it is morally preferable to use it to save or benefit life than simply to waste both the embryo *and* the lives it might save or ameliorate? But is the spare embryo rightly to be thought of as "condemned to death"?

Certainly if the embryo is not to be implanted either now or in the future then it is condemned never to become a person (if it is frozen indefinitely it may perhaps not be straightforwardly *moribund* either).[34] But might not a host mother be found or come forward to give the lie to the claim that the embryo is either moribund or condemned to refrigerated limbo? For if a woman were to say "You may implant that embryo into me, I will carry it to term" then, although the embryo might have been "condemned to death", an eleventh hour reprieve seems possible.

Where such an eleventh hour reprieve appears it will not of course be true that the embryo will inevitably die and if it will not die it cannot be claimed that its organs and experimental possibilities will go to waste. But of course if it is not morally wrong to kill the embryo, then it may be killed despite the appearance of such a reprieve; and if it is killed in these circumstances then unless the organs and so on are utilised to benefit lives in being, they will be wasted. It would only fail to be permissible to kill the embryo in these circumstances if one could not do so either without the permission of any would-be repriever or unless other consents are necessary.

Consent

Who has the right to determine the fate of the embryo fertilised *in vitro*?

In the case of a normal pregnancy there is of course no question of aborting the foetus against the will of the mother; this is partly because such a course would involve a physical assault upon the mother. Now if this mother has an abortion, who is to determine what happens to the aborted foetus? If for example medical researchers want the foetus for experiments, is the mother's consent required? We are inclined, I suppose, to think that the answer to this question is "yes". Who else if not the mother should decide such an issue? But suppose the foetus were aborted alive, late in pregnancy, and could survive; should the mother be asked whether she wishes it kept alive or not? We cannot answer this question without knowing whether or not we are morally obliged to save the life of such a foetus. If we are obliged to save its life, if we are not entitled to kill it, then the mother cannot give the licence that morality will not grant.

If, as has been the argument of this paper, we are *not* morally required to preserve the life of such a foetus then again, why should we turn to the mother? Has she not already abdicated responsibility for the foetus by opting for abortion? We should turn to her only to see whether this is so. And of course if

[34] See Edwards and Purdy, p. 362, where Trounson makes use of this very point.

IN VITRO FERTILIZATION   231

she hasn't thus abdicated responsibility for the foetus, perhaps because the abortion is being performed to preserve her own health and not because she doesn't want the baby, then the case is different. In this case, if the foetus can live it must be restored to the mother – this will be a case of premature birth.

Where the aborted foetus cannot live or is already dead, again why should we turn to the mother for a decision as to what should be done with the foetus? If experimenters ask her for and are given permission to experiment on the foetus this permission will not absolve them from the responsibility of deciding *for themselves* whether such a course of action is ethically sound. And if she withholds permission, we must ask what gives her the right to decide that others should not benefit from the research or from transplantation? This would be another case for transplantation orders.

Property Rights

The only candidate for such a right vested in the mother is the claim that she has a property right in the foetus, deriving presumably from a view about the ownership of things growing either inside or on the surface of one's own body. This might well seem to be obviously the most basic and the most secure form of ownership possible. But there are obstacles to the idea that the foetus is owned by the mother simply in virtue of its growing inside her. There seem to be powerful exceptions to the general theory that such things are simply owned by the "owner" of the relevant body, at least in any absolute sense. For example, deadly and infectious viruses and so on may grow on or in someone's body but it is not clear that they are owned in any sense that would preclude society's right to kill or otherwise dispose of them against the will of the "owner" where the social utility of their destruction is clear. It is also worth noting that any claim that the mother owned her foetus would seem to confirm that it cannot be considered a person because, since the abolition of slavery at least, it is generally agreed that persons cannot be owned.

We may conclude that even in the unlikely event of our being satisfied that the mother's relation to the embryo or foetus is one of ownership, we are not forced to accept that we may not vary such property rights where, as in the cases we are considering, there are clear gains in terms of lives to be saved and improvements to be made in the quality of lives in being.

To sum up this discussion of the fate of the embryo, the situation seems to be that where the foetus is aborted and can survive, then if the mother wants it to live it must be treated as a premature birth and restored to her. If she does not want it to live she has no right that it be killed wastefully rather than used for experiments or transplants. The same is true of the embryo in vitro, except in this case there is no mother. No woman has a right that the egg she has donated be implanted. She has only a, perhaps contractual, right that it be implanted in *her* if she wants it.

Conclusion

It looks then strongly as though if the ends we purpose are themselves morally sound we may pursue them by experimenting on or with the human embryo and by using tissue, cells and organs from embryos to benefit the lives of persons in being. Further, there is no moral virtue in killing or allowing embryos to die when they could rather be used to benefit us all and there is less virtue in allowing human cadavers to go to waste, when we could, with, say, transplantation orders or the like, save very many lives.

As we have seen, the objections to these conclusions must show either that the embryo is the sort of creature that is morally entitled to the same concern, respect and protection as are persons or that, failing this, there are other moral reasons why we should not experiment on or take tissue from such embryos. We have seen that neither of these objections holds and we must now turn to the remaining question, that of whether, despite the moral acceptability of these practices, to embark upon them somehow involves stepping onto a slippery slope of depravity.

                                    IV

THE SLIPPERY SLOPE

In the first part of this essay we reviewed a series of possibilities from the present to the reasonably foreseeable future and stopped short with Edwards's prognosis that *in vitro* embryology might well open the way to transplant procedures that would have surmounted the greatest risk, that of tissue rejection. We stopped however at a point which is artificially short although as we have seen, it is a point which is reached by morally justifiable paths. We must now explore the related questions of whether we are morally obliged to stick at that point and that of whether the gradient has become willy-nilly so steep that if we go so far we will be unable to prevent ourselves from going further.

We should perhaps start by getting a clearer look at what lies in wait for us when we leave the nursery slopes:

CLONING

Cloning human beings would involve removing the nucleus of the fertilised egg cell (which contains the hereditary genetic material) and replacing it with the nucleus of a cell taken from the adult whom it is wished to clone. The resulting embryo would be the "identical twin"[35] of the adult from whom the replacement cell nucleus was obtained. It would exactly replicate the genetic

[35] We should note that clones may not ever be the *exact* replicas of the cell donor since some genetic material is carried in the cytoplasm. (A cell consists of nucleus plus cytoplasm.)

IN VITRO FERTILIZATION 233

make-up of the adult and so its tissue and organs would be "customised" to match exactly that of its adult "progenitor". It could then be grown to whatever stage was appropriate for development of the tissue or organs required for (or potentially required for) its adult "twin".

The possibilities now become both mind and morality boggling although it must be emphasised that these are not immediate possibilities and it is unclear how far off they are.

As we have seen, some tissue and some cells can be taken from the embryo *in vitro*. For the rest, the embryo would have to be grown, perhaps still *in vitro* if substitutes could be found for the mother's blood supply and other essential features of the womb, or perhaps in a surrogate mother. Here paths divide. Along one the foetus (and perhaps the neonate) would be grown until the organs or other tissue had reached a maturity sufficient for transplantation. Along the other, it might be possible to remove cells from the foetus as soon as they became distinct as potential organ tissue. It might then be possible to grow the organs themselves *in vitro* to the stage at which they could be used for transplantation. Both paths, of course, terminate in the death of the foetus or neonate.

There is one set of further possibilities we must consider and here the gradient, on what many will regard as a very slippery slope, becomes positively precipitous. The possibilities I have in mind while extreme are extremely interesting both for the light they shed on the issues involved and for the sharp focus they give to the argument. Let us then examine the terrain at the bottom of the slippery slope, or at least as far down it as is presently visible.

Organ Banks

One way in which adults could ensure for themselves a secure supply of appropriate organs for transplant when needed would be to clone themselves and grow the resulting clones, perhaps to adult size, for transplantation of organs as and when needed. The clone could be in all respects an identical adult and of course if it were it might well claim the right to be a recipient of the "original's" organs rather than a donor of its own. To overcome this "problem" originals might arrange for the brain of the clone to be destroyed as soon as it was differentiated in the embryo or enough of the brain to prevent the development of consciousness. The clone could be nourished and perhaps even exercised and in the event of complete disaster to the original body his or her brain could be transplanted to the clone rather than the organs transplanted to the original and life could continue. An endless supply of such clones at different stages of development could then keep the original going as long as its brain lasted. There might be a problem about the identity of the resultant beings or series of beings but they would (presumably) regard an identity crisis as less of a crisis than extinction.

The Mad Dictator Problem

A fear that is perhaps worth recording is that recently expressed by Oliver Gillie[36] that these techniques might "open the way for a self-infatuated millionaire or a mad dictator to produce hundreds of copies of himself". Such self-infatuated individuals would have to be mad to suppose that anything of value to them could be thus gained. For one thing "the best guess scientifically would be that the product of cloning would be less like the source than would be two identical twins"[37] because both physical characteristics and psychological and social characteristics also would be exposed to different time frames.

GENETIC ENGINEERING

The techniques we have been considering also open the way to the possibility of influencing human evolution. But how and to what ends should this power be exercised? Clifford Grobstein puts the dilemma like this:

> ... many would be reassured to know that the intent of any intervention in human reproduction would be to benefit individuals and not to "improve" the species as a whole. Though these two are linked, in contemporary thinking the first is generally understood and accepted, the second is burdened by suspicion and fraught with uncertainties as to how "improvement" will be defined and by whom.
>
> It would also be reassuring to know that defects that *limit* self-realisation are the legitimate target; that conservation and fuller fruition of humanity as we know it is the goal, not the "engineering" of new forms of human life.[38]

Worries about the engineering of new forms of life may be real enough but the possibility of "specializing" in existing forms may be equally disturbing.

Artificial Parthenogenesis

> Cloning may be possible with female as well as with male diploid nuclei, including a diploid nucleus from the egg donor. In the last case the product would be a female twin of the egg donor. By continued and exclusive application of the technique, an almost totally female and genetically homogenous society could be created and perpetuated. The number of required males, as in the case of breeding bulls, would only have to be sufficient to provide sperm to activate the eggs. Even that requirement could be eliminated if human eggs could be activated parthenogenetically. This occurs

---

[36] Oliver Gillie, "Microscopic Life", *The Sunday Times*, 3rd October 1982.

[37] Clifford Grobstein, *From Chance to Purpose* (London, 1981).

[38] Grobstein, (1982).

naturally in many animals but not regularly in any mammals. It can also be induced artificially in frogs and some mammals but with no normal offspring so far resulting in the latter case. If it could be accomplished externally, regularly and reliably on human eggs, it would open at least a formal option for a totally female society.[39]

This prospect might be very attractive to a certain stamp of feminist and disturbing as such a prospect would be to many, it is far from obvious that there are convincing moral arguments against the voluntary establishment of such a society. And if, for example, all the women in the world voluntarily decided that in future they would "bring forth women children only" it is not clear that anyone, let alone any man, would have the right to force them to do otherwise.

The resolution of the dilemmas raised by the possibilities of genetic engineering are far too large an undertaking to be attempted here, but it is important to bear such possibilities in mind when considering what the policy of society should be towards *in vitro* fertilization and the bio-technology it generates and utilises. For if we are on a slippery slope and it is towards such scenarios we are sliding, it is our attitude to them which will determine whether we set forth with skates or crampons.

It would perhaps be prudent to emphasise again that the possibilities we have just been considering are most certainly not yet even possible and perhaps may never be. But even fifty years is a long time in science, as the last fifty years have shown, and we should be clear as to what our policy should be in the face of such "possibilities". It will not be my purpose here to sift the cases one by one and review their general merits and defects. Some general conclusions however can safely be drawn.

SLIPPERY SLOPES AGAIN

The first is that slopes are only slippery if they catch us unawares and we have strayed onto them inadequately equipped. It is up to us to decide not what we can countenance but what we ought to pursue. We would be both irrational and immoral if we cut ourselves off from options we clearly perceive to be the beneficial products of the procedures now being developed because we fear that we will be insufficiently resolute to resist the dangers. We do not outlaw effective contraception because we fear that to practice population control is to step onto a slope that leads inexorably to the extinction of the human race.

The Principle of the Dangerous Precedent

In any event the idea that we can turn our backs on a slippery slope and thus avoid its dangers is an illusion. We are in fact only able to identify slippery

---

[39] Grobstein, (1981). p. 130. See also Edwards and Purdy, p. 382 for information on the same possibility.

slopes when we are already on them. What we can always do is decide in which direction to go and constantly review our decisions in the light of new information and revisions in our thinking. The feared slippery slope is just a variant of the well-known principle of the dangerous precedent so effectively lampooned by Cornford at the turn of the century:

> *The Principle of the Dangerous Precedent* is that you should not now do an admittedly right action for fear you, or your equally timid successors, should not have the courage to do right in some future case, which *ex hypothesi* is essentially different, but superficially resembles the present one. Every public action which is not customary, either is wrong, or, if it is right, is a dangerous precedent. It follows that nothing should ever be done for the first time.[40]

The artificiality of the dilemma of the so-called "slippery slope" is precisely as identified by Cornford. It is irrationally self-defeating if we declined to permit work which is in no way immoral and which can benefit us all, merely because we fear that at some future time we will not have the courage to object to work that *is* immoral. The arguments of this paper indicate that it is not morally wrong to fertilise the human egg externally *in vitro* nor are there sound objections to our permitting researchers to end the lives of spare embryos nor to experiment upon, nor use cells, tissue or organs from them, so long as this does not involve pain or suffering to the embryo. If we can thereby learn much that is of benefit to us and eventually use such embryonic material to repair or prolong the lives of children or adults, the lives of persons, then we should clearly do so.

Whether we should permit, for example, the growing of clones to adult maturity as living organ banks in the way described earlier, is a question we can address separately (though not here), and we are in no way committed to a particular answer simply in virtue of our assenting to work on the embryo. It may be difficult to find convincing arguments against the realization of such a possibility[41] but again, the fear that we might not be able to find such arguments is not relevant to our assessment of the morality of *in vitro* embryology.

What Should We Do?

One conclusion that the various commissions reviewing the ethics of *in vitro* fertilization ought to come to is that no obstacles should be put in the way of work on the human embryo, provided that pain and suffering can be avoided. 'Embryo', for these purposes, should be defined in the same way as I have used the term in this paper, to cover all the stages of development from fertilization

---

[40] F. M. Cornford, *op. cit.*, p. 23.
[41] See my "The Survival Lottery", *Philosophy* 50 (1975).

IN VITRO FERTILIZATION 237

right through the nine months of normal growth to the point where, were the embryo developing *in vivo*, it would be born. This would be a sensible and safe first conclusion to reach for although "birth" is an arbitrary point of no moral significance, it is a point which errs comfortably on the safe side. Nine months of development leave the human embryo far short of the emergence of anything that could be called a person, far short of the capacity for valuing its own life and all the capacities that would be involved in such valuing.

Permitting work on the human embryo up until the end of the third trimester of development would allow most of the current and reasonably projected research to proceed while leaving us time to review the moral and social implications of further developments. We should be clear, however, that the arguments we have been reviewing indicate that any moral objections to beneficial work on and use of even human non-persons who do not suffer in the process would be objections to the side-effects or extrinsic features of such work rather than objections to the work as such.

The cases that must be surveyed in order to map *that* terrain adequately, cases of the sort examined briefly at the beginning of this section, require a more detailed assessment than can be given here. It is not clear at first glance, however, whether such possibilities as living cell, tissue and organ banks which involve development beyond the third trimester, cloning, genetic engineering to "improve" human beings, artificial parthenogenesis and the like, would involve a slide or an ascent on the slope or axis of morality.[42]

University of Manchester

[42] I am greatly indebted to Rodney Harris, M.D., F.R.C.P., F.R.C.Path., Professor of Medical Genetics, University of Manchester, for his detailed comments and suggestions. The errors that remain are, of course, mine. Thanks are also due to the Editors of *The Philosophical Quarterly* for many helpful suggestions.

The Philosophical Quarterly Vol. 33 No. 132

IN VITRO FERTILIZATION: THE ETHICAL ISSUES (II)

BY MARY WARNOCK

By way of introduction, I must explain the rather unusual nature of this paper. It is unusual, at least, as a paper to appear in a learned journal. I write it as a commentator on John Harris's paper, but also as one who is involved at a practical level in the subjects he discusses. I do not believe that anyone, reading his paper, would doubt that he explores in it an area of morality in which the law has a right and a duty to involve itself. The kinds of decisions he outlines must be taken, not in the private, but in the public sphere. Indeed (pp. 236–7) he explicitly offers advice to the various committees now sitting to consider the problems of *in vitro* fertilization on the conclusions they should come to. I, therefore, being chairman of one of those committees, must necessarily look at his arguments, not merely as a philosophical colleague, but as the recipient of his advice. My comments on his paper, offering as they do no solutions, but only an attempt at further analysis, must be understood to proceed from someone who has a practical interest in the subject: How is the Minister to be advised?

There is another point to be made in explanation of my paper. I hope I shall, in the pages of a learned journal, be taken to be speaking for myself, and not for my committee, who have not yet had time to make up their minds on the questions of principle confronting them. If, in a year or so, when we jointly report, we come to conclusions different from those I here suggest, that will show only that chairmen do not, and should not, dictate theories to their committees.

I shall not comment on the factual outline of present practice and future possibilities with which Harris begins his paper. It seems to me a good introduction to the subject. Moreover, I agree with his judgement (p. 227) that "By far the most significant of the new moral dilemmas posed by *in vitro* fertilization techniques are the questions of experiments on and use of tissues from embryos".

I will start with a consideration of the second section of his paper, and the questions he there raises. First he asks, when does life begin? and secondly, when does life begin to matter morally? (p. 222). Quite rightly, in my view, he rejects the first of these questions as either unanswerable or unintelligible, or unanswerable because unintelligible. I would add that it is amazing how many people still raise the question 'When does life begin?' as if the answer to it were a matter of fact, to which we cannot yet supply an answer, but only because we have not enough evidence to settle it. There are still, for example, theologians, who speak in terms of the "probability" that life begins at this stage or that. However, I suspect that it is gradually becoming more acceptable to say that the question of life is not central. There is a perfectly good sense in which a sperm or an egg may be said to have life, even though neither could produce another life unless they were brought together and fertilised, and further environmental conditions were provided. If the question is narrowed, so that it means "When does *new* life begin?", it is, I think beginning to be understood that even this is a matter not so much for empirical investigation as for definition. Do we mean by a "new" life an organism which could survive on its own? Do we mean one that could move? Do we mean one which could be spatially distinguished from other organisms? Do we mean something which, though it could not survive by itself, could yet be distinguished genetically from other things in the biological world? Questions like these could lead, among other things, to the hopeless and confusing task of counting "lives". Are Siamese twins one "life" or two? What about those cases where, *in utero*, two foetuses begin to develop separately and then rejoin themselves, so that only one baby, not identical twins, is born? Were there at first two "lives" here, which somehow became one "life", or was there only one all the time? Such considerations seem to make the question of what counts as a new life unanswerable in principle. Moreover, unless we wish, for doctrinal purposes, to be able accurately to count lives or souls, the answer we give to the puzzles seems to make very little difference to anything. And so John Harris rightly moves to his second question, as that which has practical importance, namely the question 'When does life begin to have moral significance?'.

This question, central to the debate about *in vitro* fertilization, and especially to the way in which we may use "spare" embryos, is generally posed in the form "When does an embryo become a person?". And this is how Harris presents it.

Locke understood very well that the word "person" is not a biological, but a forensic term.[1] It is therefore a matter of decision at what moment, for legal or moral purposes, an individual is to be described as a person. There is a very great difficulty here. We have on our hands a concept quite difficult to make understood. I take it to be a matter of fact that whether or not someone (or indeed some corporate body) is to be deemed a person is something that has to be *decided*. It cannot be settled simply by observation or investigation of the individual or body in question. To settle it, we need to know the criteria that have been established for settling such cases, or we need to establish new criteria for ourselves. But to say that something is a matter for decision or

[1] Locke, *Essay Concerning Human Understanding*, Book II, ch. 27, para. 26.

240   MARY WARNOCK

judgement is not to say that it is "arbitrary", or that it might as well be settled
by lottery or the blindfold sticking in of a pin. There is a tendency in the
general public to confuse these concepts, and to suppose that if the designation of something as a person is not a straightforward matter of observation,
then whether it is so described or not must necessarily be decided by chance or
by peculiar whim. It is difficult to persuade people that there may be good
judgements or bad, well-grounded or ill-grounded decisions. The question
'How can I discover whether this embryo is a person?' is nonsensical, and is
different from the question 'Ought I to count this embryo as a person?'. But to
say this does not entail that there is no proper way to answer the second
question.

Of course, to say that whether or not someone is a person rests on decision
may have undesirable consequences. For the criteria of the decision may
themselves be unacceptable. For example, there is an influential school of
paediatricians who tend to make the question whether or not a new-born
infant is to be thought of as a person turn on whether or not the parents of the
infant want him to survive?[2] Now there are obviously difficult problems
confronting a doctor who has to decide whether to attempt to keep alive a very
precarious or damaged neonate whose parents do not want him to survive. But
the suggestion that these questions can be settled by determining whether the
infant is or is not a person, and that this in turn depends on the attitude to him
of his parents seems to introduce a criterion which, if more widely applied,
could lead to consequences generally agreed to be immoral. For why should
the criterion of "wantedness" apply to neonates alone? If it is really a criterion
of personhood, then it almost must have more general application. So if it
applies to infants why not to all children? If to children, why not to senile and
dependent adults? Admittedly this is a version of the "slippery slope" argument about which, on the whole, I share Harris's scepticism; but this is a slope
upon which we need never set foot, if we do not accept the premise that a
person becomes such only if he is a "wanted" person.

Harris, while not drawing particular attention to the element of decision in
finding an answer to the question 'Is he a person?', nevertheless offers his own
criterion of personhood with the strong suggestion that others may try, if they
so wish, to establish different criteria. His own criteria are fairly wide, and
result in a definition: (p. 225) "A person will . . . be any individual capable of
valuing its own life". This definition, as he sees, will exclude neonates as well
as all foetuses from the category of persons, as well, presumably as the
profoundly mentally handicapped and the senile. He attempts to remedy this
by suggesting that those who "want to live" may be deemed to value their own
lives. But this is an extraordinarily confusing concept. Does he mean to

[2] William A. Silverman, "Mismatched Attitudes about Neonatal Death", *Hastings Center
Report*, II (1981).

suggest that only those who *say* they want to live, if asked, are to be held to value their lives and so to qualify? This would now exclude not only infants but those of suicidal tendencies as well. But if he means less than this, then it seems that new-born babies (whom he explicitly excludes) may well be thought to want to live, as indeed may all living creatures, even sea anemones, who after all do their poor best to preserve themselves in life.

I believe that we would do better to remove the concept 'person' altogether from the debate. It is both confusing and redundant. Since it is a word both in legal and in common use, its deployment in this context lends a spurious exactitude to the argument, as if something had been settled by deciding when to call someone a person. But nothing has. The question 'Is he a person?' is in effect only another way of asking "May I or may I not do what I like with him?". It is agreed that the appropriateness or otherwise of the word 'person' is a matter of decision. Would it not be less confusing, therefore, to go straight to the main decision, namely the decision how we ought to treat him? The concept 'person' is introduced because a person is held to be the bearer of certain rights, which determine the treatment he may demand from others. But if he is agreed to have rights, this is because certain moral principles which create these rights are agreed. These principles lay down how people ought to be treated. It would therefore be better to discuss the principles themselves, rather than the rights which they confer, or the characteristics of those upon whom they are conferred. This argument is exactly parallel with that used by Frey in his book on animals' rights, in which he argues for going directly to the moral principles, rather than confusingly approaching them by way of the "status" of animals as rights bearers.[3]

But, it may be argued, we need some intermediary term. For how we treat someone is to be settled by considering who or what he *is*. There is no such thing as "right treatment" with no specific object. And with this I agree. But I would rather ask whether or not the object of treatment was a full human being than whether or not he was a person. 'Human' is a biological term, and simply distinguishes humans from other animals. And it seems to me of paramount importance that we, being human, should recognise that there are ways of treating our fellow humans that are right and other ways that are wrong. This is a moral principle, the very principle, in fact, upon which the demand for rights depends. It is part of our humanity that we should regard fellow members of the species as in a special relation to ourselves. I do not, of course, hold that this simple principle settles all the problems of how we should treat embryos. For it is clear that there are some members of the species so far from full development, so nearly just collections of cells, that they do not require full human treatment. To take an extreme case, I do not suppose that anyone would demand special treatment for spontaneously aborted human foetuses.

---

[3] R. G. Frey, *Interests and Rights: the case against animals* (Oxford, 1980).

242   MARY WARNOCK

It would be totally impractical, and totally absurd to suggest such a thing. Most such foetuses live and die without our even knowing it, still less respecting their existence. Nevertheless, however far from full humanity a foetus may be, we would do well to remember that it is a *human* foetus.

Harris (p. 224) rejects this line of argument. "We are looking", he says, "for the basis of our belief that it is morally right to choose to save the life of a person rather than a dog where both cannot be saved and that this choice is not merely a form of species prejudice, arbitrary but understandable". My suggestion, then, would be regarded by him as "speciesism", and thus arbitrary and ultimately unjustifiable. I would argue, on the other hand, that the concept of "speciesism" as a form of prejudice is absurd. Far from being arbitrary, it is a supremely important moral principle. If someone did *not* prefer to save a human rather than a dog or a fly, we would think him in need of justification. It is not prejudice to work for the survival of one's own species; nor is it culpable injustice to accord to one's own species a privileged position with regard to resources and care. That we are capable of taking an interest in the survival of other species, and can concern ourselves with their well-being, while they cannot be supposed to have such a concern for us, does not entail that we, alone among animals, are not interested *primarily* in our own species. To live in a universe in which we were genuinely species-indifferent would be impossible, or if not impossible, then in the highest degree undesirable. I do not, therefore, regard a preference for humanity as "arbitrary", nor do I see it as standing in need of any other justification than that we ourselves are human. I am not persuaded by arguments that turn on the question 'How would you treat intelligent beings from other planets?' If such beings exist and if one day our descendants come to know them, then the question of how our descendants treat them might well turn on the new creatures' concept of the human race. If both species were equally aware of the other's right to exist, then doubtless it would be time to negotiate, and a contract of equal rights might be drawn up. But as to all that, I am prepared to wait and see.

The point comes to have practical significance if we consider the question of experiments for the advancement of knowledge, to which I shall be returning later. It seems self-evident, as part of the preferential treatment due to humans, that, if experiments on living creatures are shown to be necessary, as I do not doubt that they often are, experiments on animals other than humans should be preferred wherever possible, unless the humans in question can themselves consent to be the subject of experiment. This is not of course to say that we should not take the utmost care to conduct experiments on animals with the least possible suffering to them. But that is a different question.

If it is decided, then, to abandon the word 'person' and stick to the words 'human being' how do we decide whether an embryo or a fertilised egg is *sufficiently* human to warrant protection? The alternative to thinking of it as

IN VITRO FERTILIZATION   243

human, as I have suggested above, is to think of it as "just a collection of cells". This is not in itself tremendously helpful, for of course a determined reductionist could argue that I (and everybody else) was "just a collection of cells". However, there is, I believe some justification for so considering the newly fertilised egg, and *not* so considering an adult human creature. But before I come on to this crucial point, I would like to introduce a new way of looking at the matter, not very clearly isolated in Harris's paper, though it is, I think, a recurrent theme in it. This is the Utilitarian argument.

For those who are Utilitarian moralists there seem, at first sight, to be very few problems about *in vitro* fertilization, or about the use of spare embryos fertilised *in vitro*, and either stored for future implantation, or used for research. There must, here as elsewhere, be a simple calculation. Do the benefits of the procedures outweigh the disadvantages? Put simply like this the answer seems obviously affirmative. Some of the great benefits, especially with regard to avoiding the birth of severely handicapped children, were outlined at the beginning of Harris's paper. And events move fast in this kind of world. Other gains may even now be in the process of being made actual. If we could have absolute and conclusive proof that embryos, in their earliest stages of development, are incapable of experiencing pain (and this seems overwhelmingly probable, given the connexion between the experience of pain and the development of the cerebral cortex) then there seems to be little to put in the balance on the negative side to outweigh the great gains. For these gains would be not only in the prevention of handicapping conditions, but in pure knowledge of foetal development, and in the provision of "spare" organs for those who might need them. Such are the Utilitarian arguments put forward by Dr Edwards, a powerful and persuasive advocate of both the therapeutic and the research use of *in vitro* fertilization. He recognises that his position is strictly Utilitarian, in the philosophical sense of the term.[4] Harris, as it seems to me, is equally deploying Utilitarian arguments in his paper. That the therapeutic use of *in vitro* fertilization is so justified is something he takes for granted. If someone is distressed by infertility, then, in certain cases, *in vitro* fertilization is a means of remedying the condition and therefore to maximising human happiness, while not causing any further unhappiness. Therefore it is right. The same is true where the birth of a baby needs to be postponed, or where it is essential to determine the sex of a baby. All these are plainly therapeutic or "medical" arguments. But equally, again on Utilitarian grounds, the benefits of foetal research far outweigh the disadvantages, and therefore, as it leads to beneficial consequences (or may do so), it should be regarded as ethically justified. My only criticism of his argument, thus inter-

---

[4] I rely here on points raised in discussion with Dr Edwards. But see also R. G. Edwards, "Fertilization of human eggs *in vitro*: morals, ethics and the law", *The Quarterly Review of Biology* 49 (1975).

244MARY WARNOCK

preted, is that, as I have suggested already, he confuses it unnecessarily by introducing the concept of 'a person'. If a foetus does not suffer pain, what does it matter whether it is a person or not? On the felicific calculus, pleasure and pain alone are the criteria to be used in determining the rightness of an act. There seems, then, to be no question left to ask in the present case. We can bypass the whole difficult and controversial area of the definition of 'person'.

However, even for Utilitarians, perhaps not all problems are solved by this kind of calculation. Even if more neurophysiological research put it completely beyond question that foetuses feel no pain (and I must emphasise that it would already be generally agreed that they do not) there is the separate question of how far it is right, in the felicific calculus, to take into account the feelings of outrage that some people may experience, if research on embryos is encouraged. I come here to a point not of theoretical interest only, but of extreme practical importance for anyone concerned with public morality, and with the relation between morality and the law.

The question has been referred to as that of Morality-Related Harms, and has been raised principally in connexion with the interpretation of J. S. Mill's *On Liberty*. I am not, for the present purposes, interested in the exegesis of Mill's text. But the problem can be put quite generally. If someone is a Utilitarian, and is therefore committed to the view that right action is that which gives rise to more benefit than harm, is he obliged to weigh in the balance the moral outrage or distress caused to people where a practice of which they disapprove is permitted? Put in the form of a question like those discussed in *On Liberty*, we may ask whether the state is entitled to interfere to prevent someone acting in a way that will harm others *only* in the sense that it will outrage their sensibilities or, more specifically, their moral sentiments. Ted Honderich discusses this problem in connexion with Mill in a recent article. If morality-dependent harm is thought irrelevant to the principle of utility, then, as Honderich says, "There is no possibility of intervention by the state or society to stop activities which cause or occasion only such harm. Individuals and parties are to be left with an absolute liberty so long as they occasion only such harm".[5] An embryo which was genuinely "spare", that is one which was never going to be implanted, could not be thought to be harmed by being destroyed. For it would die anyway. If it could not suffer pain then there could be no harm to *it* in using it, only to someone else. And the harm to someone else could take only the form of offence to moral feelings. On the view generally ascribed to Mill (though not by Honderich) such feelings do not "count"; and therefore the state would not be justified in intervening to stop the activity of experimenting on embryos. And this seems to accord more or less with Harris's argument. The type of problem is familiar enough. It arises

[5] Ted Honderich, "On Liberty and Morality-related harms" *Political Studies* 30 (1982).

in very many cases where the question is whether, or to what extent, the law should be interventionist, in order to protect people's possible moral scruples. Laws concerning homosexuality, pornography, public decency all have thus to balance liberty against offence.

I would like to suggest that the view generally ascribed to Mill, which I have also ascribed to Harris, be called Strict Utilitarianism. For I would argue that when we begin to take moral beliefs into account and to weigh them in the balance against future good, we are beginning to move away from Utilitarianism, towards a different moral theory altogether, perhaps towards a form of intuitionism.

What is the alternative, then, to strict Utilitarianism, as a basis for possible legislation with regard to experiments on spare embryos? An answer of some sort needs to be found to this question. For, in practical terms, there would be many people who would be unhappy to follow the strict Utilitarianism suggested by Harris. The law cannot, in practice, totally disregard people's moral feelings. But it is desirable that there should be some other principle to adduce, to use as a counter-argument to the principle of Utility.

Let us, in seeking for some alternative principle, consider one of Harris's conclusions. He suggests that what stands in the way of the use of embryos in accordance with the strict Utilitarian argument is a false belief that the mother *owns* the embryo. Once that belief has been discounted, nothing but a weighing of future benefits need prevail. He writes (p. 231): "We may conclude that even in the unlikely event of our being satisfied that the mother's relation to the embryo or foetus is one of ownership, we are not forced to accept that we may not vary such property rights where . . . there are clear gains in terms of lives to be saved and improvements to be made in the quality of lives in being". His thought is that if people can be proved to own something, then they have a *prima facie* right to determine how that thing shall be used. But either the relation between donor and fertilised egg is not one of ownership (nor is the relation between mother and aborted foetal material), or, if it is, it is ownership whose rights can be overruled. For if the mother has agreed to the abortion, as she must, then she does not want the foetus to live, and therefore can have no right to determine its use. Similarly, if she just happens to have had more eggs than one taken from her, and does not want them all to be implanted, then she cannot claim any right to determine the use of the spare fertilised eggs.

Now I believe that the question of "ownership" here introduced by Harris is a red herring, like the concept of "person". Like that concept it is introduced by him to give to the argument an appearance of exactitude which is in fact spurious. It disguises the fact that the question is a straightforward question about values. Whether or not the mother can be said to "own" her egg, or the aborted foetus, whether or not the father can be said to "own" his sperm, or the foetus that results from its fertilization with an egg, the question is: *how ought such foetuses to be treated?* And one serious consideration in the answering of this question is that which turns on the *feelings* of the parents.

The question of ownership simply need not arise. All the parallels derived from the consideration of other property, all the questions about whether it can be right to own another human being are simply irrelevant. We need not be drawn into this kind of dispute.

But, it may be said, I am surreptitiously arguing that the parents' feelings should be taken into account *because* I still think they "own" the sperm and the egg. I have begged the question by using such expressions as "his" sperm and "her" egg. I do not think so. We are quite accustomed to the use of the possessive pronoun in cases other than that of ownership. There may be many different relationships implied. I do not own "my" piano teacher or "my" doctor, nor does he own me as "his" patient. All questions about rights remain to be answered even if the words 'his' and 'hers' are intelligibly used. To what extent, then, all reference to ownership apart, should the woman's wishes be taken into account when spare embryos, or aborted foetuses are to be used? I believe that the relationship between her and the egg or the foetus or the spare embryo is such that they should be used only with her consent. If she objects to their use for experimentation, then her objection must be respected and the material not used. That she may be able to give no good reason for her attitude makes no difference. The matter turns not on her reasons but on her feelings.

This point is of the greatest importance, both practically and theoretically. It is worth considering a little further. It is quite difficult to persuade members of committees that feelings or sentiments *can* have a central role to play in moral decision-making. Such people tend to believe that a moral judgement must be rational, or else it must be based on religious dogma. Otherwise it will not count as a properly moral judgement. They find it shocking to accept that, as Hume put it, morality is "more properly felt than judged of".[6] Yet I believe that it is to offend against the concept of morality itself to refuse to take moral feelings or sentiments into account in decision-making.

It is perhaps worth distinguishing the view I am here putting forward from the view of Professor Silverman whom I quoted earlier (p. 240). He argued that a neonate became a person, and therefore worthy of respect, if and only if it was wanted by its mother. So he might argue that my supposed mother who does not wish the spare embryo derived from her egg, or the aborted foetus derived from her uterus, to be used for experiment, is, by "wanting" it, turning it into a person, and therefore worthy of respect. But this would be wrong. The mother may not "want" the embryo, in that she may specifically not want it to be implanted. She may have agreed to an abortion, and yet feel a connexion between herself and the aborted foetus which determines her attitude about how it should be used. She may in no sense feel that the bundle of cells is a

---

[6] Hume, *Treatise*, Book III, Part I, Section 2.

person, yet she may feel that, being human, it is special – not just any bundle of cells. I am not saying that all women would feel this way. I very much doubt if I would, for one. And many women are deeply interested in the advance of science and would prefer that the spare embryo or the aborted foetus should be used for the general good, or simply for the advance of knowledge. All I am arguing is that people should be given a chance to express such feelings if they have them. And if they are expressed they should be respected even though they may seem unreasonable, and incapable of justification on Utilitarian grounds. And this itself is a moral principle, indeed it is the very principle which must lie behind the right treatment of one human being by another. For, though the embryo may not feel, the other parties in the whole transaction do so. And to use an embryo for however good an end, if the mother related to it (though not by "ownership") cannot bear to contemplate the idea, is to use the mother as merely a means to an end. Similarly to extract an egg from a woman who is being operated on for some different reason, in order to fertilise it for experimental purposes would in my view be wrong unless the woman had given her permission that this should be done – and this, even though she would be in no way harmed by the extraction. To overrule strongly held views simply because an end seems good, and perhaps the views silly, is to use a human being for an end that is not her own.

In arguing for the wrongness of overruling deeply felt moral sentiments, I am plainly arguing against strict Utilitarianism. I think that my position is very like (and owes something to) that adopted by Stuart Hampshire.[7] Hampshire holds that the essence of morality is the existence of a set of not necessarily coherent or unified principles which constitute barriers against what is felt to be wrong-doing, a set of prohibitions. There are, in a society, some things which must not be done, or, if done, must not be condoned. These prohibitions operate within certain uniform areas of social life. They govern, in any society, attitudes towards human life and human death, towards the treatment of the dead, towards sexual relations, the relations of loyalty and honesty. Different societies will regard different principles as inviolable; and within a geo-graphically single society, prohibitions will gradually change from time to time. But if any society, at any given time, had *no* such principles, this would be the end of morality for that society. Utilitarianism regards all such principles as conditional, dependent for their validity on the beneficial consequences shown to follow from observing them. If there seem to be no beneficial consequences, or if there can be shown to be beneficial consequences from their breach, then they must be thrown out. Hampshire argues that, though Utilitarianism is generally the official political morality, its acceptance may well lead to a brutal counting of heads, and an insensitivity to the kind of

---

[7] "Morality and Pessimism" in *Public and Private Morality*, ed. S. Hampshire (Cambridge, 1978).

248 MARY WARNOCK

inhibitions and scruples which are at the centre of morality. "In arguing against utilitarians" he writes (*op. cit.*, p. 9), "I must dwell on the epithets usually associated with morally impossible action, on a sense of disgrace, of outrage, of horror, or baseness, of brutality, and, most important, a sense that a barrier, assumed to be firm and almost insurmountable, has been knocked over and a feeling that, if this horrible or outrageous, or squalid, or brutal, action is possible, then anything is possible and nothing is forbidden, and all restraints are threatened. Evidently these ideas have often been associated with impiety, and a belief that God, or the Gods, have been defied, and with a fear of divine anger. But they need not have these associations with the supernatural, and they may have . . . a secular setting. In the face of the doing of something that must not be done, and that is categorically excluded and forbidden morally, the fear that one may feel is the fear of human nature. . . . This fear of human nature, and sense of outrage, when a barrier is broken down, is an aspect of respect for morality itself rather than for any particular morality and for any particular set of prohibitions."

The treatment of "spare" embryos and the science-fiction possibilities that seem to lie open to us in the future plainly fall into the category of things with which morality, any morality, must be concerned. They are also things with which the law must concern itself. For though the law and morality do not have identical spheres, their spheres overlap; and where, as in this case, there is the possibility of commercial exploitation, and the establishment of "pirate" laboratories or nursing homes, there is a plain case for regulation by law. Otherwise people in general may fall victim to their fears that anything will in future be permissible. The law must, in this case, be seen to uphold and support *some* prohibitions. It is, of course, the fear that some barrier may be broken down that gives force to the "slippery slope" argument, an argument which, in its general form, is to be resisted, because of its power to prevent progress and the advance of knowledge. How then are we to proceed? How is knowledge to be increased, and at the same time human sensitivity to outrage against other humans be kept alive? For it seems to me that this is what we must aim at, namely that sensitivity to the treatment of one human being by another should increase rather than diminish with the growth of new technology. For example, no human being should use another for his own ends, however noble. Therefore, suppose that embryos could be kept alive *in vitro* for so long that they became plainly human, able to experience pain, or to perceive their environment; it would immediately become wrong that they should be used for experimental or observational purposes. It would be absolutely prohibited, too, that anaesthetics should be administered to them so that, though capable of feeling pain, they did not actually feel it. Here would be an area where there would be a total difference between treatment of humans and treatment of other animals. I believe that nearly everyone would agree that this was a barrier in no circumstances to be crossed, whatever the demands of scientific knowledge. And such barriers should be incorporated in the law.

But in one respect I agree with Harris. It is of no use to try to see too far or too precisely, into the future. What is needed is a principle, and an institution of legal restraints and surveillance, which will enable research to proceed and therapeutic techniques to be developed, but constantly watched, not merely by the medical profession and the research biologists, but by the lay as well, the stupid, the prejudiced, the sentimental, the religious and the moralistic lay. Only so, I believe, shall we ensure that those sentiments out of which morality is composed will be respected. And only if they are *not* respected shall we be in danger of hurtling down the dreaded slope. We must all of us learn, to use Jane Austen's words, "to feel as we ought".

University of Oxford

[21]

SURROGATE MOTHERING: EXPLOITATION OR EMPOWERMENT?

LAURA M. PURDY

INTRODUCTION

'Pregnancy is barbaric'[1] proclaimed Shulamith Firestone in the first heady days of the new women's movement; she looked forward to the time when technology would free women from the oppression of biological reproduction. Yet as reproductive options multiply, some feminists are making common cause with conservatives for a ban on innovations. What is going on?

Firestone argued that nature oppresses women by leaving them holding the reproductive bag, while men are free of such burden; so long as this biological inequality holds, women will never be free. (Firestone, 198–200) It is now commonplace to point out the naivety of her claim: it is not the biological difference, per se, that oppresses women, but its social significance. So we need not change biology, only attitudes and institutions.

This insight has helped us to see how to achieve a better life for women, but I wonder if it is the whole story. Has Firestone's brave claim no lesson at all for us?

Her point was that being with child is uncomfortable and dangerous, and it can limit women's lives. We have become more sensitive to the ways in which social arrangements can determine how much these difficulties affect us. However, even in feminist utopias, where sex or gender are considered morally irrelevant except where they may entail special needs, a few difficulties would remain. Infertility, for instance, would exist, as would the

---

[1] Shulamith Firestone, *The Dialectic of Sex*, (New York: Bantam Books, 1970), p. 198. A version of this paper was given at the Eastern SWIP meeting, 26 March 1988. I would like especially to thank Helen B. Holmes and Sara Ann Ketchum for their useful comments on this paper; they are, of course, in no way responsible for its perverse position! Thanks also to the editors and referees of *Bioethics* for their helpful criticisms.

desire for a child in circumstances where pregnancy is impossible or undesirable.

At present, the problem of infertility is generating a whole series of responses and solutions. Among them are high-tech procedures like IVF, and social arrangements like surrogate motherhood. Both these techniques are also provoking a storm of concern and protest. As each raises a distinctive set of issues, they need to be dealt with separately, and I shall here consider only surrogate motherhood.

One might argue that no feminist paradise would need any practice such as this. As Susan Sherwin argues, it could not countenance 'the capitalism, racism, sexism, and elitism of our culture [that] have combined to create a set of attitudes which views children as commodities whose value is derived from their possession of parental chromosomes.'[2] Nor will society define women's fulfilment as only in terms of their relationship to genetically-related children. No longer will children be needed as men's heirs or women's livelihood.

We will, on the contrary, desire relationships with children for the right reasons: the urge to nurture, teach and be close to them. No longer will we be driven by narcissistic wishes for clones or immortality to seek genetic offspring no matter what the cost. Indeed, we will have recognized that children are the promise and responsibility of the whole human community. And childrearing practices will reflect these facts, including at least a more diffuse family life that allows children to have significant relationships with others. Perhaps childbearing will be communal.

This radically different world is hard to picture realistically, even by those like myself who—I think—most ardently wish for it. The doubts I feel are fanned by the visions of so-called 'cultural feminists' who glorify traditionally feminine values. Family life can be suffocating, distorting, even deadly.[3] Yet there is a special closeness that arises from being a child's primary caretaker, just as there can be a special thrill in witnessing the unfolding of biologically-driven traits in that child. These pleasures justify risking neither the health of the child[4] nor that of the mother;

<hr>

[2] Susan Sherwin, 'Feminist Ethics and In Vitro Fertilization,' *Science, Moralty and Feminist Theory*, ed. Marsha Hanen and Kai Nielsen, *The Canadian Journal of Philosophy* supplementary volume 13, 1987, p. 277.

[3] Consider the many accounts of the devastating things parents have done to children, in particular.

[4] See L. M. Purdy 'Genetic Diseases: Can Having Children be Immoral?' *Moral Problems in Medicine*, ed. Samuel Gorovitz, (N.J.: Prentice-Hall, 1983), 377–84.

20   LAURA M. PURDY

nobody's general well-being should be sacrificed to them, nor do they warrant hugh social investments. However, they are things that, other things being equal, it would be desirable to preserve so long as people continue to have anything like their current values. If this is so, then evaluating the morality of practices that open up new ways of creating children is worthwhile.[5]

MORAL OR IMMORAL?

What is surrogate mothering exactly? Physically, its essential features are as follows: a woman is inseminated with the sperm of a man to whom she is not married. When the baby is born she relinquishes her claim to it in favour of another, usually the man from whom the sperm was obtained. As currently practiced, she provides the egg, so her biological input is at least equal to that of the man. 'Surrogate' mothering may not therefore be the best term for what she is doing.[6]

By doing these things she also acts socially—to take on the burden and risk of pregnancy for another, and to separate sex and reproduction, reproduction and childrearing, and reproduction and marriage. If she takes money for the transaction (apart from payment of medical bills), she may even be considered to be selling a baby.

The bare physical facts would not warrant the welter of accusation and counter-accusation that surrounds the practice.[7] It is the social aspects that have engendered the acrimony about exploitation, destruction of the family, and baby-selling. So far we have reached no consensus about the practice's effect on women or its overall morality.

I believe that the appropriate moral framework for addressing

[5] Another critical issue is that no feminist utopia will have a supply of 'problem' children whom no one wants. Thus the proposal often heard nowadays that people should just adopt all those handicapped, non-white kids will not do. (Nor does it 'do' now.)

[6] I share with Sara Ann Ketchum the sense that this term is not adequate, although I am not altogether happy with her suggestion that we call it 'contracted motherhood' (New Reproductive Technologies and the Definition of Parenthood: A Feminist Perspective', paper given at the 1987 *Feminism and Legal Theory Conference*, at the University of Wisconsin at Madison, summer 1987, p. 44ff.) It would be better, I think, to reserve terms like 'mother' for the social act of nurturing. I shall therefore substitute the terms 'contracted pregnancy' and 'surrogacy' (in scare quotes).

[7] This is not to say that no one would take the same view as I: the Catholic Church, for instance, objects to the masturbatory act required for surrogacy to proceed.

questions about the social aspects of contracted pregnancy is consequentialist.[8] This framework requires us to attempt to separate those consequences that invariably accompany a given act from those that accompany it only in particular circumstances. Doing this compels us to consider whether a practice's necessary features lead to unavoidable overridingly bad consequences. It also demands that we look at how different circumstances are likely to affect the outcome. Thus a practice which is moral in a feminist society may well be immoral in a sexist one. This distinction allows us to tailor morality to different conditions for optimum results without thereby incurring the charge of malignant relativism.

Before examining arguments against the practice of contracted pregnancy, let us take note of why people might favour it. First, as noted before, alleviating infertility can create much happiness. Secondly, there are often good reasons to consider transferring burden and risk from one individual to another. Pregnancy may be a serious burden or risk for one woman, whereas it is much less so for another. Some women love being pregnant, others hate it; pregnancy interferes with work for some, not for others; pregnancy also poses much higher levels of risk to health (or even life) for some than for others. Reducing burden and risk is a benefit not only for the woman involved, but also for the resulting child. High-risk pregnancies create, among other things, serious risk of prematurity, one of the major sources of handicap in babies. Furthermore, we could prevent serious genetic diseases by allowing carriers to avoid pregnancy. A third benefit of 'surrogate mothering' is that it makes possible the creation of non-traditional families. This can be a significant source of happiness to single women and gay couples.

All of the above presuppose that there is some advantage in making possible at least partially genetically-based relationships between parents and offspring. Although, as I have argued above, we might be better off without this desire, I doubt that we will

---

[8] The difficulty in choosing the 'right' moral theory to back up judgments in applied ethics, given that none are fully satisfactory continues to be vexing. I would like to reassure those who lose interest at the mere sight of consequentialist—let alone utilitarian—judgment, that there are good reasons for considering justice an integral part of moral reasoning, as it quite obviously has utility.

A different issue is raised by the burgeoning literature on feminist ethics. I strongly suspect that utilitarianism could serve feminists well, if properly applied. (For a defence of this position, see my paper 'Do Feminists Need a New Moral Theory', to be given at the University of Minnesota, Duluth, at the conference *Explorations in Feminist Ethics: Theory and Practice*, 8–9 October 1988.)

22   LAURA M. PURDY

soon be free of it. Therefore, if we can satisfy it at little cost, we should try to do so.

IS SURROGATE MOTHERING ALWAYS WRONG?

Despite the foregoing advantages, some feminists argue that the practice is *necessarily* wrong: it is wrong because it must betray women's and society's basic interests.[9]

What, if anything is wrong with the practice? Let us consider the first three acts I described earlier: transferring burden and risk, separating sex and reproduction, and separating reproduction and childrearing. Separation of reproduction and marriage will not be dealt with here.

Is it wrong to take on the burden of pregnancy for another? Doing this is certainly supererogatory, for pregnancy can threaten comfort, health, even life. One might argue that women should not be allowed to take these risks, but that would be paternalistic. We do not forbid mountain-climbing or riding a motorcycle on these grounds. How could we then forbid a woman to undertake this particular risk?

Perhaps the central issue is the transfer of burden from one woman to another. However, we frequently do just that—much more often than we recognize. Anyone who has her house cleaned, her hair done, or her clothes dry-cleaned is engaging in this procedure;[10] so is anyone who depends on agriculture or public works such as bridges.[11] To the objection that in this case the bargain includes the risk to life and limb, as well as use of time and skills, the answer is that the other activities just cited entail surprisingly elevated risk rates from exposure to toxic chemicals or dangerous machinery.[12]

Furthermore, it is not even true that contracted pregnancy merely shifts the health burden and risks associated with pregnancy from one woman to another. In some cases (infertility, for example,) it makes the impossible possible; in others (for women with potentially high-risk pregnancies) the net risk is

[9] See for example Gena Corea, *The Mother Machine*, and Christine Overall, *Ethics and Human Reproduction*, (Winchester, Mass.: Allen and Unwin, 1987).

[10] These are just a couple of examples in the sort of risky service that we tend to take for granted.

[11] Modern agricultural products are brought to us at some risk by farm workers. Any large construction project will also result in some morbidity and mortality.

[12] Even something so mundane as postal service involves serious risk on the part of workers.

lowered.[13] As we saw, babies benefit, too, from better health and fewer handicaps. Better health and fewer handicaps in both babies and women also means that scarce resources can be made available for other needs, thus benefiting society in general.

I do think that there is, in addition, something suspect about all this new emphasis on risk. Awareness of risks inherent in even normal pregnancy constitutes progress: women have always been expected to forge ahead with child bearing oblivious to risk. Furthermore, childbearing has been thought to be something women owed to men or to society at large, regardless of their own feelings about a given—or any—pregnancy. When women had little say about these matters, we never heard about risk.[14] Why are we hearing about risk only now, now that women finally have some choices, some prospect of remuneration?[15] For that matter, why is our attention not drawn to the fact that surrogacy is one of the least risky approaches to non-traditional reproduction?[16]

Perhaps what is wrong about this kind of transfer is that it necessarily involves exploitation. Such exploitation may take the form of exploitation of women by men and exploitation of the rich by the poor. This possibility deserves serious consideration, and will be dealt with shortly.

Is there anything wrong with the proposed separation of sex and reproduction? Historically, this separation—in the form of contraception—has been beneficial to women and to society as a whole. Although there are those who judge the practice immoral. I do not think we need belabour the issue here.

It may be argued that not all types of separation are morally on a par. Contraception is permissible, because it spares women's health, promotes autonomy, strengthens family life, and helps make population growth manageable. But separation of sex and reproduction apart from contraception is quite another kettle of fish: it exploits women, weakens family life, and may increase population. Are these claims true and relevant?

Starting with the last first, if we face a population problem, it

---

[13] The benefit to both high-risk women, and to society is clear. Women need not risk serious deterioration of health or abnormally high death rates.

[14] See Laura Purdy, 'The Morality of New Reproductive Technologies', *The Journal of Social Philosophy*, (Winter 1987), pp. 38–48.

[15] For elaboration of this view, consider Jane Ollenburger and John Hamlin, ' "All Birthing Should be Paid Labor"—A Marxist Analysis of the Commodification of Motherhood', *On the Problem of Surrogate Parenthood: Analyzing the Baby M Case*, ed. Herbert Richardson, (Lewistong, N.Y.: The Edwin Mellen Press, 1987).

[16] Compare the physical risk with that of certain contraceptive technologies, and high-tech fertility treatments like IVF.

24   LAURA M. PURDY

would make sense to rethink overall population policy, not exploit the problems of the infertile.[17] If family strengthing is a major justification for contraception, we might point out that contracted pregnancy will in some cases do the same. Whether or not having children can save a failing marriage, it will certainly prevent a man who wants children from leaving a woman incapable of providing them. We may bewail his priorities, but if his wife is sufficiently eager for the relationship to continue it would again be paternalistic for us to forbid 'surrogacy' in such circumstances. That 'surrogacy' reduces rather than promotes women's autonomy may be true under some circumstances, but there are good grounds for thinking that it can also enhance autonomy. It also remains to be shown that the practice systematically burdens women, or one class of women. In principle, the availability of new choices can be expected to nourish rather than stunt women's lives, so long as they retain control over their bodies and lives. The claim that contracted pregnancy destroys women's individuality and constitutes alienated labour, as Christine Overall argues, depends not only on a problematic Marxist analysis, but on the assumption that other jobs available to women are seriously less alienating.[18]

Perhaps what is wrong here is that contracted pregnancy seems to be the other side of the coin of prostitution. Prostitution is sex without reproduction; 'surrogacy' is reproduction without sex. But it is difficult to form a persuasive argument that goes beyond mere guilt by association. Strictly speaking, contracted pregnancy is not prostitution; a broad-based Marxist definition would include it, but also traditional marriage. I think that in the absence of further argument, the force of this accusation is primarily emotional.

Perhaps the dread feature contracted pregnancy shares with prostitution is that it is a lazy person's way of exploiting their own 'natural resources'. But I suspect that this idea reveals a touchingly naive view of what it takes to be a successful prostitute, not to mention the effort involved in running an optimum pregnancy. Overall takes up this point by asserting that it

is not and cannot be merely one career choice among others. It

[17] Infertility is often a result of social arrangements. This process would therefore be especially unfair to those who already have been exposed to more than their share of toxic chemicals or other harmful conditions.

[18] Christine Overall, *Ethics and Human Reproduction*, (Winchester, Mass.: Allen & Unwin, 1987), ch. 6. Particularly problematic are her comments about women's loss of individuality, as I will be arguing shortly.

is not a real alternative. It is implausible to suppose that fond parents would want it for their daughters. We are unlikely to set up training courses for surrogate mothers. Schools holding 'career days' for their future graduates will surely not invite surrogate mothers to address the class on advantages of 'vocation'. And surrogate motherhood does not seem to be the kind of thing one would put on one's curriculum vitae. (p. 126)

But this seems to me to be a blatant *ad populum* argument.

Such an objection ought, in any case, to entail general condemnation of apparently effortless ways of life that involved any utilization of our distinctive characteristics.

We surely exploit our personal 'natural resources' whenever we work. Ditchdiggers use their bodies, professors use their minds. Overall seems particularly to object to some types of 'work': contracted pregnancy 'is no more a real job option than selling one's blood or one's gametes or one's bodily organs can be real job options.' (p. 126) But her discussion makes clear that her denial that such enterprises are 'real' jobs is not based on any social arrangements that preclude earning a living wage doing these things, but rather on the moral judgement that they are wrong. They are wrong because they constitute serious 'personal and bodily alienation'. Yet her arguments for such alienation are weak. She contends that women who work as 'surrogates' are deprived of any expression of individuality, (p. 126) are interchangeable, (p. 127) and that they have no choice about whose sperm to harbor. (p. 128) It is true that, given a reasonable environment (partly provided by the woman herself), bodies create babies without conscious effort. This fact, it seems to me, has no particular moral significance: many tasks can be accomplished in similar ways yet are not thought valueless.[19]

It is also usually true that women involved in contracted pregnancy are, in some sense, interchangeable. But the same is true, quite possibly necessarily so, of most jobs. No one who has graded mounds of logic exams or introductory ethics essays could reasonably withhold their assent to this claim, even though college teaching is one of the most autonomous careers available. Even those of us lucky enough to teach upper level courses that involve more expression of individual expertise and choice can be slotted

---

[19] Men have been getting handsome pay for sperm donation for years; by comparison with childbearing, such donation is a lark. Yet there has been no outcry about its immorality. Another double standard?

26 LAURA M. PURDY

into standardized job descriptions. Finally, it is just false that a woman can have no say about whose sperm she accepts: this could be guaranteed by proper regulation.

I wonder whether there is not some subtle devaluing of the physical by Overall. If so, then we are falling into the trap set by years of elitist equations of women, nature and inferiority.

What I think is really at issue here is the disposition of the fruit of contracted pregnancy: babies. However, it seems to be generally permissible to dispose of or barter what we produce with both our minds and our bodies—except for that which is created by our reproductive organs. So the position we are considering may just be a version of the claim that it is wrong to separate reproduction and childrearing.

Why? It is true that women normally expect to become especially attached to the product of this particular kind of labour, and we generally regard such attachment as desirable. It seems to be essential for successfully rearing babies the usual way. But if they are to be reared by others who are able to form the appropriate attachment, then what is wrong if a surrogate mother fails to form it? It seems to me that the central question here is whether this 'maternal instinct' really exists, and, if it does, whether suppressing it is always harmful.

Underlying these questions is the assumption that bonding with babies is 'natural' and therefore 'good'. Perhaps so: the evolutionary advantage of such a tendency would be clear. It would be simpleminded, however, to assume that our habits are biologically determined: our culture is permeated with pronatalist bias.[20] 'Natural' or not, whether a tendency to such attachment is desirable could reasonably be judged to depend on circumstance. When infant mortality is high[21] or responsibility for childrearing is shared by the community, it could do more harm than good. Beware the naturalistic fallacy![22]

But surely there is something special about gestating a baby. That is, after all, the assumption behind the judgement that Mary Beth Whitehead, not William Stern, had a stronger claim to Baby M. The moral scoreboard seems clear: they both had the same

[20] See Ellen Peck and Judith Senderowitz, *Pronatalism: The Myth of Mom and Apple Pie*, (New York: Thomas Y. Crowell Co., 1974).

[21] As it has been at some periods in the past: see for example information about family relationships in Philippe Ariès, *Centuries of Childhood: A Social History of Family Life*, trans. Robert Baldick, (New York, 1982), and Lloyd DeMause's work.

[22] Consider the arguments in chapter 8 of *Women's Work*, by Ann Oakley, (New York: Vintage Books, 1974).

genetic input, but she gestated the baby, and therefore has a better case for social parenthood.[23]

We need to be very careful here. Special rights have a way of being accompanied by special responsibilities: women's unique gestational relationship with babies may be taken as reason to confine them once more to the nursery. Futhermore, positing special rights entailed directly by biology flirts again with the naturalistic fallacy and undermines our capacity to adapt to changing situations and forge our destiny.[24]

Furthermore, we already except many varieties of such separation. We routinely engage in sending children to boarding school, foster parenting, daycare, and so forth; in the appropriate circumstances, these practices are clearly beneficial. Hence, any blanket condemnation of separating reproduction and childrearing will not wash; additional argument is needed for particular classes of cases.

John Robertson points out that for the arguments against separating reproduction and childrearing used against contracted pregnancy are equally valid—but unused—with respect to adoption.[25] Others, such as Herbert Krimmel, reject this view by arguing that there is a big moral difference between giving away an already existing baby and deliberately creating one to give away. This remains to be shown, I think. It is also argued that as adoption outcomes are rather negative, we should be wary of extending any practice that shares its essential features. In fact, there seems to be amazingly little hard information about adoption outcomes. I wonder if the idea that they are bad results from media reports of offspring seeking their biological forbears.

---

[23] One of the interesting things about the practice of contracted pregnany is that it can be argued to both strengthen and weaken the social recognition of biological relationships. On the one hand, the pregnant woman's biological relationship is judged irrelevant beyond a certain point; on the other, the reason for not valuing it is to enhance that of the sperm donor. This might be interpreted as yet another case where men's interests are allowed to overrule women's. But it might also be interpreted as a salutory step toward awareness that biological ties can and sometimes should be subordinated to social ones. Deciding which interpretation is correct will depend on the facts of particular cases, and the arguments taken to justify the practice in the first place.

[24] Science fiction, most notably John Wyndham's *The Midwich Cuckoos*, provides us with thought-provoking material.

[25] John Robertson, 'Surrogate Mothers: Not so Novel After All', *Hastings Center Report*, vol. 13, no. 5 (October 1983). This article is reprinted in *Bioethics*, ed. Rem B. Edwards and Glen C. Graber, (San Diego, California: Harcourt, Brace Jovanovich, 1988). Krimmel's article ('The Case Against Surrogate Parenting') was also orginally published in the *Hastings Center Report* and is reprinted in *Bioethics*. References here are to the latter.

28 LAURA M. PURDY

There is, in any case, reason to think that there are differences between the two practices such that the latter is likely to be more successful than the former.[26]

None of the social descriptions of surrogacy thus seem to clearly justify the outcry against the practice. I suspect that the remaining central issue is the crucial one: surrogacy is baby-selling and participating in this practice exploits and taints women.

IS SURROGACY BABY-SELLING?

In the foregoing, I deliberately left vague the question of payment in contracted pregnancy. It is clear that there is a recognizable form of the practice that does not include payment; however, it also seems clear that controversy is focusing on the commercial form. The charge is that it is baby-selling and that this is wrong.

Is paid 'surrogacy' baby-selling? Proponents deny that it is, arguing that women are merely making available their biological services. Opponents retort that as women are paid little or nothing if they fail to hand over a live, healthy child, they are indeed selling a baby. If they are merely selling their services they would get full pay, even if the child were born dead.

It is true women who agree to contracts relieving clients of responsibility in this case are being exploited. They, after all, have done their part, risked their risks, and should be paid—just like the physicians involved. Normal childbearing provides no guarantee of a live, healthy child—why should contracted pregnancy?

There are further reasons for believing that women are selling their services, not babies. Firstly, we do not consider children property. Therefore, as we cannot sell what we do not own, we cannot be selling babies. What creates confusion here is that we do think we own sperm and ova. (Otherwise, how could man sell their sperm?) Yet we do not own what they become, persons. At

[26] One major difference between adoption and contracted pregnancy is that the baby is handed over virtually at birth, thus ensuring that the trauma sometimes experienced by older adoptees is not experienced. Although children of contracted pregnancy might well be curious to know about their biological mother, I do not see this as a serious obstacle to the practice, since we could change our policy about this. There is also reason to believe that carefully-screened women undertaking a properly-regulated contracted pregnancy are less likely to experience lingering pain of separation. First, they have deliberately chosen to go through pregnancy, knowing that they will give the baby up. The resulting sense of control is probably critical to both their short- and long-term well-being. Second, their pregnancy is not the result of trauma. See also Monica B. Morris, 'Reproductive Technology and Restraints', *Transaction/SOCIETY*, March/April 1988, pp. 16–22, especially p. 18.

what point, then, does the relationship cease to be describable as 'ownership'?

Resolution of this question is not necessary to the current discussion. If we can own babies, there seems to be nothing problematic about selling them. If ownership ceases at some time before birth (and could thus be argued to be unconnected with personhood), then it is not selling of babies that is going on.

Although this response deals with the letter of the objection about babyselling, it fails to heed its spirit, which is that we are trafficking in persons, and that such trafficking is wrong. Even if we are not 'selling', something nasty is happening.

The most common analogy, with slavery, is weak. Slavery is wrong according to any decent moral theory: the institution allows people to be treated badly. Their desires and interests, whose satisfaction is held to be essential for a good life, are held in contempt. Particularly egregious is the callous disregard of emotional ties to family and self-determination generally. But the institution of surrogate mothering deprives babies of neither.[27] In short, as Robertson contends, 'the purchasers do not buy the right to treat the child . . . as a commodity or property. Child abuse and neglect laws still apply.' (p. 655)

If 'selling babies' is not the right description of what is occurring. then how are we to explain what happens when the birth mother hands the child over to others? One plausible suggestion is that she is giving up her parental right to have a relationship with the child.[28] That it is wrong to do this for pay remains to be shown. Although it would be egoistic and immoral to 'sell' an ongoing, friendly relationship, (doing so would raise questions about whether it was friendship at all), the immorality of selling a relationship with an organism your body has created but with which you do not yet have a unique social bond, is a great deal less clear.[29]

[27] There may be a problem for the woman who gives birth, as the Baby M case has demonstrated. There is probably a case for a waiting period after the birth during which the woman can change her mind.

[28] Heidi Malm suggested this position in her comment on Sara Ann Ketchum's paper 'Selling Babies and Selling Bodies: Surrogate Motherhood and the Problem of Commodification', at the Eastern Division *APA* meetings, 30 December 1987.

[29] Mary Anne Warren suggests, alternatively, that this objection could be obviated by women and children retaining some rights and responsibilities toward each other in contracted pregnancy. Maintaining a relationship of sorts might also, she suggests, help forestall and alleviate whatever negative feelings children might have about such transfers. I agree that such openness is probably a good idea in any case. (Referee's comment.)

30 LAURA M. PURDY

People seem to feel much less strongly about the wrongness of such acts when motivated by altruism; refusing compensation is the only acceptable proof of such altruism. The act is, in any case, socially valuable. Why then must it be motivated by altruistic considerations? We do not frown upon those who provide other socially valuable services even when they do not have the 'right' motive. Nor do we require them to be unpaid. For instance, no one expects physicians, no matter what their motivation, to work for beans. They provide an important service; their motivation is important only to the extent that it affects quality.

In general, workers are required to have appropriate skills, not particular motivations.[30] Once again, it seems that there is a different standard for women and for men.

One worry is that women cannot be involved in contracted pregnancy without harming themselves, as it is difficult to let go of a child without lingering concern. So far, despite the heavily-publicized Baby M case, this appears not to be necessarily true.[31]

Another worry is that the practice will harm children. Children's welfare is, of course, important. Children deserve the same consideration as other persons, and no society that fails to meet their basic needs is morally satisfactory. Yet I am suspicious of the objections raised on their behalf in these discussions: recourse to children's alleged well-being is once again being used as a trump card against women's autonomy.

First, we hear only about possible risks, never possible benefits, which, as I have been arguing, could be substantial.[32] Second, the main objection raised is the worry about how children will take the knowledge that their genetic mother conceived on behalf of another. We do not know how children will feel about having had such 'surrogate' mothers. But as it is not a completely new phenomenon we might start our inquiry about this topic with historical evidence, not pessimistic speculation. In any case, if the practice is dealt with in an honest and commonsense way, particularly if it becomes quite common (and therefore 'normal'), there is likely to be no problem. We are also hearing about the worries of existing children of women who are involved in the

---

[30] Perhaps lurking behind the objections of surrogacy is some feeling that it is wrong to earn money by letting your body work, without active effort on your part. But this would rule out sperm selling, as well as using women's beauty to sell products and services.

[31] See, for example, James Rachels, 'A Report from America: The Baby M Case', *Bioethics*, vol. 1, n. 4 (October 1987), p. 365. He reports that there have been over six hundred succesful cases; see also the above note on adoption.

[32] Among them the above mentioned one of being born healthier.

practice: there are reports that they fear their mother will give them away, too. But surely we can make clear to children the kinds of distinctions that distinguish the practice from slavery or baby-selling in the first place.

Although we must try to forsee what might harm children, I cannot help but wonder about the double standards implied by this speculation. The first double standard occurs when those who oppose surrogacy (and reproductive technologies generally) also oppose attempts to reduce the number of handicapped babies born.[33] In the latter context, it is argued that despite their problems handicapped persons are often glad to be alive. Hence it would be paternalistic to attempt to prevent their birth.

Why then do we not hear the same argument here? Instead, the possible disturbance of children born of surrogacy is taken as a reason to prevent their birth. Yet this potential problem is both more remote and most likely involves less suffering than such ailments as spina bifida, Huntington's Disease or cystic fibrosis, which some do not take to be reasons to refrain from childbearing.[34]

Considering the sorts of reasons why parents have children, it is hard to see why the idea that one was conceived in order to provide a desperately-wanted child to another is thought to be problematic. One might well prefer that to the idea that one was an 'accident', adopted, born because contraception or abortion were not available, conceived to cement a failing marriage, to continue a family line, to qualify for welfare aid, to sex-balance a family, or as an experiment in childrearing. Surely what matters for a child's well-being in the end is whether it is being raised in a loving, intelligent environment.

The second double standard involves a disparity between the interests of women and children. Arguing that surrogacy is wrong because it may upset children suggests a disturbing conception of the moral order. Women should receive consideration at least equal to that accorded children. Conflicts of interest between the two should be resolved according to the same rules we use for any other moral subjects. Those rules should never prescribe sacrificing one individual's basic interest at the mere hint of harm to another.

---

[33] To avoid the difficulties about abortion added by the assumption that we are talking about existing foetuses, let us consider here only the issue of whether certain couples should risk pregnancy.

[34] There is an interesting link here between these two aspects of reproduction, as the promise of healthier children is, I think, one of the strongest arguments for contracted pregnancy.

32 LAURA M. PURDY

In sum, there seems to be no reason to think that there is anything necessarily wrong with 'surrogate mothering', even the paid variety. Furthermore, some objections to it depend on values and assumptions that have been the chief building blocks of women's inequality. Why are some feminists asserting them? Is it because 'surrogacy' as currently practiced often exploits women?

IS 'SURROGATE MOTHERING' WRONG IN CERTAIN SITUATIONS?

Even if 'surrogate mothering' is not necessarily immoral, circumstances can render it so. For instance, it is obviously wrong to coerce women to engage in the practice. Also, certain conditions are unacceptable. Among them are clauses in a contract that subordinate a woman's reasonable desires and judgements to the will of another contracting party,[35] clauses legitimating inadequate pay for the risks and discomforts involved, and clauses that penalize her for the birth of a handicapped or dead baby through no fault of her own. Such contracts are now common.[36]

One popular solution to the problem of such immoral contracts is a law forbidding all surrogacy agreements; their terms would then be unenforceable. But I believe that women will continue to engage in surrogate mothering, even if it is unregulated, and this approach leaves them vulnerable to those who change their mind, or will not pay. Fair and reasonable regulations are essential to prevent exploitation of women. Although surrogate mothering may seem risky and uncomfortable to middle-class persons safely ensconced in healthy, interesting, relatively well-paid jobs, with adequate regulation it becomes an attractive option for some women. That these women are more likely than not to be poor is no reason to prohibit the activity.

As I suggested earlier, poor women now face substantial risks in the workplace. Even a superficial survey of hazards in occupations available to poor women would give pause to those who would prohibit surrogacy on the grounds of risk.[37]

Particularly shocking is the list of harmful substances and conditions to which working women are routinely exposed. For

[35] What this may consist of naturally requires much additional elucidation.

[36] See Susan Ince, 'Inside the Surrogate Industry', *Test-Tube Women*, ed. Rita Arditti, Renate Duelli Klein, and Shelley Minden, (London: Pandora Press, 1984).

[37] See, for example, Jeanne Mager Stellman, *Women's Work, Women's Health*, (New York: Pantheon 1977).

instance, cosmeticians and hairdressers, dry cleaners and dental technicians are all exposed to carcinogens in their daily work. (Stellman, Appendixes 1 and 2) Most low-level jobs also have high rates of exposure to toxic chemicals and dangerous machinery, and women take such jobs in disproportionate numbers. It is therefore unsurprising that poor women sicken and die more often than other members of society.[38]

This is not an argument in favour of adding yet another dangerous option to those already facing such women. Nor does it follow that the burdens they already bear justify the new ones. On the contrary, it is imperative to clean up dangerous workplaces. However, it would be utopian to think that this will occur in the near future: We must therefore attempt to improve women's lot under existing conditions. Under these circumstances it would be irrational to prohibit surrogacy on the grounds of risk when women would instead have to engage in still riskier pursuits.

Overall's emphatic assertion that contracted pregnancy is not a 'real choice' for women is unconvincing. Her major argument, as I suggested earlier, is that it is an immoral, alienating option. But she also believes that such apparently expanded choices simply mask an underlying contraction of choice. (p. 124) She also fears that by 'endorsing an uncritical freedom of reproductive choice, we may also be implicitly endorsing all conceivable alternatives that an individual might adopt; we thereby abandon the responsibility for evaluating substantive actions in favour of advocating merely formal freedom of choice.' (p. 125) Both worries are, as they stand, unpersuasive.

As I argued before, there is something troubling here about the new and one-sided emphasis on risk. If nothing else, we need to remember that contracted pregnancy constitutes a low-tech approach to a social problem, one which would slow the impetus toward expensive and dangerous high-tech solutions.[39]

A desire for children on the part of those who normally could not have them is not likely to disappear anytime soon. We could discount it, as many participants in debate about new reproduc-

<hr>

[38] See George L. Waldbott, *Health Effects of Environmental Pollutants*, (St. Louis: The C.V. Mosby Co., 1973); Nicholas Ashford, *Crisis in the Workplace: Occupational Disease and Injury*, (Cambridge: MIT Press, 1976); *Cancer and the Worker*, The New York Academy of Science, 1977); *Environmental Problems in Medicine*, ed. William D. McKee, (Springfield, Ill.: Charles C. Thomas, 1977).

[39] These are the ones most likely to put women in the clutches of the paternalistic medical establishment. Exploitation by commercial operations such as that of Noel Keane could be avoided by tight regulation or prohibition altogether of for-profit enterprises.

34   LAURA M. PURDY

tive technologies do. After all, nobody promised a rose garden to infertile couples, much less to homosexuals or to single women. Nor is it desirable to propagate the idea that having children is essential for human fulfilment.

But appealing to the sacrosancity of traditional marriage or of blood ties to prohibit otherwise acceptable practices that would satisfy people's desires hardly makes sense, especially when those practices may provide other benefits. Not only might contracted pregnancy be less risky and more enjoyable than other jobs women are forced to take, but there are other advantages as well. Since being pregnant is not usually a full-time occupation, 'surrogate mothering' could buy time for women to significantly improve their lot: students, aspiring writers, and social activists could make real progress toward their goals.

Women have until now done this reproductive labour for free.[40] Paying women to bear children should force us all to recognize this process as the socially useful enterprise that it is, and children as socially valuable creatures whose upbringing and welfare are critically important.

In short, 'surrogate mothering' has the potential to empower women and increase their status in society. The darker side of the story is that it also has frightening potential for deepening their exploitation. The outcome of the current warfare over control of new reproductive possibilities will determine which of these alternatives comes to pass.

Department of Philosophy
Hamilton College, Clinton, N.Y.

[40] The implications of this fact remain to be fully understood; I suspect that they are detrimental to women and children, but that this is a topic for another paper.

Artificial Means of Reproduction and Our Understanding of the Family

by Ruth Macklin

The new reproductive technologies force us to rethink the concepts 'mother,' 'father,' 'family.' As we draw analogies to traditional patterns, we must distinguish between ethical and conceptual questions.

It is an obvious truth that scientific and technologic innovations produce changes in our traditional way of perceiving the world around us. We have only to think of the telescope, the microscope, and space travel to recall that heretofore unimagined perceptions of the macrocosm and the microcosm have become commonplace. Yet it is not only perceptions, but also conceptions of the familiar that become altered by advances in science and technology. As a beginning student of philosophy, I first encountered problems in epistemology generated by scientific knowledge: If physical objects are really composed of molecules in motion, how is it that we perceive them as solid? Why is it that objects placed on a table don't slip through the empty spaces between the molecules? If the mind is nothing but

electrical processes occurring in the brain, how can we explain Einstein's ability to create the special theory of relativity or Bach's ability to compose the Brandenburg Concertos?

Now questions are being raised about how a variety of modes of artificial means of reproduction might alter our conception of the family. George Annas has observed:

> Dependable birth control made sex without reproduction possible....Now medicine is closing the circle...by offering methods of reproduction without sex: including artificial insemination by donor (AID), in vitro fertilization (IVF), and surrogate embryo transfer (SET). As with birth control, artificial reproduction is defended as life-affirming and loving by its proponents, and denounced as unnatural by its detractors.[1]

Opponents of artificial reproduction have expressed concerns about its effects on the family. This concern has centered largely but not entirely on surrogacy arrangements. Among the objections to surrogacy made by the Roman Catholic Church is the

charge that "the practice of surrogate motherhood is a threat to the stability of the family."[2] But before the consequences for the family of surrogacy arrangements or other new reproductive practices can be assessed, we need to inquire into our understanding of the family. Is there a single, incontrovertible conception of the family? And who are the "we" presupposed in the phrase, "our understanding"? To begin, I offer three brief anecdotes.

The first is a remark made by a long-married, middle-aged man at a wedding. The wedding couple were both about forty. The bride had been married and divorced once, the groom twice. During a light-hearted discussion about marriage and divorce, the middle-aged man remarked: "I could never divorce my wife. She's family!"

The second is a remark made by a four-year-old boy. I had just moved to the neighborhood and was getting to know the children. The four-year-old, named Mikey, was being tormented by a five-year-old named Timmy. I asked Mikey, "Is Timmy your brother?" Mikey replied: "Not any more. Not the way he acts!"

The third story appears in a case study presented as part of a bioethics project on everyday dilemmas in nursing home life. A resident, Mrs. Finch, is a constant complainer who seeks more choices and independence than the nursing home allows. A social worker at the home talked to Mrs. Finch about her adaptation, suggesting that she think of the residents and staff group as a large family where "we all make allowances for each other" and "we all pull our weight." Mrs. Finch responded that she is in the nursing home because she needs health care. She already has a family and does not want another one.

In my commentary on the case of Mrs. Finch, I gave an analysis that suggests some of the complexities in understanding the concept of the family. I wrote:

> Mrs. Finch is quite right to reject the social worker's suggestion that the nursing home be viewed as "a large family." A family is a well-defined social and cultural institution. People may choose to "adopt" unrelated persons into their own family.

Ruth Macklin is professor of bioethics, Albert Einstein College of Medicine, Bronx, N.Y.

5

and biologically related family members may choose to "disown" one of their members (which doesn't sever the kinship ties, though it may sever relations). But an organization or institution does not become a "family" because members or residents are exhorted to treat each other in the way family members should. The social worker's well-intended chat with Mrs. Finch is an exhortation to virtue rather than a proper reminder about the resident's obligations to her new "family."[3]

The Biological Concept of Family

It is possible, of course, to settle these conceptual matters simply and objectively by adopting a biological criterion for determining what counts as a family. According to this criterion, people who are genetically related to one another would constitute a family, with the type and degree of relatedness described in the manner of a family tree. This sense of *family* is important and interesting for many purposes, but it does not and cannot encompass everything that is actually meant by *family*, nor does it reflect the broader cultural customs and kinship systems that also define family ties.

What makes the first anecdote amusing is the speaker's deliberate use of the biological sense of *family* in a nonbiological context, that is, the context of being related by marriage. In saying that he could never divorce his wife because "she's family," he was conjuring up the associations normally connected with biologically related family and transferring those associations to a person related by the convention of marriage. In a society in which the divorce rate hovers around 50 percent, being a family member related by marriage is often a temporary state of affairs.

What makes the second anecdote amusing is Mikey's denial, based solely on Timmy's behavior, that his biologically related sibling was his brother. When two people are biologically related, they cannot wave away that kinship relation on grounds of their dislike of the other's character or conduct. They can sever their relationship, but not their genetic relatedness. Whether family members ought to remain loyal to one another, regardless of how they act,

is an ethical question, not a conceptual one.

The third story also relies on the biological notion of family. Mrs. Finch construed the concept literally when she insisted that she already had a family and "didn't need another one." When I observed in my commentary that a family is a well-defined social and cultural institution, I meant to rebut the social worker's implication that anything one wants to call a family can thereby become a family. Yet considered from a moral perspective, our conception of the family does draw on notions of what members owe to one another in a functional understanding of the family:

Families should be broadly defined to include, besides the traditional biological relationships, those committed relationships between individuals which fulfill the functions of family.[4]

It seems clear that we need a richer concept than that of biological relatedness to flesh out our understanding of the family. Although the biological concept is accurate in its delineation of one set of factors that determine what is a family, it fails to capture other significant determinants.

Newly developed artificial means of reproduction have rendered the term *biological* inadequate for making some critical conceptual distinctions, along with consequent moral decisions. The capability of separating the process of producing eggs from the act of gestation renders obsolete the use of the word *biological* to modify the word *mother*. The techniques of egg retrieval, in vitro fertilization (IVF), and gamete intrafallopian transfer (GIFT) now make it possible for two different women to make a biological contribution to the creation of a new life. It would be a prescriptive rather than a descriptive definition to maintain that the egg donor should properly be called the biological mother. The woman who contributes her womb during gestation—whether she is acting as a surrogate or is the intended rearing mother—is also a biological mother. We have only to reflect on the many ways that the intrauterine environment and maternal behavior during pregnancy can

influence fetal and later child development to acknowledge that a gestating woman is also a biological mother. I will return to this issue later in considering how much genetic contributions should count in disputed surrogacy arrangements.

Additional Determinants of the Meaning of *Family*

In addition to the biological meaning, there appear to be three chief determinants of what is meant by *family*. These are law, custom, and what I shall call subjective intentions. All three contribute to our understanding of the family. The effect of artificial means of reproduction on our understanding of the family will vary, depending on which of these three determinants is chosen to have priority. There is no way to assign a priori precedence to any one of the three. Let me illustrate each briefly.

Law as a Determinant of Family. Legal scholars can elaborate with precision and detail the categories and provisions of family law. This area of law encompasses legal rules governing adoption, artificial insemination by donor, foster placement, custody arrangements, and removal of children from a home in which they have been abused or neglected. For present purposes, it will suffice to summarize the relevant areas in which legal definitions or decisions have determined what is to count as a family.

Laws governing adoption and donor insemination stipulate what counts as a family. In the case of adoption, a person or couple genetically unrelated to a child is deemed that child's legal parent or parents. By this legal rule, a new family is created. The biological parent or parents of the child never cease to be genetically related, of course. But by virtue of law, custom, and usually emotional ties, the adoptive parents become the child's family.

The Uniform Parentage Act holds that a husband who consents to artificial insemination by donor (AID) of his wife by a physician is the legal father of the child. Many states have enacted laws in conformity with this legal rule. I am not aware of any laws that have been enacted making an analogous stipulation in the case of egg donation, but it is reasonable to assume that there will be symmetry of reasoning and legislation.

Commenting on the bearing of family law on the practice of surrogacy, Alexander M. Capron and Margaret J. Radin contend that the "legal rules of greatest immediate relevance" to surrogacy are those on adoption. These authors identify a number of provisions of state laws on adoption that should apply in the case of surrogacy. The provisions include allowing time for a "change of heart" period after the agreement to release a child, and prohibition of agreements to relinquish parental rights prior to the child's birth.[5]

Capron and Radin observe that in the context of adoption, "permitting the birth mother to reclaim a child manifests society's traditional respect for biological ties."[6] But how does this observation bear on artificial reproduction where the biological tie can be either genetic or gestational?

Consider first the case of the gestational surrogate who is genetically unrelated to the child. Does society's traditional respect for biological ties give her or the genetic mother the right to "reclaim" (or claim in the first place) the child? Society's traditional respect is more likely a concern for genetic inheritance than a recognition of the depth of the bond a woman may feel toward a child she has given birth to.

Secondly, consider the case of egg donation and embryo transfer to the wife of the man whose sperm was used in IVF. If the sperm donor and egg recipient were known to the egg donor, could the donor base her claim to the child on "society's traditional respect for biological ties"? As I surmised earlier, it seems reasonable to assume that any laws enacted for egg donation will be similar to those now in place for donor insemination. In the latter context, society's traditional respect for biological ties gave way to other considerations arising out of the desire of couples to have a child who is genetically related to at least one of the parents.

Custom as a Determinant of Family. The most telling examples of custom as a determinant of family are drawn from cultural anthropology. Kinship systems and incest taboos dictated by folkways and mores differ so radically that few generalizations are possible.

Ruth Benedict writes: "No known people regard all women as possible mates. This is not in an effort, as is so often supposed, to prevent inbreeding in our sense, for over great parts of the world it is an own cousin, often the daughter of one's mother's brother, who is the predestined spouse."[7] In contrast, Benedict notes, some incest taboos are

extended by a social fiction to include vast numbers of individuals who have no traceable ancestors in common....This social fiction receives unequivocal expression in the terms of relationship which are used. Instead of distinguishing lineal from collateral kin as we do in the distinction between father and uncle, brother and cousin, one term means literally "man of my father's group (relationship, locality, etc.) or his generation."... Certain tribes of eastern Australia use an extreme form of this so-called classificatory kinship system. Those whom they call brothers and sisters are all those of their generation with whom they recognize any relationship.[8]

One anthropologist notes that "the family in all societies is distinguished by a stability that arises out of the fact that it is based on marriage, that is to say, on socially sanctioned mating entered into with the assumption of permanency."[9] If we extend the notion of socially sanctioned mating to embrace socially sanctioned procreation, it is evident that the new artificial means of reproduction call for careful thought about what should be socially sanctioned before policy decisions are made.

Subjective Intention as a Determinant of Family. This category is most heterogeneous and amorphous. It includes a variety of ways in which individuals—singly, in pairs, or as a group—consider themselves a family even if their arrangement is not recognized by law or custom. Without an accompanying analysis, I list here an array of examples, based on real people and their situations.

• A homosexual couple decides to solidify their relationship by taking matrimonial vows. Despite the fact that their marriage is not recognized by civil law, they find an ordained minister who is willing to perform the marriage ceremony. Later they apply to be foster parents of children with AIDS whose biological parents have died or abandoned them. The foster agency accepts the couple. Two children are placed in foster care with them. They are now a family.

• A variation on this case: A lesbian couple has a long-term monogamous relationship. They decide they want to rear a child. Using "turkey-baster" technology, one of the women is inseminated, conceives, and gives birth to a baby. The three are now a family, with one parent genetically related to the child.

• Pat Anthony, a forty-seven-year-old grandmother in South Africa, agreed to serve as gestational surrogate for her own daughter. The daughter had had her uterus removed, but could still produce eggs and wanted more children. The daughter's eggs were inseminated with her husband's sperm, and the resulting embryos implanted in her own mother. Mrs. Anthony gave birth to triplets when she was forty-eight. She was the gestational mother and the genetic grandmother of the triplets.

• Linda Kirkman was the gestational mother of a baby conceived with a sister's egg and destined to live with the infertile sister and her husband. Linda Kirkman said, "I always considered myself her aunt." Carol Chan donated eggs so that her sister Susie could bear and raise a child. Carol Chan said: "I could never regard the twins as anything but my nephews." The two births occurred in Melbourne within weeks of each other.[10]

My point in elucidating this category of heterogeneous examples is to suggest that there may be entirely subjective yet valid elements that contribute to our understanding of the family, family membership, or family relationships. I believe it would be arbitrary and narrow to rule out all such examples by fiat. The open texture of our language leaves room for conceptions of family not recognized by law or preexisting custom.

Posing the question, Who counts as family? Carol Levine replies: "The answer to this apparently simple

Hastings Center Report, January-February 1991

He said: "Your family—they are very angry."

I looked up at him, wondering what he could mean. "I know very little of families," I said.

"I had none," he said, "though I used to think of them a lot...when I was younger."

"I don't follow you," I said. "What family?"

He looked down, with the slight brief smile of puzzlement that was so like his slight brief smile of pleasure. "When I came in from the theater, your sibling—the one with the metallic yellow flesh—was angry at your black sister; finally she took her outside while the rest of you watched."

"George—my...?" I looked up. "Nea...? [...] They're not even from our world. George and Nea are Thants. They're friends of Dyeth." But when it dawned on me, I laughed out loud. "You thought we were a family...?" Then I smiled. "Suddenly some of the things you've been saying begin to make sense. No, the Dyeths are very much our own nurture stream—at least that's the translation of the northern evelmi's term for it. This particular nurture stream has been bubbling along for seven ripples now. There're only two older streams in the area—one at the tracer collective and one at the nematode farm. And I wouldn't be all that upset if ours went on for seventeen or twenty-seven more. [...] I was adopted by the Dyeths when I was a baby— from some infant exchange in the north; but most of my sisters come from even farther south. Small Maxa was semisomed from some neuroplasm that an evelm grandmother of mine, N'yom, donated to a bioengineering experiment many many years ago and that was just taken out of suspension about a decade and a half back—though of course most of Maxa's chromosome sequence was taken from humans. But in the genetic sense she's part evelm. Still, there is no egg-and-sperm relation between any of our parents and any of this generation of children, nor between any of my sisters—human or evelm—and each other." [...] I moved, planning to speak. But he stood, with me, before words came. And walked with me as I started to walk. (Thus faith is rewarded.) "Rhyonon was a Family world, wasn't it? [...] At least someone told me that it was about to fall over in that direction."

From Samuel R. Delaney,
Stars in My Pocket Like Grains of Sand
(New York: Bantam Books, 1984), pp. 214-15.

question is by no means easy. It depends on why the question is being asked and who is giving the answer."[11] Levine's observation, made in the context of AIDS, applies equally well to the context of artificial means of reproduction.

The Gestational versus the Genetic Mother

One critical notion rendered problematic by the new technological capabilities of artificial reproduction is the once-simple concept of a mother. The traditional concept is complicated by the possibility that a woman can gestate a fetus genetically unrelated to her. This prospect has implications both for public policy and our understanding of the family. The central policy question is, How much should genetic relatedness count in disputed surrogacy arrangements?

A Matter of Discovery or Decision? Which criterion—genetic or gestational—should be used to determine who is the "real" mother? I contend that this question is poorly formulated. Referring to the "real" mother implies that it is a matter of discovery, rather than one calling for a decision. To speak of "the real x" is to assume that there is an underlying metaphysical structure to be probed by philosophical inquiry. But now that medical technology has separated the two biological contributions to motherhood, in place of the single conjoint role provided by nature, some decisions will have to be made.

One decision is conceptual, and a second is moral. The conceptual question is: Should a woman whose contribution is solely gestational be termed a mother of the baby? We may assume, by analogy with our concept of paternity, that the woman who makes the genetic contribution in a surrogacy arrangement can properly be termed a mother of the baby. So it must be decided whether there can be only one mother, conceptually speaking, or whether this technological advance calls for new terminology.

Conceptual decisions often have implications beyond mere terminology. A decision not to use the term *mother* (even when modified by the

Hastings Center Report. January-February 1991

adjective *gestational*) to refer to a woman who acts in this capacity can have important consequences for ethics and public policy. As a case in point, the Wayne County Circuit Court in Michigan issued an interim order declaring a gamete donor couple to be the biological parents of a fetus being carried to term by a woman hired to be the gestational mother. Upon birth, the court entered an order that the names of the ovum and sperm donors be listed on the birth certificate, rather than that of the woman who gave birth, who was termed by the court a "human incubator."[12]

The ethical question posed by the separation of biological motherhood into genetic and gestational components is, Which role should entitle a woman to a greater claim on the baby, in case of dispute? Since the answer to this question cannot be reached by discovery, but is, like the prior conceptual question, a matter for decision, we need to determine which factors are morally relevant and which have the greatest moral weight. To avoid begging any ethical questions by a choice of terminology, I use the terms *genetic mother* and *gestational mother* to refer to the women who make those respective contributions. And instead of speaking of the "real" mother, I'll use the phrase *primary mother* when referring to the woman presumed to have a greater claim on the child.

Morally Relevant Factors. The possibilities outlined below are premised on the notion that surrogacy contracts are voidable. I take this to mean that no legal presumption is set up by the fact that there has been a prior contract between the surrogate and the intended rearing parents. From an ethical perspective, that premise must be argued for independently, and convincing arguments have been advanced by a number of authors.[13] If we accept the premise that a contractual provision to relinquish a child born of a surrogacy agreement has no legal force, the question then becomes, Is there a morally relevant distinction between the two forms of surrogacy with respect to a claim on the child? Who has the weightiest moral claim when a surrogate is unwilling to give

the baby up after its birth? Where should the moral presumption lie? The question may be answered in one of three ways.

1. Gestation. According to this position, whether a woman is merely the gestational surrogate, or also contributes her genetic material, makes no difference in determining moral priorities. In either case, the surrogate is the primary mother because the criterion is gestation.

The gestational position is adopted by George Annas and others who have argued that the gestational mother should be legally presumed to have the right and responsibility to rear the child. One reason given in support of this presumption is "the greater biological and psychological investment of the gestational mother in the child."[14] This is referred to as "sweat equity." A related yet distinct reason is "the biological reality that the mother at this point has contributed more to the child's development, and that she will of necessity be present at birth and immediately thereafter to care for the child."[15]

The first reason focuses on what the gestational mother deserves, based on her investment in the child, while the second reason, though mentioning her contribution, also focuses on the interests of the child during and immediately after birth. Annas adds that "to designate the gestational mother, rather than the genetic mother, the legal or 'natural mother' would be protective of children."[16]

2. Genetics. In surrogacy arrangements, it is the inseminating male who is seen as the father, not the husband of the woman who acts as a surrogate. This is because the genetic contribution is viewed as determinative for fatherhood. By analogy, the woman who makes the genetic contribution is the primary mother. This position sharply distinguishes between the claim to the child made by the two different types of surrogate. It makes the surrogate who contributes her egg as well as her womb the primary (or sole) mother. But now recall the fact that in AID, the law recognizes the husband of the inseminated woman as the father—proof that laws can be made to go either way.

This position was supported by the court in *Smith & Smith v. Jones & Jones*, on grounds of the analogy with paternity. The court said: "The donor of the ovum, the biological mother, is to be deemed, in fact, the natural mother of this infant, as is the biological father to be deemed the natural father of this child."[17]

Legal precedents aside, is there a moral reason that could be invoked in support of this position? One possibility is "ownership" of one's genetic products. Since each individual has a unique set of genes, people might be said to have a claim on what develops from their own genes, unless they have explicitly relinquished any such claims. This may be a metaphorical sense of ownership, but it reflects the felt desire to have genetically related children—the primary motivation behind all forms of assisted reproduction.

Another possible reason for assigning greater weight to the genetic contribution is the child-centered position. Here it is argued that it is in children's best interest to be reared by parents to whom they are genetically related. Something like this position is taken by Sidney Callahan. She writes:

The most serious ethical problems in using third-party donors in alternative reproduction concern the well-being of the potential child....A child who has donor(s) intruded into its parentage will be cut off from its genetic heritage and part of its kinship relations in new ways. Even if there is no danger of transmitting unknown genetic disease or causing physiological harm to the child, the psychological relationship of the child to its parents is endangered—with or without the practice of deception and secrecy about its origins.[18]

Additional considerations lending plausibility to this view derive from data concerning adopted children who have conducted searches for their biological parents, and similar experiences of children whose birth was a result of donor insemination and who have sought out their biological fathers. In the case of gestational surrogacy, the child is genetically related to both of the intended rearing parents. However, there is no data to suggest whether children born of gestational mothers

Medical Ethics

Hastings Center Report. January-February 1991

might someday begin to seek out those women in a quest for their "natural" or "real" mothers.

3. Gestation and genetics. According to this position, the surrogate who contributes both egg and womb has more of a claim to being the primary mother than does the surrogate who contributes only her womb. Since the first type of surrogate makes both a genetic and a gestational contribution, in case of a dispute she gets to keep the baby instead of the biological father, who has made only one contribution. But this does not yet settle the question of who has a greater moral claim to the infant in cases where the merely gestational surrogate does not wish to give up the baby to the genetic parents. To determine that, greater weight must be given either to the gestational component or to the genetic component.

Subsidiary Views. One may reject the notion that the only morally relevant considerations are the respective contributions of each type of surrogate. Another possible criterion draws on the biological conception of family, and thus takes into account the contribution of the genetic father. According to this position, two genetic contributions count more than none. This leads to three subsidiary views, in addition to the three main positions outlined above.

4. Gestational surrogates have less of a moral claim to the infant than the intended parents, both of whom have made a genetic contribution. This is because two (genetic) contributions count more than one (gestational) contribution. This view, derived from "society's traditional respect for biological ties," gives greatest weight to the concept of family based on genetic inheritance.

5. A woman who contributes both egg and womb has a claim equal to that of the biological father, since both have made genetic contributions. If genetic contribution is what determines both "true" motherhood and fatherhood, the policy implications of this view are that each case in which a surrogate who is both genetic and gestational mother wishes to keep the baby would have to go to court and be settled in the

manner of custody disputes.

As a practical suggestion, this model is of little value. It throws every case of this type of surrogacy—the more common variety—open to this possibility, which is to move backwards in public policy regarding surrogacy.

6. However, if genetic and gestational contributions are given equal weight, but it is simply the number of contributions that counts, the artificially inseminated surrogate has the greater moral claim since she has made two contributions—genetic and gestational—while the father has made only one, the genetic contribution.

What can we conclude from all this about the effects of artificial means of reproduction on the family and on our conception of the family? Several conclusions emerge, although each requires a more extended elaboration and defense than will be given here.

A broad definition of *family* is preferable to a narrow one. A good candidate is the working definition proposed by Carol Levine: "Family members are individuals who by birth, adoption, marriage, or declared commitment share deep personal connections and are mutually entitled to receive and obligated to provide support of various kinds to the extent possible, especially in times of need."[19]

Some of the effects of the new reproductive technologies on the family call for the development of public policy, while others remain private, personal matters to be decided within a given family. An example of the former is the determination of where the presumptions should lie in disputed surrogacy arrangements, whose rights and interests are paramount, and what procedures should be followed to safeguard those rights and interests. An example of the latter is disclosure to a child of the facts surrounding genetic paternity or maternity in cases of donor insemination or egg donation, including the identity of the donor when that is known. These are profound moral decisions, about which many people have strong feelings, but they are not issues to be addressed by public policy.

It is not at all clear that artificial

modes of reproduction threaten to produce greater emotional difficulties for family members affected, or pose more serious ethical problems, than those already arising out of long-standing practices such as adoption and artificial insemination. The analogy is often made between the impact on women who serve as surrogates and those who have lost their biological offspring in other ways.

Warning of the dangers of surrogacy, defenders of birth mothers have related the profound emotional trauma and lasting consequences for women who have given their babies up for adoption. One such defender is Phyllis Chesler, a psychologist who has written about the mother-infant bond and about custody battles in which mothers have lost their children to fathers. Dr. Chesler reports that many women never get over having given up their child for adoption. Their decision "leads to thirty to forty years of being haunted."[20] Chesler contends that the trauma to women who have given up their babies for adoption is far greater than that of incest, and greater than that felt by mothers who have lost custody battles for their children.

Additional evidence of the undesirable consequences for birth mothers of adoption is provided by Alison Ward, a woman who serves as an adoption reform advocate. Having given up her own daughter for adoption in 1967, she found and was reunited with her in 1980. Ms. Ward said to an audience assembled to hear testimony on surrogacy:

I think that you lack the personal experience I have: that of knowing what it is like to terminate your parental rights and go for years not knowing if your child is dead or alive. All the intellectual and philosophical knowledge in the world cannot begin to touch having to live your life as a birthparent. Last Sunday was Mother's Day. It seems ironic, as our country gives such lip service to the values of motherhood and the sanctity of the bond between mother and child, that we even consider legalizing a process [surrogacy] which would destroy all that.[21]

The effects of these practices on children are alleged to be equally profound and damaging. Scholarly studies conducted in recent years

Hastings Center Report, January-February 1991

have sought to evaluate the adjustment of children to adoption. One expert notes that "the pattern emerging from the more recent clinical and nonclinical studies that have sampled widely and used appropriate controls, generally supports the view that, on the average, adopted children are more likely to manifest psychological problems than nonadopted children."[22] The additional fact that numerous adopted children have sought to find their biological parents, despite their being in a loving family setting, suggests that psychological forces can intrude on the dictates of law or custom regarding what counts as a family. Although it is easier to keep secret from a child the circumstances surrounding artificial insemination and egg donation, such secrets have sometimes been revealed with terrible emotional consequences for everyone involved.

Alison Ward compares the impact of surrogacy on children to both situations:

There will always be pain for these children. Just as adoptive parents have learned that they cannot love the pain of their adopted children away, couples who raise children obtained through surrogacy will have to deal with a special set of problems. Donor offspring…rarely find out the truth of their origins. But, some of them do, and we must listen to them when they speak of their anguish, of not knowing who fathered them; we must listen when they tell us how destructive it is to their self esteem to find out their father sold the essence of his lineage for $40 or so, without ever intending to love or take responsibility for them. For children born of surrogacy contracts, it will be even worse: their own mothers did this to them.[23]

Phyllis Chesler paints a similarly bleak picture of the effect on children of being adopted away from their birth mothers. She contends that this has "dramatic, extreme psychological consequences." She cites evidence indicating that adopted children seem more prone to mental and emotional disorders than other children, and concludes that "children need to know their natural origins."[24]

These accounts present only one side, and there is surely another, more positive picture of parents and children flourishing in happy, healthy families that would not have existed but for adoption or artificial insemination. Yet the question remains. What follows in any case from such evidence? Is it reasonable to conclude that the negative consequences of these practices, which have altered traditional conceptions of the family, are reasons for abolishing them? Or for judging that it was wrong to institute them in the first place, since for all practical purposes they cannot be reversed? A great deal more evidence, on a much larger scale, would be needed before a sound conclusion could be reached that adoption and artificial insemination have had such negative consequences for the family that they ought never to have been socially sanctioned practices.

Similarly, there is no simple answer to the question of how artificial means of reproduction affect our understanding of the family. We need to reflect on the variety of answers, paying special attention to what follows from answering the question one way rather than another. Since there is no single, univocal concept of the family, it is a matter for moral and social decision just which determinants of "family" should be given priority.

References

1. George J. Annas, "Redefining Parenthood and Protecting Embryos," in *Judging Medicine* (Clifton, N.J.: Humana Press, 1988), p. 59. Reprinted from the *Hastings Center Report* 14, no. 5 (1984).

2. William F. Bolan, Jr., Executive Director, New Jersey Catholic Conference, "Statement of New Jersey Catholic Conference in Connection with Public Hearing on Surrogate Mothering," Commission on Legal and Ethical Problems in the Delivery of Health Care, Newark, N.J., 11 May 1988.

3. Ruth Macklin, "Good Citizen, Bad Citizen: Case Commentary," in *Everyday Ethics: Resolving Dilemmas in Nursing Home Life*, ed. Rosalie A. Kane and Arthur L. Caplan (New York: Springer, 1990), p. 65.

4. Cited in Carol Levine, "AIDS and Changing Concepts of Family," *Milbank Quarterly* 68, supp. 1 (1990): 37.

5. Alexander M. Capron and Margaret J. Radin, "Choosing Family Law over Contract Law as a Paradigm for Surrogate Motherhood," *Law, Medicine & Health Care* 16 (Spring-Summer 1988): 35.

6. Capron and Radin, "Choosing Family Law over Contract Law," p. 35.

7. Ruth Benedict, *Patterns of Culture* (New York: Mentor Books, 1934), p. 29.

8. Benedict, *Patterns of Culture*, p. 30.

9. Melville J. Herskovits, *Cultural Anthropology* (New York: Alfred A. Knopf, 1955), p. 171.

10. R. Alta Charo, "Legislative Approaches to Surrogate Motherhood," *Law, Medicine & Health Care* 16 (Spring-Summer 1988): 104.

11. Levine, "AIDS and Changing Concepts of Family," p. 35.

12. O.T.A. report, "Infertility: Medical and Social Choices," p. 284; case cited *Smith & Smith v. Jones & Jones*, 85-532014 DZ, Detroit MI, 3rd Dist. (15 March 1986), as reported in *BioLaw*, ed. James F. Childress, Patricia King, Karen H. Rothenberg, et al. (Frederick, Md.: University Publishers of America, 1986). See also George J. Annas, "The Baby Broker Boom," *Hastings Center Report* 16, no. 3 (1986): 30-31.

13. See, e.g., George J. Annas, "Death without Dignity for Commercial Surrogacy: The Case of Baby M," *Hastings Center Report*, 18, no. 2 (1988): 21-24; and Bonnie Steinbock, "Surrogate Motherhood as Prenatal Adoption," in *Surrogate Motherhood: Politics and Privacy*, ed. Larry Gostin (Bloomington: Indiana University Press, 1990), pp. 123-35.

14. Sherman Elias and George J. Annas, "Noncoital Reproduction," *JAMA* 255 (3 January 1986): 67.

15. Annas, "Death without Dignity," p. 23.

16. Annas, "Death without Dignity," p. 24.

17. Annas, "The Baby Broker Boom," p. 31.

18. "The Ethical Challenge of the New Reproductive Technology," presentation before the Task Force on New Reproductive Practices; published in John F. Monagle and David C. Thomasma, eds., *Medical Ethics: A Guide for Health Care Professionals* (Frederick, Md.: Aspen Publishers, 1987).

19. Levine, "AIDS and Changing Concepts of Family," p. 36.

20. This statement and subsequent ones attributed to Phyllis Chesler are taken from her unpublished remarks made at a public hearing on surrogacy conducted by the New Jersey Bioethics Commission, Newark, N.J., 11 May 1988, in which the author was a participant.

21. Written testimony, presented orally at the New Jersey Bioethics Commission's public hearing on surrogacy, 11 May 1988.

22. David M. Brodzinsky, "Adjustment to Adoption: A Psychosocial Perspective," *Clinical Psychology Review* 7 (1987): 29.

23. Ward, written testimony from New Jersey public hearing.

24. Chesler, oral testimony at New Jersey public hearing.

[23]

ON THE MORAL AND LEGAL STATUS
OF ABORTION

We will be concerned with both the moral status of abortion, which for our purposes we may define as the act which a woman performs in voluntarily terminating, or allowing another person to terminate, her pregnancy, and the legal status which is appropriate for this act. I will argue that, while it is not possible to produce a satisfactory defense of a woman's right to obtain an abortion without showing that a fetus is not a human being, in the morally relevant sense of that term, we ought not to conclude that the difficulties involved in determining whether or not a fetus is human make it impossible to produce any satisfactory solution to the problem of the moral status of abortion. For it is possible to show that, on the basis of intuitions which we may expect even the opponents of abortion to share, a fetus is not a person, and hence not the sort of entity to which it is proper to ascribe full moral rights.

Of course, while some philosophers would deny the possibility of any such proof,[1] others will deny that there is any need for it, since the moral permissibility of abortion appears to them to be too obvious to require proof. But the inadequacy of this attitude should be evident from the fact that both the friends and the foes of abortion consider their position to be morally self-evident. Because pro-abortionists have never adequately come to grips with the conceptual issues surrounding abortion, most if not all, of the arguments which they advance in opposition to laws restricting access to abortion fail to refute or even weaken the traditional antiabortion argument, i.e., that a fetus is a human being, and therefore abortion is murder.

These arguments are typically of one of two sorts. Either they point to the terrible side effects of the restrictive laws, e.g., the deaths due to illegal abortions, and the fact that it is poor women

---

1. For example, Roger Wertheimer, who in "Understanding the Abortion Argument" (*Philosophy and Public Affairs*, 1, No. 1 [Fall, 1971], 67-95), argues that the problem of the moral status of abortion is insoluble, in that the dispute over the status of the fetus is not a question of fact at all, but only a question of how one responds to the facts.

44   MARY ANNE WARREN

who suffer the most as a result of these laws, or else they state that
to deny a woman access to abortion is to deprive her of her right to
control her own body. Unfortunately, however, the fact that restricting access to abortion has tragic side effects does not, in itself, show
that the restrictions are unjustified, since murder is wrong regardless
of the consequences of prohibiting it; and the appeal to the right to
control one's body, which is generally construed as a property right,
is at best a rather feeble argument for the permissibility of abortion.
Mere ownership does not give me the right to kill innocent people
whom I find on my property, and indeed I am apt to be held responsible if such people injure themselves while on my property. It
is equally unclear that I have any moral right to expel an innocent
person from my property when I know that doing so will result in
his death.

Furthermore; it is probably inappropriate to describe a woman's
body as her property, since it seems natural to hold that a person is
something distinct from her property, but not from her body. Even
those who would object to the identification of a person with his
body, or with the conjunction of his body and his mind, must admit
that it would be very odd to describe, say, breaking a leg, as damaging one's property, and much more appropriate to describe it as in-
juring one*self*. Thus it is probably a mistake to argue that the right
to obtain an abortion is in any way derived from the right to own
and regulate property.

But however we wish to construe the right to abortion, we cannot hope to convince those who consider abortion a form of murder
of the existence of any such right unless we are able to produce a
clear and convincing refutation of the traditional antiabortion argument, and this has not, to my knowledge, been done. With respect
to the two most vital issues which that argument involves, i.e., the
humanity of the fetus and its implication for the moral status of
abortion, confusion has prevailed on both sides of the dispute.

Thus, both proabortionists and antiabortionists have tended to abstract the question of whether abortion is wrong to that of whether
it is wrong to destroy a fetus, just as though the rights of another
person were not necessarily involved. This mistaken abstraction has
led to the almost universal assumption that if a fetus is a human
being, with a right to life, then it follows immediately that abortion

is wrong (except perhaps when necessary to save the woman's life), and that it ought to be prohibited. It has also been generally assumed that unless the question about the status of the fetus is answered, the moral status of abortion cannot possibly be determined.

Two recent papers, one by B. A. Brody,[2] and one by Judith Thomson,[3] have attempted to settle the question of whether abortion ought to be prohibited apart from the question of whether or not the fetus is human. Brody examines the possibility that the following two statements are compatible: (1) that abortion is the taking of innocent human life, and therefore wrong; and (2) that nevertheless it ought not to be prohibited by law, at least under the present circumstances.[4] Not surprisingly, Brody finds it impossible to reconcile these two statements, since, as he rightly argues, none of the unfortunate side effects of the prohibition of abortion is bad enough to justify legalizing the *wrongful* taking of human life. He is mistaken, however, in concluding that the incompatibility of (1) and (2), in itself, shows that "the legal problem about abortion cannot be resolved independently of the status of the fetus problem" (p. 369).

What Brody fails to realize is that (1) embodies the questionable assumption that if a fetus is a human being, then of course abortion is morally wrong, and that an attack on *this* assumption is more promising, as a way of reconciling the humanity of the fetus with the claim that laws prohibiting abortion are unjustified, than is an attack on the assumption that if abortion is the wrongful killing of innocent human beings then it ought to be prohibited. He thus overlooks the possibility that a fetus may have a right to life and abortion still be morally permissible, in that the right of a woman to terminate an unwanted pregnancy might override the right of the fetus to be kept alive. The immorality of abortion is no more demonstrated by the humanity of the fetus, in itself, than the immorality of killing in self-defense is demonstrated by the fact that the as-

---

2. B. A. Brody, "Abortion and the Law," *The Journal of Philosophy,* 68, No. 12 (June 17, 1971), 357-69.

3. Judith Thomson, "A Defense of Abortion," *Philosophy and Public Affairs,* 1, No. 1 (Fall, 1971), 47-66.

4. I have abbreviated these statements somewhat, but not in a way which affects the argument.

46   MARY ANNE WARREN

sailant is a human being. Neither is it demonstrated by the *innocence* of the fetus, since there may be situations in which the killing of innocent human beings is justified.

It is perhaps not surprising that Brody fails to spot this assumption, since it has been accepted with little or no argument by nearly everyone who has written on the morality of abortion. John Noonan is correct in saying that "the fundamental question in the long history of abortion is, How do you determine the humanity of a being?" [5] He summarizes his own antiabortion argument, which is a version of the official position of the Catholic Church, as follows:

> . . . it is wrong to kill humans, however poor, weak, defenseless, and lacking in opportunity to develop their potential they may be. It is therefore morally wrong to kill Biafrans. Similarly, it is morally wrong to kill embryos.[6]

Noonan bases his claim that fetuses are human upon what he calls the theologians' criterion of humanity: that whoever is conceived of human beings is human. But although he argues at length for the appropriateness of this criterion, he never questions the assumption that if a fetus is human then abortion is wrong for exactly the same reason that murder is wrong.

Judith Thomson is, in fact, the only writer I am aware of who has seriously questioned this assumption; she has argued that, even if we grant the antiabortionist his claim that a fetus is a human being, with the same right to life as any other human being, we can still demonstrate that, in at least some and perhaps most cases, a woman is under no moral obligation to complete an unwanted pregnancy.[7] Her argument is worth examining, since if it holds up it may enable us to establish the moral permissibility of abortion without becoming involved in problems about what entitles an entity to be considered human, and accorded full moral rights. To be able to do this would be a great gain in the power and simplicity of the proabortion position, since, although I will argue that these problems can be solved at least as decisively as can any other moral problem,

---

5. John Noonan, "Abortion and the Catholic Church: A Summary History," *Natural Law Forum*, 12 (1967), 125.

6. John Noonan, "Deciding Who is Human," *Natural Law Forum*, 13 (1968), 134.

7. "A Defense of Abortion."

we should certainly be pleased to be able to avoid having to solve them as part of the justification of abortion.

On the other hand, even if Thomson's argument does not hold up, her insight, i.e., that it requires *argument* to show that if fetuses are human then abortion is properly classified as murder, is an extremely valuable one. The assumption she attacks is particularly invidious, for it amounts to the decision that it is appropriate, in deciding the moral status of abortion, to leave the rights of the pregnant woman out of consideration entirely, except possibly when her life is threatened. Obviously, this will not do; determining what moral rights, if any, a fetus possesses is only the first step in determining the moral status of abortion. Step two, which is at least equally essential, is finding a just solution to the conflict between whatever rights the fetus may have, and the rights of the woman who is unwillingly pregnant. While the historical error has been to pay far too little attention to the second step, Ms. Thomson's suggestion is that if we look at the second step first we may find that a woman has a right to obtain an abortion *regardless* of what rights the fetus has.

Our own inquiry will also have two stages. In Section I, we will consider whether or not it is possible to establish that abortion is morally permissible even on the assumption that a fetus is an entity with a full-fledged right to life. I will argue that in fact this cannot be established, at least not with the conclusiveness which is essential to our hopes of convincing those who are skeptical about the morality of abortion, and that we therefore cannot avoid dealing with the question of whether or not a fetus really does have the same right to life as a (more fully developed) human being.

In Section II, I will propose an answer to this question, namely, that a fetus cannot be considered a member of the moral community, the set of beings with full and equal moral rights, for the simple reason that it is not a person, and that it is personhood, and not genetic humanity, i.e., humanity as defined by Noonan, which is the basis for membership in this community. I will argue that a fetus, whatever its stage of development, satisfies none of the basic criteria of personhood, and is not even enough *like* a person to be accorded even some of the same rights on the basis of this resemblance. Nor, as we will see, is a fetus's *potential* personhood a threat to the morality of abortion, since, whatever the rights of

 MARY ANNE WARREN

potential people may be, they are invariably overridden in any conflict with the moral rights of actual people.

I

We turn now to Professor Thomson's case for the claim that even if a fetus has full moral rights, abortion is still morally permissible, at least sometimes, and for some reasons other than to save the woman's life. Her argument is based upon a clever, but I think faulty, analogy. She asks us to picture ourselves waking up one day, in bed with a famous violinist. Imagine that you have been kidnapped, and your bloodstream hooked up to that of the violinist, who happens to have an ailment which will certainly kill him unless he is permitted to share your kidneys for a period of nine months. No one else can save him, since you alone have the right type of blood. He will be unconscious all that time, and you will have to stay in bed with him, but after the nine months are over he may be unplugged, completely cured, that is provided that you have cooperated.

Now then, she continues, what are your obligations in this situation? The antiabortionist, if he is consistent, will have to say that you are obligated to stay in bed with the violinist: for all people have a right to life, and violinists are people, and therefore it would be murder for you to disconnect yourself from him and let him die (p. 49). But this is outrageous, and so there must be something wrong with the same argument when it is applied to abortion. It would certainly be commendable of you to agree to save the violinist, but it is absurd to suggest that your refusal to do so would be murder. His right to life does not obligate you to do whatever is required to keep him alive; nor does it justify anyone else in forcing you to do so. A law which required you to stay in bed with the violinist would clearly be an unjust law, since it is no proper function of the law to force unwilling people to make huge sacrifices for the sake of other people toward whom they have no such prior obligation.

Thomson concludes that, if this analogy is an apt one, then we can grant the antiabortionist his claim that a fetus is a human being, and still hold that it is at least sometimes the case that a pregnant woman has the right to refuse to be a Good Samaritan towards the fetus, i.e., to obtain an abortion. For there is a great gap between

MORAL AND LEGAL STATUS OF ABORTION　　　　49

the claim that *x* has a right to life, and the claim that *y* is obligated to do whatever is necessary to keep *x* alive, let alone that he ought to be forced to do so. It is *y*'s duty to keep *x* alive only if he has somehow contracted a *special* obligation to do so; and a woman who is unwillingly pregnant, e.g., who was raped, has done nothing which obligates her to make the enormous sacrifice which is necessary to preserve the conceptus.

This argument is initially quite plausible, and in the extreme case of pregnancy due to rape it is probably conclusive. Difficulties arise, however, when we try to specify more exactly the range of cases in which abortion is clearly justifiable even on the assumption that the fetus is human. Professor Thomson considers it a virtue of her argument that it does not enable us to conclude that abortion is *always* permissible. It would, she says, be "indecent" for a woman in her seventh month to obtain an abortion just to avoid having to postpone a trip to Europe. On the other hand, her argument enables us to see that "a sick and desperately frightened schoolgirl pregnant due to rape may *of course* choose abortion, and that any law which rules this out is an insane law" (p. 65). So far, so good; but what are we to say about the woman who becomes pregnant not through rape but as a result of her own carelessness, or because of contraceptive failure, or who gets pregnant intentionally and then changes her mind about wanting a child? With respect to such cases, the violinist analogy is of much less use to the defender of the woman's right to obtain an abortion.

Indeed, the choice of a pregnancy due to rape, as an example of a case in which abortion is permissible even if a fetus is considered a human being, is extremely significant; for it is only in the case of pregnancy due to rape that the woman's situation is adequately analogous to the violinist case for our intuitions about the latter to transfer convincingly. The crucial difference between a pregnancy due to rape and the *normal* case of an unwanted pregnancy is that in the normal case we cannot claim that the woman is in no way responsible for her predicament; she could have remained chaste, or taken her pills more faithfully, or abstained on dangerous days, and so on. If, on the other hand, you are kidnapped by strangers, and hooked up to a strange violinist, then you are free of any shred of responsibility for the situation, on the basis of which it could be argued that you are obligated to keep the violinist alive. Only when her pregnancy is due to rape is a woman clearly just as nonresponsible.[8]

Consequently, there is room for the antiabortionist to argue that in the normal case of unwanted pregnancy a woman has, by her own actions, assumed responsibility for the fetus. For if x behaves in a way which he could have avoided, and which he knows involves, let us say, a 1 percent chance of bringing into existence a human being, with a right to life, and does so knowing that if this should happen then that human being will perish unless x does certain things to keep him alive, then it is by no means clear that when it does happen x is free of any obligation to what he knew in advance would be required to keep that human being alive.

The plausibility of such an argument is enough to show that the Thomson analogy can provide a clear and persuasive defense of a woman's right to obtain an abortion only with respect to those cases in which the woman is in no way responsible for her pregnancy, e.g., where it is due to rape. In all other cases, we would almost certainly conclude that it was necessary to look carefully at the particular circumstances in order to determine the extent of the woman's responsibility, and hence the extent of her obligation. This is an extremely unsatisfactory outcome, from the viewpoint of the opponents of restrictive abortion laws, most of whom are convinced that a woman has a right to obtain an abortion regardless of how and why she got pregnant.

Of course a supporter of the violinist analogy might point out that it is absurd to suggest that forgetting her pill one day might be sufficient to obligate a woman to complete an unwanted pregnancy. And indeed it *is* absurd to suggest this. As we will see, the moral right to obtain an abortion is not in the least dependent upon the extent to which the woman is responsible for her pregnancy. But unfortunately, once we allow the assumption that a fetus has full moral rights, we cannot avoid taking this absurd suggestion seriously.

---

8. We may safely ignore the fact that she might have avoided getting raped, e.g., by carrying a gun, since by similar means you might likewise have avoided getting kidnapped, and in neither case does the victim's failure to take all possible precautions against a highly unlikely event (as opposed to reasonable precautions against a rather likely event) mean that he is morally responsible for what happens.

MORAL AND LEGAL STATUS OF ABORTION 51

Perhaps we can make this point more clear by altering the violinist story just enough to make it more analogous to a normal unwanted pregnancy and less to a pregnancy due to rape, and then seeing whether it is still obvious that you are not obligated to stay in bed with the fellow.

Suppose, then, that violinists are peculiarly prone to the sort of illness the only cure for which is the use of someone else's bloodstream for nine months, and that because of this there has been formed a society of music lovers who agree that whenever a violinist is stricken they will draw lots and the loser will, by some means, be made the one and only person capable of saving him. Now then, would you be obligated to cooperate in curing the violinist if you had voluntarily joined this society, knowing the possible consequences, and then your name had been drawn and you had been kidnapped? Admittedly, you did not promise ahead of time that you would, but you did deliberately place yourself in a position in which it might happen that a human life would be lost if you did not. Surely this is at least a prima facie reason for supposing that you have an obligation to stay in bed with the violinist. Suppose that you had gotten your name drawn deliberately; surely *that* would be quite a strong reason for thinking that you had such an obligation.

It might be suggested that there is one important disanalogy between the modified violinist case and the case of an unwanted pregnancy, which makes the woman's responsibility significantly less, namely, the fact that the fetus *comes into existence* as the result of the result of the woman's actions. This fact might give her a right to refuse to keep it alive, whereas she would not have had this right had it existed previously, independently, and then as a result of her actions become dependent upon her for its survival.

My own intuition, however, is that x has no more right to bring into existence, either deliberately or as a foreseeable result of actions he could have avoided, a being with full moral rights (y), and then refuse to do what he knew beforehand would be required to keep that being alive, than he has to enter into an agreement with an existing person, whereby he may be called upon to save that person's life, and then refuse to do so when so called upon. Thus, x's responsibility for y's existence does not seem to lessen his obligation to keep y alive, if he is also responsible for y's being in a situation in which only he can save him.

52   MARY ANNE WARREN

Whether or not this intuition is entirely correct, it brings us back once again to the conclusion that once we allow the assumption that a fetus has full moral rights it becomes an extremely complex and difficult question whether and when abortion is justifiable. Thus the Thomson analogy cannot help us produce a clear and persuasive proof of the moral permissibility of abortion. Nor will the opponents of the restrictive laws thank us for anything less; for their conviction (for the most part) is that abortion is obviously *not* a morally serious and extremely unfortunate, even though sometimes justified act, comparable to killing in self-defense or to letting the violinist die, but rather is closer to being a morally neutral act, like cutting one's hair.

The basis of this conviction, I believe, is the realization that a fetus is not a person, and thus does not have a full-fledged right to life. Perhaps the reason why this claim has been so inadequately defended is that it seems self-evident to those who accept it. And so it is, insofar as it follows from what I take to be perfectly obvious claims about the nature of personhood, and about the proper grounds for ascribing moral rights, claims which ought, indeed, to be obvious to both the friends and foes of abortion. Nevertheless, it is worth examining these claims, and showing how they demonstrate the moral innocuousness of abortion, since this apparently has not been adequately done before.

II

The question which we must answer in order to produce a satisfactory solution to the problem of the moral status of abortion is this: How are we to define the moral community, the set of beings with full and equal moral rights, such that we can decide whether a human fetus is a member of this community or not? What sort of entity, exactly, has the inalienable rights to life, liberty, and the pursuit of happiness? Jefferson attributed these rights to all *men,* and it may or may not be fair to suggest that he intended to attribute them *only* to men. Perhaps he ought to have attributed them to all human beings. If so, then we arrive, first, at Noonan's problem of defining what makes a being human, and, second, at the equally vital question which Noonan does not consider, namely, What reason is there for identifying the moral community with the set of all human beings, in whatever way we have chosen to define that term?

MORAL AND LEGAL STATUS OF ABORTION 53

1. *On the Definition of 'Human'*

One reason why this vital second question is so frequently over-looked in the debate over the moral status of abortion is that the term 'human' has two distinct, but not often distinguished, senses. This fact results in a slide of meaning, which serves to conceal the fallaciousness of the traditional argument that since (1) it is wrong to kill innocent human beings, and (2) fetuses are innocent human beings, then (3) it is wrong to kill fetuses. For if 'human' is used in the same sense in both (1) and (2) then, whichever of the two senses is meant, one of these premises is question-begging. And if it is used in two different senses then of course the conclusion doesn't follow.

Thus, (1) is a self-evident moral truth,[9] and avoids begging the question about abortion, only if 'human being' is used to mean something like "a full-fledged member of the moral community." (It may or may not also be meant to refer exclusively to members of the species *Homo sapiens.*) We may call this the *moral* sense of 'human'. It is not to be confused with what we will call the *genetic* sense, i.e., the sense in which *any* member of the species is a human being, and no member of any other species could be. If (1) is acceptable only if the moral sense is intended, (2) is non-question-begging only if what is intended is the genetic sense.

In "Deciding Who is Human," Noonan argues for the classification of fetuses with human beings by pointing to the presence of the full genetic code, and the potential capacity for rational thought (p. 135). It is clear that what he needs to show, for his version of the traditional argument to be valid, is that fetuses are human in the moral sense, the sense in which it is analytically true that all human beings have full moral rights. But, in the absence of any argument showing that whatever is genetically human is also morally human, and he gives none, nothing more than genetic humanity can be demonstrated by the presence of the human genetic code. And, as we will see, the *potential* capacity for rational thought can at most show that an entity has the potential for *becoming* human in the moral sense.

---

9. Of course, the principle that it is (always) wrong to kill innocent human beings is in need of many other modifications, e.g., that it may be permissible to do so to save a greater number of other innocent human beings, but we may safely ignore these complications here.

54   MARY ANNE WARREN

2. *Defining the Moral Community*

Can it be established that genetic humanity is sufficient for moral humanity? I think that there are very good reasons for not defining the moral community in this way. I would like to suggest an alternative way of defining the moral community, which I will argue for only to the extent of explaining why it is, or should be, self-evident. The suggestion is simply that the moral community consists of all and only *people,* rather than all and only human beings; [10] and probably the best way of demonstrating its self-evidence is by considering the concept of personhood, to see what sorts of entity are and are not persons, and what the decision that a being is or is not a person implies about its moral rights.

What characteristics entitle an entity to be considered a person? This is obviously not the place to attempt a complete analysis of the concept of personhood, but we do not need such a fully adequate analysis just to determine whether and why a fetus is or isn't a person. All we need is a rough and approximate list of the most basic criteria of personhood, and some idea of which, or how many, of these an entity must satisfy in order to properly be considered a person.

In searching for such criteria, it is useful to look beyond the set of people with whom we are acquainted, and ask how we would decide whether a totally alien being was a person or not. (For we have no right to assume that genetic humanity is necessary for personhood.) Imagine a space traveler who lands on an unknown planet and encounters a race of beings utterly unlike any he has ever seen or heard of. If he wants to be sure of behaving morally toward these beings, he has to somehow decide whether they are people, and hence have full moral rights, or whether they are the sort of thing which he need not feel guilty about treating as, for example, a source of food.

How should he go about making this decision? If he has some anthropological background, he might look for such things as religion, art, and the manufacturing of tools, weapons, or shelters, since these factors have been used to distinguish our human from

---

10. From here on, we will use 'human' to mean genetically human, since the moral sense seems closely connected to, and perhaps derived from, the assumption that genetic humanity is sufficient for membership in the moral community.

MORAL AND LEGAL STATUS OF ABORTION 55

our prehuman ancestors, in what seems to be closer to the moral than the genetic sense of 'human'. And no doubt he would be right to consider the presence of such factors as good evidence that the alien beings were people, and morally human. It would, however, be overly anthropocentric of him to take the absence of these things as adequate evidence that they were not, since we can imagine people who have progressed beyond, or evolved without ever developing, these cultural characteristics.

I suggest that the traits which are most central to the concept of personhood, or humanity in the moral sense, are, very roughly, the following:

(1) consciousness (of objects and events external and/or internal to the being), and in particular the capacity to feel pain;

(2) reasoning (the *developed* capacity to solve new and relatively complex problems);

(3) self-motivated activity (activity which is relatively independent of either genetic or direct external control);

(4) the capacity to communicate, by whatever means, messages of an indefinite variety of types, that is, not just with an indefinite number of possible contents, but on indefinitely many possible topics;

(5) the presence of self-concepts, and self-awareness, either individual or racial, or both.

Admittedly, there are apt to be a great many problems involved in formulating precise definitions of these criteria, let alone in developing universally valid behavioral criteria for deciding when they apply. But I will assume that both we and our explorer know approximately what (1)-(5) mean, and that he is also able to determine whether or not they apply. How, then, should he use his findings to decide whether or not the alien beings are people? We needn't suppose that an entity must have *all* of these attributes to be properly considered a person; (1) and (2) alone may well be sufficient for personhood, and quite probably (1)-(3) are sufficient. Neither do we need to insist that any one of these criteria is *necessary* for personhood, although once again (1) and (2) look like fairly good candidates for necessary conditions, as does (3), if 'activity' is construed so as to include the activity of reasoning.

56   MARY ANNE WARREN

All we need to claim, to demonstrate that a fetus is not a person, is that any being which satisfies *none* of (1)-(5) is certainly not a person. I consider this claim to be so obvious that I think anyone who denied it, and claimed that a being which satisfied none of (1)-(5) was a person all the same, would thereby demonstrate that he had no notion at all of what a person is—perhaps because he had confused the concept of a person with that of genetic humanity. If the opponents of abortion were to deny the appropriateness of these five criteria, I do not know what further arguments would convince them. We would probably have to admit that our conceptual schemes were indeed irreconcilably different, and that our dispute could not be settled objectively.

I do not expect this to happen, however, since I think that the concept of a person is one which is very nearly universal (to people), and that it is common to both proabortionists and antiabortionists, even though neither group has fully realized the relevance of this concept to the resolution of their dispute. Furthermore, I think that on reflection even the antiabortionists ought to agree not only that (1)-(5) are central to the concept of personhood, but also that it is a part of this concept that all and only people have full moral rights. The concept of a person is in part a moral concept; once we have admitted that *x* is a person we have recognized, even if we have not agreed to respect, *x*'s right to be treated as a member of the moral community. It is true that the claim that *x* is a *human being* is more commonly voiced as part of an appeal to treat *x* decently than is the claim that *x* is a person, but this is either because 'human being' is here used in the sense which implies personhood, or because the genetic and moral senses of 'human' have been confused.

Now if (1)-(5) are indeed the primary criteria of personhood, then it is clear that genetic humanity is neither necessary nor sufficient for establishing that an entity is a person. Some human beings are not people, and there may well be people who are not human beings. A man or woman whose consciousness has been permanently obliterated but who remains alive is a human being which is no longer a person; defective human beings, with no appreciable mental capacity, are not and presumably never will be people; and a fetus is a human being which is not yet a person, and which therefore cannot coherently be said to have full moral rights. Citizens of the next century should be prepared to recognize highly advanced, self-aware

MORAL AND LEGAL STATUS OF ABORTION 57

robots or computers, should such be developed, and intelligent inhabitants of other worlds, should such be found, as people in the fullest sense, and to respect their moral rights. But to ascribe full moral rights to an entity which is not a person is as absurd as to ascribe moral obligations and responsibilities to such an entity.

3. *Fetal Development and the Right to Life*

Two problems arise in the application of these suggestions for the definition of the moral community to the determination of the precise moral status of a human fetus. Given that the paradigm example of a person is a normal adult human being, then (1) How like this paradigm, in particular how far advanced since conception, does a human being need to be before it begins to have a right to life by virtue, not of being fully a person as of yet, but of being *like* a person? and (2) To what extent, if any, does the fact that a fetus has the *potential* for becoming a person endow it with some of the same rights? Each of these questions requires some comment.

In answering the first question, we need not attempt a detailed consideration of the moral rights of organisms which are not developed enough, aware enough, intelligent enough, etc., to be considered people, but which resemble people in some respects. It does seem reasonable to suggest that the more like a person, in the relevant respects, a being is, the stronger is the case for regarding it as having a right to life, and indeed the stronger its right to life is. Thus we ought to take seriously the suggestion that, insofar as "the human individual develops biologically in a continuous fashion ... the rights of a human person might develop in the same way." [11] But we must keep in mind that the attributes which are relevant in determining whether or not an entity is enough like a person to be regarded as having some of the same moral rights are no different from those which are relevant to determining whether or not it is fully a person—i.e., are no different from (1)-(5)—and that being genetically human, or having recognizably human facial and other physical features, or detectable brain activity, or the capacity to survive outside the uterus, are simply not among these relevant attributes.

---

11. Thomas L. Hayes, "A Biological View," *Commonweal*, 85 (March 17, 1967), 677-78; quoted by Daniel Callahan, in *Abortion, Law, Choice, and Morality* (London: Macmillan & Co., 1970).

58   MARY ANNE WARREN

Thus it is clear that even though a seven- or eight-month fetus has features which make it apt to arouse in us almost the same powerful protective instinct as is commonly aroused by a small infant, nevertheless it is not significantly more personlike than is a very small embryo. It is *somewhat* more personlike; it can apparently feel and respond to pain, and it may even have a rudimentary form of consciousness, insofar as its brain is quite active. Nevertheless, it seems safe to say that it is not fully conscious, in the way that an infant of a few months is, and that it cannot reason, or communicate messages of indefinitely many sorts, does not engage in self-motivated activity, and has no self-awareness. Thus, in the *relevant* respects, a fetus, even a fully developed one, is considerably less personlike than is the average mature mammal, indeed the average fish. And I think that a rational person must conclude that if the right to life of a fetus is to be based upon its resemblance to a person, then it cannot be said to have any more right to life than, let us say, a newborn guppy (which also seems to be capable of feeling pain), and that a right of that magnitude could never override a woman's right to obtain an abortion, at any stage of her pregnancy.

There may, of course, be other arguments in favor of placing legal limits upon the stage of pregnancy in which an abortion may be performed. Given the relative safety of the new techniques of artifically inducing labor during the third trimester, the danger to the woman's life or health is no longer such an argument. Neither is the fact that people tend to respond to the thought of abortion in the later stages of pregnancy with emotional repulsion, since mere emotional responses cannot take the place of moral reasoning in determining what ought to be permitted. Nor, finally, is the frequently heard argument that legalizing abortion, especially late in the pregnancy, may erode the level of respect for human life, leading, perhaps, to an increase in unjustified euthanasia and other crimes. For this threat, if it is a threat, can be better met by educating people to the kinds of moral distinctions which we are making here than by limiting access to abortion (which limitation may, in its disregard for the rights of women, be just as damaging to the level of respect for human rights).

Thus, since the fact that even a fully developed fetus is not personlike enough to have any significant right to life on the basis of its personlikeness shows that no legal restrictions upon the stage

MORAL AND LEGAL STATUS OF ABORTION 59

of pregnancy in which an abortion may be performed can be justified on the grounds that we should protect the rights of the older fetus; and since there is no other apparent justification for such restrictions, we may conclude that they are entirely unjustified. Whether or not it would be *indecent* (whatever that means) for a woman in her seventh month to obtain an abortion just to avoid having to postpone a trip to Europe, it would not, in itself, be *immoral,* and therefore it ought to be permitted.

4. *Potential Personhood and the Right to Life*

We have seen that a fetus does not resemble a person in any way which can support the claim that it has even some of the same rights. But what about its *potential,* the fact that if nurtured and allowed to develop naturally it will very probably become a person? Doesn't that alone give it at least some right to life? It is hard to deny that the fact that an entity is a potential person is a strong prima facie reason for not destroying it; but we need not conclude from this that a potential person has a right to life, by virtue of that potential. It may be that our feeling that it is better, other things being equal, not to destroy a potential person is better explained by the fact that potential people are still (felt to be) an invaluable resource, not to be lightly squandered. Surely, if every speck of dust were a potential person, we would be much less apt to conclude that every potential person has a right to become actual.

Still, we do not need to insist that a potential person has no right to life whatever. There may well be something immoral, and not just imprudent, about wantonly destroying potential people, when doing so isn't necessary to protect anyone's rights. But even if a potential person does have some prima facie right to life, such a right could not possibly outweigh the right of a woman to obtain an abortion, since the rights of any actual person invariably outweigh those of any potential person, whenever the two conflict. Since this may not be immediately obvious in the case of a human fetus, let us look at another case.

Suppose that our space explorer falls into the hands of an alien culture, whose scientists decide to create a few hundred thousand or more human beings, by breaking his body into its component cells, and using these to create fully developed human beings, with, of course, his genetic code. We may imagine that each of these newly

created men will have all of the original man's abilities, skills, knowledge, and so on, and also have an individual self-concept, in short
that each of them will be a bona fide (though hardly unique) person.
Imagine that the whole project will take only seconds, and that its
chances of success are extremely high, and that our explorer knows
all of this, and also knows that these people will be treated fairly.
I maintain that in such a situation he would have every right to
escape if he could, and thus to deprive all of these potential people
of their potential lives; for his right to life outweighs all of theirs
together, in spite of the fact that they are all genetically human, all
innocent, and all have a very high probability of becoming people
very soon, if only he refrains from acting.

Indeed, I think he would have a right to escape even if it were
not his life which the alien scientists planned to take, but only a year
of his freedom, or, indeed, only a day. Nor would he be obligated
to stay if he had gotten captured (thus bringing all these people-
potentials into existence) because of his own carelessness, or even
if he had done so deliberately, knowing the consequences. Regardless
of how he got captured, he is not morally obligated to remain in
captivity for *any* period of time for the sake of permitting any number of potential people to come into actuality, so great is the margin
by which one actual person's right to liberty outweighs whatever
right to life even a hundred thousand potential people have. And it
seems reasonable to conclude that the rights of a woman will outweigh by a similar margin whatever right to life a fetus may have by
virtue of its potential personhood.

Thus, neither a fetus's resemblance to a person, nor its potential
for becoming a person provides any basis whatever for the claim that
it has any significant right to life. Consequently, a woman's right to
protect her health, happiness, freedom, and even her life,[12] by terminating an unwanted pregnancy, will always override whatever right
to life it may be appropriate to ascribe to a fetus, even a fully developed one. And thus, in the absence of any overwhelming social
need for every possible child, the laws which restrict the right to
obtain an abortion, or limit the period of pregnancy during which

---

12. That is, insofar as the death rate, for the woman, is higher for
childbirth than for early abortion.

MORAL AND LEGAL STATUS OF ABORTION 61

an abortion may be performed, are a wholly unjustified violation of a woman's most basic moral and constitutional rights.[13]

MARY ANNE WARREN

SONOMA STATE COLLEGE,
CALIFORNIA

---

13. My thanks to the following people, who were kind enough to read and criticize an earlier version of this paper: Herbert Gold, Gene Glass, Anne Lauterbach, Judith Thomson, Mary Mothersill, and Timothy Binkley.

[24]

PETER SINGER &
KAREN DAWSON

IVF Technology and the
Argument from Potential

I

In many respects the current debate about embryo experimentation resembles the older debate about abortion. Although one central argument *for* abortion—the claim that a woman has the right to control her own body—is not directly applicable in the newer context, the argument *against* embryo experimentation remains essentially the same as the argument against abortion. This argument has two forms, one relying on the claim that from the moment of fertilization the embryo is entitled to protection because it *is* a human being, and the other asserting instead that the embryo is entitled to protection because from the moment of fertilization it is a *potential* human being.[1]

The first form of this argument will not concern us here;[2] our focus is on the argument from potential. Those who use this argument against embryo experimentation frequently describe the potential of the early *in vitro* embryo in terms identical with those used in the context of the abortion debate to describe the potential of the early embryo inside the female body. Teresa Iglesias, for example, writes: "We know that a new human

This work was supported by a National Health and Medical Research Council of Australia Special Initiative Grant to Professor J. Swan, Dr. M. Brumby, Dr. H. Kuhse, and Professor L. Waller. We thank all four for their helpful comments, and we thank also Michaelis Michael, whose unpublished paper on the argument from potential spurred us to clarify our own ideas, as well as the Editors of *Philosophy & Public Affairs*, who forced us to confront additional objections to our argument.

1. For examples of the popular arguments against embryo experimentation, see *Test-Tube Babies*, ed. William Walters and Peter Singer (Melbourne: Oxford University Press, 1982), chap. 4.

2. One of us has discussed the argument previously: see Peter Singer, *Practical Ethics* (Cambridge: Cambridge University Press, 1979), chap. 6.

individual organism with the internal potential to develop into an adult, given nurture, comes into existence as a result of the process of fertilisation at conception."[3] But can the familiar claims about the potential of the embryo in the uterus be applied to the embryo in culture in the laboratory? Or does the new technology lead to an embryo with a different potential from that of embryos made in the old way? Asking this question leads us to probe the meaning of the term 'potential'. This probing will raise doubts about whether it is meaningful to talk of the potential of an entity independently of the context in which that entity exists and independently of the probability that that entity will develop in a specific way. In particular, we will argue that while the notion of potential may be relatively clear in the context of a naturally occurring process such as the development of an embryo inside a female body, this notion becomes far more problematic when it is extended to a laboratory situation, in which *everything* depends on our knowledge and skills, and on what we decide to do. This line of argument will lead us to the conclusion that there is no coherent notion of potential which allows the argument from potential to be applied to embryos in laboratories in the way those who invoke the argument are seeking to apply it.

We begin by considering how recent developments in reproductive technology force us to revise some previously universal truths about embryos. Before Robert Edwards began the research which was to lead to the IVF (*in vitro* fertilization) procedure, no one had observed a viable human embryo prior to the stage at which it implants in the wall of the uterus. In the normal process of reproduction inside the body, the embryo, or 'pre-embryo' as it is now sometimes called, remains unattached for the first seven to fourteen days. As long as such embryos existed only inside the woman's body, there was no way of observing them during that period. The very existence of the embryo could not be established until after implantation.

Under these circumstances, once the existence of an embryo was known, that embryo had a good chance of becoming a person, unless its development was deliberately interrupted. The probability that such an embryo would become a person was therefore very much greater than the probability that an egg in a fertile woman would unite with sperm from that woman's partner and lead to a child. It was also considerably greater than the chance that an as yet unimplanted embryo would become a child.

---

3. Teresa Iglesias, "*In Vitro* Fertilisation: The Major Issues," *Journal of Medical Ethics* 10 (1984): 36.

89 *IVF Technology and the
Argument from Potential*

There was also, in those pre-IVF days, a further important difference
between any embryo, whether implanted or not, and the egg and sperm.
Whereas the embryo inside the female body has some definite chance (we
shall consider later how great a chance) of developing into a child *unless*
a deliberate human act interrupts its growth, the egg and sperm can develop into a child *only* if there *is* a deliberate human act. So in the one
case, all that is needed for the embryo to have a prospect of realizing its
potential is for those involved to refrain from stopping it; in the other case,
they have to carry out a positive act. The development of the embryo inside
the female body can therefore be seen as a mere unfolding of a potential
that is inherent in it. The development of the separated egg and sperm is
more difficult to regard in this way, because no further development will
take place unless the couple have sexual intercourse or use artificial insemination. (This is, to be sure, an oversimplification, for it takes no account of the positive acts involved in childbirth; but it is close enough for
our purposes.)

Now consider what has happened as a result of the success of IVF. The
procedure involves removing one or more eggs from a woman's ovary,
placing them in culture medium in a glass dish, and then adding sperm to
the culture. In the more proficient laboratories, this leads to fertilization in
about 80 percent of the eggs thus treated. The embryo can then be kept in
culture for two to three days, while it grows and divides into two, four, and
then eight cells. At about this stage, if the embryo is to have any prospect
of developing into a child, it must be transferred to a woman's uterus. Although the transfer itself is a simple procedure, it is after the transfer that
things are most likely to go wrong: for reasons which are not fully understood, with even the most successful IVF teams the probability that a
given embryo which has been transferred to the uterus will actually implant there and lead to a continuing pregnancy is always less than 20 percent, and generally no more than 10 percent.[4] (Figures quoted for pregnancies per transfer procedure may be higher, but this is because it is
common to transfer more than one embryo; for our purposes the important figure is the probability that any given embryo will result in a child.)
We should also note that if the embryo is allowed to continue to grow in
culture much beyond the eight-cell stage, it is less likely to implant when

4. For these figures, see Ian Johnston, "IVF: The Australian Experience," a paper presented at the Royal College of Gynaecologists and Obstetricians Study Group on AID and
IVF, November 1984, reprinted in *Hansard*, Commonwealth of Australia, Senate, Select
Committee on the Human Embryo Experimentation Bill, 1985, report of hearings of 26 February 1986 (Canberra: Commonwealth Government Printer, 1986), pp. 560–87.

transferred. Embryos can be grown in the laboratory to the later blastocyst stage, when the cells are arranged as a hollow sphere and those which will form the embryo proper have become distinct from those which will form the extraembryonic membranes, that is, the chorion and the amnion. The blastocyst may then develop further, to the point at which it consists of hundreds of cells. No pregnancies, however, have resulted from embryos transferred at so late a stage of development. Nor, as yet, is there any prospect of keeping embryos alive and developing *in vitro* until they become viable infants. So although Edwards has reported keeping an embryo alive in culture for nine days,[5] with our present state of knowledge, such an embryo has zero probability of becoming a person.

In summary, then, before the advent of IVF, it would have been true to say of any normal human embryo known to us that, unless it was deliberately interfered with, it would most likely develop into a person. The process of IVF, however, leads to the creation of embryos which cannot develop into a person unless there is some deliberate human act (the transfer to the uterus) and which even then, in the best of circumstances, will most likely *not* develop into a person.

The upshot of all this is that IVF has reduced the difference between what can be said about the embryo and what can be said about the egg and sperm, considered jointly. Before IVF, any normal human embryo known to us had a far greater chance of becoming a child than any egg and sperm prior to fertilization. But with IVF, there is a much more modest difference in the probability that a child will result from a two-cell embryo in a glass dish and the probability that a child will result from an egg and some sperm in a glass dish. To be specific, if we assume that the laboratory's fertilization rate is 80 percent and its rate of pregnancy per embryo transferred is 10 percent, then the probability that a child will result from a given embryo is 10 percent, and the probability that a child will result from an egg which has been placed in a culture medium to which sperm has been added is 8 percent.

II

It has occasionally been suggested that there is no difference between the potential of the embryo, on the one hand, and the potential of the egg and

5. Robert Edwards and Patrick Steptoe. *A Matter of Life* (London: Sphere, 1981), p. 146.

91   *IVF Technology and the*
                                Argument from Potential

sperm when still separate, but considered jointly, on the other hand.[6] But there has been little analysis of the notion of potential in the context of the *in vitro* embryo, and the suggestions made have not succeeded in dispelling the intuitive idea that there is a major difference between the potential of the embryo and the potential of the pair of gametes. To provide this analysis, we must ask what we mean when we refer to the embryo as a potential person.

An obvious place to begin our search for the meaning of this claim is the dictionary definition of the word 'potential'. The *Oxford English Dictionary* offers several meanings of the term, of which the following seems to be the most relevant to our present concerns: "Possible as opposed to actual; existing *in posse* or in a latent or undeveloped state, capable of coming into being or action; latent." Following the dictionary definition, it would seem that *at the least* we must mean that it is *possible* for the embryo to become a person. Possibility is a necessary condition for potentiality (whether it is also a sufficient condition is not something we need consider here). But what sort of possibility?

Philosophers commonly distinguish between logical possibility and physical possibility. It is logically possible, but physically impossible, for the authors of this paper to jump over the Empire State Building. It is both logically and physically possible for us to jump over a brick. It is not logically possible for anyone to be a biological parent without having any children.

Since something is logically impossible only if its assertion involves a contradiction, it is not logically impossible for a human blastocyst in a laboratory to develop into a person. But then, it is not logically impossible for a human egg to develop into a person either—parthenogenesis happens often in some species, and no logical contradiction is involved in imagining it happening in our species. So those who claim that the human embryo is a potential person, whereas the human egg is not, cannot appeal to the mere fact that it is logically possible for the embryo to become a person.

The sense of 'possibility' that lies behind these claims that the embryo, but not the egg, is a potential person must, therefore, be real, physical possibility. We must, however, further refine the relevant sense of physical

6. See, for example, Helga Kuhse and Peter Singer, "The Moral Status of the Embryo," in *Test-Tube Babies*, ed. Walters and Singer, pp. 56–63, and John Robertson, "Extracorporeal Embryos and the Abortion Debate," *Journal of Contemporary Health Law and Policy* 2 (1986): 63.

possibility. Does it refer to what is physically possible given the present state of our knowledge and technology? In that case, the eight-cell embryo in the laboratory may be a potential person, but a late-stage blastocyst in the laboratory, consisting of hundreds of cells, cannot be a potential person; we know that if we attempt to transfer such a blastocyst, it will simply be discharged from the uterus without implanting. This yields the result that two blastocysts, to all appearances identical in their internal properties, have entirely different potentials: one, because it has resulted from natural intercourse and has implanted in the uterus, is a potential person, while the other one is not because it is in a laboratory culture.

Such a result is counterintuitive, for it means that while the eight-cell embryo in the laboratory is a potential human being, the embryo loses that status simply by continuing to develop in the laboratory. But perhaps we could come to accept such a view. There are analogous situations in which we would also say that a being has lost the potential it once had. Imagine, for instance, a doctor monitoring a risky pregnancy. The doctor might observe a healthy fetus at one stage during the pregnancy, and say: "Yes, we have a potential person there." Gradually, however, the condition of the fetus may deteriorate to such an extent that it is evident that it will die before reaching the point at which a caesarean delivery could offer any hope of producing a viable infant. The doctor might then say that the potential for personhood has been lost.

This account of potentiality may appear to confuse potential with probability. So far, however, we have been doing no more than exploring a *minimum* necessary condition, suggested by the dictionary definition, for X to have the potential to become Y. That minimum condition is that it be *possible* for X to become Y. Once we accept that it is a present physical possibility, and not logical possibility, that is meant here, we cannot disregard the differences between the eight-cell embryo in the laboratory and those blastocysts which consist of hundreds of cells. These differences do mean that, given our present state of knowledge and technology, it is possible for the former to become a person, but quite impossible, in the relevant physical sense, for the blastocyst just described to become a person. If physical possibility in our present state of knowledge and technology is a necessary condition for potentiality, it follows that the blastocyst in the laboratory is not a potential person.

Given the implications of this view, it might be said that the relevant sense of 'physically possible' should *not* refer to the present state of our

IVF Technology and the
Argument from Potential

knowledge and technology. If we should one day discover how to induce late blastocysts to implant, or if we should perfect laboratory development to such an extent that embryos can develop into infants without ever being transferred to a woman—the process known as ectogenesis—then late blastocysts in laboratories will be able to become people. Perhaps this is all the 'possibility' that is needed for an embryo to be a potential person.

This may indeed be the sense of 'possibility' which lies behind a proper attribution of potential; but it cannot help those who wish to distinguish the potential of the embryo from that of the egg alone. For if it is true that we may one day discover how to induce late blastocysts to implant, it is also true that we may one day discover how to induce parthenogenetic development in the human egg. (Scientists putting human eggs in culture media for IVF have reported seeing, on rare occasions, the beginnings of parthenogenetic development.)[7] So the same sense of 'possibility' which would allow the late embryo to be a potential person would also allow every human egg to be a potential person.

At one stage in the development of reproductive technology—roughly from 1983 until 1985—it might have been argued that the late blastocyst had a genuine possibility of becoming a person in a way that the egg did not. In 1983, human embryos were first successfully preserved by freezing, in a manner which made it possible for them to continue normal development after thawing. Until 1985, however, there was no known way of freezing human eggs which did not cause them damage so severe as to make continued development impossible. A blastocyst could therefore have been frozen to await discovery either of a technique for implanting it successfully in a uterus or of the means of developing it to viability in an artificial womb. A human egg could not have been frozen to await the development of a means of inducing parthenogenesis. Since 1985, however, it has been possible to freeze eggs as well as embryos. So if the combination of freezing and the possibility of future discoveries means that a laboratory blastocyst is a potential person, the same combination must now mean that an unfertilized egg in a laboratory is also a potential person.

Unraveling the notion of potential is leading us in an unexpected direction, and one which will not be welcomed by those who oppose experimentation on human embryos while permitting experimentation on hu-

7. R. Edwards, and also A. Trounson, "Discussion on the Growth of Human Embryos *in Vitro*," in *Human Conception in Vitro*, ed. R. Edwards and J. Purdy (London: Academic Press, 1982), pp. 219-33.

man eggs.[8] The problem, however, is not with the analysis we have proposed, but with the attempt to develop a notion of potential which supports the idea that there is a sharp distinction between the potential of the embryo and that of either the separate egg or the egg and sperm when separate but considered jointly. Is there any way in which the notion can be restored to something more suitable to those purposes?

In a discussion of parthenogenesis, Warren Quinn suggests that in this situation the environmental agent producing parthenogenetic development can be treated as a prefertilization entity that is incorporated into the 'zygote' at the onset of development.[9] In this way, he seeks to preserve the view that even if parthenogenesis occurs, the egg alone is not a potential person; it becomes a potential person only when parthenogenetic development has been triggered. But Quinn's suggestion does not succeed in marking a distinction between the egg and the embryo. For the embryo also needs a specific environment if it is to develop; and if the particular environment which leads to parthenogenesis is allowed to count as an entity for the purposes of denying potential to the egg on its own outside that environment, then the particular environment which leads to development of the embryo must also be allowed to count as an entity, and we should deny potential to the embryo on its own outside that environment.

One might try to defend Quinn's analysis by claiming that the embryo has an *inherent* potential to develop into a person, whereas the egg needs an *external* trigger if it is to develop. At first glance, this appears promising; but on closer scrutiny the promise evaporates. Both the egg and the embryo have an internal genetic code which can, in the right environment, lead to the development of a human being. True, in the embryo the forty-six chromosomes are already present, whereas in the egg the twenty-three chromosomes which are present will need to duplicate themselves to form the forty-six chromosomes necessary for further development. But in neither case does additional genetic information have

8. As was recommended by the Victorian Government's Committee to Consider the Social, Ethical and Legal Issues Arising from *In Vitro* Fertilization, chaired by Professor Louis Waller. See the committee's *Report on the Disposition of Embryos Produced by In Vitro Fertilization* (Melbourne: Victorian Government Printing Office, August 1984). The subsequent Victorian legislation, the Infertility (Medical Procedures) Act of 1984, sec. 6, incorporates these recommendations by tightly restricting embryo experimentation while explicitly exempting experimentation on human ova.

9. Warren Quinn, "Abortion: Identity and Loss," *Philosophy & Public Affairs* 13, no. 1 (Winter 1984): 28.

95   *IVF Technology and the*
                                       Argument from Potential

to be supplied from an external source. In both cases, on the other hand, a great deal else does have to come from outside. In the case of the embryo in the uterus, this includes all the nutrients needed for growth; and of course in the case of the embryo in the laboratory, it also includes skilled human intervention to transfer the embryo to a uterus. In the case of the egg, skilled human intervention would also be required to induce parthenogenetic development. The difference seems to be one of degree rather than of kind.

It might be said that the induction of parthenogenesis marks a more radical change than that caused by the provision of nutrients because it marks the beginning of a new individual, and that in this respect parthenogenesis and fertilization are alike, while the subsequent stages of growth and development have a different, and lesser, significance. But why should we regard the egg after parthenogenesis as a different individual from the egg before parthenogenesis? The following reason can be offered: before either fertilization or parthenogenesis, the egg could develop into any number of different people, because it could be fertilized by any number of different sperm or develop parthenogenetically. After fertilization or parthenogenesis, the developing embryo can become only one person. (Because of the possibility of twinning this is not strictly true, but the contrast between an indefinite range of possibilities and a very limited range of possibilities remains.)

In our view the fact that the embryo, but not the egg, has a uniquely determined potential does not suffice to show that the embryo is a different individual from the egg, or that it, but not the egg, is a potential person. Consider the analogy of a block of marble, rough-hewn from the quarry. In the hands of Michelangelo, it is a potential David, or a Moses, or a Pietà. Later, when the sculptor has chiseled it into the rough outline of a standing youthful figure, it can only become a David. Certainly, by working the marble in this way, Michelangelo has taken its development a stage further. The stage is significant because now the marble has the potential to become only one kind of sculpture (though of course there is still scope for great variation in many important details). Yet the marble is continuous in space and time with the original block. It is not a different piece of marble. That original block, we can now see, had the potential to be a David all along, and the fact that at an earlier stage it could also have become something else does not count against the claim that, even then, it was a potential David. Similarly, fertilization or parthenogenesis takes the development of the egg a stage further, but the potential of the egg is retained. The resulting embryo now has the potential to become only one kind of person (though here too there is still scope for great variation in many important details).[10] Yet the egg had the potential to become this person all along, just as it had the potential to become, in different circumstances, any one of a wide range of other people. Potentiality is one thing; uniqueness is something quite different.

Although we have used the possibility of parthenogenetic development as a means of illustrating some of the problems of attempts to separate the potential of the late blastocyst from the potential of the human egg, our general analysis of the notion of potential does not rely on this. We could equally well have returned to the simpler case of the egg and sperm together in their culture medium prior to the occurrence of fertilization. For all the senses of 'possibility' that we have considered, it is no less possible for the egg and sperm in the laboratory to develop into a person than it is for the laboratory embryo, also in its culture medium, to develop into a person. One could even say the same about the egg alone, treating the presence of sperm as part of the environment necessary for further development, just as the presence of nutrients is necessary for the further development of the embryo.

A more promising approach to distinguishing the potential of the embryo from the potential of the egg and sperm in their culture medium is to acknowledge openly a link between potential and probability, by relating potential not to the bare *possibility* of the embryo's becoming a person, but rather to the *probability* that this will happen. This has the inevitable result that potential ceases to be an all-or-nothing matter, and becomes a matter of degree. Traditional defenders of the right to life of the embryo have been reluctant to introduce degrees of potential into the debate, because once the notion is accepted, it seems undeniable that the early embryo is less a potential person than the later embryo or the fetus. This could easily be understood as leading to the conclusion that the prohibition against destroying the early embryo is less stringent than the prohibition against destroying the later embryo or fetus. Nevertheless, some defenders of the argument from potential have invoked probability and degrees of potential. Among those who have spoken most openly of prob-

10. On the range still possible after fertilization, see Karen Dawson, "Fertilisation and Moral Status: A Scientific Perspective," *Journal of Medical Ethics* 13 (1987).

97   *IVF Technology and the
Argument from Potential*

ability are the Roman Catholic theologian John Noonan and the philosopher Werner Pluhar. As Noonan puts it:

> As life itself is a matter of probabilities, as most moral reasoning is an estimate of probabilities, so it seems in accord with the structure of reality and the nature of moral thought to found a moral judgment on the change in probabilities at conception. . . . Would the argument be different if only one out of ten children conceived came to term? Of course this argument would be different. This argument is an appeal to probabilities that actually exist, not to any and all states of affairs which may be imagined. . . . If a spermatozoon is destroyed, one destroys a being which had a chance of far less than 1 in 200 million of developing into a reasoning being, possessed of the genetic code, a heart and other organs, and capable of pain. If a fetus is destroyed, one destroys a being already possessed of the genetic code, organs and sensitivity to pain, and one which had an 80 percent chance of developing further into a baby outside the womb who, in time, would reason.[11]

Pluhar is almost as explicit:

> if we allow a mere potential for simple consciousness to give rise to a prima facie right to life, then it seems that we must accord a similar right to the staggering number of gamete pairs that likewise have some such potential. . . . Clearly, however, the gamete pair's potential is vastly lower than that of the insentient fetus: even given absence of interference plus at most a modest amount of assistance, the probability of a given gamete pair's producing the individual that it has some potential to produce is so vanishingly small as to be totally negligible in practice.[12]

If, following Noonan and Pluhar, we take the probability that an embryo will become a reasoning being (or, in Pluhar's case, become sentient) as relevant to the potential of the embryo to become a person, it must follow that the potential of the laboratory embryo currently diminishes after the eight-cell stage, when the probability that the transferred embryo will result in a pregnancy begins to decline; and by the late blastocyst stage, on this view, the laboratory embryo has no potential at all. This may well be

11. John T. Noonan, Jr., "An Almost Absolute Value in History," in *The Morality of Abortion*, ed. J. T. Noonan, Jr. (Cambridge: Harvard University Press, 1970), pp. 56–57.

12. Werner Pluhar, "Abortion and Simple Consciousness," *Journal of Philosophy* 74 (1977): 167.

an implication which opponents of embryo experimentation are happy to accept; they may say that this loss of the potential to become a person is one reason why it is wrong to keep human embryos alive in laboratories, or perhaps even why it is wrong to create them *in vitro* at all.

Accepting that there are degrees of potential associated with probability does, however, have other consequences which are less likely to be congenial to opponents of embryo experimentation. For on this view, contrary to what Noonan and Pluhar claim, the distinction between the potential of the embryo in culture and the potential of the gametes in the laboratory before fertilization becomes a difference of degree, and not a marked difference at that. Fertilization is, as we have seen, one of the relatively reliable steps in the *in vitro* fertilization procedure, with success rates commonly around 80 percent. Thus if we base degrees of potential on the probability that a person will ultimately result from an embryo, we cannot treat as crucially significant the line between the stage at which we have a set of gametes and the stage at which we have an embryo. At least so far as potential is concerned, the division between the stage at which we have an embryo in the laboratory and the stage at which we have an embryo implanted in the uterus is much more significant. Insofar as the argument from potential is important to the morality of experimenting on or disposing of an entity, we cannot support the prohibition of experimenting on or disposing of embryos while remaining unconcerned about how eggs and sperm are treated.

There are two possible replies to this argument. The first claims that to speak of the potential of the egg and sperm while they are still separate is nonsense, because they are two discrete entities, and hence cannot have a single potential. The second reply is Noonan's; it asserts that the distinction between embryo and gametes does mark a sharp distinction in probability, because the probability that an embryo will become a child is very great, whereas the probability that any *one* sperm will participate in fertilization is 1 in 200 million. We will consider these replies in turn.

The first reply fails because there is no reason why an entity with potential must consist of a single object, rather than of two or more discrete objects. There is, for instance, nothing problematic about the statement (made, let us assume, shortly before the battle of El Alamein) "Montgomery's army has the potential to defeat Rommel's army."[13] Yet Montgom-

13. The example is taken from a letter by Brian Scarlett (*Journal of Medical Ethics* 10

99

*IVF Technology and the
Argument from Potential*

ery's army consisted of thousands of discrete individuals, spread over many miles of desert. We can even speak of the potential of entities which are spread across the entire planet—as Noah might have spoken of the potential of the raindrops falling all over the world to cause a great flood. So why should there be any problem about speaking of the potential of a set of gametes in a glass dish?

Noonan's reply faces several problems. One has been raised by Mark Strasser.[14] Why, Strasser asks, does Noonan focus on the probability that a given single sperm will participate in fertilization, and not on the probability of fertilization by any one of the sperm? This would, of course, provide a very different result: in the case of a normally fertile woman who has sexual intercourse without contraception during that part of her cycle when she is most likely to be fertile, the probability that fertilization will occur and result in a child is not greatly different from the probability that the newly fertilized egg will result in a child—certainly not different by the orders of magnitude Noonan suggests. Similarly, Noonan does not discuss the probability that the *egg*, rather than the sperm, will participate in fertilization. This also would give a very different result.

Even if Noonan can provide an answer to Strasser's objection, his position has, like other claims about the potential of embryos, become much more difficult to maintain in the light of new knowledge and new developments in reproductive technology. The initial difficulty is that Noonan's figures for embryo survival even in the uterus are no longer regarded as accurate. At the time Noonan wrote, the estimate of pregnancy loss was based on clinically recognized or stable, ongoing pregnancies. These pregnancies are about six to eight weeks after fertilization—embryonic heartbeat is detectable, menses has ceased, and enzyme assays will give reliable results indicating pregnancy. Currently such pregnancies are associated with a 15 percent loss through spontaneous abortion.[15] Though the total pregnancy wastage rate remains largely unknown, recent technical advances allowing earlier recognition of pregnancy suggest that this figure is an underestimate of total loss and represents an oversimplifica-

---

[1984]: 217–18) arguing, in a different context, against the views of Peter Singer and Helga Kuhse on the potential of the embryo.

14. Mark Strasser. "Noonan on Contraception and Abortion." *Bioethics* 1, no. 2 (April 1987): 199–205.

15. J. Grudzinskas and A. Nysenbaum. "Failure of Human Pregnancy after Implantation." *Annals of the New York Academy of Science* 442 (1985): 39–44.

tion of the real situation.[16] Estimates of the natural wastage at various stages of pregnancy can now be taken into account, and they provide startlingly different figures from those supplied by Noonan. If pregnancy is diagnosed before implantation (within fourteen days of fertilization) the estimated chance of a birth resulting is 25 to 30 percent.[17] After implantation this chance increases initially to between 40 and 60 percent,[18] and it is not until six weeks' gestation that the chance of birth occurring increases to between 85 and 90 percent.[19]

Noonan claimed that his argument is "an appeal to probabilities that actually exist, not to any and all states of affairs which may be imagined." We have now seen that the real probabilities are very different from what Noonan believed them to be. Once we substitute the real probabilities, Noonan's argument no longer supports the moment of fertilization as the time at which the embryo gains a significantly different moral status. Indeed, if we were to require an 80 percent probability of further development into a baby—the figure used in the passage from Noonan quoted above—we would have to wait until about six weeks after fertilization before the embryo would have the significance Noonan wants to claim for it. If, on the other hand, we simply look for the moment at which the chance of birth resulting becomes close to or better than 50 percent, that time would seem to be around the moment of implantation.

To cope with the development of IVF, some readjustment of the parts of Noonan's argument pertinent to gametes is also necessary. Most importantly, the figures for embryo survival are very different when we consider the laboratory embryo rather than the embryo implanted in a uterus; an embryo survival rate of 10 percent would be relatively optimistic, even in a proficient laboratory. In addition, Noonan estimates the probability that any one sperm will participate in fertilization as 1 in 200 million, based on the number of sperm in a male ejaculate. In IVF, however, only about 50,000 sperm are used to fertilize an egg, increasing greatly the chances that any one sperm will fertilize the egg.[20]

16. Ibid.

17. C. Roberts and C. Lowe, "Where Have All the Conceptions Gone?" *Lancet,* 1975, 1:498–99.

18. J. Muller et al., "Fetal Loss after Implantation," *Lancet,* 1980, 2:554–56.

19. D. Braunstein, "Chorionicgonadotrophin (HCG) and HCG-like Substances in Human Tissue and Bacteria," in *Pregnancy Proteins: Biology, Chemistry and Clinical Application,* ed. J. Grudzinskas et al. (London: Academic Press, 1982), pp. 39–49.

20. M. Mahadevan and G. Baker, "Assessment and Preparation of Semen for *In Vitro* Fer-

101 *IVF Technology and the Argument from Potential*

Perhaps Noonan's claim that there is a sharp difference between the embryo and the sperm, based on the probability of proceeding to the next stage of development, could survive these changes in the figures. The relevant figure for the embryo *in vitro* is now 1 in 10, and for the sperm participating in *in vitro* fertilization, about 1 in 50,000. This is still a very marked difference. The difference virtually disappears, however, if we focus on the egg rather than the sperm, or if, as Strasser suggests, we consider the prospects of a birth resulting not from a *given* sperm, but from *any* of the sperm in the seminal fluid.

In any case, the argument faces still one more difficulty. Scientists are at present on the brink of trying out a new means of overcoming male infertility caused by a low sperm count or sperm which is insufficiently motile. The egg will be removed and cultured as in the normal *in vitro* procedure, but instead of adding a drop of seminal fluid containing about 50,000 sperm, a single sperm will be microinjected under the outer membrane of the egg. This procedure has already been carried out with human gametes, although no attempt has been made to produce a pregnancy from the resulting zygote.[21] Problems may arise in the use of the technique to overcome male infertility, but assuming that it is successful, the unique genetic blueprint of the individual-to-be will be determined before fertilization; it will, to be precise, be determined at the moment when the single sperm has been selected for microinjection. So if we compare the probability that the embryo will become a person with the probability that the egg, together with the single sperm about to be microinjected into the egg, will become a person, we will be unable to find any sharp distinction between the two. Even the genetic blueprint will have been determined in both cases.

III

An Australian Senate Select Committee has recently discussed the question of the potential of the embryo in the context of human embryo experimentation. Its report, *Human Embryo Experimentation in Australia*, consists of a majority report signed by the chairman, Senator Michael

tilization," in *Clinical In Vitro Fertilization*, ed. C. Wood and A. Trounson (New York: Springer, 1984), pp. 99-116.

21. Personal communication from Dr. Ismail Kola, Centre for Early Human Development, Monash University.

Tate, with four other senators, and a dissenting report signed by two senators.[22] The majority report seems to take the notion of the potential of the laboratory embryo as unproblematic, stating that it works from the premise that "the embryo may be properly described as genetically new human life organised as a distinct entity oriented towards further development."[23] The majority clearly did not regard the egg in a similar light, for whereas they recommended the prohibition of destructive experimentation on human embryos, they made no such recommendation regarding experimentation on human eggs. They also made recommendations designed to reduce the incidence of embryo freezing, in view of the high risk of mortality for frozen embryos, encouraging instead the development and use of egg freezing.[24]

The dissenting report from Senators Rosemary Crowley and Olive Zakharov took a radically different view of potential:

> Any object or thing has an infinite number of possible future courses. For a non-sentient or inanimate thing, e.g. a rock, the particular future outcome that actually happens is determined by forces outside of itself. An embryo is like a rock in this respect—it cannot make decisions for itself. Its future is decided by others. It has potential only in virtue of decisions by others about it. If there is a clearly defined responsible party or parties their decisions determine the embryo's potential and that becomes the embryo's potential.[25]

This is a bold departure from the conventional view of potential, although it is not a great distance from the view that the potential of an entity to become a person is related to the probability that the entity will become a person. But Crowley and Zakharov have noticed something that is overlooked by straightforward attempts to identify potentiality with probability, and that is the role of human decision.

As we noticed earlier, whereas the embryo inside the female body has some definite chance of developing into a child unless a deliberate human act interrupts its growth, the egg and sperm can develop into a child only

22. Senate Select Committee on the Human Embryo Experimentation Bill. *Human Embryo Experimentation in Australia* (Canberra: Australian Government Publishing Service. 1986).

23. Ibid., para. 3.27.

24. Ibid., para. 5.13.

25. Ibid., para. D20.

        IVF Technology and the
Argument from Potential

if there is a deliberate human act; *and in this respect the IVF embryo in the laboratory is like the egg and sperm, and not like the embryo in the human body.*

Lurking in the background of discussions of the potential of the embryo is the idea that there is a 'natural' course of events, governed by the 'inherent' potential of the embryo, or as the majority report of the Senate committee might have put it, resulting from the "organization of the embryo as an entity oriented towards further development." For if it were not for this notion of a 'natural' course of events, why would the Senate committee not have noticed that the human egg is also "genetically new human life organised as a distinct entity oriented towards further development"? After all, the egg is human, not from any other animal, and it is also alive, not dead. Moreover, what the egg needs to continue its development is a sperm, just as what the embryo needs is a suitable environment, nutrients, and so on. Neither can develop without an external element, and both can develop with the right external element.[26] If we set aside the idea that the embryo will develop 'naturally' as opposed to the egg, which will develop only if a sperm is placed in proximity to it, what difference in terms of "orientation towards further development" remains?

We have seen, however, that this notion of 'natural' development—development not requiring the assistance of a deliberate human act—has no application to the IVF embryo. Hence those who wish to use the potential of the IVF embryo as a ground for protecting it cannot appeal to this notion of natural development; and for this reason, they find themselves in difficulty in explaining why the embryo in the laboratory has a potential greatly different from that of either the egg alone or the egg and sperm considered jointly. Crowley and Zakharov are correct to point to the crucial role played by human decision in determining the future of the embryo, and to focus, as they do in their dissenting report, on the question of who should have the responsibility of making this decision. (They conclude that it should be the woman or the gamete donors.)

The view of Crowley and Zakharov that an embryo has potential only in virtue of decisions by others about it amounts to the rejection of our common notion of potential, for it makes potential relative to the wishes and acts of human decision makers. Such a rejection of the common notion is

26. This point parallels that made in our earlier discussion of Quinn.

strongly supported by the difficulties we have found with it in examining a range of arguments which invoke the potential of the embryo as a reason for according it a special moral status, different from that of the egg or of the egg and sperm when separate but considered jointly. Whether these arguments succeed in establishing that in the normal reproductive situation the embryo has a potential different from that of the egg and sperm is a question we have left open. But even if these arguments are applicable to the normal situation, they cannot validly be applied to *in vitro* embryos and eggs and sperm. The new reproductive technology makes it necessary for us to think again about how our established views about the potential of the human embryo should be applied to the embryo in a laboratory.

[25]

SOUNDING BOARD

OF MICE BUT NOT MEN

Problems of the Randomized Clinical Trial

As medicine has become increasingly scientific and less accepting of unsupported opinion or proof by anecdote, the randomized controlled clinical trial has become the standard technique for changing diagnostic or therapeutic methods. The use of this technique creates an ethical dilemma.[1,2] Researchers participating in such studies are required to modify their ethical commitments to individual patients and do serious damage to the concept of the physician as a practicing, empathetic professional who is primarily concerned with each patient as an individual. Researchers using a randomized clinical trial can be described as physician-scientists, a term that expresses the tension between the two roles. The physician, by entering into a relationship with an individual patient, assumes certain obligations, including the commitment always to act in the patient's best interests. As Leon Kass has rightly maintained, "the physician must produce unswervingly the virtues of loyalty and fidelity to his patient."[3] Though the ethical requirements of this relationship have been modified by legal obligations to report wounds of a suspicious nature and certain infectious diseases, these obligations in no way conflict with the central ethical obligation to act in the best interests of the patient medically. Instead, certain nonmedical interests of the patient are preempted by other social concerns.

The role of the scientist is quite different. The clinical scientist is concerned with answering questions — i.e., determining the validity of formally constructed hypotheses. Such scientific information, it is presumed, will benefit humanity in general. The clinical scientist's role has been well described by Dr. Anthony Fauci, director of the National Institute of Allergy and Infectious Diseases, who states the goals of the randomized clinical trial in these words: "It's not to deliver therapy. It's to answer a scientific question so

PROSPECTIVE authors should consult "Information for Authors," which appears in the first issue of each month and may be obtained from the *Journal* office.

ARTICLES with original material are accepted for consideration with the understanding that, except for abstracts, no part of the data has been published, or will be submitted for publication elsewhere, before appearing here.

MATERIAL printed in the *Journal* is covered by copyright. No part of this publication may be reproduced without written permission. The *Journal* does not hold itself responsible for statements made by any contributor.

STATEMENTS or opinions expressed in the *Journal* reflect the views of the author(s) and do not represent official policy of the Massachusetts Medical Society unless so stated.

ALTHOUGH all advertising material accepted is expected to conform to ethical medical standards, acceptance does not imply endorsement by the *Journal*.

SUBSCRIPTION PRICES: Pounds sterling drawn on U.K. banks only: £80 per year (interns, residents, and students £52 per year). Send payments and correspondence to: NEJM, Saxon Way, Melbourn, Royston, Herts SG8 6NJ, U.K. Please include current mailing label with renewal order. In Japan, ¥27,800 per year (interns, residents, and students ¥18,000 per year). Send orders to: Nankodo Co., Ltd., 42-6, Hongo 3-chome, Bunkyo-Ku, Tokyo 113, Japan.

EDITORIAL OFFICES: 10 Shattuck St., Boston, MA 02115-6094, USA.

Telephone: (617) 734-9800.   FAX: (617) 734-4457.

BUSINESS AND SUBSCRIPTION OFFICES: 1440 Main St., Waltham, MA 02154-1649, USA.   FAX: (617) 893-0413.

1586   THE NEW ENGLAND JOURNAL OF MEDICINE   May 30, 1991

that the drug can be available for everybody once you've established safety and efficacy."[4] The demands of such a study can conflict in a number of ways with the physician's duty to minister to patients. The study may create a false dichotomy in the physician's opinions: according to the premise of the randomized clinical trial, the physician may only know or not know whether a proposed course of treatment represents an improvement; no middle position is permitted. What the physician thinks, suspects, believes, or has a hunch about is assigned to the "not knowing" category, because knowing is defined on the basis of an arbitrary but accepted statistical test performed in a randomized clinical trial. Thus, little credence is given to information gained beforehand in other ways or to information accrued during the trial but without the required statistical degree of assurance that a difference is not due to chance. The randomized clinical trial also prevents the treatment technique from being modified on the basis of the growing knowledge of the physicians during their participation in the trial. Moreover, it limits access to the data as they are collected until specific milestones are achieved. This prevents physicians from profiting not only from their individual experience, but also from the collective experience of the other participants.

The randomized clinical trial requires doctors to act simultaneously as physicians and as scientists. This puts them in a difficult and sometimes untenable ethical position. The conflicting moral demands arising from the use of the randomized clinical trial reflect the classic conflict between rights-based moral theories and utilitarian ones. The first of these, which depend on the moral theory of Immanuel Kant (and seen more recently in neo-Kantian philosophers, such as John Rawls[5]), asserts that human beings, by virtue of their unique capacity for rational thought, are bearers of dignity. As such, they ought not to be treated merely as means to an end; rather, they must always be treated as ends in themselves. Utilitarianism, by contrast, defines what is right as the greatest good for the greatest number — that is, as social utility. This view, articulated by Jeremy Bentham and John Stuart Mill, requires that pleasures (understood broadly, to include such pleasures as health and well-being) and pains be added together. The morally correct act is the act that produces the most pleasure and the least pain overall.

A classic objection to the utilitarian position is that according to that theory, the distribution of pleasures and pains is of no moral consequence. This element of the theory severely restricts physicians from being utilitarians, or at least from following the theory's dictates. Physicians must care very deeply about the distribution of pain and pleasure, for they have entered into a relationship with one or a number of individual patients. They cannot be indifferent to whether it is these patients or others that suffer for the general benefit of society. Even though society might gain

from the suffering of a few, and even though the doctor might believe that such a benefit is worth a given patient's suffering (i.e., that utilitarianism is right in the particular case), the ethical obligation created by the covenant between doctor and patient requires the doctor to see the interests of the individual patient as primary and compelling. In essence, the doctor–patient relationship requires doctors to see their patients as bearers of rights who cannot be merely used for the greater good of humanity.

As Fauci has suggested,[4] the randomized clinical trial routinely asks physicians to sacrifice the interests of their particular patients for the sake of the study and that of the information that it will make available for the benefit of society. This practice is ethically problematic. Consider first the initial formulation of a trial. In particular, consider the case of a disease for which there is no satisfactory therapy — for example, advanced cancer or the acquired immunodeficiency syndrome (AIDS). A new agent that promises more effectiveness is the subject of the study. The control group must be given either an unsatisfactory treatment or a placebo. Even though the therapeutic value of the new agent is unproved, if physicians think that it has promise, are they acting in the best interests of their patients in allowing them to be randomly assigned to the control group? Is persisting in such an assignment consistent with the specific commitments taken on in the doctor–patient relationship? As a result of interactions with patients with AIDS and their advocates, Merigan[6] recently suggested modifications in the design of clinical trials that attempt to deal with the unsatisfactory treatment given to the control group. The view of such activists has been expressed by Rebecca Pringle Smith of Community Research Initiative in New York: "Even if you have a supply of compliant martyrs, trials must have some ethical validity."[4]

If the physician has no opinion about whether the new treatment is acceptable, then random assignment is ethically acceptable, but such lack of enthusiasm for the new treatment does not augur well for either the patient or the study. Alternatively, the treatment may show promise of beneficial results but also present a risk of undesirable complications. When the physician believes that the severity and likelihood of harm and good are evenly balanced, randomization may be ethically acceptable. If the physician has no preference for either treatment (is in a state of equipoise[7,8]), then randomization is acceptable. If, however, he or she believes that the new treatment may be either more or less successful or more or less toxic, the use of randomization is not consistent with fidelity to the patient.

The argument usually used to justify randomization is that it provides, in essence, a critique of the usefulness of the physician's beliefs and opinions, those that have not yet been validated by a randomized clinical trial. As the argument goes, these not-yet-validated

Vol. 324   No. 22   THE NEW ENGLAND JOURNAL OF MEDICINE   1587

beliefs are as likely to be wrong as right. Although physicians are ethically required to provide their patients with the best available treatment, there simply is no best treatment yet known.

The reply to this argument takes two forms. First, and most important, even if this view of the reliability of a physician's opinions is accurate, the ethical constraints of an individual doctor's relationship with a particular patient require the doctor to provide individual care. Although physicians must take pains to make clear the speculative nature of their views, they cannot withhold these views from the patient. The patient asks from the doctor both knowledge and judgment. The relationship established between them rightfully allows patients to ask for the judgment of their particular physicians, not merely that of the medical profession in general. Second, it may not be true, in fact, that the not-yet-validated beliefs of physicians are as likely to be wrong as right. The greater certainty obtained with a randomized clinical trial is beneficial, but that does not mean that a lesser degree of certainty is without value. Physicians can acquire knowledge through methods other than the randomized clinical trial. Such knowledge, acquired over time and less formally than is required in a randomized clinical trial, may be of great value to a patient.

Even if it is ethically acceptable to begin a study, one often forms an opinion during its course — especially in studies that are impossible to conduct in a truly double-blinded fashion — that makes it ethically problematic to continue. The inability to remain blinded usually occurs in studies of cancer or AIDS, for example, because the therapy is associated by nature with serious side effects. Trials attempt to restrict the physician's access to the data in order to prevent such unblinding. Such restrictions should make physicians eschew the trial, since their ability to act in the patient's best interests will be limited. Even supporters of randomized clinical trials, such as Merigan, agree that interim findings should be presented to patients to ensure that no one receives what seems an inferior treatment.[6] Once physicians have formed a view about the new treatment, can they continue randomization? If random assignment is stopped, the study may be lost and the participation of the previous patients wasted. However, if physicians continue the randomization when they have a definite opinion about the efficacy of the experimental drug, they are not acting in accordance with the requirements of the doctor–patient relationship. Furthermore, as their opinion becomes more firm, stopping the randomization may not be enough. Physicians may be ethically required to treat the patients formerly placed in the control group with the therapy that now seems probably effective. To do so would be faithful to the obligations created by the doctor–patient relationship, but it would destroy the study.

To resolve this dilemma, one might suggest that the patient has abrogated the rights implicit in a doctor–patient relationship by signing an informed-consent form. We argue that such rights cannot be waived or abrogated. They are inalienable. The right to be treated as an individual deserving the physician's best judgment and care, rather than to be used as a means to determine the best treatment for others, is inherent in every person. This right, based on the concept of dignity, cannot be waived. What of altruism, then? Is it not the patient's right to make a sacrifice for the general good? This question must be considered from both positions — that of the patient and that of the physician. Although patients may decide to waive this right, it is not consistent with the role of a physician to ask that they do so. In asking, the doctor acts as a scientist instead. The physician's role here is to propose what he or she believes is best medically for the specific patient, not to suggest participation in a study from which the patient cannot gain. Because the opportunity to help future patients is of potential value to a patient, some would say physicians should not deny it. Although this point has merit, it offers so many opportunities for abuse that we are extremely uncomfortable about accepting it. The responsibilities of physicians are much clearer; they are to minister to the current patient.

Moreover, even if patients could waive this right, it is questionable whether those with terminal illness would be truly able to give voluntary informed consent. Such patients are extremely dependent on both their physicians and the health care system. Aware of this dependence, physicians must not ask for consent, for in such cases the very asking breaches the doctor–patient relationship. Anxious to please their physicians, patients may have difficulty refusing to participate in the trial the physicians describe. The patients may perceive their refusal as damaging to the relationship, whether or not it is so. Such perceptions of coercion affect the decision. Informed-consent forms are difficult to understand, especially for patients under the stress of serious illness for which there is no satisfactory treatment. The forms are usually lengthy, somewhat legalistic, complicated, and confusing, and they hardly bespeak the compassion expected of the medical profession. It is important to remember that those who have studied the doctor–patient relationship have emphasized its empathetic nature.

> [The] relationship between doctor and patient partakes of a peculiar intimacy. It presupposes on the part of the physician not only knowledge of his fellow men but sympathy. . . . This aspect of the practice of medicine has been designated as the art; yet I wonder whether it should not, most properly, be called the essence.[9]

How is such a view of the relationship consonant with random assignment and informed consent? The Physician's Oath of the World Medical Association affirms the primacy of the deontologic view of patients' rights: "Concern for the interests of the subject must always prevail over the interests of science and society."[10]

1588   THE NEW ENGLAND JOURNAL OF MEDICINE   May 30, 1991

Furthermore, a single study is often not considered sufficient. Before a new form of therapy is generally accepted, confirmatory trials must be conducted. How can one conduct such trials ethically unless one is convinced that the first trial was in error? The ethical problems we have discussed are only exacerbated when a completed randomized clinical trial indicates that a given treatment is preferable. Even if the physician believes the initial trial was in error, the physician must indicate to the patient the full results of that trial.

The most common reply to the ethical arguments has been that the alternative is to return to the physician's intuition, to anecdotes, or to both as the basis of medical opinion. We all accept the dangers of such a practice. The argument states that we must therefore accept randomized, controlled clinical trials regardless of their ethical problems because of the great social benefit they make possible, and we salve our conscience with the knowledge that informed consent has been given. This returns us to the conflict between patients' rights and social utility. Some would argue that this tension can be resolved by placing a relative value on each. If the patient's right that is being compromised is not a fundamental right and the social gain is very great, then the study might be justified. When the right is fundamental, however, no amount of social gain, or almost none, will justify its sacrifice. Consider, for example, the experiments on humans done by physicians under the Nazi regime. All would agree that these are unacceptable regardless of the value of the scientific information gained. Some people go so far as to say that no use should be made of the results of those experiments because of the clearly unethical manner in which the data were collected. This extreme example may not seem relevant, but we believe that in its hyperbole it clarifies the fallacy of a utilitarian approach to the physician's relationship with the patient. To consider the utilitarian gain is consistent neither with the physician's role nor with the patient's rights.

It is fallacious to suggest that only the randomized clinical trial can provide valid information or that all information acquired by this technique is valid. Such experimental methods are intended to reduce error and bias and therefore reduce the uncertainty of the result. Uncertainty cannot be eliminated, however. The scientific method is based on increasing probabilities and increasingly refined approximations of truth.[11] Although the randomized clinical trial contributes to these ends, it is neither unique nor perfect. Other techniques may also be useful.[12]

Randomized trials often place physicians in the ethically intolerable position of choosing between the good of the patient and that of society. We urge that such situations be avoided and that other techniques of acquiring clinical information be adopted. For example, concerning trials of treatments for AIDS, Byar et al.[13] have said that "some traditional approaches to the clinical-trials process may be unnecessarily rigid and unsuitable for this disease." In this case, AIDS is not what is so different; rather, the difference is in the presence of AIDS activists, articulate spokespersons for the ethical problems created by the application of the randomized clinical trial to terminal illnesses. Such arguments are equally applicable to advanced cancer and other serious illnesses. Byar et al. agree that there are even circumstances in which uncontrolled clinical trials may be justified: when there is no effective treatment to use as a control, when the prognosis is uniformly poor, and when there is a reasonable expectation of benefit without excessive toxicity. These conditions are usually found in clinical trials of advanced cancer.

The purpose of the randomized clinical trial is to avoid the problems of observer bias and patient selection. It seems to us that techniques might be developed to deal with these issues in other ways. Randomized clinical trials deal with them in a cumbersome and heavy-handed manner, by requiring large numbers of patients in the hope that random assignment will balance the heterogeneous distribution of patients into the different groups. By observing known characteristics of patients, such as age and sex, and distributing them equally between groups, it is thought that unknown factors important in determining outcomes will also be distributed equally. Surely, other techniques can be developed to deal with both observer bias and patient selection. Prospective studies without randomization, but with the evaluation of patients by uninvolved third parties, should remove observer bias. Similar methods have been suggested by Royall.[12] Prospective matched-pair analysis, in which patients are treated in a manner consistent with their physician's views, ought to help ensure equivalence between the groups and thus mitigate the effect of patient selection, at least with regard to known covariates. With regard to unknown covariates, the security would rest, as in randomized trials, in the enrollment of large numbers of patients and in confirmatory studies. This method would not pose ethical difficulties, since patients would receive the treatment recommended by their physician. They would be included in the study by independent observers matching patients with respect to known characteristics, a process that would not affect patient care and that could be performed independently any number of times.

This brief discussion of alternatives to randomized clinical trials is sketchy and incomplete. We wish only to point out that there may be satisfactory alternatives, not to describe and evaluate them completely. Even if randomized clinical trials were much better than any alternative, however, the ethical dilemmas they present may put their use at variance with the primary obligations of the physician. In this regard,

Vol. 324   No. 22   THE NEW ENGLAND JOURNAL OF MEDICINE

Angell cautions, "If this commitment to the patient is attenuated, even for so good a cause as benefits to future patients, the implicit assumptions of the doctor–patient relationship are violated."[14] The risk of such attenuation by the randomized trial is great. The AIDS activists have brought this dramatically to the attention of the academic medical community. Techniques appropriate to the laboratory may not be applicable to humans. We must develop and use alternative methods for acquiring clinical knowledge.

University of Chicago
Chicago, IL 60637-1470   SAMUEL HELLMAN, M.D.

Harvard University
Cambridge, MA 02138   DEBORAH S. HELLMAN, M.A.

REFERENCES

1. Hellman S. Randomized clinical trials and the doctor–patient relationship: an ethical dilemma. Cancer Clin Trials 1979; 2:189-93.
2. *Idem.* A doctor's dilemma: the doctor-patient relationship in clinical investigation. In: Proceedings of the Fourth National Conference on Human Values and Cancer. New York, March 15–17, 1984. New York: American Cancer Society, 1984:144-6.
3. Kass LR. Toward a more natural science: biology and human affairs. New York: Free Press. 1985:196.
4. Palca J. AIDS drug trials enter new age. Science 1989; 246:19-21.
5. Rawls J. A theory of justice. Cambridge, Mass.: Belknap Press of Harvard University Press. 1971:183-92, 446-52.
6. Merigan TC. You can teach an old dog new tricks — how AIDS trials are pioneering new strategies. N Engl J Med 1990; 323:1341-3.
7. Freedman B. Equipoise and the ethics of clinical research. N Engl J Med 1987; 317:141-5.
8. Singer PA, Lantos JD, Whitington PF, Broelsch CE, Siegler M. Equipoise and the ethics of segmental liver transplantation. Clin Res 1988; 36:539-45.
9. Longcope WT. Methods and medicine. Bull Johns Hopkins Hosp 1932; 50:4-20.
10. Report on medical ethics. World Med Assoc Bull 1949; 1:109, 111.
11. Popper K. The problem of induction. In: Miller D. ed. Popper selections. Princeton, N.J.: Princeton University Press, 1985:101-17.
12. Royall RM. Ethics and statistics in randomized clinical trials. Stat Sci 1991; 6(1):52-62.
13. Byar DP, Schoenfeld DA, Green SB. et al. Design considerations for AIDS trials. N Engl J Med 1990; 323:1343-8.
14. Angell M. Patients' preferences in randomized clinical trials. N Engl J Med 1984; 310:1385-7.

[26]

SPECIAL ARTICLE

EQUIPOISE AND THE ETHICS OF CLINICAL RESEARCH

BENJAMIN FREEDMAN, PH.D.

Abstract The ethics of clinical research requires equipoise — a state of genuine uncertainty on the part of the clinical investigator regarding the comparative therapeutic merits of each arm in a trial. Should the investigator discover that one treatment is of superior therapeutic merit, he or she is ethically obliged to offer that treatment. The current understanding of this requirement, which entails that the investigator have no "treatment preference" throughout the course of the trial, presents nearly insuperable obstacles to the ethical commencement or completion of a controlled trial and may also contribute to the termination of trials because of the failure to enroll enough patients.

I suggest an alternative concept of equipoise, which would be based on present or imminent controversy in the clinical community over the preferred treatment. According to this concept of "clinical equipoise," the requirement is satisfied if there is genuine uncertainty within the expert medical community — not necessarily on the part of the individual investigator — about the preferred treatment. (N Engl J Med 1987; 317: 141-5.)

THERE is widespread agreement that ethics requires that each clinical trial begin with an honest null hypothesis.[1,2] In the simplest model, testing a new treatment B on a defined patient population P for which the current accepted treatment is A, it is necessary that the clinical investigator be in a state of genuine uncertainty regarding the comparative merits of treatments A and B for population P. If a physician knows that these treatments are not equivalent, ethics requires that the superior treatment be recommended. Following Fried, I call this state of uncertainty about the relative merits of A and B "equipoise."[3]

Equipoise is an ethically necessary condition in all cases of clinical research. In trials with several arms, equipoise must exist between all arms of the trial; otherwise the trial design should be modified to exclude the inferior treatment. If equipoise is disturbed during the course of a trial, the trial may need to be terminated and all subjects previously enrolled (as well as other patients within the relevant population) may have to be offered the superior treatment. It has been rigorously argued that a trial with a placebo is ethical only in investigating conditions for which there is no known treatment[2]; this argument reflects a special application of the requirement for equipoise. Although equipoise has commonly been discussed in the special context of the ethics of randomized clinical trials,[4,5] it is important to recognize it as an ethical condition of all controlled clinical trials, whether or not they are randomized, placebo-controlled, or blinded.

The recent increase in attention to the ethics of research with human subjects has highlighted problems associated with equipoise. Yet, as I shall attempt to show, contemporary literature, if anything, minimizes those difficulties. Moreover, there is evidence that concern on the part of investigators about failure to satisfy the requirements for equipoise can doom a trial

as a result of the consequent failure to enroll a sufficient number of subjects.

The solutions that have been offered to date fail to resolve these problems in a way that would permit clinical trials to proceed. This paper argues that these problems are predicated on a faulty concept of equipoise itself. An alternative understanding of equipoise as an ethical requirement of clinical trials is proposed, and its implications are explored.

Many of the problems raised by the requirement for equipoise are familiar. Shaw and Chalmers have written that a clinician who "knows, or has good reason to believe," that one arm of the trial is superior may not ethically participate.[6] But the reasoning or preliminary results that prompt the trial (and that may themselves be ethically mandatory)[7] may jolt the investigator (if not his or her colleagues) out of equipoise before the trial begins. Even if the investigator is undecided between A and B in terms of gross measures such as mortality and morbidity, equipoise may be disturbed because evident differences in the quality of life (as in the case of two surgical approaches) tip the balance.[3-5,8] In either case, in saying "we do not know" whether A or B is better, the investigator may create a false impression in prospective subjects, who hear him or her as saying "no evidence leans either way," when the investigator means "no controlled study has yet had results that reach statistical significance."

Late in the study — when P values are between 0.05 and 0.06 — the moral issue of equipoise is most readily apparent,[9,10] but the same problem arises when the earliest comparative results are analyzed.[11] Within the closed statistical universe of the clinical trial, each result that demonstrates a difference between the arms of the trial contributes exactly as much to the statistical conclusion that a difference exists as does any other. The contribution of the last pair of cases in the trial is no greater than that of the first. If, therefore, equipoise is a condition that reflects equivalent evidence for alternative hypotheses, it is jeopardized by the first pair of cases as much as by the last. The investigator who is concerned about the ethics of recruitment after

From the McGill Centre for Medicine, Ethics and Law, McGill University, Lady Meredith Bldg., 1110 Pine Ave. W., Montreal, PQ H3A 1A3, Canada, where reprint requests should be addressed to Dr. Freedman.

Supported in part by a research grant from the Social Sciences and Humanities Research Council of Canada.

142   THE NEW ENGLAND JOURNAL OF MEDICINE   July 16, 1987

the penultimate pair must logically be concerned after the first pair as well.

Finally, these issues are more than a philosopher's nightmare. Considerable interest has been generated by a paper in which Taylor et al.[12] describe the termination of a trial of alternative treatments for breast cancer. The trial foundered on the problem of patient recruitment, and the investigators trace much of the difficulty in enrolling patients to the fact that the investigators were not in a state of equipoise regarding the arms of the trial. With the increase in concern about the ethics of research and with the increasing presence of this topic in the curricula of medical and graduate schools, instances of the type that Taylor and her colleagues describe are likely to become more common. The requirement for equipoise thus poses a practical threat to clinical research.

Responses to the Problems of Equipoise

The problems described above apply to a broad class of clinical trials, at all stages of their development. Their resolution will need to be similarly comprehensive. However, the solutions that have so far been proposed address a portion of the difficulties, at best, and cannot be considered fully satisfactory.

Chalmers' approach to problems at the onset of a trial is to recommend that randomization begin with the very first subject.[11] If there are no preliminary, uncontrolled data in support of the experimental treatment B, equipoise regarding treatments A and B for the patient population P is not disturbed. There are several difficulties with this approach. Practically speaking, it is often necessary to establish details of administration, dosage, and so on, before a controlled trial begins, by means of uncontrolled trials in human subjects. In addition, as I have argued above, equipoise from the investigator's point of view is likely to be disturbed when the hypothesis is being formulated and a protocol is being prepared. It is then, before any subjects have been enrolled, that the information that the investigator has assembled makes the experimental treatment appear to be a reasonable gamble. Apart from these problems, initial randomization will not, as Chalmers recognizes, address disturbances of equipoise that occur in the course of a trial.

Data-monitoring committees have been proposed as a solution to problems arising in the course of the trial.[13] Such committees, operating independently of the investigators, are the only bodies with information concerning the trial's ongoing results. Since this knowledge is not available to the investigators, their equipoise is not disturbed. Although committees are useful in keeping the conduct of a trial free of bias, they cannot resolve the investigators' ethical difficulties. A clinician is not merely obliged to treat a patient on the basis of the information that he or she currently has, but is also required to discover information that would be relevant to treatment decisions. If interim results would disturb equipoise, the investigators are obliged to gather and use that information. Their

agreement to remain in ignorance of preliminary results would, by definition, be an unethical agreement, just as a failure to call up the laboratory to find out a patient's test results is unethical. Moreover, the use of a monitoring committee does not solve problems of equipoise that arise before and at the beginning of a trial.

Recognizing the broad problems with equipoise, three authors have proposed radical solutions. All three think that there is an irresolvable conflict between the requirement that a patient be offered the best treatment known (the principle underlying the requirement for equipoise) and the conduct of clinical trials; they therefore suggest that the "best treatment" requirement be weakened.

Schafer has argued that the concept of equipoise, and the associated notion of the best medical treatment, depends on the judgment of patients rather than of clinical investigators.[14] Although the equipoise of an investigator may be disturbed if he or she favors B over A, the ultimate choice of treatment is the patient's. Because the patient's values may restore equipoise, Schafer argues, it is ethical for the investigator to proceed with a trial when the patient consents. Schafer's strategy is directed toward trials that test treatments with known and divergent side effects and will probably not be useful in trials conducted to test efficacy or unknown side effects. This approach, moreover, confuses the ethics of competent medical practice with those of consent. If we assume that the investigator is a competent clinician, by saying that the investigator is out of equipoise, we have by Schafer's account said that in the investigator's professional judgment one treatment is therapeutically inferior — for that patient, in that condition, given the quality of life that can be achieved. Even if a patient would consent to an inferior treatment, it seems to me a violation of competent medical practice, and hence of ethics, to make the offer. Of course, complex issues may arise when a patient refuses what the physician considers the best treatment and demands instead an inferior treatment. Without settling that problem, however, we can reject Schafer's position. For Schafer claims that in order to continue to conduct clinical trials, it is ethical for the physician to offer (not merely accede to) inferior treatment.

Meier suggests that "most of us would be quite willing to forego a modest expected gain in the general interest of learning something of value."[15] He argues that we accept risks in everyday life to achieve a variety of benefits, including convenience and economy. In the same way, Meier states, it is acceptable to enroll subjects in clinical trials even though they may not receive the best treatment throughout the course of the trial. Schafer suggests an essentially similar approach.[5,14] According to this view, continued progress in medical knowledge through clinical trials requires an explicit abandonment of the doctor's fully patient-centered ethic.

These proposals seem to be frank counsels of desperation. They resolve the ethical problems of equi-

Vol. 317   No. 3   THE NEW ENGLAND JOURNAL OF MEDICINE   143

poise by abandoning the need for equipoise. In any event, would their approach allow clinical trials to be conducted? I think this may fairly be doubted. Although many people are presumably altruistic enough to forgo the best medical treatment in the interest of the progress of science, many are not. The numbers and proportions required to sustain the statistical validity of trial results suggest that in the absence of overwhelming altruism, the enrollment of satisfactory numbers of patients will not be possible. In particular, very ill patients, toward whom many of the most important clinical trials are directed, may be disinclined to be altruistic. Finally, as the study by Taylor et al.[12] reminds us, the problems of equipoise trouble investigators as well as patients. Even if patients are prepared to dispense with the best treatment, their physicians, for reasons of ethics and professionalism, may well not be willing to do so.

Marquis has suggested a third approach. "Perhaps what is needed is an ethics that will justify the conscription of subjects for medical research," he has written. "Nothing less seems to justify present practice."[4] Yet, although conscription might enable us to continue present practice, it would scarcely justify it. Moreover, the conscription of physician investigators, as well as subjects, would be necessary, because, as has been repeatedly argued, the problems of equipoise are as disturbing to clinicians as they are to subjects. Is any less radical and more plausible approach possible?

THEORETICAL EQUIPOISE VERSUS CLINICAL EQUIPOISE

The problems of equipoise examined above arise from a particular understanding of that concept, which I will term "theoretical equipoise." It is an understanding that is both conceptually odd and ethically irrelevant. Theoretical equipoise exists when, overall, the evidence on behalf of two alternative treatment regimens is exactly balanced. This evidence may be derived from a variety of sources, including data from the literature, uncontrolled experience, considerations of basic science and fundamental physiologic processes, and perhaps a "gut feeling" or "instinct" resulting from (or superimposed on) other considerations. The problems examined above arise from the principle that if theoretical equipoise is disturbed, the physician has, in Schafer's words, a "treatment preference" — let us say, favoring experimental treatment B. A trial testing A against B requires that some patients be enrolled in violation of this treatment preference.

Theoretical equipoise is overwhelmingly fragile; that is, it is disturbed by a slight accretion of evidence favoring one arm of the trial. In Chalmers' view, equipoise is disturbed when the odds that A will be more successful than B are anything other than 50 percent. It is therefore necessary to randomize treatment assignments beginning with the very first patient, lest equipoise be disturbed. We may say that theoretical equipoise is balanced on a knife's edge.

Theoretical equipoise is most appropriate to one-dimensional hypotheses and causes us to think in those terms. The null hypothesis must be sufficiently simple and "clean" to be finely balanced: Will A or B be superior in reducing mortality or shrinking tumors or lowering fevers in population P? Clinical choice is commonly more complex. The choice of A or B depends on some combination of effectiveness, consistency, minimal or relievable side effects, and other factors. On close examination, for example, it sometimes appears that even trials that purport to test a single hypothesis in fact involve a more complicated, portmanteau measure — e.g., the "therapeutic index" of A versus B. The formulation of the conditions of theoretical equipoise for such complex, multidimensional clinical hypotheses is tantamount to the formulation of a rigorous calculus of apples and oranges.

Theoretical equipoise is also highly sensitive to the vagaries of the investigator's attention and perception. Because of its fragility, theoretical equipoise is disturbed as soon as the investigator perceives a difference between the alternatives — whether or not any genuine difference exists. Prescott writes, for example, "It will be common at some stage in most trials for the survival curves to show visually different survivals," short of significance but "sufficient to raise ethical difficulties for the participants."[16] A visual difference, however, is purely an artifact of the research methods employed: when and by what means data are assembled and analyzed and what scale is adopted for the graphic presentation of data. Similarly, it is common for researchers to employ interval scales for phenomena that are recognized to be continuous by nature — e.g., five-point scales of pain or stages of tumor progression. These interval scales, which represent an arbitrary distortion of the available evidence to simplify research, may magnify the differences actually found, with a resulting disturbance of theoretical equipoise.

Finally, as described by several authors, theoretical equipoise is personal and idiosyncratic. It is disturbed when the clinician has, in Schafer's words, what "might even be labeled a bias or a hunch," a preference of a "merely intuitive nature."[14] The investigator who ignores such a hunch, by failing to advise the patient that because of it the investigator prefers B to A or by recommending A (or a chance of random assignment to A) to the patient, has violated the requirement for equipoise and its companion requirement to recommend the best medical treatment.

The problems with this concept of equipoise should be evident. To understand the alternative, preferable interpretation of equipoise, we need to recall the basic reason for conducting clinical trials: there is a current or imminent conflict in the clinical community over what treatment is preferred for patients in a defined population P. The standard treatment is A, but some evidence suggests that B will be superior (because of its effectiveness or its reduction of undesirable side effects, or for some other reason). (In the rare case when the first evidence of a novel therapy's superiority would be entirely convincing to the clinical community, equipoise is already disturbed.) Or there is a split in the clinical community, with some clinicians favoring A and others favoring B. Each side recognizes that the opposing side has evidence to support its position, yet each still thinks that overall its own view is correct. There exists (or, in the case of a novel therapy, there may soon exist) an honest, professional disagreement among expert clinicians about the preferred treatment. A clinical trial is instituted with the aim of resolving this dispute.

At this point, a state of "clinical equipoise" exists. There is no consensus within the expert clinical community about the comparative merits of the alternatives to be tested. We may state the formal conditions under which such a trial would be ethical as follows: at the start of the trial, there must be a state of clinical equipoise regarding the merits of the regimens to be tested, and the trial must be designed in such a way as to make it reasonable to expect that, if it is successfully concluded, clinical equipoise will be disturbed. In other words, the results of a successful clinical trial should be convincing enough to resolve the dispute among clinicians.

A state of clinical equipoise is consistent with a decided treatment preference on the part of the investigators. They must simply recognize that their less-favored treatment is preferred by colleagues whom they consider to be responsible and competent. Even if the interim results favor the preference of the investigators, treatment B, clinical equipoise persists as long as those results are too weak to influence the judgment of the community of clinicians, because of limited sample size, unresolved possibilities of side effects, or other factors. (This judgment can necessarily be made only by those who know the interim results — whether a data-monitoring committee or the investigators.)

At the point when the accumulated evidence in favor of B is so strong that the committee or investigators believe no open-minded clinician informed of the results would still favor A, clinical equipoise has been disturbed. This may occur well short of the original schedule for the termination of the trial, for unexpected reasons. (Therapeutic effects or side effects may be much stronger than anticipated, for example, or a definable subgroup within population P may be recognized for which the results demonstrably disturb clinical equipoise.) Because of the arbitrary character of human judgment and persuasion, some ethical problems regarding the termination of a trial will remain. Clinical equipoise will confine these problems to unusual or extreme cases, however, and will allow us to cast persistent problems in the proper terms. For example, in the face of a strong established trend, must we continue the trial because of others' blind fealty to an arbitrary statistical bench mark?

Clearly, clinical equipoise is a far weaker — and more common — condition than theoretical equipoise. Is it ethical to conduct a trial on the basis of clinical equipoise, when theoretical equipoise is disturbed?

Or, as Schafer and others have argued, is doing so a violation of the physician's obligation to provide patients with the best medical treatment?[4,5,14] Let us assume that the investigators have a decided preference for B but wish to conduct a trial on the grounds that clinical (not theoretical) equipoise exists. The ethics committee asks the investigators whether, if they or members of their families were within population P, they would not want to be treated with their preference, B? An affirmative answer is often thought to be fatal to the prospects for such a trial, yet the investigators answer in the affirmative. Would a trial satisfying this weaker form of equipoise be ethical?

I believe that it clearly is ethical. As Fried has emphasized,[3] competent (hence, ethical) medicine is social rather than individual in nature. Progress in medicine relies on progressive consensus within the medical and research communities. The ethics of medical practice grants no ethical or normative meaning to a treatment preference, however powerful, that is based on a hunch or on anything less than evidence publicly presented and convincing to the clinical community. Persons are licensed as physicians after they demonstrate the acquisition of this professionally validated knowledge, not after they reveal a superior capacity for guessing. Normative judgments of their behavior — e.g., malpractice actions — rely on a comparison with what is done by the community of medical practitioners. Failure to follow a "treatment preference" not shared by this community and not based on information that would convince it could not be the basis for an allegation of legal or ethical malpractice. As Fried states: "[T]he conception of what is good medicine is the product of a professional consensus." By definition, in a state of clinical equipoise, "good medicine" finds the choice between A and B indifferent.

In contrast to theoretical equipoise, clinical equipoise is robust. The ethical difficulties at the beginning and end of a trial are therefore largely alleviated. There remain difficulties about consent, but these too may be diminished. Instead of emphasizing the lack of evidence favoring one arm over another that is required by theoretical equipoise, clinical equipoise places the emphasis in informing the patient on the honest disagreement among expert clinicians. The fact that the investigator has a "treatment preference," if he or she does, could be disclosed; indeed, if the preference is a decided one, and based on something more than a hunch, it could be ethically mandatory to disclose it. At the same time, it would be emphasized that this preference is not shared by others. It is likely to be a matter of chance that the patient is being seen by a clinician with a preference for B over A, rather than by an equally competent clinician with the opposite preference.

Clinical equipoise does not depend on concealing relevant information from researchers and subjects, as does the use of independent data-monitoring commit-

Vol. 317 No. 3 THE NEW ENGLAND JOURNAL OF MEDICINE 145

tees. Rather, it allows investigators, in informing subjects, to distinguish appropriately among validated knowledge accepted by the clinical community, data on treatments that are promising but are not (or, for novel therapies, would not be) generally convincing, and mere hunches. Should informed patients decline to participate because they have chosen a specific clinician and trust his or her judgment — over and above the consensus in the professional community — that is no more than the patients' right. We do not conscript patients to serve as subjects in clinical trials.

THE IMPLICATIONS OF CLINICAL EQUIPOISE

The theory of clinical equipoise has been formulated as an alternative to some current views on the ethics of human research. At the same time, it corresponds closely to a preanalytic concept held by many in the research and regulatory communities. Clinical equipoise serves, then, as a rational formulation of the approach of many toward research ethics; it does not so much change things as explain why they are the way they are.

Nevertheless, the precision afforded by the theory of clinical equipoise does help to clarify or reformulate some aspects of research ethics; I will mention only two.

First, there is a recurrent debate about the ethical propriety of conducting clinical trials of discredited treatments, such as Laetrile.[17] Often, substantial political pressure to conduct such tests is brought to bear by adherents of quack therapies. The theory of clinical equipoise suggests that when there is no support for a treatment regimen within the expert clinical community, the first ethical requirement of a trial — clinical equipoise — is lacking; it would therefore be unethical to conduct such a trial.

Second, Feinstein has criticized the tendency of clinical investigators to narrow excessively the conditions and hypotheses of a trial in order to ensure the validity of its results.[18] This "fastidious" approach purchases scientific manageability at the expense of an inability to apply the results to the "messy" conditions of clinical practice. The theory of clinical equipoise adds some strength to this criticism. Overly "fastidious" trials, designed to resolve some theoretical question, fail to satisfy the second ethical requirement of clinical research, since the special conditions of the trial will render it useless for influencing clinical decisions, even if it is successfully completed.

The most important result of the concept of clinical equipoise, however, might be to relieve the current crisis of confidence in the ethics of clinical trials. Equipoise, properly understood, remains an ethical condition for clinical trials. It is consistent with much current practice. Clinicians and philosophers alike have been premature in calling for desperate measures to resolve problems of equipoise.

I am indebted to Robert J. Levine, M.D., and to Harold Merskey, D.M., for their valuable suggestions.

REFERENCES

1. Levine RJ. Ethics and regulation of clinical research. 2nd ed. Baltimore. Urban & Schwarzenberg, 1986.
2. *Idem*. The use of placebos in randomized clinical trials. IRB: Rev Hum Subj Res 1985; 7(2):1-4.
3. Fried C. Medical experimentation: personal integrity and social policy. Amsterdam: North-Holland Publishing, 1974.
4. Marquis D. Leaving therapy to chance. Hastings Cent Rep 1983; 13(4):40-7.
5. Schafer A. The ethics of the randomized clinical trial. N Engl J Med 1982; 307:719-24.
6. Shaw LW, Chalmers TC. Ethics in cooperative clinical trials. Ann NY Acad Sci 1970; 169:487-95.
7. Hollenberg NK, Dzau VJ, Williams GH. Are uncontrolled clinical studies ever justified? N Engl J Med 1980; 303:1067:
8. Levine RJ, Lebacqz K. Some ethical considerations in clinical trials. Clin Pharmacol Ther 1979; 25:728-41.
9. Klimt CR, Canner PL. Terminating a long-term clinical trial. Clin Pharmacol Ther 1979; 25:641-6.
10. Veatch RM. Longitudinal studies, sequential designs and grant renewals: what to do with preliminary data. IRB: Rev Hum Subj Res 1979; 1(4):1-3.
11. Chalmers T. The ethics of randomization as a decision-making technique and the problem of informed consent. In: Beauchamp TL, Walters L, eds. Contemporary issues in bioethics. Encino, Calif.: Dickenson, 1978:426-9.
12. Taylor KM, Margolese RG. Soskolne CL. Physicians' reasons for not entering eligible patients in a randomized clinical trial of surgery for breast cancer. N Engl J Med 1984; 310:1363-7.
13. Chalmers TC. Invited remarks. Clin Pharmacol Ther 1979; 25:649-50.
14. Schafer A. The randomized clinical trial: for whose benefit? IRB: Rev Hum Subj Res 1985; 7(2):4-6.
15. Meier P. Terminating a trial — the ethical problem. Clin Pharmacol Ther 1979; 25:633-40.
16. Prescott RJ. Feedback of data to participants during clinical trials. In: Tagnon HJ, Staquet MJ, eds. Controversies in cancer: design of trials and treatment. New York: Masson Publishing, 1979:55-61
17. Cowan DH. The ethics of clinical trials of ineffective therapy. IRB: Rev Hum Subj Res 1981; 3(5):10-1.
18. Feinstein AR. An additional basic science for clinical medicine. II. The limitations of randomized trials. Ann Intern Med 1983; 99:544-50.

[27]

Xenotransplantation and Speciesism

P. Singer

PROLOGUE

IN The Netherlands a few years ago, an observer reported on the lives of some people confined in a new kind of institution. These people were not at all impaired physically, but intellectually they were well below the normal human level; they could not speak, although they made noises and gestures. In standard institutions, they had tended to spend much of their time making repetitive movements, and rocking their bodies to and fro. This institution was an unusual one, in that its policy was to allow the inmates the maximum possible freedom to live their own lives and form their own community. This freedom extended even to sexual relationships, which led to pregnancy, birth, and child rearing.

The observer's report was long and detailed, and I can only give you a few relevant highlights. First, the behavior of the inmates under these circumstances was far more varied than in the more conventional institutional settings. They rarely spent time alone, and they appeared to have no difficulty in understanding each other's gestures and grunts. They were physically active, spending a lot of time outside, where they had access to about two acres of relatively natural forest, surrounded by a wall. They cooperated in many of these activities, including on one occasion—to the consternation of the supervisors—an attempt to escape that involved carrying a large fallen branch to one of the walls, and propping it up as a kind of ladder that made it possible to climb over the wall.

The observer was particularly interested in what he called the "politics" of the community. A defined leader soon emerged. His leadership—and it was always a "he"—depended, however, on the support of other members of the group. The leader had privileges, but also, it seemed, obligations. He had to cultivate the favor of others by sharing food and other treats. Fights would develop from time to time, but they would usually be followed by some conciliatory gestures, so that the loser could be readmitted into the society of the leader. If the leader became isolated, and allowed the others to form a coalition against him, his days as leader were numbered.

A simple ethical code could also be detected within the community. Its two basic rules, the observer commented, could be summed up as "one good turn deserves another," and "an eye for an eye and a tooth for a tooth." The breach of one of these rules apparently led to a sense of being wronged. For example when N was fighting with L, P came to L's assistance. Later, N attacked P, who gestured to L for assistance, but L did nothing. After the fight between P and N was over, N then furiously attacked L.

The mothers were with one exception competent at nursing and rearing their children. The mother-child relationships were close, and lasted many years. The death of a baby led to prolonged grieving behavior. Because sexual relationships were not monogamous, it was not always possible to tell who the father of the child was, and in fact fathers did not play a significant role in the rearing of the children.

In view of the very limited mental capacities that these inmates had been considered to possess, the observer was impressed by instances of behavior that clearly showed planning, and a high degree of self-awareness. In one example, two young mothers were having difficulty in stopping their small children from fighting. An older mother, a considerable authority figure in the community, was dozing nearby. One of the younger mothers woke her, and pointed to the squabbling children. The older mother made the appropriate noises and gestures, and the children, suitably intimidated, stopped fighting. The older mother then went back to her nap. On another occasion, after a fight, it was noticeable that the loser limped badly when in the presence of the victor, but not when alone; presumably by pretending to be more seriously hurt than he really was, he hoped for some kind of sympathy, or at least mercy, from his conqueror. A good deal of deceit also focused around sexual relationships, and to observers of human nature, this will come as no surprise. Although, as already mentioned, sexual relationships were not monogamous, there were occasions on which flirtations, leading up to sexual intercourse, were conducted with a good deal of discretion, so as not to attract the notice of a leader who would have been likely to claim exclusive sexual rights over one of his favorites.

In order to see just how far ahead these people could think, the observer devised an ingenious test of problem-solving ability. One inmate was presented with two series of five locked clear plastic boxes, each of which opened with a different key. One series of five boxes led to a food treat, whereas the other series led to an empty box. It was necessary to begin by choosing one of the two boxes that were the first in each series; and to succeed, one had to work through the five boxes to see which initial choice would lead one to the box with the treat. The inmate was able to succeed in this complex task.

Now I would like you to consider a proposal. Suppose

From the Centre for Human Bioethics, Clayton, Melbourne, Victoria 3168, Australia.

Address reprint requests to Peter Singer, Centre for Human Bioethics, Clayton, Melbourne, Victoria 3168, Australia.

that in view of the scarcity of organs for medical purposes, it was proposed to select some members of the community I have just described, give them an anesthetic, and then remove their hearts for transplantation into human beings whose mental capacities were normal, but who were suffering from a diseased heart and could only survive with a transplant. What would you think of such a proposal?

My guess is that your reaction to this proposal might vary according to the mental image you formed of the inmates of the community just described. I referred to them as "people," and I believe that the use of this term is justifiable, in view of the long philosophical tradition that, since at least the 17th century British philosopher John Locke, has been prepared to apply the term "person" to a rational and self-conscious being, irrespective of whether that being was a member of our own species. If, however, you were led by my use of that term to assume that the people I have described were human beings suffering from some intellectual disability, you will probably have been shocked at the suggestion that we consider killing them in order to make use of their hearts. But in fact the description was not one of human beings, but of chimpanzees, living in the Amsterdam Zoo.[1] If you were able to guess this, you may not have been so shocked by the proposal. But why not? Should we be any less disturbed by the proposal, now that we know that it is not members of our own species who will be killed? That is the question I shall explore.

The exploration is in two parts. I begin with a summary statement of the principles of animal liberation, as I understand them. I shall then turn to the specific issue of the use of animals as organ donors.

ANIMALS AND ETHICS

Animal liberation is a new movement, dating back to the mid-1970s, and growing out of the same period of ferment that gave rise to feminism and modern green politics. Until that time, though there were many animal welfare groups and anticruelty societies, they were built on the assumption that the welfare of nonhuman animals deserves protection *only* when *our* interests are not at stake. Animals remained "lower creatures." Human beings were seen as quite distinct from, and infinitely superior to, all forms of animal life. If our interests conflict with theirs, it is always their interests that have to give way.

Animal liberationists question the right of our species to assume that *our* interests must always prevail. They want to extend the basic moral ideas of equality and rights—which we apply to all *human* beings—to animals as well.

At first this sounds crazy. Obviously animals cannot have equal rights to vote, or to free speech. But the kind of equality that animal liberationists wish to extend to animals is a special kind: *equal consideration of interests*. And the basic right that animals should have is the right to equal consideration. This sounds like a difficult idea, but essentially it means that if an animal feels pain, the pain

matters as much as it does when a human feels pain—if the pains hurt just as much. *Pain is pain*, whatever the species of being that experiences it.

Many people make a sharp distinction between humans and other animals. They say that all human beings are infinitely more valuable than any animals of any other species. But they don't give reasons for this view. When you think about it, it is not difficult to see that there is no morally important feature which *all* human beings possess, and *no* nonhuman animals have.

To a dispassionate Martian, it would be amusing to see how determinedly the human species, or more specifically the Western element of that species, has tried to distance itself from the other species with which it shares the planet. Only humans, we used to say, are made in the image of God, and only humans have an immortal soul. When it became apparent that those ideas lacked any basis in reason or science, we switched to saying things like: "Only humans can use tools." Then we found that chimpanzees use sticks for digging out insects, some seals will use rocks in order to break open shellfish, and various birds use thorns or small sticks to probe insects out of bark. So we said: "Only humans *make* tools." Then we discovered that chimpanzees do shape their sticks, by stripping off leaves and small branches until they get the right kind of implement for the task. So we switched ground and said: "Only humans use language"—just before several studies proved that chimpanzees and gorillas could learn hundreds of signs in the sign language used by the deaf, and could communicate in quite complex ways. Of course, we then upped the requirements for what it was to use language. . . and so the story goes.

But all of these attempts at drawing lines are really quite irrelevant to the question of justifying the things we do to animals. After all, even if no animals could use tools, or communicate by means of signs or words, we could not use these abilities to draw a line between *all* humans and the nonhuman animals. For there are many humans, too, who cannot use tools and have no language. All humans under 3 months of age, for a start. And even if they are excluded, on the grounds that they have the potential to learn to use tools and to speak, there are other human beings who do not have this potential. Sadly, some humans are born with brain damage so severe that they will never be able to use a tool or learn any form of language.

If it would be absurd to give animals the right to vote, it would be no less absurd to give that right to infants or to severely retarded human beings. Yet we still give equal consideration to their interests. We don't raise them for food, or test new cosmetics in their eyes. Nor should we. But we do these things to nonhuman animals who show greater abilities in using tools, or learning language, or doing any of the other things that use those capacities of reason that we like to believe distinguish humans from animals.

Once we understand this, it is easy to see the belief that all humans are somehow infinitely more valuable than any animal for what it is: a prejudice. Sadly, such prejudices are not unusual. Racists have a similar prejudice in favor of their own race, and sexists have the same type of prejudice in favor of their own sex.

Speciesism is logically parallel to racism and sexism. Speciesists, racists, and sexists all say: the boundary of my own group is also the boundary of my concern. Never mind what you are like, if you are a member of my group, you are superior to all those who are not members of my group. The speciesist favors a larger group than the racist, and so has a large circle of concern; but all of these prejudices are equally wrong. They all use an arbitrary and morally irrelevant fact—membership of a race, sex, or species—as if it were morally crucial.

The only acceptable limit to our moral concern is the point at which there is no awareness of pain or pleasure, and no preferences of any kind. That is why pigs have rights, but lettuces don't. Pigs can feel pain, and pleasure. Lettuces can't.

Until now the human species, especially so-called "Western civilization," has regarded our planet as a resource to be plundered for its own immediate benefit. The animal liberation movement, together with much of the environment movement, is seeking to change this attitude; to get us to see that we share the planet with other species, and that we have no God-given right to exploit them for our benefit. The change is a fundamental one, and one that threatens all the major economic forces in our society. It will not be brought about quickly or easily. But the effects of change are already visible, and the movement is growing. It rests on an argument that is so simple, and so plainly sound, that it can only continue to spread.

ANIMALS AND ORGAN DONATION

The idea of using animals as a source for organ donation is an example of speciesism, premised as it is on the idea that animals are things for us to use as best suits our own interests, without much concern for the interests of the animals themselves. Perhaps the easiest way to see this is to ask yourself the following question: why should we be prepared to accept the use of organs from animals, but not be prepared to take them from human infants who are, and always will be, less intellectually developed than the nonhuman animals?

The human infants I have in mind fall into two categories. First, there are the anencephalics—those born with no brain, other than perhaps some brain stem. Next are the cortically dead—infants who, perhaps as a result of a brain hemorrhage soon after birth, have irreversibly lost all function in their cortex. At a recent conference at Melbourne's Royal Children's Hospital, I heard a pediatrician tell of a time when, in the hospital's intensive care ward, he had two young patients. One was healthy in every respect except one—an irreparable and lethal heart defect. The only possible treatment was a heart transplant, but no suitable donor was available, nor likely to become avail-

able. (In Australia, with a population of only 16 million, it is very rare to be able to find a suitable donor for an infant with a heart defect.) The other infant in the ward had suffered a massive brain hemorrhage and was cortically dead. The thought crossed the mind of the pediatrician, that if he could take the heart from the cortically dead baby, he could save the other one, and at least one of his patients would survive. He thought that if he asked the parents, they might see this as a way of salvaging some good out of the tragedy that had befallen their baby. But he knew that he could not do this; though a cortically dead baby can never become conscious, it is not legally dead, and to cut out its heart is, under present law, clearly murder. So the pediatrician could see that the inevitable result was going to be that both babies would die; and that is indeed what happened.

What kind of ethic can tell us that it is all right to rear sentient animals in barren cages that give them no decent life at all, and then kill them to take their organs, while refusing to permit us to take the organ of a human being who is not, and never can be, even minimally conscious? Obviously, a speciesist ethic. And that is essentially what is wrong with the present situation. My objection is not that we value the life of a normal, self-aware human being, one with a vivid awareness of the future and a desire to continue to be around next week, next month and next year, ahead of the life of an animal who lacks self-awareness and is incapable of any such future-oriented desires. Such an evaluation can be defended, without invoking an arbitrary preference for our own species. My objection is to the fact that we disregard the interests of nonhuman animals by ranking them as less worthy of our concern and respect than *any* member of our own species, no matter how limited in capacities and potential.

I therefore suggest that, before you endorse or accept the use of animals as organ sources, you ask yourself whether you are prepared to endorse or accept the use of anencephalic and cortically dead human infants. I know that there are some who do endorse this, or at least some part of it. Arthur Caplan, for instance, has persuasively argued in favor of the use of organs from fetuses and anencephalic infants.[2] He does not extend his argument to cortically dead infants. I am not sure why; perhaps he is troubled by the difficulty of establishing that cortical death really has occurred, and I know that there is still room for debate on this topic. That may be a reason for not implementing the proposal to use organs from the cortically dead until further careful study of current methods of diagnosing this state, but such obstacles have never deterred philosophers from considering the issues in a hypothetical manner, on the assumption that the technical difficulties can be overcome.

Another reason for reluctance to use cortically dead infants, even if there are no doubts about diagnosis, is that, while the cortex may be dead, the infants are, by any normal definition of the term, not dead. They are warm, pink, they breathe, sometimes unaided, they respond to touch, and so on. Of course, those who are legally brain dead satisfy many of these criteria too, although they do not breathe without assistance. But cortical death is not brain death, and I am not proposing that a cortically dead infant should be thought of, legally, ethically, or in any other sense, as a dead human being. After all, when we take a heart from a baboon, it is a warm, pink (underneath the fur) breathing animal we are killing in order to remove the heart. So if we are prepared to kill a baboon in an attempt to save the life of a human being, why aren't we prepared to kill a human being, with no potential that comes even near to equalling that of the baboon, for the same purpose?

I can think of only two ways in which someone might try to defend the view that it is better to kill the baboon than the cortically dead infant. One is that the parents of the infant may be upset by what happens to their infant in a way that the parents of the baboon will not be. Now we should not ignore the fact that baboons are mammals, and baboon mothers may and probably do suffer considerably when their infants are taken from them. But even if we overlook this fact, it remains the case that often—as in the case I mentioned—the human parents of the cortically dead infant would welcome the opportunity for some good to emerge from the death of their child. We know that this feeling has been expressed by the parents of anencephalic infants, when the possibility of the infant becoming a donor was raised.[3] So this objection does not apply to all cases in which the organs of a cortically dead infant might be used to save a life.

The second way of defending the view that it is better to kill the baboon than the cortically dead infant is by a frank defense of speciesism. This has been attempted by some of my recent critics—among them, Jeffrey Gray, Head of the Department of Psychology at the Institute of Psychiatry, University of London.[4-6] Gray's defense of speciesism is, in essence, that just as we properly give preference to our own children over the children of strangers, so we may properly give preference to the interests of members of our own species over the interests of members of other species. In passing, I note that Gray and others who use this kind of argument do not, for obvious reasons, make use of an intermediate step that, in other times and places, would surely have been seized on as further evidence of the case in favor of speciesism. Some of us can easily imagine our forefathers saying, just a generation or two ago: "Just as we properly give preference to the interests of members of our own race over the interests of members of other races. . ."

I agree, naturally, that parents are likely to prefer the interests of their own children to those of strangers. No doubt this preference has a biological basis. I also agree that it can be morally justifiable, under certain circumstances. Similarly, humans are likely to prefer the interests of members of their own species to those of members of other species. Maybe this too has a biological basis. But so

what? The question is not why this preference exists, but whether this preference is justifiable.

The preference for the interests of our children can be defended on the grounds that, in recognizing the special duty of parents to look after their interests, we are promoting the greater overall welfare of children. Children thrive best in a family environment—not in large institutions, looked after by impersonal bureaucrats. Thus our support for the idea that parents should look after their own children before they look after the children of strangers works for the good of children as a whole. If we look at the fate of animals today, whether in the wild, in laboratories, or in factory farms, we cannot think that putting the interests of members of our own species ahead of the interests of members of other species works out better for all sentient beings. This naked bias in favor of our own is simply a reflection of our power over the other animals and our lack of consideration of their interests.

So the second defense of our preference for killing a baboon rather than a cortically dead infant in order to obtain a heart is no more successful than the first. I conclude that this preference is indefensible. That does not, of course, prove that it is always wrong to kill a baboon in order to obtain a heart with which one can save a human life. It might be that it is justifiable to kill both cortically dead infants *and* baboons in order to do this, or it might be that it is justifiable to kill neither, or it might be that it is justifiable to kill cortically dead infants but *not* to kill baboons. How we answer these questions, now, might also depend on the prospects of success of the transplant in each case. But if we imagine that the transplants had a very high chance of saving a life in each case, and we assume also that the parents of the infant have freely consented to the donation of the heart, then my own preference would certainly be to use the cortically dead infant before using the baboon, and I would base this preference on the higher level of awareness of the baboon.

There is, however, a more difficult question for me to answer. Suppose that we need a heart for a child who is, apart from the heart defect, healthy and much loved by her parents. Suppose that there are no anencephalic or cortically dead infant hearts available. Suppose it is a question of killing a baboon and taking her heart, or allowing the child to die? What do I say then?

Before I answer, one observation. A society that accepts the rearing of pigs in miserable conditions in intensive farms, and then allows them to be killed just because some people prefer pork to tofu, would be very odd indeed if it did not accept imposing similar suffering and death on baboons in order to save the life of a human being. That is why I have spent so much of this talk trying to put the issue of xenotransplantation in the context of a nonspeciesist ethic, one that takes seriously the interests of nonhuman animals. If anyone thinks that it is wrong to attempt to use the body parts of animals for transplantation purposes, but alright to use them for breakfast, then their way of thinking has nothing in common with mine.

Now what do I say about the case of the child or the baboon? I find it genuinely difficult. As I have already suggested, it is not speciesist to prefer the life of a being who is self-aware, and sees herself as existing over time, and who is capable of having complex future desires, to the life of a being who lacks these capacities. And it may be that a child does have these capacities and a baboon does not have them, or does not have them to nearly as high a degree. It *may* also be true that the family of the child will suffer more intensely and for a longer period if she dies than any of the baboon's family group will suffer if it dies. So considering the hypothetical choice from this perspective alone, it seems defensible to kill the baboon to save the child. At the same time, choosing the child over the baboon reinforces the attitude that animals are just things for us to use—and this is an attitude that we should strive to change. That is one reason why I do not want to see us come to rely on organs from animals as a cheap way of overcoming our health problems. Another reason is that, while in the example just given I have compared simply the death of the child with the death of a baboon, in the real world we can expect that, once organs from baboons become suitable for use in humans, there will be large colonies of baboons kept in whatever conditions can most economically be devised, as long as they are compatible with keeping the baboons alive and their organs usable. Finally, let us remember that, if we are prepared to use a baboon as a source of organs, we should be prepared to use a human of equal or inferior capacities, as long as there is no family who has greater ties to the human than the family of the baboon has to the baboon.

In a world that needlessly rears several billion animals in factory farms each year and then kills them to satisfy a mere preference of taste, it is difficult to argue persuasively against the rearing and slaughter of a few thousand animals so that their organs can be used to save people's lives. That, however, is not a reason for using animals; it is, rather, a reason for changing our views about animals. In a better world, a world that cared properly for the interests of animals, we would do our utmost to avoid choices that pit the essential interests of animals against our own, so that the issue of "the child or the baboon" does not arise. This might involve more effective ways of obtaining organs from humans who are brain dead, or cortically dead. It might involve the development of artificial organs. Or it might involve using our limited medical resources to educate people in looking after the organs with which they were born. These are ethically preferable paths to pursue.

I shall end with a quotation from Isaac Bashevis Singer, one of the great writers of our time. The passage epitomizes what is wrong with the attitude to other animals that allows us to think of them as just so much beef, or bacon—or a reservoir of hearts and kidneys:

As often as Herman had witnessed the slaughter of animals and fish, he always had the same thought: in their behavior toward creatures, all men were Nazis. The smugness with which man could do with other species as he pleased exemplified the most extreme racist theories, the principle that might is right.[7]

REFERENCES

1. de Waal F: Chimpanzee Politics. London: Jonathan Cape, 1982

2. Caplan A: Bioethics 1:119, 1987

3. Caplan A: Bioethics 1:128, 1987

4. Gray JA: Behav Brain Sci 13:22, 1990

5. Gray JA: Behav Brain Sci 14:759, 1991

6. Gray JA: Psychologist 4:196, 1991

7. Singer IB: Enemies, a Love Story. New York: Farrar, Straus, & Giroux, 1972

[28]

Bioethics ISSN 0269-9702
Volume 7 Number 2/3 1993

IS GENE THERAPY A FORM OF EUGENICS?

JOHN HARRIS

Eugenic A. *adj.* Pertaining or adapted to the production of
fine offspring. B. *sh.* in *pl.* The science which treats of this.
(*The Shorter Oxford English Dictionary* Third Edition 1965).

It has now become a serious necessity to better the breed of
the human race. The average citizen is too base for the
everyday work of modern civilization. Civilised man has
become possessed of vaster powers than in old times for
good or ill but has made no corresponding advance in wits
and goodness to enable him to conduct his conduct rightly.
(Sir Francis Galton)

If, as I believe, gene therapy is in principle ethically sound except
for its possible connection with eugenics then there are two obvious
ways of giving a simple and straightforward answer to a question
such as this. The first is to say "yes it is, and so what?" The second
is to say "no it isn't so we shouldn't worry". If we accept the first
of the above definitions we might well be inclined to give the first
of our two answers. If on the other hand, we accept the sort of gloss
that Ruth Chadwick gives on Galton's account, "those who are
genetically weak should simply be discouraged from reproducing",
either by incentives or compulsory measures, we get a somewhat
different flavour, and one which might incline a decent person who
favours gene therapy towards the second answer.

The nub of the problem turns on how we are to understand the
objective of producing "fine children". Does "fine" mean "as fine
as children normally are", or does it mean "as fine as a child can
be"? Sorting out the ethics of the connection between gene therapy
and eugenics seems to involve the resolution of two morally significant
issues. The first is whether or not there is a relevant moral distinction between attempts to remove or repair dysfunction on the one
hand and measures designed to enhance function on the other, such
that it would be coherent to be in favour of curing dysfunction but

IS GENE THERAPY A FORM OF EUGENICS?   179

against enhancing function? The second involves the question of whether gene therapy as a technique involves something specially morally problematic.

THE MORAL CONTINUUM

Is it morally wrong to wish and hope for a fine baby girl or boy? Is it wrong to wish and hope that one's child will not be born disabled? I assume that my feeling that such hopes and wishes are not wrong is shared by every sane decent person. Now consider whether it would be wrong to wish and hope for the reverse? What would we think of someone who hoped and wished that their child would be born with disability? Again I need not spell out the answer to these questions.

But now let's bridge the gap between thought and action, between hopes and wishes and their fulfilment. What would we think of someone who, hoping and wishing for a fine healthy child, declined to take the steps necessary to secure this outcome when such steps were open to them?

Again I assume that unless those steps could be shown to be morally unacceptable our conclusions would be the same.

Consider the normal practice at I.V.F. clinics where a woman who has had say, five eggs fertilised *in vitro*, wishes to use some of these embryos to become pregnant. Normal practice would be to insert two embryos or at most three. If pre-implantation screening had revealed two of the embryos to possess disabilities of one sort or another, would it be right to implant the two embryos with disability rather than the others? Would it be right to choose the implantation embryos randomly? Could it be defensible for a doctor to override the wishes of the mother and implant the disabled embryos rather than the healthy ones – would we applaud her for so doing?[1]

The answer that I expect to all these rhetorical questions will be obvious. It depends however on accepting that disability is somehow disabling and therefore undesirable. If it were not, there would be no motive to try to cure or obviate disability in health care more generally. If we believe that medical science should try to cure disability where possible, and that parents would be wrong to withhold from their disabled children cures as they become available, then we will be likely to agree on our answers to the rhetorical questions posed.

[1] The argument here follows that of my paper "Should We Attempt to Eradicate Disability" to be published in the Proceedings of the Fifteenth International Wittgenstein Symposium.

180 JOHN HARRIS

WHAT IS DISABILITY?

It is notoriously hard to give a satisfactory definition of disability although I believe we all know pretty clearly what we mean by it. A disability is surely a physical or mental condition we have a strong rational preference not to be in, it is, more importantly, a condition which is in some sense a 'harmed condition'.[2] I have in mind the sort of condition in which if a patient presented with it unconscious in the casualty department of a hospital and the condition could be easily and immediately reversed, but not reversed unless the doctor acts without delay, a doctor would be negligent were she not to attempt reversal. Or, one which, if a pregnant mother knew that it affected her fetus and knew also she could remove the condition by simple dietary adjustment, then to fail to do so would be to knowingly harm her child.[3]

To make clearer what's at issue here let's imagine that as a result of industrial effluent someone had contracted a condition that she felt had disabled or harmed her in some sense. How might she convince a court say, that she had suffered disability or injury?

The answer is obvious but necessarily vague. Whatever it would be plausible to say in answer to such a question is what I mean (and what is clearly meant) by disability and injury. It is not possible to stipulate exhaustively what would strike us as plausible here, but we know what injury is and we know what disability or incapacity is. If the condition in question was one which set premature limits on their lifespan – made their life shorter than it would be with treatment, or was one which rendered her specially vulnerable to infection, more vulnerable than others, we would surely recognise that she had been harmed and perhaps to some extent disabled. At the very least such events would be plausible candidates for the description "injuries" or "disabilities".

Against a background in which many people are standardly protected from birth or before against pollution hazards and infections and have their healthy life expectancy extended, it would surely be plausible to claim that failure to protect in this way constituted an injury and left them disabled. Because of their vulnerability to infection and to environmental pollutants there would be places it was unsafe for them to go and people with whom they could not freely consort. These restrictions on liberty are surely at least *prima facie* disabling as is the increased relative vulnerability.

---

[2] See my discussion of the difference between harming and wronging in my *Wonderwoman & Superman: The Ethics of Human Biotechnology*. Oxford, 1992. Chapter 4.

[3] This goes for relatively minor conditions like the loss of a finger or deafness and also for disfiguring conditions right through to major disability like paraplegia.

IS GENE THERAPY A FORM OF EUGENICS? 181

These points are crucial because it is sometimes said that while we have an obligation to cure disease – to restore normal functioning – we do not have an obligation to enhance or improve upon a normal healthy life, that enhancing function is permissive but could not be regarded as obligatory. But, what constitutes a normal healthy life, is determined in part by technological and medical and other advances (hygiene, sanitation etc.) It is normal now for example to be protected against tetanus, the continued provision of such protection is not merely permissive. If the AIDS pandemic continues unabated and the only prospect, or the best prospect, for stemming it's advance is the use of gene therapy to insert genes coding for antibodies to AIDS, I cannot think that it would be coherent to regard making available such therapy as permissive rather than mandatory.[4]

If this seems still too like normal therapy to be convincing, suppose genes coding for repair enzymes which would not only repair radiation damage or damage by other environmental pollutants but would also prolong healthy life expectancy could be inserted into humans. Again, would it be permissible to let people continue suffering such damage when they could be protected against it? Would it in short be O.K. to let them suffer?

It is not normal for the human organism to be self-repairing in this way, this must be eugenic if anything is. But if available, its use would surely, like penicillin before it, be more than merely permissive.

Of course, there will be unclarity at the margins but at least this conception of disability captures and emphasises the central notion that a disability is disabling in some sense, that it is a harm to those who suffer, it, and that to knowingly disable another individual or leave them disabled when we could remove the disability is to harm that individual.[5]

This is not an exhaustive definition of disability but it is a way of thinking about it which avoids certain obvious pitfalls. First it does not define disability in terms of any conception or normalcy. Secondly it does not depend on *post hoc* ratification by the subject of the condition – it is not a prediction about how the subject of the condition will feel. This is important because we need an account of disability we can use for the potentially self-conscious; gametes, embryos, fetuses and neonates and for the temporarily unconscious, which does not wait upon subsequent ratification by the person concerned.

---

[4] In this sense the definition of disability is like that of "poverty".

[5] See my more detailed account of the relationship between harming and wronging in my *Wonderwoman & Superman* Oxford University Press, Oxford 1992 Chapter 4.

182 JOHN HARRIS

With this account in mind we can extract the sting from at least one dimension of the charge that attempts to produce fine healthy children might be wrongful. Two related sorts of wrongfulness are often alleged here. One comes from some people and groups of people with disability or from their advocates. The second comes from those who are inclined to label such measures as attempts at eugenic control.

It is often said by those with disability or by their supporters[6] that abortion for disability, or failure to keep disabled infants alive as long as possible, or even positive infanticide for disabled neonates, constitutes discrimination against the disabled as a group, that it is tantamount to devaluing them as persons, to devaluing them in some existential sense. Alison Davis identifies this view with utilitarianism and comments further that "(i)t would also justify using me as a donor bank for someone more physically perfect (I am confined to a wheel-chair due to spina bifida) and, depending on our view of relative worth, it would justify using any of us as a donor if someone of the status of Einstein or Beethoven, or even Bob Geldof, needed one of our organs to survive".[7] This is a possible version of utilitarian-ism of course, but not I believe one espoused by anyone today. On the view assumed here and which I have defended in detail elsewhere,[8] all persons share the same moral status whether disabled or not. To decide not to keep a disabled neonate alive no more con-stitutes an attack on the disabled than does curing disability. To set the badly broken legs of an unconscious casualty who cannot consent does not constitute an attack on those confined to wheelchairs. To prefer to remove disability where we can is not to prefer non-disabled individuals as persons. To reiterate, if a pregnant mother can take steps to cure a disability affecting her fetus she should certainly do so, for to fail to do so is to deliberately handicap her child. She is not saying that she prefers those without disability as persons when she says she would prefer not to have a disabled child.

The same is analogously true of charges of eugenics in related circumstances. The wrong of practising eugenics is that it involves the assumption that "those who are genetically weak should be discouraged from reproducing" or are less morally important than other persons and that compulsory measures to prevent them repro-ducing might be defensible.

---

[6] Who should of course include us all.

[7] Davis 1988. p. 150.

[8] See my *The Value of Life*, Routledge, London 1985 & 1990 Ch.1 and my "Not all babies should be kept alive as long as possible" in Raanan Gillon and Anne Lloyd Eds. *Principles of Health Care Ethics*, John Wiley & Sons, Chichester, in press, publication 1993.

IS GENE THERAPY A FORM OF EUGENICS? 183

It is not that the genetically weak should be discouraged from reproducing but that everyone should be discouraged from reproducing children who will be significantly harmed by their genetic constitution.[9]

Indeed, gene therapy offers the prospect of enabling the genetically weak to reproduce and give birth to the genetically strong. It is to this prospect and to possible objections to it that we must now turn.

In so far as gene therapy might be used to delete specific genetic disorders in individuals or repair damage that had occurred genetically or in any other way it seems straightforwardly analogous to any other sort of therapy and to fail to use it would be deliberately to harm those individuals whom its use would protect.

It might thus, as we have just noted, enable individuals with genetic defects to be sure of having healthy rather than harmed children and thus liberate them from the terrible dilemma of whether or not to risk having children with genetic defects.

Suppose now that it becomes possible to use gene therapy to introduce into the human genome genes coding for antibodies to major infections like AIDS, Hepatitis B, Malaria and others, or coding for repair enzymes which could correct the most frequently occurring defects caused by radiation damage, or which could retard the ageing process and so lead to greater healthy longevity, or which might remove predispositions to heart disease, or which would destroy carcinogens or maybe permit human beings to tolerate other environmental pollutants?[10]

I have called individuals who might have these protections built into their germ line a "new breed".[11] It might be possible to use somatic cell therapy to make the same changes. I am not here intersted in the alleged moral differences between germ line and somatic line therapy, though elsewhere I have argued strongly that there is no morally relevant difference.[12] The question we must address is whether it would be wrong to fail to protect individuals in ways like these which would effectively enhance their function rather than cure dysfunction, which would constitute improvements in human individuals or indeed to the human genome, rather than simple (though complex in another sense and sophisticated) repairs? I am assuming

---

[9] I use the term "weak" here to echo Chadwick's use of the term. I take "genetically weak" to refer to those possessing a debilitating genetic condition or those who will inevitably pass on such a condition. All of us almost certainly carry some genetic abnormalities and are not thereby rendered "weak".

[10] Here I borrow freely from my *Wonderwoman & Superman: The Ethics of Human Biotechnology* Oxford University Press 1992. Chapter 9, where I discuss all these issues in greater depth than is possible here.

[11] Ibid.

[12] Ibid Chapter 8.

184 JOHN HARRIS

of course that the technique is tried, tested and safe.

To answer this question we need to know whether to fail to protect individuals whom we could protect in this way would constitute a harm to them.[13] The answer seems to be clearly that it would. If the gene therapy could enhance prospects for healthy longevity then just as today, someone who had a life expectancy of fifty years rather than one of seventy would be regarded as at a substantial disadvantage, so having one of only seventy when others were able to enjoy ninety or so would be analogously disadvantageous. However even if we concentrate on increased resistance, or reduced susceptibility, to disease there would still be palpable harms involved. True, to be vulnerable is not necessarily to suffer the harm to which one is vulnerable, although even this may constitute some degree of psychological damage. However the right analogy seems here to be drawn from aviation.

Suppose aircraft manufacturers could easily build in safety features which would render an aircraft immune to, or at least much less susceptible to, a wide range of aviation hazards. If they failed to do so we would regard them as culpable whether or not a particular aircraft did in fact succumb to any of these hazards in the course of its life. They would in short be like a parent who failed to protect her children from dangerous diseases via immunization or our imagined parent who fails to protect through gene therapy.

I hope enough has been said to make clear that where gene therapy will effect improvements to human beings or to human nature that provide protections from harm or the protection of life itself in the form of increases in life expectancy ('death postponing' is after all just 'life saving' redescribed) then call it what you will, eugenics or not, we ought to be in favour of it. There is in short no moral difference between attempts to cure dysfunction and attempts to enhance function where the enhancement protects life or health.

WHAT SORTS OF ENHANCEMENT PROTECT HEALTH?

I have drawn a distinction between attempts to protect life and health and other uses of gene therapy. I have done so mostly for the sake of brevity and to avoid the more contentious area of so-called cosmetic or frivolous uses of gene therapy. Equally and for analogous reasons I have here failed to distinguish between gene therapy on the germ line and gene therapy on the somatic line. I avoid contention here not out of distaste for combat but simply because to deploy

---

[13] For an elaboration on the importance of this distinction see my discussion of 'the wrong of wrongful life' in *Wonderwoman & Superman* Chapter 4.

IS GENE THERAPY A FORM OF EUGENICS?   185

the arguments necessary to defend cosmetic uses of gene therapy would take up more space than I have available now. Elsewhere I have deployed these arguements.[14] However, the distinction between preservation of life and health or normal medical uses and other uses of gene therapy is difficult to draw and it is worth here just illustrating this difficulty.

The British Governments' "Committee on the Ethics of Gene Therapy" in its report to Parliament attempted to draw this distinction. The report, known by the surname of its chairman as *The Clothier Report* suggested "in the current state of knowledge it would not be acceptable to attempt to change traits not associated with disease".[15] This was an attempt to rule out so called cosmetic uses of gene therapy which would include attempts to manipulate intelligence.[16]

Imagine two groups of mentally handicapped or educationally impaired children. In one the disability is traceable to a specific disease state or injury, in the other it has no obvious cause. Suppose now that gene therapy offered the chance of improving the intelligence of children generally and those in both these groups in particular. Those who think that using gene therapy to improve intelligence is wrong because it is not a dimension of health care would have to think that neither group of children should be helped and those, like Clothier, who are marginally more enlightened would have to think that it might be ethical to help children in the first group but not those in the second.[17]

I must now turn to the question of whether or not gene therapy as a technique is specially morally problematic.

WHAT'S WRONG WITH GENE THERAPY?

Gene therapy may of course be scientifically problematic in a number of ways and in so far as these might make the procedure unsafe we would have some reason to be suspicious of it. However these problems are ethically uninteresting and I shall continue to assume that gene therapy is tried and tested from a scientific perspective. What else might be wrong with it?

One other ethical problem for gene therapy has been suggested

[14] Ibid. Chapter 7.

[15] *Report of the Committee on the Ethics of Gene Therapy*, presented to Parliament by Command of Her Majesty, January 1992. London HMSO para.4.22.

[16] In fact intelligence is unlikely to prove responsive to such manipulation because of its multifactorial nature.

[17] There would be analogous problems about attempts to block the use of gene therapy to change things like physical stature and height since it might be used in the treatment of achondroplasia or other forms of dwarfism.

186   JOHN HARRIS

and it deserves the small space left. Ruth Chadwick has given massive importance to the avoidance of doubt over ones genetic origins. Chadwick suggests that someone:

> who discovers that her parents had an extra gene or genes added . . . may suffer from what today in the 'problem pages' is called an 'identity crisis' . . . Part of this may be an uncertainty about her genetic history. We have stressed the importance of this knowledge, and pointed out that when one does not know where 50 per cent of one's genes come from, it can cause unhappiness.[18]

Chadwick then asks whether this problem can be avoided if only a small amount of genetic make-up is involved. Her answer is equivocal but on balance she seems to feel that "we must be cautious about producing a situation where children feel they do not really belong anywhere, because their genetic history is confused."[19] This sounds mild enough until we examine the cash value of phrases like "can cause unhappiness" or "be cautious" as Chadwick uses them.

In discussing the alleged unhappiness caused by ignorance of 50 per cent of one's genetic origin, Chadwick argued strongly that such unhappiness was so serious that "it seems wise to restrict artificial reproduction to methods that do not involve donation of genetic material. This rules out AID, egg donation, embryo donation and partial surrogacy".[20]

In elevating doubt about one's genetic origin to a cause of unhappiness so poignant that it would be better that a child who might experience it had never been born, Chadwick ignores entirely the (in fact false) truism that while motherhood is a fact paternity is always merely a hypothesis. It is a wise child indeed that knows her father and since such doubt might reasonably cloud the lives of a high proportion of the population of the world, we have reason to be sceptical that its effects are so terrible that people should be prevented from reproducing except where such doubt can be ruled out.

The effect of Chadwick's conclusion is to deny gay couples and single people the possibility of reproducing. Chadwick denies this suggesting "they are not being denied the opportunity to have children. If they are prepared to take the necessary steps ('the primitive sign of wanting is trying to get') their desire to beget can be satisfied." What are we to make of this? It seems almost self-consciously mischievous. In the first place gay couples and single women resorting

---

[18] Ruth Chadwick *Ethics, Reproduction and Genetic Control*, Routledge, London, 1987. page 126.
[19] Ibid. page 127.
[20] Ibid. page 39.

IS GENE THERAPY A FORM OF EUGENICS? 187

to what must, *ex hypothesi*, be distasteful sex with third parties merely for procreational purposes, are unlikely to preserve the identity of their sexual partners for the benefit of their offspring's alleged future peace of mind. If this is right then doubt over genetic origin will not be removed. Since Chadwick is explicitly addressing public policy issues she should in consistency advocate legislation against such a course of action rather than recommend it.

But surely, if we are to comtemplate legislating against practices which give rise to doubt about genetic origins we would need hard evidence not only that such practices harm the resulting children but that the harm is of such high order that not only would it have been better that such children had never been born but also better that those who want such children should suffer the unhappiness consequent on a denial of their chance to have children using donated genetic material?

Where such harm is not only unavoidable but is an inherent part of sexual reproduction and must affect to some degree or other a high percentage of all births, it is surely at best unkind to use the fear of it as an excuse for discriminating against already persecuted minorities in the provision of reproductive services.

Where, as in the case of gene therapy, such donated[21] material also protects life and health or improves the human condition we have an added reason to welcome it.

Centre for Social Ethics and Policy
University of Manchester

NOTES

This paper was presented at the Inaugural Congress of the International Association of Bioethics, Amsterdam, The Netherlands, 5-7th October 1992. I am grateful to the audience at that meeting and particularly to Dan Brock, Norman Daniels, Raanan Gillon, Douglas Maclean and Maurice de Wachter for helpful comments.

[21] I use the term 'donated' here but I do not mean to rule out commerce in such genetic material. See *My Wonderwoman & Superman*. Chapter 6.

[29]

The Case for Involuntary Hospitalization of the Mentally Ill

BY PAUL CHODOFF, M.D.

*The author examines three points of view on the
question of society's right to involuntarily hospitalize
a mentally ill individual. The "abolitionists" oppose
involuntary hospitalization entirely; the medical model
psychiatrists support the need for commitment under
certain circumstances and so do the civil liberties
lawyers, but by different standards. The author
believes that with the current overreliance on the
dangerousness standard, we are witnessing a
pendular swing in which the rights of the mentally ill to
be treated and protected are being set aside in the rush
to give them their freedom. He favors a return to the
use of medical criteria by psychiatrists, albeit with
constructive legal safeguards.*

I WILL BEGIN this paper with a series of vignettes designed to illustrate graphically the question that is my focus: under what conditions, if any, does society have the right to apply coercion to an individual to hospitalize him against his will, by reason of mental illness?

Case 1. A woman in her mid 50s, with no previous overt behavioral difficulties, comes to believe that she is worthless and insignificant. She is completely preoccupied with her guilt and is increasingly unavailable for the ordinary demands of life. She eats very little because of her conviction that the food should go to others whose need is greater than hers, and her physical condition progressively deteriorates. Although she will talk to others about herself, she insists that she is not sick, only bad. She refuses medication, and when hospitalization is suggested she also refuses that on the grounds that she would be taking up space that otherwise could be occupied by those who merit treatment more than she.

Case 2. For the past 6 years the behavior of a 42-year-old woman has been disturbed for periods of 3 months or longer. After recovery from her most recent episode she has been at home, functioning at a borderline level. A month ago she again started to withdraw from her environment. She pays increasingly less attention to her bodily needs, talks very little, and does not respond to questions or attention from those about her. She lapses into a mute state and lies in her bed in a totally passive fashion. She does not respond to other people, does not eat, and does not void. When her arm is

Revised version of a paper presented at a symposium sponsored by
Georgetown University Law School, October 6, 1975.

Dr. Chodoff is Clinical Professor of Psychiatry, George Washington
University School of Medicine. He is also in private practice at 1904
R St., N.W., Washington, D.C. 20009.

raised from the bed it remains for several minutes in the position in which it is left. Her medical history and a physical examination reveal no evidence of primary physical illness.

Case 3. A man with a history of alcoholism has been on a binge for several weeks. He remains at home doing little else than drinking. He eats very little. He becomes tremulous and misinterprets spots on the wall as animals about to attack him, and he complains of "creeping" sensations in his body, which he attributes to infestation by insects. He does not seek help voluntarily, insists there is nothing wrong with him, and despite his wife's entreaties he continues to drink.

Case 4. Passersby and station personnel observe that a young woman has been spending several days at Union Station in Washington, D.C. Her behavior appears strange to others. She is finally befriended by a newspaper reporter who becomes aware that her perception of her situation is profoundly unrealistic and that she is, in fact, delusional. He persuades her to accompany him to St. Elizabeths Hospital, where she is examined by a psychiatrist who recommends admission. She refuses hospitalization and the psychiatrist allows her to leave. She returns to Union Station. A few days later she is found dead, murdered, on one of the surrounding streets.

Case 5. A government attorney in his late 30s begins to display pressured speech and hyperactivity. He is too busy to sleep and eats very little. He talks rapidly, becomes irritable when interrupted, and makes phone calls all over the country in furtherance of his political ambitions, which are to begin a campaign for the Presidency of the United States. He makes many purchases, some very expensive, thus running through a great deal of money. He is rude and tactless to his friends, who are offended by his behavior, and his job is in jeopardy. In spite of his wife's pleas he insists that he does not have the time to seek or accept treatment, and he refuses hospitalization. This is not the first such disturbance for this individual; in fact, very similar episodes have been occurring at roughly 2-year intervals since he was 18 years old.

Case 6. Passersby in a campus area observe two young women standing together, staring at each other, for over an hour. Their behavior attracts attention, and eventually the police take the pair to a nearby precinct station for questioning. They refuse to answer questions and sit mutely, staring into space. The police request some type of psychiatric examination but are informed by the city attorney's office that state law (Michigan) allows persons to be held for observation only if they appear obviously dangerous to themselves or others. In this case, since the women do not seem homicidal or suicidal, they do not qualify for observation and are released.

Less than 30 hours later the two women are found on the floor of their campus apartment, screaming and writhing in pain with their clothes ablaze from a self-made pyre. One woman recovers; the other dies. There is no conclusive evidence that drugs were involved (1).

Most, if not all, people would agree that the behavior described in these vignettes deviates significantly from even elastic definitions of normality. However, it is clear that there would not be a similar consensus on how to react to this kind of behavior and that there is a considerable and increasing ferment about what attitude the organized elements of our society should take toward such individuals. Everyone has a stake in this important issue, but the debate about it takes place principally among psychiatrists, lawyers, the courts, and law enforcement agencies.

Points of view about the question of involuntary hospitalization fall into the following three principal groups: the "abolitionists," medical model psychiatrists, and civil liberties lawyers.

THE ABOLITIONISTS

Those holding this position would assert that in none of the cases I have described should involuntary hospitalization be a viable option because, quite simply, it should never be resorted to under any circumstances. As Szasz (2) has put it, "we should value liberty more highly than mental health no matter how defined" and "no one should be deprived of his freedom for the sake of his mental health." Ennis (3) has said that the goal "is nothing less than the abolition of involuntary hospitalization."

Prominent among the abolitionists are the "anti-psychiatrists," who, somewhat surprisingly, count in their ranks a number of well-known psychiatrists. For them mental illness simply does not exist in the field of psychiatry (4). They reject entirely the medical model of mental illness and insist that acceptance of it relies on a fiction accepted jointly by the state and by psychiatrists as a device for exerting social control over annoying or unconventional people. The anti-psychiatrists hold that these people ought to be afforded the dignity of being held responsible for their behavior and required to accept its consequences. In addition, some members of this group believe that the phenomena of "mental illness" often represent essentially a tortured protest against the insanities of an irrational society (5). They maintain that society should not be encouraged in its oppressive course by affixing a pejorative label to its victims.

Among the abolitionists are some civil liberties lawyers who both assert their passionate support of the magisterial importance of individual liberty and react with repugnance and impatience to what they see as the abuses of psychiatric practice in this field—the commitment of some individuals for flimsy and possibly self-serving reasons and their inhuman warehousing in penal institutions wrongly called "hospitals."

The abolitionists do not oppose psychiatric treatment when it is conducted with the agreement of those being treated. I have no doubt that they would try to gain the consent of the individuals described earlier to undergo treatment, including hospitalization. The psychiatrists in this group would be very likely to confine their treatment methods to psychotherapeutic efforts to influence the aberrant behavior. They would be unlikely to use drugs and would certainly eschew such somatic therapies as ECT. If efforts to enlist voluntary compliance with treatment failed, the abolitionists would not employ any means of coercion. Instead, they would step aside and allow social, legal, and community sanctions to take their course. If a human being should be jailed or a human life lost as a result of this attitude, they would accept it as a necessary evil to be tolerated in order to avoid the greater evil of unjustified loss of liberty for others (6).

THE MEDICAL MODEL PSYCHIATRISTS

I use this admittedly awkward and not entirely accurate label to designate the position of a substantial number of psychiatrists. They believe that mental illness is a meaningful concept and that under certain conditions its existence justifies the state's exercise, under the doctrine of parens patriae, of its right and obligation to arrange for the hospitalization of the sick individual even though coercion is involved and he is deprived of his liberty. I believe that these psychiatrists would recommend involuntary hospitalization for all six of the patients described earlier.

The Medical Model

There was a time, before they were considered to be ill, when individuals who displayed the kind of behavior I described earlier were put in "ships of fools" to wander the seas or were left to the mercies, sometimes tender but often savage, of uncomprehending communities that regarded them as either possessed or bad. During the Enlightenment and the early nineteenth century, however, these individuals gradually came to be regarded as sick people to be included under the humane and caring umbrella of the Judeo-Christian attitude toward illness. This attitude, which may have reached its height during the era of moral treatment in the early nineteenth century, has had unexpected and ambiguous consequences. It became overextended and partially perverted, and these excesses led to the reaction that is so strong a current in today's attitude toward mental illness.

However, reaction itself can go too far, and I believe that this is already happening. Witness the disastrous consequences of the precipitate dehospitalization that is occurring all over the country. To remove the protective mantle of illness from these disturbed people is to expose them, their families, and their communities to consequences that are certainly maladaptive and possibly irreparable. Are we really acting in accordance with their best interests when we allow them to "die with their rights on" (1) or when we condemn

CASE FOR INVOLUNTARY HOSPITALIZATION

them to a "preservation of liberty which is actually so destructive as to constitute another form of imprisonment" (7)? Will they not suffer "if [a] liberty they cannot enjoy is made superior to a health that must sometimes be forced on them" (8)?

Many of those who reject the medical model out of hand as inapplicable to so-called "mental illness" have tended to oversimplify its meaning and have, in fact, equated it almost entirely with organic disease. It is necessary to recognize that it is a complex concept and that there is a lack of agreement about its meaning. Sophisticated definitions of the medical model do not require only the demonstration of unequivocal organic pathology. A broader formulation, put forward by sociologists and deriving largely from Talcott Parsons' description of the sick role (9), extends the domain of illness to encompass certain forms of social deviance as well as biological disorders. According to this definition, the medical model is characterized not only by organicity but also by being negatively valued by society, by "nonvoluntariness," thus exempting its exemplars from blame, and by the understanding that physicians are the technically competent experts to deal with its effects (10).

Except for the question of organic disease, the patients I described earlier conform well to this broader conception of the medical model. They are all suffering both emotionally and physically, they are incapable by an effort of will of stopping or changing their destructive behavior, and those around them consider them to be in an undesirable sick state and to require medical attention.

Categorizing the behavior of these patients as involuntary may be criticized as evidence of an intolerably paternalistic and antitherapeutic attitude that fosters the very failure to take responsibility for their lives and behavior that the therapist should uncover rather than encourage. However, it must also be acknowledged that these severely ill people are not capable at a conscious level of deciding what is best for themselves and that in order to help them examine their behavior and motivation, it is necessary that they be alive and available for treatment. Their verbal message that they will not accept treatment may at the same time be conveying other more covert messages—that they are desperate and want help even though they cannot ask for it (11).

Although organic pathology may not be the only determinant of the medical model, it is of course an important one and it should not be avoided in any discussion of mental illness. There would be no question that the previously described patient with delirium tremens is suffering from a toxic form of brain disease. There are a significant number of other patients who require involuntary hospitalization because of organic brain syndrome due to various causes. Among those who are not overtly organically ill, most of the candidates for involuntary hospitalization suffer from schizophrenia or one of the major affective disorders. A growing and increasingly impressive body of evidence points to the presence of an important genetic-biological factor in these conditions; thus, many of them qualify on these grounds as illnesses.

Despite the revisionist efforts of the anti-psychiatrists, mental illness *does* exist. It does not by any means include all of the people being treated by psychiatrists (or by nonpsychiatrist physicians), but it does encompass those few desperately sick people for whom involuntary commitment must be considered. In the words of a recent article, "The problem is that mental illness is not a myth. It is not some palpable falsehood propagated among the populace by power-mad psychiatrists, but a cruel and bitter reality that has been with the human race since antiquity" (12, p.1483).

Criteria for Involuntary Hospitalization

Procedures for involuntary hospitalization should be instituted for individuals who require care and treatment because of diagnosable mental illness that produces symptoms, including marked impairment in judgment, that disrupt their intrapsychic and interpersonal functioning. All three of these criteria must be met before involuntary hospitalization can be instituted.

1. *Mental illness*. This concept has already been discussed, but it should be repeated that only a belief in the existence of illness justifies involuntary commitment. It is a fundamental assumption that makes aberrant behavior a medical matter and its care the concern of physicians.

2. *Disruption of functioning*. This involves combinations of serious and often obvious disturbances that are both intrapsychic (for example, the suffering of severe depression) and interpersonal (for example, withdrawal from others because of depression). It does not include minor peccadilloes or eccentricities. Furthermore, the behavior in question must represent symptoms of the mental illness from which the patient is suffering. Among these symptoms are actions that are imminently or potentially dangerous in a physical sense to self or others, as well as other manifestations of mental illness such as those in the cases I have described. This is not to ignore dangerousness as a criterion for commitment but rather to put it in its proper place as one of a number of symptoms of the illness. A further manifestation of the illness, and indeed, the one that makes involuntary rather than voluntary hospitalization necessary, is impairment of the patient's judgment to such a degree that he is unable to consider his condition and make decisions about it in his own interests.

3. *Need for care and treatment*. The goal of physicians is to treat and cure their patients; however, sometimes they can only ameliorate the suffering of their patients and sometimes all they can offer is care. It is not possible to predict whether someone will respond to treatment; nevertheless, the need for treatment and the availability of facilities to carry it out constitute essential preconditions that must be met to justify requir-

ing anyone to give up his freedom. If mental hospital patients have a right to treatment, then psychiatrists have a right to ask for treatability as a front-door as well as a back-door criterion for commitment (7). All of the six individuals I described earlier could have been treated with a reasonable expectation of returning to a more normal state of functioning.

I believe that the objections to this formulation can be summarized as follows.

1. The whole structure founders for those who maintain that mental illness is a fiction.

2. These criteria are also untenable to those who hold liberty to be such a supreme value that the presence of mental illness per se does not constitute justification for depriving an individual of his freedom; only when such illness is manifested by clearly dangerous behavior may commitment be considered. For reasons to be discussed later, I agree with those psychiatrists (13, 14) who do not believe that dangerousness should be elevated to primacy above other manifestations of mental illness as a sine qua non for involuntary hospitalization.

3. The medical model criteria are "soft" and subjective and depend on the fallible judgment of psychiatrists. This is a valid objection. There is no reliable blood test for schizophrenia and no method for injecting grey cells into psychiatrists. A relatively small number of cases will always fall within a grey area that will be difficult to judge. In those extreme cases in which the question of commitment arises, competent and ethical psychiatrists should be able to use these criteria without doing violence to individual liberties and with the expectation of good results. Furthermore, the possible "fuzziness" of some aspects of the medical model approach is certainly no greater than that of the supposedly "objective" criteria for dangerousness, and there is little reason to believe that lawyers and judges are any less fallible than psychiatrists.

4. Commitment procedures in the hands of psychiatrists are subject to intolerable abuses. Here, as Peszke said, "It is imperative that we differentiate between the principle of the process of civil commitment and the practice itself" (13, p. 825). Abuses can contaminate both the medical and the dangerousness approaches, and I believe that the abuses stemming from the abolitionist view of no commitment at all are even greater. Measures to abate abuses of the medical approach include judicial review and the abandonment of indeterminate commitment. In the course of commitment proceedings and thereafter, patients should have access to competent and compassionate legal counsel. However, this latter safeguard may itself be subject to abuse if the legal counsel acts solely in the adversary tradition and undertakes to carry out the patient's wishes even when they may be destructive.

Comment

The criteria and procedures outlined will apply most appropriately to initial episodes and recurrent attacks of mental illness. To put it simply, it is necessary to find a way to satisfy legal and humanitarian considerations and yet allow psychiatrists access to initially or acutely ill patients in order to do the best they can for them. However, there are some involuntary patients who have received adequate and active treatment but have not responded satisfactorily. An irreducible minimum of such cases, principally among those with brain disorders and process schizophrenia, will not improve sufficiently to be able to adapt to even a tolerant society.

The decision of what to do at this point is not an easy one, and it should certainly not be in the hands of psychiatrists alone. With some justification they can state that they have been given the thankless job of caring, often with inadequate facilities, for badly damaged people and that they are now being subjected to criticism for keeping these patients locked up. No one really knows what to do with these patients. It may be that when treatment has failed they exchange their sick role for what has been called the impaired role (15), which implies a permanent negative evaluation of them coupled with a somewhat less benign societal attitude. At this point, perhaps a case can be made for giving greater importance to the criteria for dangerousness and releasing such patients if they do not pose a threat to others. However, I do not believe that the release into the community of these severely malfunctioning individuals will serve their interests even though it may satisfy formal notions of right and wrong.

It should be emphasized that the number of individuals for whom involuntary commitment must be considered is small (although, under the influence of current pressures, it may be smaller than it should be). Even severe mental illness can often be handled by securing the cooperation of the patient, and certainly one of the favorable effects of the current ferment has been to encourage such efforts. However, the distinction between voluntary and involuntary hospitalization is sometimes more formal than meaningful. How "voluntary" are the actions of an individual who is being buffeted by the threats, entreaties, and tears of his family?

I believe, however, that we are at a point (at least in some jurisdictions) where, having rebounded from an era in which involuntary commitment was too easy and employed too often, we are now entering one in which it is becoming very difficult to commit anyone, even in urgent cases. Faced with the moral obloquy that has come to pervade the atmosphere in which the decision to involuntarily hospitalize is considered, some psychiatrists, especially younger ones, have become, as Stone (16) put it, "soft as grapes" when faced with the prospect of committing anyone under any circumstances.

THE CIVIL LIBERTIES LAWYERS

I use this admittedly inexact label to designate those members of the legal profession who do not in principle reject the necessity for involuntary hospitalization but who do reject or wish to diminish the importance of medical model criteria in the hands of psychiatrists. Accordingly, the civil liberties lawyers, in dealing with the problem of involuntary hospitalization, have enlisted themselves under the standard of dangerousness, which they hold to be more objective and capable of being dealt with in a sounder evidentiary manner than the medical model criteria. For them the question is not whether mental illness, even of disabling degree, is present, but only whether it has resulted in the probability of behavior dangerous to others or to self. Thus they would scrutinize the cases previously described for evidence of such dangerousness and would make the decision about involuntary hospitalization accordingly. They would probably feel that commitment is not indicated in most of these cases, since they were selected as illustrative of severe mental illness in which outstanding evidence of physical dangerousness was not present.

The dangerousness standard is being used increasingly not only to supplement criteria for mental illness but, in fact, to replace them entirely. The recent Supreme Court decision in *O'Connor v. Donaldson* (17) is certainly a long step in this direction. In addition, "dangerousness" is increasingly being understood to refer to the probability that the individual will inflict harm on himself or others in a specific physical manner rather than in other ways. This tendency has perhaps been carried to its ultimate in the *Lessard v. Schmidt* case (18) in Wisconsin, which restricted suitability for commitment to the "extreme likelihood that if the person is not confined, he will do immediate harm to himself or others." (This decision was set aside by the U.S. Supreme Court in 1974.) In a recent Washington, D.C., Superior Court case (19) the instructions to the jury stated that the government must prove that the defendant was likely to cause "substantial physical harm to himself or others in the reasonably foreseeable future."

For the following reasons, the dangerousness standard is an inappropriate and dangerous indicator to use in judging the conditions under which someone should be involuntarily hospitalized. Dangerousness is being taken out of its proper context as one among other symptoms of the presence of severe mental illness that should be the determining factor.

1. To concentrate on dangerousness (especially to others) as the sole criterion for involuntary hospitalization deprives many mentally ill persons of the protection and treatment that they urgently require. A psychiatrist under the constraints of the dangerousness rule, faced with an out-of-control manic individual whose frantic behavior the psychiatrist truly believes to be a disguised call for help, would have to say, "Sorry, I would like to help you but I can't because you haven't threatened anybody and you are not suicidal." Since psychiatrists are admittedly not very good at accurately predicting dangerousness to others, the evidentiary standards for commitment will be very strin-

gent. This will result in mental hospitals becoming prisons for a small population of volatile, highly assaultive, and untreatable patients (14).

2. The attempt to differentiate rigidly (especially in regard to danger to self) between physical and other kinds of self-destructive behavior is artificial, unrealistic, and unworkable. It will tend to confront psychiatrists who want to help their patients with the same kind of dilemma they were faced with when justification for therapeutic abortion on psychiatric grounds depended on evidence of suicidal intent. The advocates of the dangerousness standard seem to be more comfortable with and pay more attention to the factor of dangerousness to others even though it is a much less frequent and much less significant consequence of mental illness than is danger to self.

3. The emphasis on dangerousness (again, especially to others) is a real obstacle to the right-to-treatment movement since it prevents the hospitalization and therefore the treatment of the population most amenable to various kinds of therapy.

4. Emphasis on the criterion of dangerousness to others moves involuntary commitment from a civil to a criminal procedure, thus, as Stone (14) put it, imposing the procedures of one terrible system on another. Involuntary commitment on these grounds becomes a form of preventive detention and makes the psychiatrist a kind of glorified policeman.

5. Emphasis on dangerousness rather than mental disability and helplessness will hasten the process of deinstitutionalization. Recent reports (20, 21) have shown that these patients are not being rehabilitated and reintegrated into the community, but rather, that the burden of custodialism has been shifted from the hospital to the community.

6. As previously mentioned, emphasis on the dangerousness criterion may be a tactic of some of the abolitionists among the civil liberties lawyers (22) to end involuntary hospitalization by reducing it to an unworkable absurdity.

DISCUSSION

It is obvious that it is good to be at liberty and that it is good to be free from the consequences of disabling and dehumanizing illness. Sometimes these two values are incompatible, and in the heat of the passions that are often aroused by opposing views of right and wrong, the partisans of each view may tend to minimize the importance of the other. Both sides can present their horror stories—the psychiatrists, their dead victims of the failure of the involuntary hospitalization process, and the lawyers, their Donaldsons. There is a real danger that instead of acknowledging the difficulty of the problem, the two camps will become polarized, with a consequent rush toward extreme and untenable solutions rather than working toward reasonable ones.

The path taken by those whom I have labeled the

PAUL CHODOFF

abolitionists is an example of the barren results that ensue when an absolute solution is imposed on a complex problem. There are human beings who will suffer greatly if the abolitionists succeed in elevating an abstract principle into an unbreakable law with no exceptions. I find myself oppressed and repelled by their position, which seems to stem from an ideological rigidity which ignores that element of the contingent immanent in the structure of human existence. It is devoid of compassion.

The positions of those who espouse the medical model and the dangerousness approaches to commitment are, one hopes, not completely irreconcilable. To some extent these differences are a result of the vantage points from which lawyers and psychiatrists view mental illness and commitment. The lawyers see and are concerned with the failures and abuses of the process. Furthermore, as a result of their training, they tend to apply principles to classes of people rather than to take each instance as unique. The psychiatrists, on the other hand, are required to deal practically with the singular needs of individuals. They approach the problem from a clinical rather than a deductive stance. As physicians, they want to be in a position to take care of and to help suffering people whom they regard as sick patients. They sometimes become impatient with the rules that prevent them from doing this.

I believe we are now witnessing a pendular swing in which the rights of the mentally ill to be treated and protected are being set aside in the rush to give them their freedom at whatever cost. But is freedom defined only by the absence of external constraints? Internal physiological or psychological processes can contribute to a throttling of the spirit that is as painful as any applied from the outside. The "wild" manic individual without his lithium, the panicky hallucinator without his injection of fluphenazine hydrochloride and the understanding support of a concerned staff, the sodden alcoholic—are they free? Sometimes, as Woody Guthrie said, "Freedom means no place to go."

Today the civil liberties lawyers are in the ascendancy and the psychiatrists on the defensive to a degree that is harmful to individual needs and the public welfare. Redress and a more balanced position will not come from further extension of the dangerousness doctrine. I favor a return to the use of medical criteria by psychiatrists—psychiatrists, however, who have been chastened by the buffeting they have received and are quite willing to go along with even strict legal safeguards as long as they are constructive and not tyrannical.

REFERENCES

1. Treffert DA: The practical limits of patients' rights. Psychiatric Annals 5(4):91–96, 1971
2. Szasz T: Law, Liberty and Psychiatry. New York, Macmillan Co, 1963
3. Ennis B: Prisoners of Psychiatry. New York, Harcourt Brace Jovanovich, 1972
4. Szasz T: The Myth of Mental Illness. New York, Harper & Row, 1961
5. Laing R: The Politics of Experience. New York, Ballantine Books, 1967
6. Ennis B: Ennis on 'Donaldson'. Psychiatric News, Dec 3, 1975, pp 4, 19, 37
7. Peele R, Chodoff P, Taub N: Involuntary hospitalization and treatability. Observations from the DC experience. Catholic University Law Review 23:744–753, 1974
8. Michels R: The Right to Refuse Psychotropic Drugs. Hastings Center Report. Hastings-on-Hudson, NY, Hastings Institute of Health and Human Values, 1973
9. Parsons T: The Social System. New York, Free Press, 1951
10. Veatch RM: The medical model: its nature and problems. Hastings Center Studies 1(3):59–76, 1973
11. Katz J: The right to treatment—an enchanting legal fiction? University of Chicago Law Review 36:755–783, 1969
12. Moore MS: Some myths about "mental illness." Arch Gen Psychiatry 32:1483–1497, 1975
13. Peszke MA: Is dangerousness an issue for physicians in emergency commitment? Am J Psychiatry 132:825–828, 1975
14. Stone AA: Comment on Peszke MA: Is dangerousness an issue for physicians in emergency commitment? Ibid, 829–831
15. Siegler M, Osmond H: Models of Madness, Models of Medicine. New York, Macmillan Co, 1974
16. Stone A: Lecture for course on The Law, Litigation, and Mental Health Services. Adelphi, Md, Mental Health Study Center, September 1974
17. O'Connor v Donaldson, 43 USLW 4929 (1975)
18. Lessard v Schmidt, 349 F Supp 1078, 1092 (ED Wis 1972)
19. In re Johnnie Hargrove. Washington, DC, Superior Court Mental Health number 506-75, 1975
20. Rachlin S, Pam A, Milton J: Civil liberties versus involuntary hospitalization. Am J Psychiatry 132:189–191, 1975
21. Kirk SA, Therrien ME: Community mental health myths and the fate of former hospitalized patients. Psychiatry 38:209–217, 1975
22. Dershowitz AA: Dangerousness as a criterion for confinement. Bulletin of the American Academy of Psychiatry and the Law 2:172–179, 1974

SOUNDING BOARD

WHEN COMPETENT PATIENTS MAKE IRRATIONAL CHOICES

In recent years, physicians and patients have tended to move toward shared decision making. Although it sounds reasonable on the surface that patients and physicians should collaborate in making decisions about medical care, surprisingly little attention has been given to the complex and troubling issues that can arise. In particular, what does shared decision making imply for a physician's responsibilities when an apparently competent patient's choice appears to be irrational? A discussion of this issue requires a taxonomy of the different sources and forms of irrational decision making. We believe such a taxonomy should include the bias toward the present and near future, the belief that "it won't happen to me," the fear of pain or the medical experience, patients' values or wants that make no sense, framing effects, and conflicts between individual and social rationality. Our main aim here is to develop this taxonomy and thus to bring out some of the theoretical and practical obstacles involved in distinguishing between a patient's irrational choices, which the physician may seek to change, and merely unusual choices that should be respected. To avoid any misunderstanding, we emphasize at the outset that even the irrational choices of a competent patient must be respected if the patient cannot be persuaded to change them.

Shared Decision Making between Physician and Patient

Historically, the professional ideal of the physician–patient relationship held that the physician directed care and made decisions about treatment; the patient's principal role was to comply with "doctor's orders." Although this paternalistic approach often took account of the patient's general preferences and attitudes toward treatment, it gave the patient only a minimal role in making decisions. When faced with

Prospective authors should consult "Information for Authors," which appears in the first issue of each month and may be obtained from the *Journal* office.

Articles with original material are accepted for consideration with the understanding that, except for abstracts, no part of the data has been published, or will be submitted for publication elsewhere, before appearing here.

Material printed in the *Journal* is covered by copyright. No part of this publication may be reproduced without written permission. The *Journal* does not hold itself responsible for statements made by any contributor.

Statements or opinions expressed in the *Journal* reflect the views of the author(s) and do not represent official policy of the Massachusetts Medical Society unless so stated.

Although all advertising material accepted is expected to conform to ethical medical standards, acceptance does not imply endorsement by the *Journal*.

Subscription Prices: Pounds sterling drawn on U.K. banks only: £75 per year (interns, residents, and students £51 per year). Send payments and correspondence to: NEJM, Saxon Way, Melbourn, Royston, Herts SG8 6NJ, U.K. Please include current mailing label with renewal order. In Japan, ¥25,000 per year (interns, residents, and students ¥17,000 per year). Send orders to: Nankodo Co., Ltd., 42-6, Hongo 3-chome, Bunkyo-Ku, Tokyo 113, Japan.

Editorial Offices: 10 Shattuck St., Boston, MA 02115-6094, USA. Telephone: (617) 734-9800.   FAX: (617) 734-4457.

Business and Subscription Offices: 1440 Main St., Waltham, MA 02154-1649, USA.   FAX: (617) 893-0413.

what appeared to be a patient's irrational choices or preferences, physicians were encouraged by this approach to overlook or override them as not being in the patient's true interests.

Challenged by a number of forces within and outside the medical profession during the past two or three decades, the paternalistic approach has generally been replaced by the concept of shared decision making, in which both physicians and patients make active and essential contributions.[1] Physicians bring their medical training, knowledge, and expertise — including an understanding of the available treatment alternatives — to the diagnosis and management of patients' conditions. Patients bring a knowledge of their own subjective aims and values, through which the risks and benefits of various treatment options can be evaluated. With this approach, selecting the best treatment for a particular patient requires the contributions of both parties.[2]

This description of the division of labor oversimplifies the complexities of the roles and contributions of physicians and patients when real decisions about treatment are made, but it does highlight the patient's new, active part in that process. Some have concluded that in shared decision making, proper respect for patient autonomy and self-determination means accepting the patient's treatment preferences however they are arrived at. We believe that such a conclusion is unwarranted, because it fails to recognize the trade-off between the sometimes conflicting values that underlie shared decision making and that are involved in respecting or seeking to change patients' choices. The first value is the well-being of patients, which can require the physician to attempt to protect them from the harmful consequences of their choices when their judgment is irrational. The second value is respecting the right of patients to make decisions about their own lives when they are able. Whenever competent patients appear to be making irrational choices about treatment that are contrary to their own well-being, the two values will be in conflict.

Distinguishing choices that are truly irrational from those that are merely unusual often requires complex, difficult, and controversial judgments. When the physician properly judges a patient's treatment choice to be irrational, attempts to change that choice through persuasion are common and proper. Noncoercive and nonmanipulative attempts to persuade patients of the irrational and harmful nature of their choices do not violate their right of self-determination. Instead, they reflect an appropriate responsibility and concern for the patients' well-being.

Sometimes, however, attempts to persuade will fail. Physicians lack both ethical and legal authority to override patients' treatment choices unilaterally. Nevertheless, in a few cases an irrational choice that cannot be changed by persuasion may reflect a sufficiently serious impairment in decision making — and the consequences of that choice may be suffi-

ciently harmful to the patient — to call the patient's competence into question. In such cases, the physician may begin an investigation of the patient's competence that can ultimately involve recourse to the courts. Since the vast majority of irrational decisions are made by apparently competent patients, we shall not address the determination of incompetence here.[3] Our concern is with the more usual cases, in which the patient's competence does not come into question. The responsibility to try to change their competent patients' irrational choices requires that physicians gain a better understanding of the different forms of irrational treatment choices and of the theoretical and practical difficulties involved in distinguishing truly irrational from merely unusual choices.

THE STANDARD OF RATIONAL DECISION MAKING

Any discussion of irrational decision making must rely on a description of rational decision making.[4] We believe it will be helpful to make that description explicit, if only in brief outline. Specifically, what is the norm of rationality that underlies the ideal of shared decision making between patients and physicians? Essentially, shared decision making entitles patients (or their surrogates if they are incompetent) to weigh the benefits and risks of alternative treatments, including the alternative of no treatment, according to their own values and to select the alternative that best promotes those values. In the language of decision theory, each patient's values will determine his or her utility function, and the rational choice will be the one that maximizes expected utility. Since treatment decisions always involve some degree of uncertainty about the beneficial and harmful effects of alternative treatments, these effects should be discounted by their probabilities (to the extent that they are known) in calculating the expected utility of various treatment alternatives. If the probabilities are not known, each patient's attitude toward risk will determine the weight given to uncertain beneficial or adverse effects.

Shared decision making requires that physicians ensure that their patients are well informed.[5] Thus, another aspect of rational decision making is that each patient has and uses correct information about relevant alternatives. This sketch of rational decision making relies ultimately on the patient's own aims and values, unless they are irrationally distorted in the ways discussed below, as the ends that guide decision making. An irrational choice is one that satisfies those aims and values less completely than another available choice.

There is a second notion of irrational decision making that deems a patient's choice irrational if it fails to promote a set of basic aims and values that belong to the physician or to standard guidelines of medical practice. Physicians who criticize a patient's choice as irrational in this sense are disagreeing with the basic aims and values by which the patient defines his or her own good, rather than arguing that the patient's choice will fail to promote those aims and values best. Since this second notion ignores the patient's own aims and values and thus fails to respect the right of self-determination, we rely here on the first account of rational and irrational choices.

FORMS OF IRRATIONAL DECISION MAKING

We now turn to common forms of irrational decision making by patients or their surrogates (and sometimes by physicians). In many treatment decisions, more than one form of irrationality affects a single choice, but we separate them here for analytical clarity.

Bias toward the Present and Near Future

The ideal of rational decision making gives equal weight to a beneficial or harmful effect whenever it occurs in a person's life, with differences determined only by the size and probability of the effect. In the case of money it is rational to apply a discount rate, because a dollar received today can earn interest and is thus worth more than a dollar received 10 years from now. Some effects of health care are similar: it is rational to prefer a restoration of function now rather than later and to prefer that a loss of function occur as far in the future as possible, so as to minimize the period of disability. Similarly, it is rational to prefer that the loss of one's life be postponed for as long as possible, at least while it remains a life worth living. For other effects of medical care — especially pain and suffering — rational choice would seem to require indifference to their timing. In particular, it is irrational to refuse to undergo a painful experience now, if by undergoing it one can avoid a much worse experience in the future. Such a refusal would amount to preferring more rather than less pain or suffering in one's life.

Yet, as doctors know, medical practice is replete with such irrational choices by patients. Some patients who continue to smoke or drink heavily or who fail to follow relatively simple steps to control moderate hypertension may not be irrational, but are simply willing to gamble that they will beat the odds. Others, however, have given inadequate weight in their present decision making to the harm they are likely to suffer in the relatively distant future. We call this a bias to the present and near future, because people commonly give disproportionate weight to securing benefits and avoiding harm in the present and near future as opposed to the more distant future.[6] The physician's task in such cases is to help the patient fully appreciate the size and seriousness of the more distant harm or benefit, so that it can play an appropriate part in the patient's decision making.

"It Won't Happen to Me"

Patients may view the nature of the risk or harm of not following medical advice differently. This is especially true for events that have a low probability of occurring.[7] However, what constitutes low probability may vary considerably from patient to patient. Furthermore, since some patients are more willing to take risks than others, it is often difficult to determine whether a patient is more of a risk taker than most or whether the patient has simply failed to give adequate weight to a low probability or a distant event. This situation is complicated by the difficulty of distinguishing among patients who, for example, ignore a risk (that is, acknowledge the risk but decide to accept it), irrationally deny the possibility that an untoward event could happen to them, have "magical" or illusory beliefs about their vulnerability to harm, or simply have a different way of viewing the medical problem.[8] Adolescents, for example, are commonly subject to feelings of invulnerability to certain harms disproportionate to the real risk of those harms.

Physicians often need to gain some understanding of their patients' general attitudes toward risk and the extent to which they are risk averse, perhaps as evidenced by their past behavior. Physicians should attempt to distinguish among the possibilities noted above. Sometimes a physician can help a patient appreciate a risk more vividly and relate it to the patient's life. However, for patients who deny a risk or have magical beliefs, a more detailed medical and scientific explanation is not likely to be helpful. In these cases, formal counseling or psychiatric evaluation may be more fruitful.

Fear of Pain or the Medical Experience

Many patients delay or will not even consider a particular treatment for fear of the perceived nature of the experience, although they may acknowledge that the treatment is clearly in their best interests. Sometimes their decision is coupled with some form of rationalization — "there's no need to do it yet," or "I'm too busy now with other things," for example. In other cases, when a dreaded experience draws near, a patient may be almost paralyzed with fear. Sometimes the fear may be focused not on pain or suffering but on other dreaded experiences, such as being "cut open" or being "put to sleep" in surgery. In still other cases, the fear of a disease such as cancer or the acquired immunodeficiency syndrome can prevent a person from making informed decisions about its treatment.

Determining when this form of irrational decision making is present is considerably complicated by the fact that no single, correct weight can be given to pain or a particular medical experience as measured against the beneficial outcomes for which the experience may be necessary. Patients differ, for example, in the degree to which they are prepared to tolerate painful treatments or conditions for the sake of other ends,[9] but these reasonable differences are difficult to distinguish from the undue weight some patients give to certain aspects of treatment because of irrational fear.

1598 THE NEW ENGLAND JOURNAL OF MEDICINE May 31, 1990

Physicians may have seen patients who in the end were grateful that they had been pressured or even forced to undergo painful or dreaded treatments. The responsibility of the physician in these cases is a difficult one — to respect the different weights people give to avoiding pain and suffering, while helping patients overcome the irrational fear that prevents them from pursuing promising treatment plans. The physician's task will often involve helping patients to distinguish whether they are experiencing a fear that they want to overcome or whether they have made a choice with which they are comfortable.

What the Patient Wants Does Not Make Sense

When competent patients decline a recommended course of treatment because of an obvious and understandable, albeit unusual, belief — Jehovah's Witnesses, for example, who refuse blood transfusions — physicians (and the courts) commonly yield to that belief. When patients request treatment that physicians believe to be ineffective — Asian patients who request "coining," for example — physicians are not obliged to provide it, but they may respect the patients' right to pursue it when medically acceptable treatment is also provided. Special difficulties arise when a seemingly competent patient wants something that does not make sense and is not attributable to a clearly recognizable religious belief or cultural preference. It can be extremely difficult in these situations for the physician to determine the basis of the patient's preference. However unusual, the more the preference seems to reflect a deeply held, enduring value that is important in the patient's life, the stronger the case for respecting it, as long as it does not require that the physician participate in useless or medically unacceptable treatment.

In other cases, what the patient does not care about makes no sense. For example, patients may state that they understand but simply do not care that death or serious disability will result from a refusal of treatment. It may be difficult to determine whether this is an authentic, although unusual, choice, or the result of a distortion of values caused by a treatable condition such as depression.

Framing Effects

It is well known that the way choices are formulated and presented, or framed, can have major effects on decisions.[10] A simple example is the presentation of a surgical treatment as "substantially extending the lives of 70 percent of the patients who select it" or as "potentially killing on the operating table 30 percent of the patients who select it." Both characterizations may be true, but which is used, or emphasized, may have a substantial effect on the rate of selection of the surgery. There is a variety of different and more subtle framing effects, one of which we illustrate below.

Studies in the psychology of choice show that losses tend to loom larger than gains in most people's deci-

sion making. Of course, whether a particular outcome is viewed as a gain or loss depends on the reference point against which the outcome is compared. Many choices in medicine can be framed in either way. For example, lowering moderate hypertension can be presented as adding months to the patient's expected life span or as a way to avoid shortening the life span because of untreated hypertension. Neither framing of the choice before the patient is wrong; each simply relies on different characterizations of the patient's present situation. Tversky and Kahneman[10] have compared the framing effects in decision making to changes in perspective in visual judgments. Which of two mountains appears to be higher, for example, depends on the position from which one views them. There is, of course, an objective standard by which the height of the mountains can be determined, but there appears to be no objectively correct way to frame many medical choices, such as that facing the patient with moderate hypertension. There are simply two different but correct ways to frame the choice, and the one that is used will influence whether some patients choose treatment. Sometimes, the best that physicians can do is present the choice in alternative ways in the hope of minimizing framing effects.

Individual versus Social Rationality

The Irrational Use of Resources

The circumstances that make individual choices rational can sometimes make the outcome of those choices irrational when viewed from a different perspective.[11] One factor fueling the intense pressure to control rapidly rising health care costs is the perception that resources are often used in circumstances in which their expected benefits do not justify their true costs. An insured patient has little or no economic incentive to weigh the true costs of medical care against its expected benefits. When patients have no out-of-pocket costs, it is rational for them to choose all the care that has any expected medical benefit, no matter how small or costly. If physicians accept the common professional norm that their obligation is to do whatever may benefit their patients, without regard to cost, then it is also rational for them to ignore the cost of care in making recommendations and decisions about treatment. The result will be the overuse of health care as compared with other goods and services whose benefits are weighed against their true costs. From the perspective of those who pay the insurance premiums (employers or the government, for example), the result is an irrational overallocation of resources to health care.

The issues raised by this form of irrational social choice involving the use of resources are very different from those involved in the forms of irrational patient choice previously discussed. It would be a mistake for physicians to seek to persuade insured patients that choosing care that is not cost effective is irrational. On the contrary, an insured patient's choice of such care is rational, but it leads to an irrational overallocation of resources to health care. Since the irrationality is not at the level of the insured patient's choice of treatment, the principal response to it cannot be at that level. A physician's failure to respect an insured patient's choice of such care on the grounds that it is irrational is not justifiable. Instead, the irrationality must be addressed where it exists — in the social and economic system of health care financing.

Public Health versus Individual Benefit

Often, physicians are concerned about the public health benefits of medical interventions, whereas their patients are not. For example, national campaigns to reduce serum cholesterol levels will clearly benefit the health of the country as a whole. However, the chance of a substantial benefit in a given patient may be very small. Consequently, some people may rationally decide that for them the benefits of the intervention do not outweigh its burdens. This distinction between community-wide and individual benefits has been called the "prevention paradox"; in it, a treatment that brings large benefits to the community may not seem worth the trouble to individual participants.[12] There is no true paradox, however. The existence of a society-wide benefit constitutes no reason to view as irrational an individual's choice to decline an intervention.

For some infectious diseases, preventing infection through the vaccination of one person (or shortening the period of transmissibility through treatment) lessens the risk of disease for others. A patient's or parent's refusal to accept immunization may be rational if the patient or parent is not concerned about the risks for others or believes that because enough of the population is immunized, the threat of the disease is minimal and the risks of immunization outweigh the benefits. In this case, for the protection of others, society may adopt mandatory immunization programs or physicians may seek to change the patient's mind. Patients do not have an unqualified right to make even rational individual choices that risk serious harm to others.

WHAT SHOULD PHYSICIANS DO?

Shared decision making respects the patient's right of self-determination but does not require that the patient's preferences be simply accepted when they are irrational. In most cases, it is appropriate for physicians to attempt to persuade competent patients to reconsider their irrational choices. However, distinguishing irrational preferences from those that simply express different attitudes, values, and beliefs can be difficult in both theory and practice. Physicians need to be sensitive to the complexity of these judgments in helping patients to make sound treatment choices. They must also bear in mind that even truly irrational choices are not sufficient to establish a patient's in-

competence and to justify overriding them. The taxonomy of irrational treatment choices we have presented here (and expand on elsewhere[13]) is meant to be a beginning guide for further consideration of the issue. More research is needed on the frequency of irrational treatment choices and their different forms, as well as on how physicians and patients can work together to overcome them.

DAN W. BROCK, PH.D.

Brown University
Providence, RI 02912   STEVEN A. WARTMAN, M.D., PH.D.

REFERENCES

1. President's Commission for the Study of Ethical Problems in Medicine and Biomedical and Behavioral Research. Making health care decisions: the ethical and legal implications of informed consent in the patient-practitioner relationship. Vol. 1. Washington, D.C.: Government Printing Office, 1982.
2. Forrow L, Wartman SA, Brock DW. Science, ethics, and the making of clinical decisions. JAMA 1988; 259:3161-7.
3. Buchanan AE, Brock DW. Deciding for others: the ethics of surrogate decisionmaking. Cambridge: Cambridge University Press, 1989.
4. Pauker SG, Kassirer JP. Decision analysis. N Engl J Med 1987; 316:250-8.
5. Katz J. Why doctors don't disclose uncertainty. Hastings Cent Rep 1984; 14(1):35-44.
6. Parfit D. Reasons and persons. Oxford: Oxford University Press, 1984.
7. Tversky A, Kahneman D. Judgment under uncertainty: heuristics and biases. Science 1974; 185:1124-31.
8. Gillick MR. Talking with patients about risk. J Gen Intern Med 1988; 3:166-70.
9. Cassell EJ. The relief of suffering. Arch Intern Med 1983; 143:522-3.
10. Tversky A, Kahneman D. The framing of decisions and the psychology of choice. Science 1981; 211:453-8.
11. Menzel PT. Medical costs, moral choices: a philosophy of health care economics in America. New Haven, Conn.: Yale University Press, 1983.
12. Rose G. Strategy of prevention: lessons from cardiovascular disease. BMJ 1981; 282:1847-51.
13. Kassirer JP, ed. Current therapy in internal medicine. 3rd ed. Philadelphia: B.C. Decker, 1990.

[31]

ON PSYCHIATRY AND SOULS:
WALKER PERCY AND THE ONTOLOGICAL
LAPSOMETER

CARL ELLIOTT*

> Who of us is not so strangely alone that it is the cool clinical touch of the
> stranger that serves best to treat his loneliness?—WALKER PERCY

> The human body is the best picture of the human soul.—LUDWIG
> WITTGENSTEIN

Psychiatry occupies a curious place among the medical disciplines. In
most disciplines, specialists can behave as if (or at least pretend that)
theirs is a specialty concerned with physiological mechanisms and facts:
facts that may be difficult to uncover, for reasons to do with the patient's
obstinance, self-deception, or ignorance, or even facts that may be mys-
teriously influenced (physiologically) by the patient's state of mind; but
facts that, nonetheless, can be explained and treated best within a framework that employs the language of medical biology.

Psychiatrists, on the other hand, have no such luxury. Unlike the
mechanisms of the body, human thought and behavior seem to resist
analysis in purely biological terms. Of course, this has not deterred psychiatrists from trying to make psychiatry more like other medical disciplines; indeed, biological psychiatry has had some remarkable successes,
and many psychiatrists optimistically hope that, sometime in the future,
psychiatry will become a science at least as exact as other medical sciences. But for now, at least, psychiatry remains clouded by the opacities
and uncertainties that mark human thought and behavior, and psychia-

This paper grew out of separate conversations with Grant Gillett and Bruce Charlton,
both of whom suggested some of its central themes. The author is also grateful to Daniel
Fort, who first introduced him to the novels of Walker Percy. This paper was written at
the University of Otago Bioethics Research Centre, Dunedin, New Zealand.

*Department of Medical Humanities, East Carolina University School of Medicine,
Brody Medical Science Building, Greenville, North Carolina 27858.

trists, unless they abandon all contact with patients, must operate within a conceptual framework that, more than any other, considers not only the language of biochemistry and neuroendocrinology but also the language of ordinary human life.

In his social satire *Love in the Ruins*, Walker Percy takes aim at many targets—American politics, Southern manners, euthanasia, sex therapy, racism, and religious fundamentalism, to name but a few. But his focus is clearest when he turns it toward the modern exaltation of science and technology that he sees manifested in the biological pretensions of present-day psychiatry. Educated as a physician, and practicing as a pathologist before he turned to literature and philosophy, Percy writes with respect for the accomplishments of science and the elegance of its methods. But he is deeply suspicious of the attitudes that science can engender. One important theme that emerges in *Love in the Ruins* is the tension between, on the one hand, the attitudes and assumptions of science, and, on the other, those that operate within the relationships between human beings.

I

Subtitled "The Adventures of a Bad Catholic at a Time Near the End of the World," *Love in the Ruins* is narrated by Tom More, an alcoholic psychiatrist and self-described "lapsed Catholic," who writes from Feliciana Parish in the Louisiana bayous at a time when apocalypse seems imminent. The reason for this imminent danger has to do with Tom More himself—or rather, with one of his inventions, which has fallen into the wrong hands. As More relates:

For I have reason to believe that within the next two hours an unprecedented fallout of noxious particles will settle hereabouts and perhaps in other places as well. It is a catastrophe whose cause and effect—and prevention—are known only to me. The effects of the evil particles are psychic rather than physical. They do not burn the skin and rot the marrow; rather do they inflame and worsen the secret ill of the spirit and rive the very self from itself. If a man is already prone to anger, he'll go mad with rage. If he lives affrighted, he'll quake with terror. If he's already abstracted from himself, he'll be sundered from himself and roam the world like Ishmael. [1].

The invention that More believes will cause this psychic fallout is the More Qualitative-Quantitative Ontological Lapsometer. The Lapsometer is a diagnostic instrument developed by More, a "stethoscope of the human soul." Just as a stethoscope or an EEG diagnoses the infirmities of the body, More's Ontological Lapsometer can measure the ills of the spirit. Alienation, angst, terror, depression, rage—"In fact," says More, "with this device in hand any physician can make early diagnoses of potential suicides, paranoiacs, impotence, stroke, anxiety and angelism/ bestialism. Think of the significance of it!"

More relates the case history of Ted Tennis, "a well-educated, somewhat abstracted graduate student who suffered from massive free-floating terror, identity crisis, and sexual impotence." "Every psychiatrist knows the type," says More: "the well-spoken slender young man who recites his symptoms with precision and objectivity—so objective that they seem to be somebody else's symptoms—and above all with that eagerness, don't you know, as if nothing would please him more than that his symptom, his dream, should turn out to be a textbook case. *Allow me to have a proper disease, Doctor*, he all but tells me."

Tennis suffers from "daytime terror and nighttime impotence." More passes the lapsometer over his head and takes a reading:

He registered a dizzy 7.6 mmv over Brodmann 32, the area of abstractive activity. Since that time I have learned that a reading over 6 generally means that a person has so abstracted himself from himself and from the world around him, seeing things as theories and himself as a shadow, that he cannot, so to speak, reenter the lovely ordinary world. Instead he orbits the world and himself. Such a person, and there are millions, is destined to haunt the human condition like the Flying Dutchman.

Because he has not yet hit on a therapeutic breakthrough for "angelism"—excessive abstraction of the self from itself"—More must rely on a rough-and-ready, short-term cure; he instructs Tennis to walk home 6 miles through the swamp. The only treatment for angelism is "recovery of the self through ordeal." And that evening, Tennis arrives home, "half-dead of fatigue, having been devoured by mosquitoes, leeches, vampire bats, tsetse flies, snapped at by alligators, moccasins, copperheads, chased by Bantu guerillas and once even cuffed about by a couple of Michigan State dropouts on a bummer who mistook him for a parent." The treatment was successful; "half-dead and stinking like a catfish, he fell into the arms of his good wife, Tanya, and made lusty love to her the rest of the night."

The source of More's worries about his Lapsometer is a mysterious, Mephistophelian character called Art Immelman, who claims to be a government liaison interested in funding More's new instrument. After a bit of tinkering, Immelman converts the Lapsometer into an instrument not only of diagnosis but also of treatment: a means of curing spiritual ills with ionizing radiation. Immelman approaches More in the hospital men's room and offers to demonstrate this new development. He aims the Lapsometer at More's "red nucleus"; More's readings jump up a few notches on the anxiety scale. He reports: "My shoulders are rounded and I am gazing at my hands clenched in my lap. At last I raise my eyes. A horrid white light streams through the frosted window and falls into the glittering porcelain basins of the urinals. It is the

Terror, but tolerable. The urinals, which are the wall variety, are shaped like skulls."

Immelman then reverses the Lapsometer, beaming negative ions at More's skull. The lapsometer hums against his head. "When I open my eyes, I am conscious first of breathing. Something in my diaphragm lets go. I realize that I've been breathing at the top of my lungs for forty-five years. . . . Then I notice a hand clenched into a fist on my knee. I open it slowly, turning it this way and that, inspecting every pore and crease. What a beautiful strong hand! The tendons! The bones! But the hand of a stranger! I have never seen it before."

Like most of Percy's novels, *Love in the Ruins* is a book about people who feel ill at ease in the world, and, perhaps more importantly, about whether it might not be still worse not to feel ill at ease. (The epigraph for Percy's first book, *The Moviegoer,* was a remark by Kierkegaard: ". . . the specific character of despair is precisely this: it is unaware of being despair.") In contrast to his other novels, however, *Love in the Ruins* is about the perils and absurdities of a certain way of looking at such problems, that of seeing spiritual ills as psychiatric disorders. To hold such a view is to misunderstand profoundly the nature of these spiritual ailments, and at least part of Percy's aim in *Love in the Ruins* is to show us why this is so.

II

It is a platitude that medicine is an art as well as a science, and the extraordinary growth of medical technology over the past half-century has prompted fear in many humanistically minded clinicians that medicine has swung much too far toward the scientific-technological. The cost of that swing has been a deteriorating relationship between physicians and patients, a shift that has left both parties uneasy about the state of present-day medical practice. As the surgeon and author Richard Selzer says: "You don't have to ask your patients anything. You order a hundred blood tests, get a hundred X-rays, hook them up to the machinery, and you don't have to look at them or ask them questions. . . . It's a different thing entirely. It's a mechanical, technical, more brilliant process, for which I am not at all suited" [2].

Nonetheless, despite the cost to the personal relationship between physicians and patients, technological medicine has had spectacular success in curing and controlling disease. And whatever the advantages of a closer understanding between doctors and patients, few of us, when faced with life-threatening or debilitating illness, would hesitate to trade that understanding for technical excellence. Its flaws notwithstanding, the biomedical approach to disease continues to achieve a sounder understanding of the ills and frailties of the human body.

Essential to this approach is a view of the human body as a mechanism. The task of biomedical science is to discover the pathophysiological mechanisms that underlie disease and dysfunction and then to devise a remedy. The task of medical practitioners is to diagnose, by observing signs and symptoms, and to treat, using the appropriate technology, the diseases and dysfunctions that underlie the problems of a particular patient. The practitioner may have other tasks—comfort, friendship, emotional support—that may or may not influence this underlying pathophysiology. Some of these tasks may be morally obligatory, no matter what their influence. But regardless of these additional tasks, modern medicine has built whatever success it has achieved largely on mechanistic foundations—the human body as a vast, elaborate, and sometimes mysterious machine.

This mechanistic approach to the human body underlies the peculiar status of psychiatry as a medical discipline. To see something mechanistically—be it a body, a brain, or a blender—is to take up a certain attitude toward it, an attitude that entails certain beliefs, preconceptions, and ways of behaving. This attitude is difficult to reconcile with much of the subject matter of psychiatry, which is concerned largely with human relationships and problems in living.

Some of these difficulties are simply the result of the assumptions that underlie science. To see something as an object of scientific inquiry is to see it as a product of causal forces, something to be tested, probed, and experimented on for the purposes of prediction and control. Most of us are able quite easily to picture the human body in this way, and even the human brain. This is not, of course, the way that we *ordinarily* see our bodies, and to see our bodies as objects of scientific inquiry may require that we suspend our ordinary attitudes. A clinician shifts from his ordinary attitude toward the body to a mechanistic one the moment he enters the examining room. But it is much more difficult to take up this scientific attitude (at least for very long) toward human behavior. No matter how hard we try to see behavior as the product of causal forces, governed by the laws of nature, and no matter how tempting such a view may be in clinically controlled, laboratory conditions, it is difficult to take the scientific attitude toward human behavior as it occurs, so to speak, in nature: people falling in love, telling stories, playing baseball, saying prayers.

A more important reason for the difficulties in reconciling psychiatry and mechanism relates to the contrast between what Strawson has called "reactive" and "objective attitudes" [3, 4]. Reactive attitudes are those attitudes that we take toward other human beings and that govern our relationships with them: "the non-detached attitudes and reactions of people directly involved with each other," such as "gratitude, resentment, forgiveness, love, and hurt feelings." Reactive attitudes are the currency of human life, and we attach great importance to them—both the attitudes that we take toward others, and the attitudes that they take toward us. As Strawson says:

We should think of the many different kinds of relationship we can have with other people—as sharers of a common interest; as members of the same family; as colleagues; as friends; as lovers; as chance parties to an enormous range of transactions and encounters. And then we should think, in each of these transactions in turn, and in others, of the kind of importance we attach to the attitudes and intentions towards us on the part of those who stand in these relationships to us, and of the kinds of *reactive* attitudes and feelings to which we are prone. [3]

Though much of ordinary life is characterized by these reactive attitudes, we are also able to take toward other human beings another sort of attitude, profoundly opposed to the first. To take an *objective* attitude toward another human being is to see him or her as an object—of social policy, of scientific inquiry, of medical treatment, or of many other things. The objective attitude may even be emotionally colored in some ways. According to Strawson, "[i]t may include repulsion or fear, it may include pity or even love, though not all kinds of love." However, to take the objective attitude is to abandon the reactive attitudes that characterize our ordinary relationships with other human beings, such as forgiveness, resentment, gratitude, and a certain sort of love. As Strawson puts it: "If your attitude toward someone is wholly objective, then though you may fight him, you cannot quarrel with him, and though you may talk to him, you cannot reason with him. You can at most pretend to quarrel, or reason, with him."

To some extent we all take the objective attitude toward human beings who are immature or mentally disordered or handicapped beyond a certain degree. We suspend, for example, our ordinary judgments of responsibility, praise, and blame. Less often, we take this attitude toward normal, mature individuals—perhaps as a way of studying them. But as Strawson notes, "what is above all interesting is the tension there is, in us, between the participant attitude and the objective attitude. One is tempted to say: between our humanity and our intelligence. But to say this would be to distort both notions."

Psychiatry straddles the border between objective and reactive attitudes, between our intelligence and our humanity. Like any other medical practitioner, the psychiatrist must look upon the patient as an object of inquiry and treatment; to do any less would be to do something other than psychiatry. But to an extent much greater than in the other medical specialties, the psychiatrist must also remain aware and take account of the reactive attitudes that characterize human life outside the therapeutic relationship. The encounter between a patient and his or her psychiatrist is a much different affair than that between, say, a patient and a surgeon. It bears a far greater resemblance, at least superficially, to those encounters that are familiar from ordinary human life. The balance between the reactive and the objective is a fragile one, and some psychiatrists are better at maintaining it than others. Many of us have had the slightly eerie experience of suspecting that we are being clinically examined during an ordinary conversation with a psychiatrist—the result of an inappropriate "I see," or "tell me more about that," or "and how did that make you feel?"

Percy's Ontological Lapsometer is comic precisely because it exploits the pretensions of the behavioral sciences toward objectivity; it objectifies those aspects of our experience that are most resistant to analysis in scientific terms. With the Lapsometer in hand, any physician can "probe the very secrets of the soul, diagnose the maladies that poison the wellsprings of man's hope" [1]. It is the same aspiration toward scientific objectivity that seems to underlie the jargon that behavioral scientists invent to describe the intercourse of ordinary life—jargon that, no matter how effective a means of communication between professionals, seems peculiarly inappropriate when we try to apply it to our own experience. As Percy says elsewhere, "Take these two sentences that I once read in a book on mental hygiene: 'The most profound of all human needs, the prime requisite for successful living, is to be emotionally inclusive. Socrates, Jesus, Buddha, St. Francis were emotionally inclusive.' These words tremble with anxiety and alienation, even though I would not deny that they are, in their own eerie way, true" [5].

The attitude of objectivity is one that all clinicians must, at certain points in the clinical encounter, take toward their patients, but for several reasons the objective attitude is a delicate one for psychiatrists. First, the means by which psychiatrists diagnose mental disorders is the same means by which they conduct the intercourse of ordinary life. Language is the psychiatrist's diagnostic instrument—the medium for objective attitudes as well as reactive. Laboratory medicine, radiology, and physical diagnosis are largely (but not, of course, entirely) outside the psychiatrist's typical diagnostic armamentarium. Psychiatric diagnosis involves an intricate interplay of words, hints, cues, and gestures, similar to the language that we all use to conduct our lives but put to a different task. As Percy states, "The psychiatrist not only enters into a conversation as other people do; he also preserves a posture of objectivity from which he takes note of the patient's behavior, and his own, according to the principles of his science" [6].

Second, the relationship between psychiatrist and patient is itself a focus of objective attitudes. The relationship of most clinicians to their patients is simply a *means* of getting at the patient's problems—a means by which to diagnose and treat. In contrast, the relationship of a psychiatrist to his or her patient is not only such a means; it is also a proper object of study. The psychiatrist is interested not only in the patient's life outside the clinic; he is also interested in the relationship that he and the patient share. This also sets the psychiatrist apart from many other behavioral scientists. Percy remarks, "The social psychologist studies the interactions of person and groups. But the psychiatrist is largely concerned with the 'interaction' between the patient and himself. And so the psychiatrist has come to be called the 'participant observer'" [6].

Third, insofar as a psychiatrist uses psychotherapy, he or she must maintain a balance between objective and reactive attitudes not only in diagnosis but also in treatment. For most nonpsychiatric practitioners, the border between objective and reactive attitudes in their treatment is clear. They treat illness or disability with drugs, surgery, radiotherapy, or whatever, and they also provide encouragement, emotional support, and guidance. Technological treatment requires an objective attitude; emotional support requires a reactive one. Both sorts of treatment and attitudes seem necessary for healing (although the reasons may sometimes be obscure). On the other hand, the psychiatrist, whose therapeutic tool may be largely or entirely psychotherapy, must treat the patient in a manner that combines both reactive and objective attitudes. The patient must be thought of as an object of treatment, but he or she cannot be thought of solely as an object; part of the reason that psychotherapy is effective is that the patient is treated as a person, a proper focus of reactive attitudes.

There is a tendency in medicine to devalue those aspects of practice that are not easily manipulated by technological means. Psychiatrists know all too well that within the typical U.S. medical school hierarchy, psychiatry falls near the bottom. Even practitioners who are very sensitive to the emotional needs of their patients tend to see this aspect of medical practice as something intuitive and scientifically soft: the so-called art of medicine. As a physician, Percy was very familar with this prejudice. "Unfortunately, there still persists in the medical profession the quaint superstition that only the visible is real. Thus the soul is not real. Uncaused terror cannot exist. Then, friend, how come you are shaking?" [1]

In psychiatry itself there is much controversy over whether to embrace a biological or a psychodynamic model of psychiatric practice. Implicit in a biological model is the assumption that most or many psychiatric disorders are the result of neurochemical abnormalities and that psychiatric research will eventually discover a way of rectifying these abnormalities, probably by chemical means. Percy's Ontological Lapsometer parodies the biological approach by taking it to its logical extension—electrochemically measuring the human soul, treating its ailments with ionized "heavy sodium."

A prominent U.S. psychiatrist, Samuel Guze, recently wrote: "[T]here is no such thing as a psychiatry which is too biological" [7]. By this he meant to respond to the criticism that a biologically based psychiatry was in some way inadequate or incomplete, and he followed his assertion with a broad sketch of the way in which all of human life, culture, and society can be thought of as the result of vast, complex permutations of human brain function. In one sense Guze is certainly right; if we view biology as the study of life, then the charge that psychiatry can be too biological would be an odd one. But surely to defend biological psychiatry on these grounds is to miss the point of the criticism.

Biological psychiatry has come into its own largely as a result of greater scientific knowledge about neurotransmitter function and the development of psychopharmacological agents: the phenothiazines, tricyclic antidepressants, lithium, and the MAO inhibitors. The impressive results of these investigations into brain function have meant that psychiatrically disordered patients now have a far greater chance of being successfully treated than they had in the past. But the aim of most critics of biological psychiatry, including Percy, is not to challenge the results of biological investigation, now or in the future; nor is it to question the therapeutic worth of psychopharmacological agents. Rather, the point of the criticism is to question whether the subject matter of psychiatry can be completely and fully explained in biological terms.

Psychiatry certainly has to do with things such as dopamine and acetylcholine—but it also has to do with things like worrying, teasing, and grieving, with getting married, losing a job, and joining the marines. The problem for biological psychiatry is to explain things like the latter in terms of the former. Now, it is no doubt possible to devise an explanation of some sort—to account for the notion of "worry" in terms of brain function, in the same way that it may be possible to account for my experience of listening to Tommy Dorsey's rendering of "I'm Getting Sentimental over You" in terms of its effects on my ears, my acoustic nerves, and my brain. But the point is that an explanation of a biological sort, simply by virtue of its being biological, will not be able to account for all of the subject matter of psychiatry—at least not in the way that we wish to have it explained.

Much philosophical history has been built on the difficulties that emerge when we try to explain phenomena of one sort with the vocabulary of another. Percy was himself well aware of the troubled history of the philosophy of mind—of the difficulties of explaining the mind with the vocabulary of the brain, of explaining free will within the framework of causal laws. In *Love in the Ruins* More puts up his Lapsometer as the culmination of this history: "the first hope of bridging the dread chasm that has rent the soul of Western man ever since the famous philosopher Descartes ripped body loose from mind and turned the very soul into a ghost that haunts its own house" [1].

But it is not at all clear whether biological psychiatry can ever realize its implicit agenda—treating all psychiatric disorders by correcting neurochemical function. One reason is that even if we know all that there is to know about neurochemistry, we cannot explain everything about human behavior that is relevant to psychiatric disorders within the vocabulary of neurochemistry. Much of our interest in and knowledge of human behavior derives from a context much wider than neurochemistry: the context of human life and culture. Neurochemical and anatomical explanations are obviously related to psychological, anthropological, and humanistic explanations, and they do seem, in some sense, more basic—but it would be naive to assume that all other descriptions of human life can ultimately be reduced to the vocabulary of brain function [8].

For one thing, psychiatry is concerned with the human being not only as an object but also as a subject of experience. Psychiatrists have the difficult task of reconciling what they know about human beings, so to speak, from "the outside"—their behavior, their neuroanatomy and neurophysiology, their language—with what it is like to be a human being "from the inside." It is debatable whether combining the subjective and the objective points of view is conceptually possible [9]. But it is clear that the subjective point of view cannot be discounted. Biological psychiatrists are in danger of forgetting that our interest in psychiatry arises largely from our interest in what it is like to be a human being.

A second problem for biological psychiatry is the fact that much of the vocabulary by which we describe and understand human mental life is logically interwoven into a much wider context than that of brain events [10]. It is impossible to understand beliefs, desires, and intentions—not to mention fear, hope, love, and anxiety—apart from the broader setting in which they occur. These are concepts that have evolved within a certain form of human life, and they make sense only against the backdrop of that life. Speaking of fear and remorse apart from the setting of human life is as unintelligible as speaking of bishops and checkmates apart from the game of chess. The concept "checkmate" is interwoven with a variety of other concepts, such as "king," "chessboard," "game," and "rule," to the extent that some understanding of all of them is necessary for an understanding of any of them. In like fashion, the concept of "fear" or "remorse" or "love" will not be intelligible without some understanding of the setting in which people feel "fear" or "remorse," or "love," and the vast array of related concepts with which they are intertwined.

A third problem is simply thast scientific explanations are often causal ones, and our interest in human behavior is not always an interest in causes. Suppose that I encounter, as I once did as a medical student, a patient whom I believe to be psychotic, and who has been brought to the hospital by the police for attending classical music concerts in his pajamas, without a ticket, drinking Johnny Walker Black Label Scotch whisky. When he is interviewed, I notice that he has a shirt pocket full of shaving cream, which he eats from time to time. I ask him about the reason he has been brought to the hospital; he walks over to the attending psychiatrist and begins to tug gently on this man's necktie. I probe further, and he says something to the effect: "Black is black? Reds are trump. I can't tell—yes or no?"

Now this patient's behavior and his bizarre speech may or may not eventually be explainable causally—in terms of genetics, neurochemistry, environmental factors, and so on. But even if this information allowed me to identify the causes of his actions and predict them infallibly, I will still not have understood his behavior or his speech; they will still not be intelligible to me. Understanding his behavior is more than understanding what caused it; it is placing his actions in some sort of wider context, establishing some sort of communicative link, seeing what it might be like to be in his situation, establishing some sort of kinship with him, understanding his reasons for acting and answering as he did (if he can be said to have reasons). This is why psychotic behavior seems so intriguing and mysterious: not because we do not understand its causes, but because it appears so disconcertingly alien [11]. We cannot understand the severely psychotic because we cannot take the same sort of attitude toward them as we do toward ordinary human beings.

In his *Philosophical Investigations*, Wittgenstein makes the remark: "My attitude towards him is an attitude towards a soul. I am not of the *opinion* that he has a soul" [12]. A least part of what Wittgenstein is getting at with this cryptic comment is that our attitudes toward and relationships with other human beings are of a certain character, and that this character is different from that of our attitudes toward other things or beings. Our attitudes toward persons are attitudes toward souls. This does not mean that we have any beliefs about an immaterial substance that distinguishes humans from other beings—"I am not of the *opinion* that he has a soul"—but it does mean that we have certain ways of describing and understanding human behavior that are distinct from our ways of describing and understanding anything else.

To understand another "soul" is partly, of course, to understand the relationships that human beings enter into with each other—as friends, rivals, colleagues, confessors—and the sorts of activities that characterize those relationships—playing, celebrating, pretending, cheating. But it is also to understand those aspects of human life that we often call, for lack of a better word, spiritual. To speak of the spiritual, of souls, is to speak not only of the religious but also of those things that surround a unique part of human life—that part of life where we speak of reverence and transcendence, and of alienation, meaninglessness, and absurdity. A person's soul is not just his mind, or his brain, or even his psyche; it is his self. Soul implies—among other things—depth, moral constitution, one's true nature. Thus, when Percy speaks of treating the ailments of the soul, he is not simply speaking metaphorically; "spiritual illness" is the best description of an aspect of human life recognizable to all of us.

Like those in most theoretical disciplines, psychiatrists are often tempted to consider their subject within the simplest possible conceptual framework. Thus some psychiatrists are inclined to think of psychiatric problems as a peculiar set of biological problems; others, like the so-called anti-psychiatrists, argue that psychiatric problems are no more than the problems of life. Most psychiatrists realize that the truth falls somewhere between these two extremes. Most psychiatric problems are not simply medical, or even social or psychological. In Harry Stack Sullivan's words, "psychiatry deals with living" [13]—and so psychiatric problems are also spiritual problems, ailments of the soul. It may be that these problems are the inevitable consequence of human existence: of the sort of life in which one is able to step back and compare the way life is and the way one would like it to be. Perhaps psychiatrists are no better equipped to treat such problems than anyone else. But these ailments of the soul are so closely tied to the problems that psychiatrists encounter that they cannot be ignored. In Percy's words, these ailments are "the new plague, the modern Black Death, the current hermaphroditism of the spirit, namely: More's syndrome, or: chronic angelism-bestialism that rives soul from body and sets it orbiting the great world as the spirit of abstraction whence it takes the form of beasts, swans and bulls, werewolves, blood-suckers, Mr. Hydes, or just poor lonesome ghost locked in its own machinery" [1].

REFERENCES

1. Percy, W. *Love in the Ruins.* New York: Farrar, Straus & Giroux, 1971.
2. Joseph, P. An interview with Richard Selzer. *Med. Humanities Rev.* 5:24–40, 1991.
3. Strawson, P. Freedom and Resentment. In *Freedom and Resentment and Other Essays.* London: Methuen, 1974.
4. Gillett, G. "Reactive and objective attitudes in psychiatry," unpublished manuscript, 1990.
5. Percy, W. The man on the train. In *The Message in the Bottle.* New York: Farrar, Straus & Giroux, 1975.
6. Percy, W. The symbolic structure of interpersonal process. In *The Message in the Bottle.* New York: Farrar, Straus & Giroux, 1975.
7. Guze, S. Biological psychiatry: is there any other kind? *Psychol. Med.* 19: 315–323, 1989.
8. Charlton, B. A critique of biological psychiatry. *Psychol. Med.* 20:3–6, 1990.

9. NAGEL, T. "What is it like to be a bat?" *Mortal Questions.* Cambridge: Cambridge Univ. Press, 1979.
10. DILMAN, I. Wittgenstein on the soul. In *Understanding Wittgenstein.* London: Macmillan, 1974.
11. JOHNSTON, P. *Wittgenstein and Moral Philosophy.* London: Macmillan, 1989.
12. WITTGENSTEIN, L. *Philosophical Investigations,* translated by G. E. M. ANSCOMBE. New York: Macmillan, 1958.
13. SULLIVAN, H. S. *The Interpersonal Theory of Psychiatry.* London: Tavistock, 1955.

GNATCATCHER BY LEATHERWOOD CREEK

Airy treetop wheezer,
Peevish eye-ringed screamer,
Frantic small-feathered scolder
Flipping anger with energetic throat
And tail to us harmless stoneskippers
Wading in near, pristine stream;
Darting to teacup nest
Of inner bark, lichens, tendrils dried,
Entangled, mortared by insect down
And spiderweb, saddled
Aback a beech limb so high
We should never have noticed
Up there in our water play
Had she not told us
Where she and spotted eggs live.

ERIC L. DYER

British Journal of Psychiatry (1993), **162**, 801–810

Philosophy and Practice

Concepts of Disease and the Abuse of Psychiatry in the USSR

K. W. M. FULFORD, A. Y. U. SMIRNOV and E. SNOW

There is a strong prima facie case linking the abuse of psychiatry with difficulties about the concept of mental illness. However, a survey of recent Soviet literature showed that the concept of disease employed in the former USSR (where abuse was for a time widespread) was similar to its counterparts in the UK and USA in being strongly scientific in nature. A number of factors – legal, bureaucratic and professional – are important in abuse becoming widespread. These, however, fail to explain why psychiatry, rather than physical medicine, should be vulnerable to abuse. It is here that the concept of disease could be important. A scientific model of disease suggests that a significant vulnerability factor is the relatively underdeveloped status of psychiatry as a science. This leaves room for poor standards of scientific work in clinical research and practice, factors which are recognised as important in the Soviet case. In addition to the scientific element, there is an evaluative element of meaning in the concept of disease. Hence a second vulnerability factor could be the evaluatively problematic nature of judgements of mental illness. It is concluded that a failure to recognise this factor greatly increases the vulnerability of psychiatry, not only to gross abuses, but also to inadvertent misuses of involuntary treatment in everyday practice. This conclusion, far from undermining the role of science in psychiatry, is a step towards clarifying its proper role.

With glasnost and perestroika has come official acknowledgement of recent abuses of psychiatry in the former USSR. The issues here are not yet fully resolved (Merskey & Shafran, 1986; Smulevitch, 1989; Shafran *et al*, 1989). But under new legislation, introduced by the Supreme Council of the former Soviet Union under Chairman Gorbachov in 1988, the special hospitals for the criminally insane were transferred from the Ministry of Internal Affairs to the Ministry of Health Care, and many political 'patients' were released. Moreover, a number of psychiatrists have now been prosecuted for false diagnoses (though not of political dissidents) (Koryagin, 1989; *New Scientist*, 1990).

It is well recognised that psychiatry is vulnerable to abuse. In historical times, and in many cultures, the diagnosis of mental illness has been misused, sometimes for personal, sometimes for political ends (Wing, 1978). More recently, allegations of abuse have been made in a number of countries other than the Soviet Union. The motivation for abuse has varied. In Japan, for example, it seems to have been for profit rather than for politics (Totsuka, 1990). But the continuing vulnerability of psychiatry to abuse makes it timely to see what lessons can be learned from the Soviet experience.

The causes of abuse of psychiatry are complex and various. Besides plain corruption, they include social and political pressures, poor standards of clinical training and practice, inadequate procedural checks and balances, and a weak legislature. Factors such as these were certainly important in the Soviet case

(Bloch & Chodoff, 1977). However, they fail to explain the essential vulnerability of psychiatry to abuse. They explain the 'how' but not the 'why' of abuse. They explain how abuse can become widespread in a given case, but they do not explain why psychiatry, rather than some other area of medicine, should be vulnerable to abuse in the first place.

It is the 'why' question we will be specifically concerned with in this paper. Furthermore, we will be concerned with this question mainly from a conceptual point of view. There is a strong prima facie case for believing that conceptual issues may be important. Bloch & Reddaway (1977, ch. 1), for example, cite problems in conceptualising mental illness, and the correspondingly ill-defined boundaries of psychiatry, as key factors in the origins of the abuse of psychiatry in the USSR. Similarly, in relation to particular psychiatric diagnoses, a number of authors have criticised the Soviet use both of particular disease categories such as 'sluggish schizophrenia' and of individual symptoms, such as 'reformist delusions' (Bloch & Reddaway, 1977, ch. 8). Yet the actual connections between the difficulties raised by these concepts and the abuse of psychiatry have generally been left unexamined. This is perhaps the more surprising given the extent of the debate about mental illness in the West (Clare, 1979). We return to this debate later; but what it amounts to is whether psychiatry as a whole is no more than an abuse of the authority of medicine. Much of this argument actually turns on the conceptual question of whether mental illness is a valid extension of the concept of physical illness (Fulford, 1989, ch. 1).

The relevant literature

There is no foolproof or final method for exploring the meanings of the concepts employed in a given area of discourse (Fulford, 1990). Direct linguistic analysis of ordinary usage is perhaps the most reliable approach but was beyond the resources of this study. We undertook instead a sample review of the published literature. Even this presented many difficulties, however. There are no computer-based search facilities in the USSR, and many interesting papers are indeed published in collections for circulation mainly between academic departments. In addition, as in the West, much important material appears not in academic journals but in books, and is thus even less readily accessible to comprehensive review.

Nonetheless, we believe we were able to achieve at least a representative picture from the following sources.

(a) The *Index Medicus* MEDLINE search facility, employing the categories 'concept', 'illness', 'disease', and 'mental illness', appearing either in the title or the subsidiary classification of topics. MEDLINE covers each of the major international Russian language journals including:

(i) the *Journal of the Academy of Medical Science (Vestnik Academii Meditsinskiich Nauk SSSR)*; this journal, rather like the *Lancet* or the *Journal of the American Medical Association*, takes most of the important theoretical papers

(ii) the *Journal of Neuropathology and Psychiatry (Zhurnal Nevropathologii & Psichiatrii)*, roughly equivalent to a combined *British Journal of Psychiatry* and *Journal of Mental Sciences* (psychiatry shared a journal with neurology in the USSR)

(iii) *Soviet Medicine (Sovetskaia Meditsina)* and *Clinical Medicine (Klinicheskaya Meditsina)*, both of which publish review articles and discussion papers, some being consciously intended for Western consumption

(iv) *Archives of Pathology (Archiv Patologii)*, the journal in which the anatomist 1. V. Davydovskii published his influential ideas on the concept of disease.

(b) The general index of the Moscow State Central Medical Library (under the Ministry of Health Care) employing similar categories as for the MEDLINE search.

(c) The folio collection of Samizdat (underground) literature in the Slavonic reading room of the Bodleian Library, Oxford. This material includes a complete copy of all the Samizdat literature from the USSR collected by Munich Radio between 1975 and 1989.

Translation presented no special difficulties, beyond those arising from any attempted transfer of difficult ideas between two languages and cultures. Many key papers are available, at least in summary form, in both Russian and English, and two of us (AYUS and ES) are bilingual.

Findings

We examined the Soviet literature from two main aspects: firstly, from an aspect of simple publication statistics – that is the number of publications and their locations – these being taken to be measures respectively of the level and distribution of interest in the subject; secondly, from an aspect of content – the actual ideas expressed. Our principal finding was that in both respects the Soviet literature was similar to the corresponding literature in the West.

The overall pattern of publications on the concepts of illness and disease in the USSR was found to have run broadly parallel with that in the West. The most influential author was the pathologist, Davydovskii, whose ideas on the concept of disease appeared first in 1962, corresponding approximately with a period of growing interest in these concepts in the West, as well as in the USSR (Akhmedzhanov & Lifshits, 1968; Sil-vestrov, 1968; Aleksakhina, 1968). A second phase of publication, much of which centred around a paper by Vasilenko (1972), followed in the early 1970s (Akhmedzhanov & Lifshits, 1971; Akhmedzhanov, 1973; Vail, 1973; Sarkisov, 1973; Kagermazov, 1973; Vasilenko, 1976). In the 1980s, articles continued to appear, though less frequently (Vlasiuk, 1980; Pavlenko, 1980; Petlenko *et al*, 1984), with a brief upturn towards the end of the decade (Vlasov, 1988; IL-in, 1988; Petrov & Petrov, 1989). There were considerably fewer publications overall in the Soviet literature. However, this is a reflection of the smaller volume of publications in the USSR generally.

Davydovskii's views were published in his influential textbook *Problems of Causality in Medicine* (1962) and in the *Archives of Pathology* (Davydovskii & Silvestrov, 1966). This was during the Kruschev era, a period of partial liberalisation following the fall of Stalin. It was at this time that psychiatric repression of dissidents first became widespread (Koryagin, 1989). Vasilenko's papers, and the literature he provoked, although not directly concerned with abuse, coincided with growing concern among many Soviet psychiatrists, as well as in the West, about the political manipulation of psychiatry in the USSR.

The Samizdat literature was concerned largely with political protest. Psychiatry is widely criticised: there are many accounts of false diagnosis, and calls for reform, but little discussion of conceptual issues. This, of course, stands in contrast to the corresponding anti-psychiatric and anti-medical literature in the West, much of which, as we noted earlier, actually turned on the validity of the concept of mental illness.

Davidovskii was an anatomist and his views on disease, which became the basis of the dominant Soviet school of thought, were strongly biological. Arguing against the view of certain Marxist-Leninist philosophers that disease is essentially a social phenomenon, he noted that there are no external agents (not even infections) which cause disease in all cases (e.g. Davidovskii, 1962, p. 12). It is rather the internal condition of the organism which determines whether or not disease develops when it comes into contact with a pathogen (e.g. Davidovskii, 1962, p. 32). Disease is thus a reaction of the organism to a pathogen, the form of which is governed by such factors as inherited predisposition, age, sex, and previous exposure. Social factors are among the agents which may provoke certain diseases. Similarly, social adaptation may be impaired by disease. But disease is primarily a biological phenomenon, the criteria for which are predominantly anatomical and functional in nature.

The literature in the early 1970s takes up the issue of the criteria of disease in more detail, and this theme continues through to the 1980s. In Vasilenko's 1972 paper, for example, a specifically pathological 'reaction' of the organism is identified with disturbance of functioning. This is in turn defined partly by reference to the normal operation of particular functional systems (e.g. Sarkisov, 1973), partly by reference to the goals of the organism as a whole (e.g. Kagermazov, 1973). Again, social criteria of disturbance of functioning are discussed (e.g. Akhmedzhanov, 1973; Petlenko *et al*, 1984), but the overall emphasis is still on the essentially biological nature of disease. The disease reaction is, at root, a disturbance of bodily structure and functioning (Vasilenko, 1976; Vlasov, 1988; Petrov & Petrov, 1989).

Discussion

As already noted, the most striking feature of the Soviet literature on the concept of disease is its similarity to the corresponding medical literature in the West. The parallel publication statistics suggest that interest in this subject was as lively in the USSR as elsewhere. The Soviet and Western literatures were similar in content also. However, there was more emphasis in the Soviet literature on the reactivity of the organism. Yet the central themes of biological adaptation, of norms of bodily structure and functioning, and of scientific analysis, all echo the so-called 'medical' model that has been favoured by most medical authors in the West (e.g. Roth & Kroll, 1986).

At first sight these similarities are not only striking but remarkable. As noted at the start of this paper, there is a strong prima facie case for a connection between the disease concepts employed in psychiatry and abuse. If the connection is there, however, and important, should we not expect the disease concepts employed respectively in the USSR and the West to be different? After all, much of the anti-psychiatric literature in the West has been based on the premis that mental illness is really a social-evaluative rather than biological-scientific concept. Szasz (1960) was among those who led the field in this respect, emphasising the relatively value-laden nature of mental illness. This, he and others suggested, showed that psychiatric treatment as a whole is no more than a means of social control. Similarly, even among the pro-psychiatry lobby there have been expressions of concern about social criteria of illness. Aubrey Lewis (1955), for example, recognising social causes and consequences of illness, argued, like Davydovskii, against an exclusively social definition of health. A number of doctors, including some who have been concerned with the abuse of psychiatry, have pointed out the difficulties involved in defining disease (Merskey, 1986). But most medical commentators, concerned with the more value-laden nature of mental illness compared with physical illness, have sought simply to 'tidy up' the concept of mental illness by defining it, as they take physical disease concepts to be defined, in terms of purely factual criteria of biological functioning (Boorse, 1975; Kendell, 1975).

What conclusions are to be drawn, therefore, from the finding that Soviet concepts of disease, far from being defined socially, were if anything more exclusively and explicitly biological than their counterparts in the West? Does this mean that the prima facie case notwithstanding, the concept of disease is after all irrelevant to the abuse of psychiatry? There are other possibilities. One is that it is the concept of mental disease, or mental illness, rather than the concept of disease as a whole, that is relevant. This would be consistent with the arguments in the debate about mental illness in the West. Another is that it is only certain sub-categories of mental disease, or particular diagnostic entities, that are relevant. We will consider both these possibilities before returning to the concept of disease, and to two lessons that we believe may be drawn from the Soviet experience.

The concept of mental illness

A first possible explanation, then, for the similarity between Soviet and Western concepts of disease, is that the vulnerability of psychiatry to abuse arises from some feature of the concept specifically of mental illness. This explanation depends on the idea that while the rest of Soviet medicine had been operating with strongly biological criteria of disease, the criteria employed in psychiatry might have been, say, social in nature.

Such an account would certainly be consistent with the position of many anti-psychiatric authors. Szasz's (1960) arguments, for instance, amount to the view that the concept of mental illness is defective precisely because it is different from the concept of physical illness (Fulford, 1989, ch. 1). Furthermore, the particular difference between mental illness and physical illness upon which this argument relies is directly relevant to the case of abuse. For the abuse of psychiatry is an ethical issue; and the key difference between mental illness and physical illness, the difference that gives Szasz's argument its purchase, is that mental illness is a more value-laden concept (Boorse, 1975). As we noted a moment ago, this is why pro-psychiatry authors have sought to 'tidy up' the concept by defining it in purely biological terms.

In the case of Soviet psychiatry, however, there is simply no evidence to support the underlying contention on which this explanation rests. On the contrary, in the Soviet literature as in much of the medical literature in the West, it was generally assumed that mental and physical disease are essentially similar. Snezhnevsky, for example, possibly the most influential Soviet psychiatrist over this period, and one of those whose names are linked with the term 'sluggish schizophrenia', emphasised the biological nature of mental disease (Snezhnevsky, 1971; Snezhnevsky & Vartanyan, 1970). Moreover, he worked closely with Davidovskii, the two actually publishing a joint paper in 1972.

The relevance of particular diagnostic categories

The Soviet system of classification of mental disorders, as employed during the 1960s and 1970s, was different in certain respects from that employed in the West. Furthermore, particular diagnoses ('sluggish schizophrenia', 'paranoid personality reaction'), and indeed particular symptoms ('reformist delusion'), were often associated with cases of abuse (Bloch & Reddaway, 1977). There is thus a clear possibility that the relevant conceptual differences between Soviet and Western psychiatry arise from their respective classifications of mental disorder (Reich, 1991). The same overall concepts of health and disease, and the same concept of mental disease, might thus have been employed, with the abuse of psychiatry arising only from the use of particular diagnostic categories.

Closer inspection shows, however, that differences in psychiatric nosology, although important, are not in themselves sufficient to explain the abuse of psychiatry in the USSR. There are several reasons for this. In the first place, the differences between Soviet and Western classifications of mental disorders are relatively minor, the two systems indeed being derived from common roots in German phenom-enology. Second, the differences, such as they are, are not of a kind that are immediately relevant to abuse: there is more emphasis, for example, in the Soviet classification both on the time course of mental disorders and on their aetiology, but this is firmly within the biological-scientific framework already described. Third, as to the particular diagnostic categories just mentioned, although these figured prominently in cases of abuse, each has its counterpart in the West. Thus, the relatively broad criteria for schizophrenia employed over this period in the USSR have been implicated in abuse (Bloch & Reddaway, 1977), but broad criteria were employed at this time also in the USA (World Health Organization, 1973). The particular criteria employed were indeed different to some extent in the USSR. However, in the International Pilot Study of Schizophrenia, patients diagnosed in Moscow as suffering from sluggish schizophrenia were not found to be normal by Western criteria but reallocated to other disease categories (manic or depressive psychoses and depressive neuroses – World Health Organization, 1973). Broad criteria certainly provide scope for overdiagnosis. But as Wing (1978) noted, the category of sluggish schizophrenia is similar, at least in the description given by Snezhnevsky, to the Western concept of 'latent schizophrenia' (included, for example, in the World Health Organization's ICD–9, published in 1978). Similarly, 'paranoid reactions' are described in Western textbooks in similar terms to those used in the USSR (for example, in the influential third edition of Mayer-Gross *et al*, published in 1969).

The similarities between Soviet and Western diagnostic concepts is illustrated most clearly by the specific symptom of 'reformist delusions'. This has been criticised on various grounds. It has been said that it is only a symptom, while psychiatric diagnoses, such as schizophrenia, should be based on syndromes (Merskey & Shafran, 1986). However, while this is true of schizophrenia, Western psychiatry recognises a range of monosymptomatic delusional disorders, not indeed as varieties of schizophrenia, but as severe mental illnesses in their own right – for example, the Othello syndrome defined by delusions of infidelity (Vauhkonen, 1968). Then again, the symptom has been criticised for its political content (Merskey & Shafran, 1986). But in Western psychiatry, delusions with a political theme are common in a wide variety of mental conditions. Moreover, following Jaspers (1913), and as both Wing (1978) and Bloch & Reddaway (1977) make clear, it is not the content but the form of a belief that is relevant to its status as a delusion. This was indeed emphasised by Snezhnevsky himself in his account of schizophrenia (1971).

The question that is raised by these considerations is what the criteria for delusional beliefs should be. There are philosophical grounds for believing that the criteria to be found in most textbooks are inadequate (Fulford, 1989, ch. 10). In the present case, this is suggested by the fact that where sufficiently detailed records are available, it is just these textbook criteria that were employed in cases of abuse. In Shimanov's account of his 'diagnostic' interviews, for example, it seems that his psychiatrist considered his beliefs (religious beliefs in this case) to be delusional because (consistently with textbook criteria) they appeared in the absence of understandable psychological precursors and were culturally atypical (Bloch & Reddaway, 1977, p. 166). However, the essential point to be taken from all this is that if the issue is indeed one of criteria – if the issue is the criteria by which pathological beliefs (beliefs that are symptoms of mental illness) should be marked out from those that are simply false or merely deviant – then we are brought back by reformist delusions to the central importance of the concept of disease.

The relevance of the concept of disease

We return, therefore, to the possibility that the concept of disease is indeed relevant in some way to the abuse of psychiatry. Before considering this directly, however, we should remind ourselves first of the significance of other factors – political, medico-legal and professional. Such factors, as noted at the start of this paper, were significant in the Soviet case; a relatively bureaucratic administrative and political framework, an absence of judicial review, and a hierarchical medical profession, are among the factors noted in the Samizdat literature and emphasised by Bloch & Reddaway (1977). The essential conservatism of Soviet attitudes was indeed reflected even in the literature on the medical concepts. Criticisms of the dominant view were generally deferential. There was little in the way of open debate, even about the concept of mental illness. There was no anti-establishment literature corresponding to the anti-psychiatric and anti-medical literature of the 1960s and 1970s in the West. Even the Samizdat literature, concerned as it was mainly with political protest, is largely silent on conceptual issues. All this contrasts sharply with the post-perestroika situation. There is now a vigorous anti-psychiatric literature, not, admittedly, from the medical establishment, but appearing in newspapers and magazines. This literature, moreover, like the corresponding anti-medical literature in the 1960s and 1970s in the West, has been strongly critical not only of the institutions and treatment methods of psychiatry, but also of its diagnostic concepts (Novikov, 1988; Gluzman, 1989; Vilensky, 1990).

If social and political factors are important, however, we have still to explain the essential vulnerability of psychiatry to abuse. As we put it earlier, these factors explain the 'how' of abuse but not the 'why' – why psychiatry rather than physical medicine. Concentrating then on the 'why' question, we believe that the striking similarity between the concepts of health and disease in the USSR and the West, far from showing these concepts to be irrelevant, suggests two lessons from the Soviet experience: one concerned with the scientific content of the concept of disease; the other arising from its logical status as a value term.

The scientific content of the concept of disease

The first lesson to be drawn from the similarity between Soviet and Western concepts of disease is that an exclusively scientific model of disease is in itself not a sufficient protection against the abuse of psychiatry. As we saw earlier, a number of authors have argued to the effect that the vulnerability of psychiatry to abuse arises from its relatively underdeveloped status as a science compared with other medical disciplines. What is shown by the Soviet experience, however, is that the conventional response to this which we noted above – the attempted construction of a purely biological-scientific medical 'model' of disease – is not sufficient to protect psychiatry from abuse, Soviet concepts of disease being if anything even more firmly biological and scientific than those employed in the West.

This should not be taken to imply that good science is any less relevant to good practice in psychiatry than in other areas of medicine. On the contrary, diagnosis in psychiatry, as in medicine generally, should be based on accurate and reliable observations combined with a knowledge of clearly defined syndromes and causal relationships established by objective scientific means. The importance of this is underscored by the fact that, in the present state of the development of scientific psychiatry, diagnosis is largely dependent on subjective reports of symptoms rather than on clinical signs and laboratory test results. Such symptoms provide more scope for dissimulation – that is for simply pretending (whether as patient or doctor) that a symptom is present when it is not. This leaves psychiatrists, as in the Soviet case, vulnerable to political and other pressures to make diagnoses of mental illness against their better clinical judgement (Bloch & Chodoff, 1977, ch. 8).

An important vulnerability factor, therefore, for the abuse of psychiatry, is the subjective nature of the observations on which psychiatric diagnosis currently depends. A purely scientific conception of disease, however, would imply that factors of this kind are not only important but sufficient to explain the vulnerability of psychiatry to abuse. But is this really so? After all, with appropriate clinical training the symptoms of mental illness, although subjective, can be identified as reliably as those of physical illness (Clare, 1979). Moreover, the psychiatric profession in the USSR, through its most influential public figures, argued consistently and openly that while mistakes are always possible, a majority of those dissidents who had been diagnosed as mentally ill really were so (Schmidt *et al*, 1973). It would be easy, especially with hindsight, to be sceptical of such avowals – to believe that the leaders of psychiatry in the Soviet Union were involved in no more than propaganda. Yet if this were so, if there were this much room for manoeuvre, it would point rather directly to the limitations of a purely biological-scientific understanding of the concepts of disease as a protection against the abuse of psychiatry.

The logical status of disease as a value term

If science is not sufficient, something more is required to reduce the vulnerability of psychiatry to abuse. This is the second lesson to be drawn from the Soviet experience: diagnosis in medicine depends not just on the facts but on the interpretation that

is placed on the facts. This may seem uncontentious. However, recast this interpretive element in an explicitly non-scientific form, and the positive lesson to be drawn from the Soviet experience is then seen to be that diagnosis in medicine may depend not just on scientific but also on evaluative considerations.

We are thus led back to one of the key issues noted earlier in the debate about mental illness, namely what significance should be attached to the more overtly evaluative connotations of mental illness compared with physical illness. The Soviet experience tends to undermine the positions of both main protagonists on this issue. It undermines the supporters of mental illness for the reasons noted in the last section. The firmly biological-scientific stance of Soviet psychiatry shows that, so far at least as abuse is concerned, attempts to 'tidy up' the concept of mental illness to make it more 'scientific', as the concept of physical illness is supposed to be, are not sufficient. But it also undermines the position of the opponents of mental illness. This is more surprising. At first sight it might seem that any abuse of psychiatry endorses the claims of Szasz and others that the concept of mental illness (being an evaluative concept) is an illegitimate extension of the (supposedly scientific) concept of physical illness. Yet the very pervasiveness of the abuse of psychiatry in the USSR raises in a most acute form the central difficulty with this claim. It begs the question why so apparently radical an extension of the concept of physical illness should have had any plausibility in the first place.

The Soviet experience suggests a third possibility, however. This is that disease concepts in general (physical as well as mental) might be essentially evaluative in nature. Medical sociologists have long argued that lay concepts of disease are value-laden (Sedgwick, 1973). Moreover, there are philosophical arguments to suggest that even in technical contexts (as in medical diagnosis) disease, despite appearances, is an evaluative notion (Fulford, 1989, ch. 2 & 3). There are difficult philosophical issues here. Understood in this way, indeed, the debate about mental illness is a forme fruste of a central debate in ethical theory, the so-called 'is-ought' debate. This debate, which is about the overall logical relationship between facts and values, runs back at least as far as the 18th-century empiricist philosopher David Hume (Warnock, 1967). If the basic idea is right, however, if disease really is an evaluative concept, then the effect of an exclusively scientific interpretation of its meaning (as in the USSR) can be shown actually to increase, rather than decrease, the vulnerability of psychiatry to abuse.

The argument to this conclusion has been set out in detail elsewhere (Fulford, 1989). It runs from the fact that the criteria by which we evaluate typical symptoms of mental illness (such as anxiety) are inherently and legitimately diverse compared with those by which we evaluate typical symptoms of physical illness (such as pain). To put the point another way, people disagree about what is good or bad, welcome or unwelcome, in respect of anxiety to a greater extent than in respect of pain. For most people, anything except the mildest of pain is at best a necessary evil. On the other hand, while some people avoid anxiety, others actively seek it out: they invite the 'buzz' of fear, for example in horror films, or parachute jumping. Thus, where pain is a narrow-band experience, evaluatively speaking, with little scope for individual variation in the way in which it is evaluated, anxiety is a broad-band experience.

Notice that this is not a matter of perception as such – of varying thresholds for the symptom in question, or differing degrees of tolerance. What is material is rather the greater variation in our evaluations (on a scale of good and bad) of a given experience of anxiety compared with a given experience of pain. Notice, too, that this has nothing to do with the absence of scientific criteria: our evaluations are a matter of our psychological make-up. Notice, finally, that this is nothing to do with disease specifically. It is true of our evaluations of anxiety and pain respectively, whether or not on a given occasion they are symptoms of disease. But what this in turn means is that if a diagnosis of disease indeed entails a (negative) value judgement, then there will be greater scope for legitimate disagreement about the diagnosis of mental illness than about the diagnosis of physical illness. A second vulnerability factor, therefore, and one to which the Soviet experience points, is the wider variation in our evaluations of the phenomena by which mental illnesses are typically constituted, compared with those by which physical illnesses are typically constituted.

The difference between mental illness and physical illness in the respective strengths of their evaluative connotations provides further support for this idea. Thus, as Hare (1963), Urmson (1950), and others have pointed out, the evaluative connotations even of all-purpose value terms such as good and bad, vary with context. For a non-medical example, 'good' used of pictures has overtly evaluative connotations whereas used of, for instance, apples, its connotations are mainly descriptive (it implies clean-skinned, sweet, etc.). This is because the criteria for good apples are relatively settled or agreed upon (most people in most contexts consider clean-skinned, sweet etc., apples to be good). Hence, where good is used of apples, as against pictures, its evaluative

connotations are largely eclipsed by the descriptive criteria for the value judgement it expresses. Transferring this argument to medicine then, it can be seen that if disease is a value term, physical illness (with its predominantly descriptive connotations) would be like 'good' used of apples, while mental illness (with its more marked evaluative connotations) would be like 'good' used of pictures.

There is clearly more to be said about all this. A full account would have to consider a wider range of symptoms, both mental and physical; it would have to examine the differences between illness and disease (used here as synonyms); and it would have to consider these terms not just as value terms but as terms expressing a particular kind of value (Fulford, 1989, ch. 8). This last point is especially relevant. Much of the debate about mental illness is concerned, not so much with whether the conditions ordinarily thought of as mental illnesses are bad conditions, as with whether they are bad conditions of a kind legitimately regarded as diseases. The debate, as in the Soviet case, is mad versus bad, or sad, or merely foolish.

However, taking the argument even in this preliminary form, it can be seen how it helps to explain the Soviet experience. On the view now presented, a key difference between physical illness and mental illness is simply the degree to which the criteria for the value judgement expressed by 'disease' are settled or agreed upon in the two cases. On this view, therefore, the interpretive element in the diagnosis of physical illness (to the extent that this involves a value judgement) will generally be uncontentious and hence can be ignored. As a practical simplification, the diagnosis of physical illness can usually be treated as though it were a purely descriptive scientific procedure. By the same token, however, since we tend to differ in the criteria by which we evaluate the symptoms of mental illness, then this same diagnostic simplification will be dangerously misleading in psychiatry. To suppose, on the model of physical illness, that the diagnosis of mental illness is solely a matter of establishing the facts, is actually to deny the very element of evaluation that in this case leads to difficulty. It is to the implications of this for avoiding abuse that we turn in the final part of this discussion.

Implications for avoiding abuse

The view that diagnosis in medicine involves (in part) evaluation may appear to make medical diagnosis a matter merely of personal preferences. As noted earlier, this is what lies behind traditional objections to the idea that health might be a social rather than biological concept. If diagnosis is even in part a matter of evaluation, then it may seem that there is no right or wrong in diagnosis, and hence that the way is left wide open for abuse. Given however the (outline) account in the last section of the way in which value judgements come into medical diagnosis, it can be seen that this would be mistaken.

In the first place, in all those areas of diagnosis (especially in physical medicine) in which the evaluative element is uncontentious, it may safely be ignored. This is the 'practical simplification' noted in the preceding section. There is a view in the philosophy of science to the effect that even scientific concepts are really value-laden (Hesse, 1980); and in ethics too, some have argued that there are no value-free facts from which to proceed (Williams, 1985). It is not arguments of this kind with which we have been concerned here, however. We have assumed that there is at least a part of science which is purely descriptive and that this is important in medicine. But we have argued that the concept of disease involves both descriptive and evaluative elements of meaning. The effect of this is not to undermine the importance of descriptive science in medicine, but to clarify its proper role.

In the second place, as Kopelman (1990) has argued, even where the evaluative element in diagnosis is contentious, the effect of acknowledging it is to reduce, not to increase, the scope for abuse. This is because making this element explicit shows the checks and balances provided by an appropriate political and medico-legal framework for psychiatric diagnosis in a quite different light. The biological-scientific view of the medical concepts entails the idea that this framework is a stop-gap measure, necessary only to the extent that psychiatry is under-developed as a science. Viewed in this way, the involvement of social workers, let alone lawyers, in psychiatry is regarded merely as an unfortunate, if for the time being necessary, encumbrance to the exercise of medical authority.

Recognising the essentially evaluative nature of the medical concepts, on the other hand, shows lay, or non-medical, opinion to be an essential component of good clinical practice in psychiatry. If the ways in which we evaluate mental phenomena are legitimately diverse compared with physical phenomena, then we are all at risk, if not of deliberate abuses of psychiatry, at least of inadvertent misuses (Fulford, 1991). It is true that where the evaluative element in psychiatric diagnosis is genuinely contentious, it may not always be possible for disagreements to be resolved in the way that (in principle) matters of fact may be resolved. There is thus an important sense in which recognising the evaluative element in the medical

concepts does indeed show psychiatric diagnosis to be less determinate than it is often supposed to be (Fulford, 1993). Moreover, this will be especially so with such inherently contentious diagnoses as those involved in involuntary psychiatric treatment. But this means that it is in just these cases, cases in which the value judgements are genuinely contentious, that an open and explicit framework for diagnosis is required. The lesson from the Soviet experience therefore, is that it is by exposing our practice to what Birley (1991) has called the agora (the market place of free exchange of ideas), rather than by sheltering behind an exclusively scientific model of disease, that we can help to reduce the vulnerability of psychiatry to abuse.

Conclusions

The concept of disease used in the former USSR was close to that used in the UK and USA, both being strongly scientific in nature. This points not to conceptual factors being irrelevant to the abuse of psychiatry, but to abuse arising in part from a failure to recognise the evaluative element in the meaning of disease. This is not to say that other factors are unimportant, either in general or in the Soviet case. On the contrary, although we have been concerned specifically with the vulnerability of psychiatry to abuse – with why psychiatry rather than physical medicine should be open to abuse – a number of factors are well recognised to be important in allowing abuse to become widespread: legal, political, bureaucratic, and professional. Moreover, specifically as a vulnerability factor, the relatively under-developed state of psychiatric science is important.

However, in addition to all these factors, there is a further and less well recognised factor arising from the logical status of 'disease' as a value term. Acknowledging this implies not that the diagnosis of mental illness is (in principle) unscientific where that of physical illness is scientific, but that the value judgements involved in the diagnosis of mental illness are sometimes open and problematic where those involved in the diagnosis of physical illness are (generally) closed and unproblematic. The consequences of this for avoiding abuse are far reaching, however. Good science remains as important as ever. But instead of attempting to exclude the evaluative element from diagnoses of mental illness, by elaborating ever more exclusively scientific models of disease, we should seek rather to make this element explicit. This is not in itself sufficient to ensure that this element will be less problematic in everyday clinical work, but it is a step in the right direction.

Acknowledgements

The authors are grateful to Associate Professor Sidney Bloch, Professor Alec Jenner and Mr David Pears for their most helpful comments on an early version of this paper.

References

AKHMEDZHANOV, M. (1971) Methodological aspects of the problem of determining the basic concepts of medicine. *Journal of the Academy of Medical Science*, **26** (4), 45–50.

—— (1973) Apropos of the article of academician V. Kh. Vasilenko: "The problem of the concept of disease". *Clinical Medicine*, **51** (5), 139–142.

—— & LIFSHITS, A. M. (1971) On the discussion of the "disease" concept. *Archives of Pathology*, **30** (3), 87–90.

ALEKSAKHINA, R. I. (1968) The concept of "essence" and the question of the essence of the disease. *Journal of the Academy of Medical Science*, **23** (1), 30–34.

BIRLEY, J. L. T. (1991) Psychiatrists and citizens. *British Journal of Psychiatry*, **159**, 1–6.

BLOCH, S. & REDDAWAY, P. (1977) *Russia's Political Hospitals*. London: Gollancz.

—— & CHODOFF, P. (1991) *Psychiatric Ethics* (2nd edn). Oxford: Oxford University Press.

BOORSE, C. (1975) On the distinction between disease and illness. *Philosophy and Public Affairs*, **5**, 49–68.

CLARE, A. (1979) The disease concept in psychiatry. In *Essentials of Postgraduate Psychiatry* (eds P. Hill, R. Murray & A. Thorley). New York: Academic Press, Grune & Stratton.

DAVIDOVSKII, I. V. (1962) *Problems of Causality in Medicine*. Moscow: The State Medical Publisher.

—— & SIL-VESTROV, V. E. (1966) On the definition of "disease" concept. *Archives of Pathology*, **28** (1), 3–8.

—— & SNEZHNEVSKY, A. V. (1972) *Schizophrenia*. Moscow: News of the Academy of Medical Science.

FULFORD, K. W. M. (1989) *Moral Theory and Medical Practice*. Cambridge: Cambridge University Press.

—— (1990) Philosophy and medicine: the Oxford connection. *British Journal of Psychiatry*, **157**, 111–115.

—— (1991) The concept of disease. In *Psychiatric Ethics* (2nd edn) (eds S. Bloch & P. Chodoff), ch. 6. Oxford: Oxford University Press.

—— (1993) Dissent and dissensus: the limits of consensus formation in psychiatry. In *Consensus Formation in Health Care Ethics* (eds H. T. Have & M. Sass). Kluwer (in press).

GALANKIN, V. N. (1988) The interrelation of adaptation and disease in phylogeny and ontogeny. *Archives of Pathology*, **50** (10), 73–78.

GLUZMAN, S. (1989) On the road towards science and law. *Neolitsinskaio jazeta*, **60**, 21 May, p. 31.

HARE, R. M. (1963) Descriptivism. *Proceedings of the British Academy*, **49**, 115–134. Reprinted in *Essays on the Moral Concepts* (1972) (ed. R. M. Hare). London: Macmillan Press.

HESSE, M. (1980) *Revolutions and Reconstructions in the Philosophy of Science*. Brighton: Harvester Press.

IL-IN, B. M. (1988) The concept of human health. *Journal of the Academy of Medical Science*, **4**, 15–18.

JASPERS, K. (1913) Causal and "meaningful" connexions between life history and psychosis. In *Themes and Variations in European Psychiatry* (1974) (eds S. R. Kirsch & M. Shepherd), ch. 5. Bristol: Wright & Sons.

KAGERMAZOV, U. A. (1973) Concepts of "norm", "health" and "disease". *Journal of the Academy of Medical Science*, **28** (9), 16–22.

KENDELL, R. E. (1975) The concept of disease and its implications for psychiatry. *British Journal of Psychiatry*, **127**, 305–315.

KOPELMAN, L. M. (1990) On the evaluative nature of competency and capacity judgements. *International Journal of Law and Psychiatry*, **13**, 309–329.

KORYAGIN, A. (1989) The involvement of soviet psychiatry in the persecution of dissenters. *British Journal of Psychiatry*, **154**, 336–340.

LEWIS, A. J. (1955) Health as a social concept. *British Journal of Sociology*, **4**, 109–124.

MAYER-GROSS, W., SLATER, E. & ROTH, M. (1969) *Clinical Psychiatry*. London: Baillière, Tindall & Cassell.

MERSKEY, H. (1986) Variable meanings for the definition of disease. *Journal of Medicine and Philosophy*, **11**, 215–232.

—— & SHAFRAN, B. (1986) Political hazards in the diagnosis of sluggish schizophrenia. *British Journal of Psychiatry*, **148**, 247–256.

NEW SCIENTIST (1990) Soviet psychiatrists paid to issue false diagnoses. *New Scientist*, 17 February, p. 19.

NOVIKOV, A. (1988) Investigations of the 'closed' themes. *Komsomolsuaia Pravda*, **164**, 16 July, p. 14.

PAVLENKO, S. M. (1980) Systems approach to the study of the problem of nosology and the concept of sanatogenesis. *Soviet Medicine*, **10**, 93–96.

PETLENKO, V. P., STRUKOV, A. I. & KHMEL-NITSKII, O. K. (1984) The deterministic concept of human diseases. *Archives of Pathology*, **46** (10), 3–10.

PETROV, S. S. & PETROV, S. V. (1989) The content of the concepts of "etiology" and "pathogenesis". *Archives of Pathology*, **4**, 87–91.

REICH, W. (1991) Psychiatric diagnosis as an ethical problem. In *Psychiatric Ethics* (2nd edn) (eds S. Bloch & P. Chodoff), pp. 101–135. Oxford: Oxford University Press.

ROTH, M. & KROLL, J. (1986) *The Reality of Mental Illness*. Cambridge: Cambridge University Press.

SARKISOV, D. S. (1973) Apropos of the article by academician V. Kh. Vasilenko: "The problem of the concept of disease". *Clinical Medicine*, **51** (5), 143–145.

SCHMIDT, Y., MOROZOV, G., BADALYAN, L., *et al* (1973) A letter from the Presidium of the All-Union Society of Neurologists and Psychiatrists to *The Guardian*. Reprinted in *Russia's Political Hospitals* (1977) (eds S. Bloch & P. Reddaway). London: Victor Gollancz.

SEDGWICK, P. (1973) Illness – mental and otherwise. *The Hastings Studies Center Studies I*, **3**, 19–40.

SHAFRAN, B., MERSKEY, H. & ZOUBOK, B. (1989) Comments on 'slowly progressive schizophrenia' by A. B. Smulevitch. *British Journal of Psychiatry*, **155**, 174–177.

SIL-VESTROV, V. E. (1968) Definition of the "disease" concept – the key to discovery of general, particular and specific regularities of pathology. *Archives of Pathology*, **30** (3), 90–92.

SMULEVITCH, A. B. (1989) Slowly progressive schizophrenia – myth or clinical reality? *British Journal of Psychiatry*, **155**, 166–177.

SNEZHNEVSKY, A. V. (1971) The symptomatology, clinical forms and nosology of schizophrenia. In *Modern Perspectives in World Psychiatry* (ed. J. G. Howells). New York: Brunner/Mazel.

—— & VARTANYAN, M. (1970) The forms of schizophrenia and their biological correlates. In *Biochemistry, Schizophrenia and Affective Illnesses* (ed. H. E. Himwich). Baltimore: Williams & Wilkins.

SZASZ, T. S. (1960) The myth of mental illness. *American Psychologist*, **15**, 113–118.

TOTSUKA, E. (1990) The history of Japanese psychiatry and the rights of mental patients. *Psychiatric Bulletin*, **14**, 193–200.

URMSON, J. O. (1950) On grading. *Mind*, **59**, 145–169.

VAIL, S. S. (1973) Some observations apropos of the article by academician V. Kh. Vasilenko: "The problem of the concept of disease". *Clinical Medicine*, **51** (5), 142–143.

VASILENKO, V. KH. (1972) The concept of disease. *Clinical Medicine*, **50** (9), 140–146.

—— (1976) Discussion about concept of disease and concomitant problems. *Clinical Medicine*, 54 (12), 114–124.

VAUHKONEN, K. (1968) *On the Pathogenesis of Morbid Jealousy, with Special Reference to the Personality Traits of, and Interaction between, Jealous Patients and their Spouses.* Copenhagen: Munksgaard.

VILENSKY, D. (1990) Psychiatry and politics. *Argumenty i Facti*, 14, 7–13.

VLASIUK, V. V. (1980) Concept of etiology as interaction. *Journal of the Academy of Medical Science*, 8, 68–74.

VLASOV, V. V. (1988) Concepts of the development of disease in the theory of internal medicine. *Soviet Medicine*, 1, 50–53.

WARNOCK, G. J. (1967) *Contemporary Moral Philosophy.* Basingstoke: Macmillan Press.

WILLIAMS, B. (1985) *Ethics and the Limits of Philosophy.* London: Fontana.

WING, J. K. (1978) *Reasoning About Madness.* Oxford: Oxford University Press.

WORLD HEALTH ORGANIZATION (1973) *Report of the International Pilot Study of Schizophrenia.* Geneva: WHO.

—— (1978) *Mental Disorders: Glossary and Guide to their Classification in Accordance with the Ninth Revision of the International Classification of Diseases* (ICD–9). Geneva: WHO.

*K. W. M. Fulford, DPhil, MRCP, MRCPsych, *Research Psychiatrist, University Department of Psychiatry, Warneford Hospital, Oxford OX3 7JX*; A. Y. U. Smirnov, MD, PhD, *Research Psychiatrist, All-Union Centre for Mental Health Research, Kashirskoye sh. 34, Moscow 115522, USSR*; E. Snow, BA(Hons), CQSW, *Senior Social Worker, Warneford Hospital, Oxford OX3 7JX*

*Correspondence

[33]

NORMAN DANIELS

The Ideal Advocate and Limited Resources

1. INTRODUCTION

Recently, a friend of mine confided to me that he is not sure he will be able to continue practicing medicine if current trends in the health care system continue. He complained that various reforms — actual and proposed — in the financing of health care make him feel that he will not be able to remain the unbiased agent or advocate for his patients. He feels he has always been such an advocate and that medical ethics requires him to be one. To represent his patient's best interests, he feels he must be free to make medical decisions aimed at the best treatments and outcome which are *medically possible* for his patient.

Of course, he knows he cannot be a completely autonomous agent. Though this was not part of his early medical training, he has learned that his patient should have the ultimate say in what is done and that he must act with his patient's informed consent. But my friend is now concerned about threats to his autonomy that come not from the patient, but from outside the doctor-patient relationship. He feels he cannot in good conscience comply with hospital pressures to discharge his Medicare patients before he thinks they are ready. He finds repugnant a recent capitation scheme proposed for physicians at his hospital. Under the plan, doctors would be financially rewarded for not ordering certain diagnoses or consultations. He insists these are threats to his "moral character" and to his "psyche" as a physician.

I do not think my friend's complaints are unfamiliar. Similar remarks can be heard in scrub rooms, hos-

pital staff meetings, and letters columns in medical journals. Many physicians believe that the 'old' retrospective fee-for-service schemes facilitated acting as the unfettered agent of the patient, but that cost-containment schemes destroy morally essential features of the doctor-patient relationship by restricting physician autonomy. I want [to] explore some general questions underlying these reactions and beliefs. Specifically, I want to address these questions: What kinds of autonomy have been granted American physicians, and how do these fit with ethical constraints on how a physician may act concerning his patient? Do the pre-cost-containment arrangements many physicians prefer institutionally embody or facilitate the ideal doctor-patient relationship? Can we, or how can we, reconcile the fact of resource limitations with the plausible view that physicians should remain neutral advocates of their patients' best interests? In answering these questions, I shall argue that we can reconcile resource limitations with what I will call the Ideal Advocate model of the doctor-patient relationship, but that doing so requires that our health care institutions be just.

2. PHYSICIAN AUTONOMY AND IDEAL ADVOCACY

It will help to analyze briefly the dimensions of autonomy traditionally claimed by U.S. physicians. We can pick out four main dimensions: (1) Whom to treat, (2) Where to practice, (3) What to specialize in, and (4) How to treat?

Unlike their colleagues in many other countries, U.S. physicians retain the power to decide *whom* they will treat. They may consider facts about the individual patient or his method of reimbursement. Choices about both *where* to practice and *what* to specialize in

From *Theoretical Medicine* 8 (1987), 69–80. © 1987 by D. Reidel Publishing Company. Reprinted by permission of Kluwer Academic Publishers.

70   RIGHTS AND RESPONSIBILITIES

are of course subject to what might be called 'market' constraints. They are subject to facts about the availability of training positions, practices to enter, indebtedness, and other factors. But few of these market constraints are themselves the results of centralized planning, and so there is an extensive, unregulated space for physicians' choice.

These first three dimensions of autonomy are similar in that they all are responsive to physician interests — some would say physicians' 'rights' — rather than patient interests. Granting these dimensions of autonomy to physicians has a major negative impact, for example, on programs to improve access to health care for underserved groups. Thus, only a minority of physicians will treat Medicaid patients. But I am not chiefly interested here in these three dimensions of autonomy. Rather, it is the fourth dimension, *clinical autonomy*, autonomy in *how* to treat, that is most directly affected by the recent cost-containment measures.

Granting physicians clinical autonomy is justified by reference to the patient's interests, not the physician's. Thus autonomy in treatment decisions is constrained by what might be called an 'ethic of advocacy (or agency)'. The autonomy we grant the physician is necessary precisely if he is to act in his patient's best interest, and for this reason it also includes some constraints on the physician. The clinical decisions must be: (A) competent: up to professional standards of care; (B) respectful of patient autonomy; (C) respectful of other patient rights, e.g., confidentiality; (D) free from consideration of the physician's interests; (E) uninfluenced by judgments about the patient's worth.

The first of these constraints, the competency constraint, is enforced by peer review and tort law. The four remaining constraints are special features of the kind of fiduciary relationship that holds between a physician, with his greater knowledge and skill, and the patient, on whose behalf the physician acts as agent or advocate. Much recent clinical medical ethics has focused on patient autonomy and rights [constraints (B) and (C)]. Because they have little to do with the problem of cost-containment, I will not talk about them here. But the "purity" constraints, as I will call constraints (D) and (E), are at the heart of the issue. Constraint (D) requires that the physician not allow consideration of his economic or career interests to influence his treatment of his patient. Constraint (E)

is interpreted by some to mean that the physician should not put a price on his patient's life — should not decide how much it is worth to save or extend a particular patient's life. More narrowly interpreted, constraint (E) bars a physician from considering facts other than medical need or likelihood of treatment success in making clinical decisions for a particular patient. I shall call the Ideal Advocate model the view that physicians should be autonomous in their clinical decision-making and pursuit of their patients' best interests, while abiding by constraints (A)–(E) of the ethic of agency.

An important loose-end remains here. Some people believe that the Ideal Advocate is necessarily also an Unrestricted Ideal Advocate. That is, the physician should be subject to no external constraints on treatments he can pursue for his patient. Our retrospective fee-for-service reimbursement schemes may have contributed to this belief. They give the appearance that no resource constraints affect clinical decision-making: just treat, and then bill. Of course, these arrangements hide the way in which rationing actually takes place, by ability to pay, that is, to buy insurance. But this form of rationing seems to leave the clinician untouched. There seem to be no direct incentives to physicians to consider their own interest or the relative worth of the patient in decisions about how to treat (though the physician can refuse to treat at all, which clearly has something to do with his interests and possibly with his assessment of patient worth). In reality, retrospective fee-for-service schemes contain incentives for physicians to treat too much. But this tendency has been viewed as a lesser evil than incentives to deny beneficial care.

Because pre-cost-containment arrangements seem to embody the virtues of the Unrestricted Ideal Advocate, many physicians may have come to think of them as the form medicine must take if it is to be morally acceptable. Similarly, because current cost-containment measures introduce a concern about resource limitations through incentives which threaten the purity constraints (D) and (E), it is easy for physicians to overgeneralize and to think that any challenge to the Unrestricted Ideal Advocate must undermine the Ideal Advocate. A glance at some history may put this issue in perspective.

3. A HISTORY LESSON

Paul Starr has recently described the rise of the American medical profession from an early period in which the medical profession lacked the cultural authority and power it now enjoys.[1] He shows that physicians did not acquire their cultural power merely because they were "healers" and society has always revered healers. He documents the ways in which physicians resisted "capture" by hospitals and other emerging institutions, because hospitals in the U.S. remained dependent on physicians for referrals. In contrast, in many European countries, physicians were often salaried employees of hospitals from early on. Consequently they too had an interest in undercutting the independence of non-hospital-based physicians. Starr also documents the ways in which physicians and their professional associations and lobbies resisted "capture" by institutions developed to improve access to health care through new financing and insurance schemes. For example, when Medicare and Medicaid were established, physicians retained the power to determine whether they would treat such patients and how many they would treat. They also retained the retrospective, fee-for-service reimbursement scheme that characterized private insurance schemes. If we add to this the control physicians retain over where they locate their practices and what specialties they enter, we arrive at a unique pattern of physician autonomy and power, one that has had a negative effect on access to care for important subgroups in the population.

By exposing the details of the idiosyncratic history that led to this result, Starr shows us that the arrangements we presently have [are] not the result of an "inner logic" or ethical necessity that characterizes the doctor-patient relationship. We should not transform features of the relationships and institutions that result from such a unique historical process into a "nature." We have not stumbled on the *natural form* of the professional-patient relationship. When we see the details of this history, we lose any inclination we might have had to believe that the autonomy and power that has been granted American physicians is based either on the inner necessities of the doctor-patient relationship or on a reasoned social calculation about how to guarantee equitable access to high-quality care at acceptable costs. Rather we see ingenious lobbying by the medical profession, strategic exercises of economic strength, and the effective use of cultural authority. The results have been a series of exasperating political compromises embedded in financing reforms throughout this century. But past political success on this uneven historical battleground is hardly a *justification* of

the institutions which grant and protect the profession's power. Might does not make right, and the peculiarities and vagaries of the historical process undermine claims that it is procedurally fair. Moreover, the very idiosyncrasy of the profession's historical success undercuts claims that "legitimate" expectations would weigh in favor of preserving the status quo.

An important feature of the history Starr documents is the way in which some physicians, we must suppose quite sincerely, made explicitly ethical arguments in favor of the broad institutional powers and authority they sought. Starr cites the code of ethics the AMA adopted in 1934 which claimed it was "unprofessional" for a physician to permit making "a direct profit" from his work: "The making of a profit from medical work is beneath the dignity of professional practice, is unfair competition with the profession at large, is harmful alike to the profession of medicine and the welfare of the people, and is against sound public policy." As Starr points out, it was unprofessional only for someone *other* than a doctor to make a profit from a physician's work. It was acceptable, however, for another doctor to make such a profit! How exquisitely refined this principle of professional ethics is! The first of ten principles for medical service adopted by the AMA in 1934 (current codes are less explicit about converting economic considerations into ethical ones) says that "All features of medical service in any method of medical practice should be under the control of the medical profession." The fifth claimed that the "medical profession alone can determine the adequacy and character" of the institutions involved in medical care, which should be construed as "but expansions of the equipment of the physician." Starr notes that "the doctors took professional authority, patient confidentiality, and free choice to require a specific set of economic relations." For example, "However the cost of medical service may be distributed . . . the immediate cost should be borne by the patient if able to pay at the time the service is rendered." Thus, as Starr concludes, "the AMA insisted that all health insurance plans accept the private physician's monopoly control of the medical market and complete authority over all aspects of medical institutions," and it did so by deriving these controls from its view of professional ethics.

Of course the fact that physicians later embraced many of the institutional arrangements which they earlier thought unethical does not mean they were morally inconsistent. Rather it suggests that their moral concerns about some features of the doctor-patient relationship had led them to make false claims about ethically acceptable institutional arrangements. Obviously, this is a pattern of which we must be wary. (I am not even considering the more cynical view that all these moral concerns are secondary to economic interests and are appealed to only to disguise bald self-interest; Starr is less generous.)

Let me summarize the argument I have been making in this historical section. First, the kinds of control physicians have in our society over whom they will treat, where they will locate, what they will specialize in, as well as the autonomy they retain within largely retrospective fee-for-service reimbursement schemes — this autonomy and power of physicians is the result of a very particular, even idiosyncratic series of historical events. When we examine the power struggles that yielded physicians these results, we find no evidence that the institutional arrangements were the product of a social consensus in which all parties agreed that the Ideal Advocate model necessitated such full-blown autonomy and powers. Second, at points in that history, some physicians sincerely believed that Ideal Advocacy did require that particular institutional arrangements be established and others opposed. Physicians later embraced institutions which they had earlier thought ethically unacceptable, suggesting that Ideal Advocacy had fewer implications for institutional arrangements than physicians had previously believed. Third, in view of this history, we should be very careful not to assume that important, morally desirable features of medical decision-making can be preserved only if we maintain the institutional arrangements with which we are familiar. These arrangements are not necessarily the historical product of respect for that moral core of the doctor-patient relationship. They have, if Starr is right, a less respectable birthright.

This history lesson brings me to a central claim. The shape of professional relationships, and thus the scope and content of professional ethics, should depend on what kinds of institutions are needed to guarantee the just distribution of the goods provided by those relationships. It is justice that should be primary here, as should other general moral principles, and professional ethics should govern roles circumscribed by just institutions. Professional ethics should not be the tail that wags the dog. Ludicrous professional codes, such as the 1934 AMA principles, are but an extreme result of reversing priorities in this way.

4. JUSTICE AND IDEAL ADVOCACY

To see how the ethic of agency and the Ideal Advocate model can fit within a just health care system, we must consider what justice requires. As we shall see, justice will require that we abandon the Unrestricted Ideal Advocate in favor of a more modest Ideal Advocate. I have provided elsewhere a detailed account of what a just health care system might look like.[6] Here I shall offer but a brief summary of that argument.

We can begin with the question, Is health care 'special'? Should we distinguish it from other goods, say video recorders, because of its special moral importance? And does that moral importance mean there are social obligations to distribute it in particular ways, ways which might not coincide with the results of market distribution? I believe the answer to all these questions is "yes".

Health care — I mean the term quite broadly — does many important things for people. Some extends lives, some reduces pain and suffering, some merely gives important information about one's condition. I have argued that a central, unifying function of health care is to maintain and restore functional organization, let us say 'functioning', that is typical or normal for our species. This central function of health care derives its moral importance from the following fact: normal functioning has a central effect on the opportunity open to an individual. More specifically, an individual's fair share of the normal opportunity range for his society is impaired when disease or disability impairs normal functioning. I believe this means there are social obligations to provide health care services that protect and restore normal functioning. In short, the principle of justice that should govern the design of health care institutions is a principle that calls for guaranteeing fair equality of opportunity.

This principle of justice has implications for access and resource allocation. It implies that there should be no financial, geographical or discriminatory barriers to a level of care which promotes normal functioning. It also implies that resources [should] be allocated in ways that are effective in promoting normal functioning. That is, we can use the effect on normal opportunity range as a crude way of ranking the moral importance of health care services. This does not mean that any technology which might have a positive impact on normal functioning for some individuals should be introduced: we must weigh new technologies against alternatives to judge the overall impact of introducing them on fair equality of opportunity—this gives a slightly new sense to the term 'opportunity cost'. The point is that social obligations to provide just health care must be met within the conditions of moderate scarcity that we face. This approach is not one which gives individuals a basic right to have all their health care needs met. Rather, there is a social obligation to provide individuals only with those services which are part of the design of a system that on the whole protects equal opportunity.

This view has implications for the autonomy and powers we might grant physicians. Specifically, institutions must give providers incentives that yield equitable access to care. This may mean restricting some of the powers now held by providers to choose whom they are willing to treat, what specialties they will enter, and where they will locate. These restrictions need violate no fundamental liberties of providers, though realistic options open to individual providers might be dramatically different from those enjoyed under current incentives. Similarly, providers will find themselves in a framework that restricts the resources that may be devoted to treating certain conditions in order that a more equitable distribution of resources overall results. There will be some things that providers cannot do for their patients—providers will not be able to be the unrestricted advocates of their patients, but will have to do the best they can for them under the restrictions that exist in the system.⁷

What is crucial to understand about these restrictions on the Ideal Advocate is their underlying justification. Under conditions of moderate resource scarcity, there will be some things we cannot do for certain classes of patients because doing them would mean we would not be able to meet the requirements of justice regarding other classes of patients. Notice that there are two central features underlying these kinds of rationing decisions. First, weighing the opportunity cost of one class of treatments or technologies against another must take place in a *closed* system. When beneficial care is denied it must be because the resources will be better used elsewhere in the system. Second, principles of justice must govern the decisions about priorities within this closed system—and thus define what counts as "better" uses of services. Thus, the just distribution of health care resources implies that we cannot implement the Unrestricted Ideal Advocate model. Rather, we can now state how the Ideal Advocate model must be qualified physicians should be the advocates of their patients, abiding by the ethic of agency, within the limits imposed by just resource allocation. The physician as Ideal Advocate cannot do things which would be unfair or unjust to other patients. This is the sense in which justice is primary, or provides the framework within which professional ethics can be elaborated.

Stringent—but just—rationing schemes need not threaten the ethic of advocacy. The purity constraint (D), which requires clinical decisions to be free from consideration of the physician's interests, is perfectly compatible with the just rationing of limited health care resources. British physicians, for example, who deny beneficial care that may be available to patients in the United States, do not do so because of any economic incentives that directly reward them for denying care.⁸ It is possible to construct institutions in which physicians pursue their patients' best interests and respect fair resource limitations without their incentive for denying care deriving from economic incentives to them.

Similarly, a physician need not violate the constraint (E) that he avoid judgments about a patient's worth. Judgments about the just distribution of health care resources must be social and public ones. For example, the fair equality of opportunity principle I described might require us to forego treatments or technologies which consume resources more effectively used elsewhere to protect opportunity. But this principled social decision does not involve the physician in making any judgments of social worth. The physician acts as a "gatekeeper," but he is abiding by a just social decision, not his own determination that it is not worth the resources to treat a particular class of patients in a particular way. Physicians can still do the best they can for their patients within the limits imposed by justice, which is all that constraints (D) and (E) require.

We can now better see why American cost-containment measures have seemed so threatening to the idea that a physician must be the advocate for his patients. Constraints on physician autonomy embodied within current cost-restraint measures carry with them no such justification grounded in requirements of justice. In the United States, there is no assurance that when a patient is required to forego beneficial treatment, say a needed day in the hospital beyond the DRG [Diagnosis Related Group] standard, the saving in resources works to the advantage of other patients whom justice requires we treat instead. Rather, services that might well benefit one patient are foregone simply because it is not profitable to treat him compared to another, and the system of incentives has no principle guiding it other than the intention of reducing 'unnecessary' services. Indeed, decisions about the dissemination of new technologies are made without the system being closed at all: opportunity costs are not considered at all, let alone by reference to a principle of justice.

The Ideal Advocate who plays the role of "gatekeeper" in a just system can nevertheless reassure himself that his denials of care are *fair*. It is because this reassurance is most definitely lacking for the U.S. physician under existing cost-containment schemes that we hear the complaints my friend expressed. When he denies beneficial care, the American physician can be rather sure that the savings will not go to more urgently needed care elsewhere in the system. He may know, for example, the savings will be returned to investors for a for-profit hospital or be consumed elsewhere in a hospital budget which has never been examined to see what implicit assumptions about health care priorities govern it. To be compelled to play the role of "gatekeeper" under these circumstances may interfere with Ideal Advocacy in a morally unacceptable way. In the long run it can erode patient confidence that physicians will act as their advocates or agents. My physician friend was right to feel threatened by cost-containment measures with such implications.

5. A PALLIATIVE FOR COST-CONSTRAINTS?

The problem with current cost-containment measures is that they are not part of an overall effort to make the U.S. health care system more just. They compromise the physician, who must deny beneficial care for reasons other than those imposed by justice. The measures fail to preserve important features of the Ideal Advocate model, especially the purity constraints on clinical decisions. These are serious flaws, and only quite basic reforms — drastic reconstructive surgery — could eliminate them. Contrary to what many physicians believe, we would have to undertake more, not less, extensive planning within our health care system, and we would have to do so with a com-

mitment to justice. In the current political climate, no one seems ready to finance such measures, yet nothing short of them can let us preserve the Ideal Advocate model and face resource scarcity at the same time.

Since I am loathe to suggest a band-aid or palliative when only major interventions will produce real reform, I hesitate to advance the following suggestion. Nevertheless, one feature of the current situation that clearly exacerbates it is that physicians have no public way of resisting pressures to deny beneficial care. They have no way to appeal what they take to be unacceptable pressures in particular cases. Physicians — and other medical personnel — need some hearing board to which they can appeal against hospital policies and third-party restrictions. It is not clear what form such a board should take, but perhaps some expanded role for hospital ethics committees is in order. Instead of merely approving plug-pulling, they might consider the ethical issues involved in decision-making under cost-constraints. This would provide a broader, more public forum in which disputes between physicians and hospital administrators might be aired. It might also provide a setting in which evidence about the effects of the cost-constraints can be gathered — effects on access and quality of care, not just on costs.

Such appeals to ethics committees are costly and may be time-consuming. And it is difficult to imagine many hospitals surrendering authority over policies to such committees. Indeed, only about 10% of all hospitals have such committees at all. In contrast, it is easy to imagine physicians trying to do quiet end-runs around the cost-constraints instead, even if it involves some compromise to integrity. But some way of protecting the physician — and ultimately the patient — against policies which are aimed at profit, not fair allocation, is definitely in order. Such boards might give us a way to monitor the cost-containment process, but they are no substitute for careful research into effects on access to care and quality of care. Unfortunately, the government which was so quick to install DRGs — without full consideration of them — has taken only small steps to measure their real effects. Funding for this research is hard to come by.

I think there is another argument for establishing a mechanism for this type of review. The measures we have so far encountered may be mild compared to what we may encounter next — especially if there is no defined forum for appeal against what we already have. I am particularly concerned that our halfway measures in the direction of cost-containment will be seen as typical failures of "regulation" and that there will be a further push to make the health care market more competitive and entrepreneurial. This would only postpone facing the problem of rationing equitably in the face of resource limitations. Hearing boards might thus offer some preventive effects. In any case, they provide another context in which the physician can attempt to abide by the Ideal Advocate model, and this may slow the erosion of physician commitment to important moral ideals.

Acknowledgment: Research for this paper was funded by grants from the National Endowment for the Humanities Basic Research Program and the Retirement Research Foundation. I am indebted to David Ozar for editorially carving this paper out of a much longer take. "Are Physicians Treating Patients Too Well?" delivered at the Loyola-Strich School of Medicine, Loyola University of Chicago, April, 1985.

NOTES

1. Paul Starr, *Social Transformation of American Medicine* (New York: Basic Books, 1982). Material in this section draws on my review of Starr's book, "Understanding Physician Power." *Philosophy and Public Affairs* 13:4, pp. 347–357.

2. Starr, *Social Transformation*, p. 216.

3. Starr, *Social Transformation*, p. 299.

4. Starr, *Social Transformation*, p. 300.

5. Starr, *Social Transformation*, p. 300.

6. Norman Daniels, *Just Health Care* (New York: Cambridge University Press, 1985).

7. For further discussion of the relationship between provider liberties and the requirements of justice, see my *Just Health Care*, Ch. 6.

8. See my "Why Saying 'No' to Patients in the United States Is so Hard," *New England Journal of Medicine* 314 (May 22, 1986), 1381–1393; also see Henry Aaron and William Schwartz, *The Painful Prescription* (Washington: Brookings Institution, 1984).

*Journal of medical ethics, 1987, **13**, 117-123*

QALYfying the value of life

John Harris   *Centre for Social Ethics and Policy, University of Manchester*

This paper argues that the Quality Adjusted Life Year or QALY is fatally flawed as a way of priority setting in health care and of dealing with the problem of scarce resources. In addition to showing why this is so the paper sets out a view of the moral constraints that govern the allocation of health resources and suggests reasons for a new attitude to the health budget.

Against a background of permanently scarce resources it is clearly crucial that such health care resources as are available be not used wastefully. This point is often made in terms of 'efficiency' and it is argued, not implausibly, that to talk of efficiency implies that we are able to distinguish between efficient and inefficient use of health care resources, and hence that we are in some sense able to measure the results of treatment. To do so of course we need a standard of measurement. Traditionally, in life-endangering conditions, that standard has been easy to find. Successful treatment removes the danger to life, or at least postpones it, and so the survival rates of treatment have been regarded as a good indicator of success (1). However, equally clearly, it is also of crucial importance to those treated that the help offered them not only removes the threat to life, but leaves them able to enjoy the remission granted. In short, gives them reasonable quality, as well as extended quantity of life.

A new measure of quality of life which combines length of survival with an attempt to measure the quality of that survival has recently (2) been suggested and is becoming influential. The need for such a measure has been thus described by one of its chief architects: 'We need a simple, versatile, measure of success which incorporates both life expectancy and quality of life, and which reflects the values and ethics of the community served. The "Quality Adjusted Life Year" (QALY) measure fulfils such a role' (3). This is a large claim and an important one, if it can be sustained its consequences for health care will be profound indeed.

Key words

QALY; equality; civil rights; efficiency; scarce resources.

There are, however, substantial theoretical problems in the development of such a measure, and more important by far, grave dangers of its misuse. I shall argue that the dangers of misuse, which partly derive from inadequacies in the theory which generates them, make this measure itself a life-threatening device. In showing why this is so I shall attempt to say something positive about just what is involved in making scrupulous choices between people in situations of scarce resources, and I will end by saying something about the entitlement to claim in particular circumstances, that resources are indeed scarce.

We must first turn to the task of examining the QALY and the possible consequences of its use in resource allocation. A task incidentally which, because it aims at the identification and eradication of a life-threatening condition, itself (surprisingly perhaps for a philosophical paper) counts also as a piece of medical research (4), which if successful will prove genuinely therapeutic.

The QALY

I. WHAT ARE QALYS?

It is important to be as clear as possible as to just what a QALY is and what it might be used for. I cannot do better than let Alan Williams, the architect of QALYs referred to above, tell you in his own words:

'The essence of a QALY is that it takes a year of healthy life expectancy to be worth one, but regards a year of unhealthy life expectancy as worth less than 1. Its precise value is lower the worse the quality of life of the unhealthy person (which is what the "quality adjusted" bit is all about). If being dead is worth zero, it is, in principle, possible for a QALY to be negative, ie for the quality of someone's life to be judged worse than being dead.

The general idea is that a beneficial health care activity is one that generates a positive amount of QALYs, and that an efficient health care activity is one where the cost per QALY is as low as it can be. A high priority health care activity is one where the cost-per-QALY is low, and a low priority activity is one where cost-per-QALY is high' (5).

The plausibility of the QALY derives from the idea that 'given the choice, a person would prefer a shorter healthier life to a longer period of survival in a state of severe discomfort and disability' (6). The idea that any rational person would endorse this preference provides the moral and political force behind the QALY. Its acceptability as a measurement of health then depends upon its doing all the theoretical tasks assigned to it, and on its being what people want, or would want, for themselves.

II. HOW WILL QALYS BE USED?

There are two ways in which QALYs might be used. One is unexceptionable and useful, and fully in line with the assumptions which give QALYs their plausibility. The other is none of these.

QALYs might be used to determine which of rival therapies to give to a particular patient or which procedure to use to treat a particular condition. Clearly the one generating the most QALYs will be the better bet, both for the patient and for a society with scarce resources. However, QALYs might also be used to determine not what treatment to give *these* patients, but which group of patients to treat, or which conditions to give priority in the allocation of health care resources. It is clear that it is this latter use which Williams has in mind, for he specifically cites as one of the rewards of the development of QALYs, their use in 'priority setting in the health care system in general' (7). It is this use which is likely to be of greatest interest to all those concerned with efficiency in the health service. And it is for this reason that it is likely to be both the most influential and to have the most far-reaching effects. It is this use which is I believe positively dangerous and morally indefensible. Why?

III. WHAT'S WRONG WITH QALYS?

It is crucial to realise that the whole plausibility of QALYs depends upon our accepting that they simply involve the generalisation of the 'truth' (8) that 'given the choice a person would prefer a shorter healthier life to a longer period of survival in a state of severe discomfort'. On this view giving priority to treatments which produce more QALYs or for which the cost-per-QALY is low, is both efficient and is also what the community as a whole, and those at risk in particular, actually want. But whereas it follows from the fact that given the choice a person would prefer a shorter healthier life to a longer one of severe discomfort, that the best treatment *for that person* is the one yielding the most QALYs, it does not follow that treatments yielding more QALYs are preferable to treatments yielding fewer where *different people* are to receive the treatments. That is to say, while it follows from the fact (if it is a fact) that I and everyone else would prefer to have, say one year of healthy life rather than three years of severe discomfort, that we value healthy existence more than uncomfortable existence for ourselves, it does not follow that where the choice is between three years of

discomfort for *me* or immediate death on the one hand, and one year of health for *you*, or immediate death on the other, that I am somehow committed to the judgement that you ought to be saved rather than me.

Suppose that Andrew, Brian, Charles, Dorothy, Elizabeth, Fiona and George all have zero life-expectancy without treatment, but with medical care, all but George will get one year complete remission and George will get seven years' remission. The costs of treating each of the six are equal but George's operation costs five times as much as the cost of the other operations. It does not follow that even if each person, if asked, would prefer seven years' remission to one for themselves, that they are all committed to the view that George should be treated rather than that they should. Nor does it follow that this is a preference that society should endorse. But it is the preference that QALYs dictate.

Such a policy does not value life or lives at all, for it is individuals who are alive, and individuals who lose their lives. And when they do the loss is principally their loss. The value of someone's life is, primarily and overwhelmingly, its value to him or her; the wrong done when an individual's life is cut short is a wrong to that individual. The victim of a murder or a fatal accident is the person who loses his life. A disaster is the greater the more victims there are, the more lives that are lost. A society which values the lives of its citizens is one which tries to ensure that as few of them die prematurely (that is when their lives could continue) as possible. Giving value to life-years or QALYs, has the effect in this case of sacrificing six lives for one. If each of the seven *wants* to go on living for as long as he or she can, if each values the prospective term of remission available, then to choose between them on the basis of life-years (quality adjusted or not), is in this case to give no value to the lives of six people.

IV. THE ETHICS OF QALYS

Although we might be right to claim that people are not committed to QALYs as a measurement of health simply in virtue of their acceptance of the idea that each would prefer to have more QALYs rather than fewer for themselves, are there good moral reasons why QALYs should none the less be accepted?

The idea, which is at the root of both democratic theory and of most conceptions of justice, that each person is as morally important as any other and hence, that the life and interests of each is to be given equal weight, while apparently referred to and employed by Williams plays no part at all in the theory of QALYs. That which is to be given equal weight is not persons and their interests and preferences, but quality-adjusted life-years. And giving priority to the manufacture of QALYs can mean them all going to a few at the expense of the interests and wishes of the many. It will also mean that all available resources will tend to be deployed to assist those who will thereby gain the maximum QALYs – the young.

V. THE FALLACY OF VALUING TIME

There is a general problem for any position which holds that time-spans are of equal value no matter who gets them, and it stems from the practice of valuing life-units (life-years) rather than people's lives.

If what matters most is the number of life-years the world contains, then the best thing we can do is devote our resources to increasing the population. Birth control, abortion and sex education come out very badly on the QALY scale of priorities.

In the face of a problem like this, the QALY advocate must insist that what he wants is to select the therapy that generates the most QALYs for those people who already exist, and not simply to create the maximum number of QALYs. But if it is people and not units of life-span that matter, if the QALY is advocated because it is seen as a moral and efficient way to fulfil our obligation to provide care for our fellows, then it does matter who gets the QALYs – because it matters how people are treated. And this is where the ageism of QALYs and their other discriminatory features become important.

VI. QALYS ARE AGEIST

Maximising QALYs involves an implicit and comprehensive ageist bias. For saving the lives of younger people is, other things being equal, always likely to be productive of more QALYs than saving older people. Thus on the QALY arithmetic we always have a reason to prefer, for example, neonatal or paediatric care to all 'later' branches of medicine. This is because any calculation of the life-years generated for a particular patient by a particular therapy, must be based on the life expectancy of that patient. The older a patient is when treated, the fewer the life-years that can be achieved by the therapy.

It is true that QALYs dictate that we prefer people, not simply who have *more life expectancy*, but rather people who have *more life expectancy to be gained from treatment*. But wherever treatment saves a life, and this will be frequently, for quite simple treatments, like a timely antibiotic, can be life-saving, it will, other things being equal, be the case that younger people have more life expectancy to gain from the treatment than do older people.

VII. AGEISM AND AID

Another problem with such a view is that it seems to imply, for example, that when looking at societies from the outside, those with a lower average age have somehow a greater claim on our aid. This might have important consequences in looking at questions concerning aid policy on a global scale. Of course it is true that a society's having a low average age might be a good indicator of its need for help, in that it would imply that people were dying prematurely. However, we can imagine a society suffering a disaster which killed off many of its young people (war perhaps) and which was consequently left with a high average age

but was equally deserving of aid despite the fact that such aid would inevitably benefit the old. If QALYs were applied to the decision as to whether to provide aid to this society or another much less populous and perhaps with less pressing problems, but with a more normal age distribution, the 'older' society might well be judged 'not worth' helping.

VIII. QALYS CAN BE RACIST AND SEXIST

If a 'high priority health care activity is one where the cost-per-QALY is low, and a low priority activity is one where cost-per-QALY is high' then people who just happen to have conditions which are relatively cheap to treat are always going to be given priority over those who happen to have conditions which are relatively expensive to treat. This will inevitably involve not only a systematic pattern of disadvantage to particular groups of patients, or to people afflicted with particular diseases or conditions, but perhaps also a systematic preference for the survival of some kinds of patients at the expense of others. We usually think that justice requires that we do not allow certain sections of the community or certain types of individual to become the victims of systematic disadvantage and that there are good moral reasons for doing justice, not just when it costs us nothing or when it is convenient or efficient, but also and particularly, when there is a price to be paid. We'll return shortly to this crucial issue of justice, but it is important to be clear about the possible social consequences of adopting QALYs.

Adoption of QALYs as the rationale for the distribution of health care resources may, for the above reasons, involve the creation of a systematic pattern of preference for certain racial groups or for a particular gender or, what is the same thing, a certain pattern of discrimination against such groups. Suppose that medical statistics reveal that say women, or Asian males, do better than others after a particular operation or course of treatment, or, that a particular condition that has a very poor prognosis in terms of QALYs afflicts only Jews, or gay men. Such statistics abound and the adoption of QALYs may well dictate very severe and systematic discrimination against groups identified primarily by race, gender or colour, in the allocation of health resources, where it turns out that such groups are vulnerable to conditions that are not QALY-efficient (9).

Of course it is just a fact of life and far from sinister that different races and genders are subject to different conditions, but the problem is that QALYs may tend to reinforce and perpetuate these 'structural' disadvantages.

IX. DOUBLE JEOPARDY

Relatedly, suppose a particular terminal condition was treatable, and would, with treatment, give indefinite remission but with a very poor quality of life. Suppose for example that if an accident victim were treated, he would survive, but with paraplegia. This might always cash out at fewer QALYS than a condition which with treatment would give a patient perfect remission for about five years after which the patient would die. Suppose that both candidates wanted to go on living as long as they could and so both wanted, equally fervently, to be given the treatment that would save their lives. Is it clear that the candidate with most QALYS on offer should always and inevitably be the one to have priority? To judge so would be to count the paraplegic's desire to live the life that was available to him as of less value than his rival's – what price equal weight to the preferences of each individual?

This feature of QALYS involves a sort of double jeopardy. QALYS dictate that because an individual is unfortunate, because she has once become a victim of disaster, we are required to visit upon her a second and perhaps graver misfortune. The first disaster leaves her with a poor quality of life and QALYS then require that in virtue of this she be ruled out as a candidate for life-saving treatment, or at best, that she be given little or no chance of benefiting from what little amelioration her condition admits of. Her first disaster leaves her with a poor quality of life and when she presents herself for help, along come QALYS and finish her off!

X. LIFE-SAVING AND LIFE-ENHANCING

A distinction, consideration of which is long overdue, is that between treatments which are life-saving (or death-postponing) and those which are simply life-enhancing, in the sense that they improve the quality of life without improving life-expectancy. Most people think, and for good as well as for prudential reasons, that life-saving has priority over life-enhancement and that we should first allocate resources to those areas where they are immediately needed to save life and only when this has been done should the remainder be allocated to alleviating non-fatal conditions. Of course there are exceptions even here and some conditions, while not life-threatening, are so painful that to leave someone in a state of suffering while we attend even to the saving of life, would constitute unjustifiable cruelty. But these situations are rare and for the vast majority of cases we judge that life-saving should have priority.

It is important to notice that QALYS make no such distinction between types of treatment. Defenders of QALYS often cite with pride the example of hip-replacement operations which are more QALY-efficient than say kidney dialysis (10). While the difficulty of choosing between treating very different groups of patients, some of whom need treatment simply to stay alive, while others need it to relieve pain and distress, is clearly very acute, and while it may be that life-saving should not *always* have priority over life-enhancement, the dangers of adopting QALYS which regard only one dimension of the rival claims, and a dubious one at that, as morally relevant, should be clear enough.

There is surely something fishy about QALYS. They can hardly form 'an appropriate basis for health service policy'. Can we give an account of just where they are deficient from the point of view of morality? We can, and indeed we have already started to do so. In addition to their other problems, QALYS and their use for priority setting in health care or for choosing not which treatment to give these patients, but for selecting which patients or conditions to treat, involve profound injustice, and if implemented would constitute a denial of the most basic civil rights. Why is this?

Moral constraints

One general constraint that is widely accepted and that I think most people would judge should govern life and death decisions, is the idea that many people believe expresses the values animating the health service as a whole. These are the belief that the life and health of each person matters, and matters as much as that of any other and that each person is entitled to be treated with equal concern and respect both in the way health resources are distributed and in the way they are treated generally by health care professionals, however much their personal circumstances may differ from that of others.

This popular belief about the values which animate the health service depends on a more abstract view about the source and structure of such values and it is worth saying just a bit about this now.

I. THE VALUE OF LIFE

One such value is the value of life itself. Our own continued existence as individuals is the *sine qua non* of almost everything. So long as we want to go on living, practically everything we value or want depends upon our continued existence. This is one reason why we generally give priority to life-saving over life-enhancing.

To think that *life is valuable*, that in most circumstances, the worst thing that can happen to an individual is that she lose her life when this need not happen, and that the worst thing we can do is make decisions, a consequence of which, is that others die prematurely, we must think that *each life is valuable*. Each life counts for one and that is why more count for more. For this reason we should give priority to saving as many lives as we can, not as many life-years (11).

One important point must be emphasised at this stage. We talk of 'life-saving' but of course this must always be understood as 'death-postponing'. Normally we want to have our death postponed for as long as possible but where what's possible is the gaining of only very short periods of remission, hours or days, these may not be worth having. Even those who are moribund in this sense can usually recognise this fact, particularly if they are aware that the cost of postponing their death for a few hours or days at the most will mean suffering or death for others. However, even brief remission can be valuable in enabling the individual to put her affairs in order, make farewells and so on, and this can be important. It is for the individual to decide whether the remission that she can be granted is worth having. This is a delicate point that needs more discussion than I can give it here. However, inasmuch as QALYs do not help us to understand the features of a short and painful remission that might none the less make that period of vital importance to the individual, perhaps in terms of making something worthwhile out of her life as a whole, the difficulties of these sorts of circumstances, while real enough, do not undermine the case against QALYs (12).

II. TREATING PEOPLE AS EQUALS

If each life counts for one, then the life of each has the same value as that of any. This is why accepting the value of life generates a principle of equality. This principle does not of course entail that we treat each person equally in the sense of treating each person *the same*. This would be absurd and self-defeating. What it does involve is the idea that we treat each person with the same concern and respect. An illustration provided by Ronald Dworkin, whose work on equality informs this entire discussion, best illustrates this point: 'If I have two children, and one is dying from a disease that is making the other uncomfortale, I do not show equal concern if I flip a coin to decide which should have the remaining dose of a drug' (13).

It is not surprising then that the pattern of protections for individuals that we think of in terms of civil rights (14) centres on the physical protection of the individual and of her most fundamental interests. One of the prime functions of the State is to protect the lives and fundamental interests of its citizens and to treat each citizen as the equal of any other. This is why the State has a basic obligation, *inter alia*, to treat all citizens as equals in the distribution of benefits and opportunities which affect their civil rights. The State must, in short, treat each citizen with equal concern and respect. The civil rights generated by this principle will of course include rights to the allocation of such things as legal protections and educational and health care resources. And this requirement that the State uphold the civil rights of citizens and deal justly between them, means that it must not choose between individuals, or permit choices to be made between individuals, that abridge their civil rights or in ways that attack their right to treatment as equals.

Whatever else this means, it certainly means that a society, through its public institutions, is not entitled to discriminate between individuals in ways that mean life or death for them on grounds which count the lives or fundamental interests of some as worth less than those of others. If for example some people were given life-saving treatment in preference to others because they had a better quality of life than those others, or more dependants and friends, or because they were considered more useful, this would amount to regarding such people as more valuable than others on that account. Indeed it would be tantamount, literally,

to sacrificing the lives of others so that they might continue to live (15).

Because my own life would be better and even of more value to me if I were healthier, fitter, had more money, more friends, more lovers, more children, more life expectancy, more everything I want, it does not follow that others are entitled to decide that because I lack some or all of these things I am less entitled to health care resources, or less worthy to receive those resources, than are others, or that those resources would somehow be wasted on me.

III. CIVIL RIGHTS

I have spoken in terms of civil rights advisedly. If we think of the parallel with our attitude to the system of criminal justice the reasons will be obvious. We think that the liberty of the subject is of fundamental importance and that no one should be wrongfully detained. This is why there are no financial constraints on society's obligation to attempt to ensure equality before the law. An individual is entitled to a fair trial no matter what the financial costs to society (and they can be substantial). We don't adopt rubrics for the allocation of justice which dictate that only those for whom justice can be cheaply provided will receive it. And the reason is that something of fundamental importance is at stake – the liberty of the individual.

In health care something of arguably greater importance is often at stake – the very life of the individual. Indeed, since the abolition of capital punishment, the importance of seeing that individuals' civil rights are respected in health care is pre-eminent.

IV. DISCRIMINATION

The only way to deal between individuals in a way which treats them as equals when resources are scarce, is to allocate those resources in a way which exhibits no preference. To discriminate between people on the grounds of quality of life, or QALY, or life-expectancy, is as unwarranted as it would be to discriminate on the grounds of race or gender.

So, the problem of choosing how to allocate scarce resources is simple. And by that of course I mean 'theoretically simple', not that the decisions will be easy to make or that it will be anything but agonisingly difficult actually to determine, however justly, who should live and who should die. Life-saving resources should simply be allocated in ways which do not violate the individual's entitlement to be treated as the equal of any other individual in the society: and that means the individual's entitlement to have his interests and desires weighed at the same value as those of anyone else. The QALY and the other bases of preference we have considered are irrelevant.

If health professionals are forced by the scarcity of resources, to choose, they should avoid unjust discrimination. But how are they to do this?

Just distribution

If there were a satisfactory principle or theory of just

distribution now would be the time to recommend its use (14). Unfortunately there is not a satisfactory principle available. The task is to allocate resources between competing claimants in a way that does not violate the individual's entitlement to be treated as the equal of any other individual – and that means her entitlement to have her fundamental interests and desires weighed at the same value as those of anyone else. The QALY and other quality-of-life criteria are, as we have seen, both dangerous and irrelevant as are considerations based on life-expectancy or on 'life-years' generated by the proposed treatment. If health professionals are forced by the scarcity of resources to choose, not *whether* to treat but *who* to treat, they must avoid any method that amounts to unjust discrimination.

I do not pretend that the task of achieving this will be an easy one, nor that I have any satisfactory solution. I do have views on how to approach a solution, but the development of those ideas is a task for another occasion (12). I will be content for the moment if I have shown that QALYs are not the answer and that efforts to find one will have to take a different direction.

I. DEFENSIVE MEDICINE

While it is true that resources will always be limited it is far from clear that resources for health care are justifiably as limited as they are sometimes made to appear. People within health care are too often forced to consider simply the question of the best way of allocating the *health care budget*, and consequently are forced to compete with each other for resources. Where lives are at stake however, the issue is a moral issue which faces the whole community, and in such circumstances, is one which calls for a fundamental reappraisal of priorities. The question should therefore be posed in terms, not of the health care budget alone, but of the *national budget* (16). If this is done it will be clearer that it is simply not true that the resources necessary to save the lives of citizens are not available. Since the citizens in question are in real and present danger of death, the issue of the allocation of resources to life-saving is naturally one of, among other things, national defence. Clearly then health professionals who require additional resources simply to save the lives of citizens, have a prior and priority claim on the defence budget.

QALYs encourage the idea that the task for health economics is to find more efficient ways of doing the wrong thing – in this case sacrificing the lives of patients who could be saved. All people concerned with health care should have as their priority defensive medicine: defending their patients against unjust and lethal policies, and guarding themselves against devices that tend to disguise the immorality of what they are asked to do.

II. PRIORITY IN LIFE-SAVING

It is implausible to suppose that we cannot deploy vastly greater resources than we do at present to save the lives of all those in immediate mortal danger. It should be only in exceptional circumstances – unforeseen and massive disasters for example – that we cannot achieve this. However, in such circumstances our first duty is to try to save the maximum number of lives possible. This is because, since each person's life is valuable, and since we are committed to treating each person with the same concern and respect that we show to any, we must preserve the lives of as many individuals as we can. To fail to do so would be to value at zero the lives and fundamental interests of those extra people we could, but do not, save. Where we cannot save all, we should select those who are not to be saved in a way that shows no unjust preference.

We should be very clear that the obligation to save as many lives as possible is *not the obligation to save as many lives as we can cheaply or economically save*. Among the sorts of disasters that force us to choose between lives, is not the disaster of overspending a limited health care budget!

There are multifarious examples of what I have in mind here and just a couple must suffice to illustrate the point. Suppose, as is often the case, providing health care in one region of a country (17) is more expensive than doing so in another, or where saving the lives of people with particular conditions, is radically more expensive than other life-saving procedures, and a given health care budget won't run to the saving of all. Then any formula employed to choose priorities should do just that. Instead of attempting to measure the value of people's lives and select which are worth saving, any rubric for resource allocation should *examine the national budget afresh* to see whether there are any headings of expenditure that are more important to the community than rescuing citizens in mortal danger. For only if all other claims on funding are plausibly more important than that, is it true that resources for life-saving are limited.

III. CONCLUSION

The principle of equal access to health care is sustained by the very same reasons that sustain both the principle of equality before the law and the civil rights required to defend the freedom of the indivual. These are rightly considered so important that no limit is set on the cost of sustaining them. Equal access to health care is of equal importance and should be accorded the same priority for analogous reasons. Indeed, since the abolition of capital punishment, due process of law is arguably of less vital importance than is access to health care. We have seen that QALYs involve denying that the life and health of each citizen is as important as that of any. If, for example, we applied the QALY principle to the administration of criminal justice we might find that those with little life expectancy would have less to gain from securing their freedom and therefore should not be defended at all, or perhaps given a jury trial only if not in competition for such things with younger or fitter fellow citizens.

A recent BBC television programme calculated (18) that if a health authority had £200,000 to spend it would get 10 QALYs from dialysis of kidney patients, 266 QALYs from hip-replacement operations or 1197 QALYs from anti-smoking propaganda. While this information is undoubtedly useful and while advice to stop smoking is an important part of health care, we should be wary of a formula which seems to dictate that such a health authority would use its resources most efficiently if it abandoned hip replacements and dialysis in favour of advice to stop smoking.

John Harris is Senior Lecturer in Philosophy in the Department of Education and Research Director of the Centre For Social Ethics and Policy, University of Manchester.

Acknowledgement

This is a revised version of a paper presented to the British Medical Association Annual Scientific Meeting, Oxford, April 1986.

As so often, I must thank my colleague Dr Mary Lobjoit for her generous medical advice. The fact that, like certain patients, I am apt to misunderstand this advice is of course my own fault. Thank are also due to Don Evans, Alan Williams and the editors of the *Journal of Medical Ethics* for helpful comments.

References and notes

(1) See the excellent discussion of the recent history of this line of thought in the Office of Health Economics publication *The measurement of health* London, 1985.

(2) Williams A. Economics of coronary artery bypass grafting. *British medical journal* 1985; 291; and his contribution to the article, Centre eight – in search of efficiency. *Health and social service journal* 1985. These are by no means the first such attempts. See reference (1).

(3) Williams A. The value of QALYs. *Health and social service journal* 1985.

(4) I mention this in case anyone should think that it is only medical scientists who do medical research.

(5) See reference (3): 3.

(6) See reference (1): 16.

(7) See reference (3): 5, and reference (3).

(8) I'll assume this can be described as 'true' for the sake of argument.

(9) I am indebted to Dr S G Potts for pointing out to me some of these statistics and for other helpful comments.

(10) For examples see reference (1) and reference (2).

(11) See Parfit D. Innumerate ethics. *Philosophy and public affairs* 1978; 7, 4. Parfit's arguments provide a detailed defence of the principle that each is to count for one.

(12) I consider these problems in more detail in my: EQALYty. In: Byrne P, ed. *King's College studies*. London: King's Fund Press, 1987/8. Forthcoming.

(13) Dworkin R. *Taking rights seriously*. London: Duckworth, 1977: 227.

(14) I do not of course mean to imply that there are such things as rights, merely that our use of the language of rights captures the special importance we attach to certain freedoms and protections. The term 'civil rights' is used here as a 'term of art' referring to those freedoms and protections that are customarily classed as 'civil rights'.

(15) For an interesting attempt to fill this gap see Dworkin R. What is equality? *Philosophy and public affairs* 1981; 4 and 5.

(16) And of course the international budget: see my *The value of life*. London: Routledge & Kegan Paul 1985: chapter 3.

(17) See Townsend P, Davidson N, eds. *Inequalities in health: the Black Report*. Harmondsworth, Penguin: 1982.

(18) BBC 1. *The heart of the matter* 1986, Oct.

Response: QALYfying the value of life

Alan Williams *University of York*

The essence of Harris's position can be encapsulated in the following three propositions:

1) Health care priorities should not be influenced by any other consideration than keeping people alive;
2) Everyone has an equal right to be kept alive if that is what they wish, irrespective of how poor their prognosis is, and no matter what sacrifices others have to bear as a consequence;
3) When allocating health care resources, we must not discriminate between people, not even according to their differential capacity to benefit from treatment.

My position, which he attacks, can be encapsulated in the following three propositions:

1) Health care priorities should be influenced by our capacity both to increase life expectation and to improve people's quality of life.
2) A particular improvement in health should be regarded as of equal value, no matter who gets it, and should be provided unless it prevents a greater improvement being offered to someone else.
3) It is the responsibility of everyone to discriminate wherever necessary to ensure that our limited resources go where they will do the most good.

At the end of the day we simply have to stand up and be counted as to which set of principles we wish to have underpin the way the health care system works.

The rest of Harris's points are really detail and I will deal with them on a subsequent occasion when I have had a chance to study his promised way forward, for that may help to dispel the very serious doubts I hold at present as to whether he realises the grave implications of the position he has adopted.

Alan Williams is Professor of Economics at the University of York.

Key words

QALY; equality; civil rights; efficiency; scarce resources.

[35]

Journal of medical ethics 1995; **21**: 91–96

Literature and medical ethics

Doing harm: living organ donors, clinical research and *The Tenth Man*

Carl Elliott *McGill University Centre for Medicine, Ethics and Law, and Montreal Children's Hospital, Canada*

Abstract

This paper examines the ethical difficulties of organ donation from living donors and the problem of causing harm to patients or research subjects at their request. Graham Greene explored morally similar questions in his novella, The Tenth Man.

Medical treatment is often painful, usually unpleasant, and sometimes genuinely harmful. The administration of pain has become a routine part of diagnosis and treatment, from blood-drawings, intravenous lines and lumbar punctures to chemotherapy, limb amputations and involuntary psychiatric confinement. Many doctors are understandably uncomfortable with this part of medicine, even when the patient agrees to it, especially when the harm is permanent or severe. Life may be short and the art long, but the art's most delicate aspect is not to shorten life further, and not to diminish it.

Although medical procedures that harm patients are ordinarily intended to serve the patient's welfare, there are two related exceptions: non-therapeutic clinical research on human subjects, and organ transplantation from living donors. The procedures are related in that living organ donation, at least in its early stages, has been an experimental therapy. They are exceptional in that both human research and living organ donation require people to take risks or undergo harm for the sake of others, rather than for themselves.

The bioethical literature of the past three decades has done a thorough job of exploring the rights of competent patients to refuse treatment, and it has struggled, not always successfully, with the question of when research or other risky procedures are justifiable on patients incompetent to consent. But it has tended to overlook a cluster of questions surrounding the opposite problem: competent people who consent to, or even request, procedures which are risky, painful or harmful. Part of the

Key words

Organ transplantation; organ donation; research ethics; medical ethics; supererogation.

reason for this neglect may be the idiom in which bioethical questions are usually scripted and rehearsed, which is not well suited to the moral backdrop against which these issues are often played out. A vocabulary of rights and autonomy can be inadequate to represent the intimate bonds of family and friends, the delicate balance between sacrifice and self-interest, and the complex, often awkward relationship between doctors and organ donors or research subjects. In a moral framework shaped by respect for patient autonomy, whether or not to undergo risk or harm can come to seem a matter solely for patients to decide. The worries that many doctors feel about exposing willing subjects to harm or great risk can be frustratingly difficult to express.

What I would like to do here is to articulate some of these worries and to take the debate beyond the terms in which it is ordinarily expressed: as a conflict between the principles of beneficence and autonomy. To do this, I draw on Graham Greene's novella about shame and redemption, *The Tenth Man*. I will suggest that the issue of doing harm to willing subjects is more complicated than philosophers often acknowledge. I conclude with some practical recommendations for approaching the problem of patients who willingly expose themselves to harm or risk.

Volunteering to be harmed

Sometimes competent adults volunteer for research or other sorts of medical procedure that are likely to harm them. Sometimes they volunteer for good reasons, other times for bad ones, but in either case a certain proportion of them are well aware of the harms they are risking and freely consent to them. One relatively common example is phase one clinical trials for chemotherapeutic drugs. Phase one trials test a drug's safety, and for chemotherapy they are generally done on patients with incurable cancer. Patients are at first given a small dose of the drug, which is increased until the patients begin to have toxic side-effects. However, with the toxicity comes only an exceedingly small chance of therapeutic benefit; for example, one study put the rate of complete remission at 0·16 per cent, and the likelihood of any objective response at all at less than 5 per cent (1).

While some people see no problem in exposing competent adults to the risk of harm as long as they are informed and willing, many others feel vaguely uneasy about it. In fact, most people can imagine some limit to the degree of risk, and the severity of the harm, to which they would be willing to allow a subject to expose him or herself. Renee Fox reported a dramatic example at a conference sponsored by the University of Utah after the total artificial heart implantation in 1982 (2). Commenting on her experience at Stanford University, Fox said that the Stanford heart transplant team had been contacted by a number of healthy volunteers who wanted to become living heart donors. The volunteers wished to donate their hearts to patients in need, knowing that this meant sacrificing their lives.

William De Vries, the surgeon who performed the first artificial heart implant at Utah, said his team also received a number of calls from healthy volunteers when their surgical team was in the process of selecting a patient for the implant. These volunteers had no medical need for an artificial heart, but nevertheless wanted to volunteer to have one implanted, apparently solely to become test subjects for the sake of medical science. Some of these volunteers were death row inmates. Another was a sixty-year-old woman who had raised her family, and evidently thought this would be a fitting way to end her life.

It might be thought that few people would approve of very dangerous cardiovascular research on healthy subjects, much less heart transplants from living donors. Yet in a moral framework whose dominant principle is respect for individual autonomy, doubts about harmful procedures are difficult to defend. The volunteers are competent and their sacrifices would clearly help people in need. We allow patients to refuse procedures, even when a refusal will be harmful. So when they *request* harmful procedures, why shouldn't we agree to perform them? John Harris, who professes to see no problem with such procedures, puts the case simply: 'Should I be permitted voluntarily to donate a vital organ like the heart? Again, if I know what I am doing then I do not see why I should not give my life to save that of another if that is what I want to do' (3).

The Tenth Man

Graham Greene's novella, *The Tenth Man*, is a subtle reminder that self-sacrifice is often more morally complicated than it seems (4). It tells the story of a French lawyer, Chavel, who is jailed by the Nazis during World War II. Chavel has been rounded up by the police for reasons unknown and

imprisoned in a cell with twenty-nine other men. Most of the men are poor, below Chavel's station in life, and this fact increases Chavel's agitation about his plight.

After a number of months a guard enters the cell and tells the prisoners that there have been some murders in the town by the resistance movement. As a result, the commanders have ordered that one man out of every ten in the camp is to be shot. In a day's time, three of the thirty prisoners in Chavel's cell will be executed. The prisoners themselves must choose which three.

The prisoners decide to draw lots, and Chavel is among the three marked to die. Unlike the other condemned men, Chavel panics. He alone among the prisoners is a wealthy man, and fear-stricken, he begins to offer all his wealth and belongings to the other prisoners, if only one of them will change places with him. To the astonishment of all, one man accepts the offer. Michel Janvier says that if Chavel will sign over his house and all his wealth to him, so that he can in turn leave it to his impoverished mother and sister, he will take Chavel's place before the firing squad. He and Chavel draw up a will, and the next day, Janvier is shot.

This exchange takes place in only the first chapter of the book, but it is the story's defining event. The exchange was freely agreed by both men and witnessed by the other prisoners. Yet even though the deal was freely made, we know that Chavel was wrong to make it. Even though we might admire Janvier for sacrificing his life in order to provide for his mother and sister, we know that Chavel was wrong to take advantage of Janvier's selflessness.

Chavel knows this as well, and his actions torment him. *The Tenth Man* is a book about guilt and shame, and its plot turns on Chavel's efforts to purge himself of the guilt that he feels about bartering for his life. After the Nazis fall and Chavel is freed from prison, he is celebrating in a bar when he sees his face in a water decanter.

'It is the face of failure. It was odd, he thought, that one failure of nerve had ingrained the face as deeply as a tramp's, but, of course, he had the objectivity to tell himself, it wasn't one failure; it was a whole lifetime of preparation for the event. An artist paints his picture not in a few hours but in all the years of experience before he takes up the brush, and it is the same with failure' (4).

Harm and autonomy

Our ordinary moral and political vocabulary makes it natural to think of exchanges involving harm, such as the exchange made by Janvier and Chavel, as questions primarily of rights, freedom and fairness. Yet very often our private reservations about harmful practices bear only a tangential relationship to these questions. That this is so can be seen in the awkward terms in which contemporary debates about harmful practices are often played out: whether people have a 'right' to act altruistically, or whether a research subject's 'freedom' is compromised by payment. In *The Tenth Man*, a prisoner objects to the deal struck by Chavel and Janvier on the grounds that it is not fair. But argued in these terms, his legitimate moral concerns are bound to be frustrated. As Janvier angrily replies: 'Why isn't it fair to let me do what I want? You'd all be rich men if you could, but you haven't the spunk. I see my chance and I take it. Fair, of course, it's fair. I'm going to die a rich man and anyone who thinks it isn't fair can rot' (4).

In a debate shaped by concepts like these, taking part in a harmful medical procedure or research protocol comes to be seen primarily as a matter of individual autonomy. Genuine worries about exposing a subject to harm are channelled into a debate about freedom of choice. When a surgical team at the University of Chicago transplanted a liver lobe from a living mother to her daughter with biliary atresia in 1989, critics of the procedure said that to offer a mother the chance to donate a liver lobe to her daughter was 'coercive', that no parent could refuse the offer (5). The bonds between parent and child are so tight, it was said, that they constrict a parent's ability to make a free choice about risking the chance of harm.

While this criticism expresses some legitimate worries, it is aimed in the wrong direction. The most worrying part of living organ donation is not freedom of choice, though there is certainly the possibility of subtle coercion in such a situation. The worrying part is the chance of harm to a healthy donor: the liver transplant procedure was a new one, the risks potentially minimal but in many respects unknown (6). That these worries about self-chosen risks should emerge disguised as concerns about free choice – the idea that a parent is *coerced* by her love for and moral obligations towards her child – says something about the central place the ethic of autonomy holds in our culture. Yet the fact is that no one would have thought to call such a choice coercive if no risk of harm were involved.

While debates over rights and freedom should not be ignored, they do not quite get at the real source of Chavel's shame, nor at what is most troubling about subjects who volunteer for harmful procedures or research protocols. An exchange can be made fairly and freely, yet still fail to be admirable or honourable. Certainly Chavel's actions were understandable; they were the actions of a desperate man, who grasped frantically at the only possible chance of surviving his imprisonment. But they were also the actions of a coward, a man who took advantage of his wealth and another man's selflessness in order to save his own skin. A person who attempted such an exchange might well be

justified in demanding that no one prevent him from making it, but as Adam Smith remarks of this type of situation, '[N]o man, I imagine, who had gone through an adventure of this kind would be fond of telling the story' (7).

Benefit from harm

To get at what is troubling about a person who knowingly and willingly consents to a harmful medical procedure, it is necessary to look not simply at the person making the decision to participate, but beyond him to the other people involved in and affected by the exchange. In many ordinary, non-medical cases, if a person chooses to risk his life or health, we feel that this is ultimately his decision to make. Miners, police officers and soldiers all take risks, often very dangerous ones. Our highest admiration, in fact, is reserved for those rare people who risk or even sacrifice themselves for the sake of others.

But while we honour self-sacrifice, we would rightly criticize a person like Chavel, who willingly *took advantage of* another person's sacrifice. And this is what is hard to avoid in many harmful medical procedures: a person who stands to gain from a volunteer's selflessness. Altruistic acts benefit other people, both directly, as with an organ recipient, and indirectly, as with the clinical researcher whose reputation is made through the fruits of his research. And while it might be admirable to risk harm to oneself, it is not admirable to encourage another person to risk harm to himself for one's own benefit (8).

The most obvious example is organ donation from living donors – of kidneys, bone marrow, and more recently, liver lobes and lungs. Though the risks associated with each of these procedures vary considerably, from very little to unknown, they are all undertaken for the good of a recipient who, unless he or she is a child, has presumably agreed to be a recipient. Accepting a sacrifice of great magnitude is not mere passive acquiescence, devoid of any moral import. If I allow someone else to risk his life or health for my sake, I am endorsing his self-sacrifice and agreeing to profit by it (9). Now, of course, if the risk to the donor were very small, as in the case of bone marrow transplantation, and the alternative were death, an offer like this would be difficult to refuse, and accepting it would surely be justified. But what if the risk were very high? What would we think of a person who would take advantage of a donor's willingness to take life-threatening risks? What would we think of a person who would accept a heart from a living donor?

Unless the circumstances were extraordinary, most of us would think very badly indeed of a person who would agree to, and take advantage of, a sacrifice of this magnitude. Like Chavel's, his would be an act of failure: a failure of courage, a lapse of moral nerve. Chavel is ashamed because his hour came; he had the chance to behave honourably; and he betrayed himself. Like Conrad's Lord Jim, he was faced with a moral test and he floundered. If an ailing patient were to take advantage of a healthy donor's voluntary self-sacrifice, it might well be understandable, but it would not be morally admirable. It would not be the sort of behaviour that we would aspire to and want to encourage.

This point also helps to explain why we often feel very differently about a person who donates an organ to a family member. Chavel's life was saved through a bargain struck with a stranger, and we rightly feel that he was wrong to take advantage of Janvier's unusual wishes. But relationships between family members are coloured by very different moral and emotional hues. Here talk of rights, obligations, respect and freedom gives way more naturally to talk of gratitude, grudges, devotion and kinship. If a father wishes to donate an organ to a child, or a sister to a brother, we can immediately understand the wish. It arises out of love. And accepting a gesture of love, even if it involves the risk of harm to the giver, is profoundly different from paying someone to harm himself, or even from endorsing self-harm from a stranger. When a person is faced with serious illness, we *expect* her family to respond, and we can identify with the impulse to undergo whatever risks or harms are necessary to help the loved one. It is a legitimate question, of course, whether or not a person who truly loves another could in good conscience allow that person to take great risks for him. But we can understand and approve of the relationship out of which such an offer and acceptance might take place. If a person offers to risk his life for a stranger, even if we admire him we feel the need for him to explain why he is willing to take such grave risks. But if a sister offers to risk her life for her brother, the explanation 'because he is my brother' will suffice.

For related reasons, it seems less problematic for a small child to be the recipient of an organ from a living donor than it is for an adult. Since a small child has no choice in the matter, unlike an adult, he cannot endorse or agree with a donor's decision to undergo risk or harm. Thus there is no worry that the recipient might be taking advantage of the donor.

It must be remembered that decisions about risking harmful procedures are always made within a web of social relationships: between family members, between strangers, between clinician and patient, researcher and subject. The nature of those relationships affects the moral standing of the decisions, as I have pointed out, but the reverse is also true: what sort of decisions we allow or encourage affects the nature of the social relationships. For example, it may be admirable for a person to place another person's interests above his own, but for doctors to encourage or endorse such

decisions by their patients might undermine the already endangered assumption that doctors put the interests of their patients first. This would probably change significantly the relationship between doctors and patients. Even those of us who resent being told by doctors how we should behave might be wary of doctors who had no qualms about doing significant harm to their patients for the benefit of someone else.

Paying for organs

The nature of the doctor-patient relationship would probably also be altered if we were to commercialise the transfer of human organs, though just how it would be altered is not easy to predict. Organ transplantation is a practice in which a relatively small proportion of people ever take part, and it fits into our cultural landscape rather awkwardly. Both the language we use to describe the prelude to organ transplantation and our customary ways of proceeding suggest that we have begun thinking of the practice, however tentatively, as a variation on gift-giving (10). We speak of 'donating' organs; promotional campaigns encourage potential blood donors to 'give the gift of life'.

However, the anthropology of a practice is altered by the exchange of money for what would otherwise be undertaken for reasons of affection, charity or duty. We make important distinctions between favours and services, gifts and merchandise (11). To put a price on organs and sell them alters, in a rather uncomfortable way, both the way we think of the organs themselves and the relationship between the organ donor and the recipient. The donor becomes a vendor, the recipient a customer, the organ a commodity, and the relationship a contract. Many doctors would be uncomfortable with this commercialized version of transplantation, even those who doubt that generosity can meet the demand for organs.

The Tenth Man also reminds us that few decisions affect only the person who makes them. Chavel eventually takes a job under an assumed name as a handyman at his old estate, which is now owned by Janvier's sister and mother. There he realizes how much his exchange has hurt Janvier's sister, who despises the unknown man whose bargaining led to her brother's death. She wonders how Janvier could have ever thought that she and her mother would have preferred the wealth they have inherited to his life.

That a person's decision to harm himself deeply affects a circle of people far beyond him seems so obvious a part of ordinary life that it seems almost trite to emphasize it here, but a recognition of this point is often strangely absent in philosophical writing. To emphasize the broader effects of a person's actions is not, of course, to deny that a person's liberty rights entitle him to harm himself if he wishes. It is rather to point out that these actions often extract a heavy toll on those who love and care about the agent, and that for this reason, they are not ethically uncomplicated. If I pay another person to harm himself for my sake, or if I agree to use him in a risky research protocol, I must recognize that my actions might very likely damage his family and friends very much. And even while I might defend that person's right to make the decision to harm himself, I would feel very awkward trying to defend myself against the criticism of his family and friends, whose resentment most of us could readily understand.

Finally, it is important to realize that the doctor is not a mere instrument of the patient's wishes. Analyses of living organ donation and risky clinical research are often simplified needlessly by a failure to acknowledge outright that the doctor is also a moral agent who should be held accountable for his actions. If a patient undergoes a harmful procedure, the moral responsibility for that action does not belong to the patient alone; it is shared by the doctor who performs it. Thus a doctor is in the position of deciding not simply whether a subject's choice is reasonable or morally justifiable, but whether *he* is morally justified in helping the subject accomplish it.

This alters the doctor's perspective in at least two important ways. First, as a moral agent, the doctor must ask not simply whether a change in a given state of affairs would be morally better, as a detached observer might ask, but whether or not he should become the *agent* of that change. Answers to these two questions need not be the same. If I were faced with a dying person in intractable pain who wanted to be a heart donor, I might well judge that all things considered, it would be better if he were to die. But this does not mean that I would be willing to kill him, or that I believe that I (or anyone) would be morally justified in doing so. It is an essential part of our notion of agency that we distinguish between that which we *do* and that which merely *happens*. It is not at all unreasonable for a doctor to think that it would be good for an event to take place but bad for him to bring it about.

To take another, slightly different example: opponents of a market trade in human organs often argue that an organ-market would exploit the poor, who would be tempted to alleviate their poverty at great risk to their health. Market defenders respond that the harms a poor person chooses to undergo should be a matter for that person himself to decide. A poor person might well think that it is better to be without a kidney than without money. But if I am the surgeon faced with doing the transplantation, this argument may still not win me over. Because even if I agree that the choice of harms should be up to the poor person himself, and that his choice to donate a kidney for money is reasonable, the fact is that *I* would not be responsible for his being poor, but I *would* be responsible for his being without a

kidney. Greene makes this point in *The Tenth Man.* What torments Chavel is not a mere event, the death of Janvier, but the fact that he, Chavel, is at least partly morally responsible for bringing that death about.

The second important way in which the doctor's perspective differs from that of a patient or a detached observer is in the balance of harms and interests that he must weigh. A potential organ donor or research subject must decide whether to weigh the interests of other people over his own. To do so would be admirable, and not to do so would still be understandable. However, the doctor is looking at a different sort of balance. He must weigh not his own interests, but the interests of one person against another: in the case of organ transplantation, the interests of a potential donor against the interests of a recipient; or in the case of non-therapeutic clinical research, the interests of a potential research subject against the potential beneficiaries of the research. This shifts the moral balance of the problem in an important way, because while we admire the person who *undergoes* harm to himself for the sake of another, we do not necessarily admire the person who *inflicts* harm on one person for the sake of another. And the latter is what the doctor must do (12).

Conclusion

How should these points shape the way we approach policy decisions on procedures that involve the likelihood of significant harm to patients? First, there is a legitimate distinction to be drawn between *allowing* a person to risk harm to himself and *encouraging* it. So, for example, even if we acknowledge the argument that a person has a right to risk harm to herself and that her action would benefit others, it does not follow that a system is justified which encourages people to harm themselves. Substantial payment to organ donors or volunteers for dangerous research arguably crosses the line between allowing and encouraging.

Second, there is obviously a difference between choosing to risk harm to oneself and choosing to aid another person in risking it. It is partly for this reason that we might admire a person who chose to risk his life or health for the sake of others, but at the same time criticize the doctor or researcher who exposed him to that risk (12). It is not unreasonable, then, for doctors to be reluctant to expose willing subjects to the risk of harm, even while acknowledging the legitimacy of a system which allows subjects to take great risks. In fact, we might be justifiably suspicious of the character of a doctor who had no such reservations.

Third, it is important to acknowledge outright that when a person chooses to risk harm to himself, very often he is risking harm to others as well. When

96 *Literature and medical ethics: Doing harm: living organ donors, clinical research and* The Tenth Man

a person suffers, those who love him suffer, and when a person dies, he is missed. Any decision to encourage or assist a person who is willing to undergo a risky or harmful procedure must take into account these broader effects. (Of course, these effects touch the circle of people surrounding the potential *beneficiary* as well as those surrounding the person taking the risk.)

Fourth, at least part of the reason why we have reservations about patients who volunteer to be harmed is the possibility that other people might be taking advantage of the volunteer's selflessness – organ recipients taking advantage of donors, researchers taking advantage of volunteers, and so on. For this reason, any system of practices in which people are likely to be harmed should be set up in ways that minimize this possibility. Of course, there is a sense in which *any* person who benefits from such a system is taking advantage of those who contribute to it, but it is possible to draw some limits. For example, it would be better to have a system of living organ transplantation in which nobody is able to make a financial profit from the procedure, including transplant surgeons and organ procurement agencies. This would limit incentives for anyone to encourage potential donors to take risks.

Carl Elliott, MD, PhD, is Assistant Professor, McGill University Faculty of Medicine, Centre for Medicine, Ethics and Law, and Clinical Ethicist, Montreal Children's Hospital, Canada.

References and notes

(1) Markham M. The ethical dilemma of phase one clinical trials. *C A – a journal for clinicians* 1986; 36, 6: 367–369.
(2) Shaw M, ed. *After Barney Clark: reflections on the Utah artificial heart program.* Austin, Texas: University of Texas Press, 1984.
(3) Harris J. *Wonderwoman and superman: the ethics of human biotechnology.* New York: Oxford University Press, 1992: 113.
(4) Greene G. *The Tenth Man.* London: Penguin, 1985.
(5) Much of this criticism was reported in the popular press. See, for example, comments by: Annas G, *New York Times* 1989 Nov 27; Colen B D, *Los Angeles Times* 1989 Dec 11; Kohrman A, *Chicago Tribune Magazine* 1990 Jan 21; Caplan A, *Knight-Ridder Newspapers* 1989 Dec 14.
(6) Singer P, Siegler M, Whitington P, *et al.* Ethics of liver transplantation with living donors. *New England journal of medicine* 1989; 321, 9: 620–622.
(7) Smith A. *The theory of moral sentiments.* Indianapolis: Liberty Classics, 1982 [originally 1759]: 333.
(8) We recognize this in non-medical situations as well. There are limits to the harms to which we allow employers to expose workers, even if the workers are aware of the harms and willing to risk them.
(9) Brecher B. The kidney trade: or, the customer is always wrong. *Journal of medical ethics* 1990; 16: 120–123.
(10) Murray T. Gifts of the body and the needs of strangers. *Hastings Center report* 1987; 2, Apr: 30–38.
(11) Campbell C. Body, self and the property paradigm. *Hastings Center report* 1992; 22, 5: 34–42.
(12) Elliott C. Constraints and heroes. *Bioethics* 1992; 6, 1: 1–11.

Journal of medical ethics, 1986, 12, 174-181

Health

R M Hare   *University of Florida, USA and White's Professor of Moral Philosophy Emeritus,
University of Oxford*

Author's abstract

*Many practical issues in medical ethics depend on an
understanding of the concept of health. The main question
is whether it is a purely descriptive or a partly evaluative or
normative concept. After posing some puzzles about the
concept, the views of C Boorse, who thinks it is descriptive,
are discussed and difficulties are found for them. An
evaluative treatment is then suggested, and used to shed
light on some problems about mental illness and to compare
and contrast it with physical illness and with political and
other deviancies which are not illnesses.*

*This paper is a shortened and revised version of the first
John Locke Lecture given to the Society of Apothecaries in
London in 1978, under the title What Can Philosophy do
for Medicine?*

The concept of health is one the understanding of
which would help with both theoretical problems in
philosophy and practical problems in medicine. The
theoretical problems arise because philosophers, at
least since Plato and Aristotle, have used what may be
called the medical analogy when discussing morality;
they have claimed that expressions such as 'good man'
behave in some ways like the expression 'healthy man',
and that if we have no difficulty in applying the latter,
we should have no more difficulty in applying the
former. Thus advocates of descriptivist ethical theories
(ie those which assimilate moral words, in respect of
their logical properties, to standardly descriptive
words like 'red' or 'triangular') often claim that since
'healthy' is a descriptive concept, so may 'good' be.
The obvious reply, for those who reject descriptivism,
is to ask whether 'healthy' is purely descriptive either;
and that is what I shall be doing in this paper.

That this discussion is of practical importance
should be clear to anybody who reflects on the bitter
disputes that have been going on recently about what is
called 'mental illness'. We have for example,
psychiatrists in the Soviet Union arraigned by their
colleagues from other countries for classing as mental

Key words

Health, illness, disease; mental illness, political deviancy;
descriptive, evaluative, normative; suffering, incapacity;
natural function; species-typical; survival; reproduction.

illness, and treating by allegedly inhumane methods,
what is really only political deviancy (1); and we have
'anti-psychiatrists' like Thomas Szasz (2) accusing
their colleagues even in the West of treating what they
call 'mental illness' as if it were the analogue of physical
illness, whereas, he says, it is nothing of the kind. We
shall never be clear about these disputes until we are
clear about the meaning of the term 'illness', whether
applied to mental or physical conditions, and about its
opposite 'health', and its near synonyms 'disease' and
'disorder'.

But even if we confine ourselves to physical health,
there are severe practical problems which would be
easier to handle if we were clearer about the concept.
Take, for example, the treatment of children born with
spina bifida, which has been much discussed recently.
Spina bifida is in the ordinary sense a disease and I
suppose an illness; but what counts as 'treatment' let
alone as 'cure' of it? If medicine is the art of healing,
how near to normality has the patient to be brought
before it can be said that the exercise of the art was
justified? And how could we answer that question,
without deciding what we mean by 'heal' and therefore
by 'health'?

I will start, as Aristotle used to (he was the son of a
doctor) by looking at some of the conceptual
difficulties (the symptoms of our ignorance of what we
are saying when we call a person healthy). Is health
perhaps the absence of disease or illness? But is illness
the same thing as disease, and health just the absence of
these, or is it something more positive? A patient can
have a disease (say diabetes), and yet not be ill if the
disease is well controlled. He will *become* ill, if he does
not observe the prescribed diet and take the prescribed
remedies; but he is not ill now. Also, we say that there
are two different diseases, if there are two different
causes (for example, when it was discovered that some
dysenteries were caused by amoebae and some by
bacilli, it was said that there were two different
diseases, amoebic and bacillary dysentery); but are
there two different illnesses? The whole notion of
counting or classifying illnesses, as opposed to
diseases, in this way is a bit strange. As we shall see,
some philosophers have made more even than this of
the difference between the concepts of disease and
illness. Professor Boorse (of whom more below)

considers the interesting suggestion that illnesses are particulars, diseases universals (3).

Doctors tend, in fact, to use neither of these words, but the more non-committal word 'condition'. They do this because it is useful to be able to describe the patient's condition without committing oneself about its aetiology, and by saying that he has a certain disease one may so commit oneself. Secondly, not all conditions are pathological, but all diseases are, by definition. If a doctor says that his patient has a certain condition, he does not presuppose that it is a bad condition to be in (the condition might, for example, be pregnancy, both normal and desired). As we shall see, this is very important for our understanding of the concepts.

Not all the conditions treated by doctors are diseases, therefore. There are even bad conditions which are not diseases, such as injuries and wounds. If I am bitten by a dog and go to the doctor for repair, I am not suffering from a disease (assuming that the dog did not carry rabies). The same is true if I am knocked down by a lorry (assuming that I have got over the shock and just require a few stitches). But if it is a virus that has attacked me, I do have a disease.

Why do the attacks of viruses count as diseases, but not the attacks of larger animals or of motor vehicles? Is it just a question of size? Or of invisibility? I believe that doctors call the attacks of intestinal and other worms diseases, though there are also more precise words like 'infestation'. If I have a tape or a guinea worm (which are quite large), do I have a disease? Does it make a difference if the worm can be seen but its eggs cannot? Or does it make a difference that the worm, although it can eventually be seen, is in some sense, while active, *inside* the patient, whereas dogs and lorries, and also lice and fleas, whose attacks are likewise not called diseases, are always outside the body? Does a disease have to be something *in* me? And in what sense of 'in'? Some skin diseases such as scabies are so called, although the organisms which cause them are in the skin, and do not penetrate the body. They penetrate the *skin* indeed; but then so does the ichneumon maggot, and the body too. Is the difference between these maggots and the scabies mite merely one of size? Or of visibility?

Or is it simply that our conceptual classification of these terms grew up before we knew as much about the causes of diseases as we do now? Now, we can actually see viruses and bacilli through microscopes; but the diseases they cause came to be called diseases before we could do this. On the other hand we could always see dogs. So perhaps we use the word 'disease' for conditions whose cause was not visible before the invention of microscopes. We must note, though, that in order to identify a condition as a disease we do not have to *know* what its cause is (think of cancer, for example). But we do have to commit ourselves to there being a cause, ascertainable in principle, of the same general sort as the causes of diseases whose aetiology we understand. Thus the names of diseases are what

logicians call 'natural kind' terms (4).

Fortunately the puzzle about why dog- bites are not diseases does not affect our main problem very much, because, whether they are diseases or not, they can certainly claim the attention and care of doctors. The patient, if he is in the army, will be 'on the sick list'. However, the puzzle that I am now coming to *is* crucial to our understanding of the role of doctors. Before we classify something as a disease, does it have to be something *bad*? Could there be a wholly beneficial disease, or one which was neither beneficial nor harmful? It seems not. But we have to be careful. If a soldier is prevented by a mild attack of malaria from being sent back to the battle in which he is very likely to be killed, it was in his interest to have the disease. The device which philosophers use for dealing with this complication is called the '*ceteris paribus* clause'. Malaria can be classified as a disease because *other things being equal*, or *in general*, it is a bad condition to be in; that does not prevent its being a good condition to be in in this soldier's particular circumstances.

But there are worse complications. Who or what does the disease have to be bad for? Consider the diseases of plants, and in particular of weeds. Let us assume for the sake of argument that the word 'disease' has the same meaning when applied to plants as it has when applied to dumb animals and to man. If I have in my garden a bad infestation of ground elder, and the ground elder plants get a disease and die out, I shall be pleased; so the disease is not a bad thing *for me*. (The same applies if in a battle the *enemy* has an outbreak of disease like the army of Sennacherib, or like the Greeks in front of Troy.) In what sense is the disease a bad thing for the ground elder? Do plants have interests, so that things can be good or bad for them? The same problems that afflict the concepts of health and disease afflict also the more general concepts of good and bad: philosophers who discuss these issues are deeply divided, as we shall see.

Conversely, there is a mildew of vines (and mildews are classified in the gardening books as diseases and not as pests) called *pourriture noble*, which actually improves the taste of the wine. Do we rightly call it a disease, because it is bad from the vine's point of view? But does the vine *have* a 'point of view' if it cannot think about the question?

There is said to be a tribe in South America in which the disease of dyschromic spirochetosis, marked by coloured spots on the skin, is so prevalent that it is accepted as normal, and those without the spots are regarded as pathological and excluded from marriage (5). In that tribe, is dyschromic spirochetosis a disease? Recently I had a painful boil removed from the middle of my back, and the report from the laboratory said that it was caused by an organism which exists normally in the bowel, but which, if it gets into the blood-stream, causes this sort of trouble. So whether this organism is pathogenic seems to depend on where it is. Are we to say that whether the spirochete I have just mentioned is pathogenic depends on whether it is on the skin of a South American Indian of that tribe or on that of a European?

If, frightened by such puzzles, we try to define the notion of disease without bringing in the notions of good and bad, we get into other difficulties. We might try, without mentioning the goodness or badness of the conditions, saying that they were diseases if they had, or were likely to have, certain specified alternative effects. For example, we might say to begin with that a condition is a disease if and only if it has a tendency to cause either pain or death or both. This obviously will not do, because a condition would be called a disease if it had a tendency to cause not pain or death, but, say, blindness. It may be said that if a disease causes blindness, it can tend to cause pain or death indirectly, because the blind are more likely to hurt themselves; but this indirect causation is irrelevant to our problem. We do not want to have to say that courage is a disease because it leads to the greater likelihood of being killed in battles.

Perhaps, in view of the blindness example, we should be moved to extend the definition a bit and say that a condition is a disease if it has a tendency to cause *suffering* (which will include pain and other kinds of suffering) or *incapacity* (which will include, as the extreme case, death; for only the dead are totally incapacitated). But then we are on a 'slide'. For what is to count as suffering or incapacity? Can we define *those* notions without bringing in the requirement that to count as an incapacity or as suffering, a condition has to be the cause of some effect which is thought of as *bad?*

I have raised enough problems, in this more or less unsystematic way, to make us think twice before swallowing too easily the arguments of writers like Szasz. He says that what has been called 'mental illness' is a 'myth'; physical illness, he says, is an established and acceptable concept, but the concept of mental illness has been invented by a false analogy with it. Szasz's ideas have led some psychiatrists to make drastic alterations in the way they treat patients; but we cannot know whether they are well founded unless we know whether we can share his assurance that the concept of *physical* health is a clear and incontestable one. I have been trying to cast some doubt on this assurance, not because I think that the concept of physical health is not perfectly viable, but rather because it may well be that, in the process of showing how it is viable, and what its definition should be, we shall discover that the notion of health so characterised *is*, after all, extensible to include mental health, for all that Szasz says. And that might make a very big difference to the practice of psychiatrists.

It is time now to be more systematic. I shall achieve this by considering first the approach to this problem of one of the parties to the philosophical dispute, and then, after pointing out some difficulties in this approach, giving my own view of the question, which is favourable to the other party, though with qualifications.

The approach I shall consider rests heavily on the notion of *natural function*. This is supposed to be a purely descriptive notion – ie, we can, it is claimed, say which functions are natural without committing ourselves as to whether they are good or bad for the organism or for anything or anybody else. Professor Boorse has suggested a definition of 'health' which well expresses this approach:

An organism is *healthy* at any moment in proportion as it is not diseased; and a *disease* is a type of internal state of the organism which:
(i) interferes with the performance of some natural function – ie, some species-typical contribution to survival and reproduction – characteristic of the organism's age; and
(ii) is not simply in the nature of the species, ie is either atypical of the species or, if typical, mainly due to environmental causes (6).

He later gives a partial defining characteristic of 'illness' which distinguishes the meaning of this term from that of 'disease':

A disease is an *illness* only if it is serious enough to be incapacitating, and therefore is
(i) undesirable for its bearer;
(ii) a title to special treatment; and
(iii) a valid excuse for normally criticisable behaviour (7).

Boorse thus distinguishes 'illness' from 'disease' by including evaluative terms like 'undesirable', 'valid' and 'title' in the definition of the latter. I have already indicated that the two terms are to be distinguished; but I do not agree with Boorse that this can be done by treating 'illness' as evaluative while keeping 'disease' descriptive; for, as I shall argue, 'disease' is evaluative too. But quite apart from this Boorse's definition of 'health' presents difficulties, of some of which he is aware.

What does 'internal' mean? As we have seen, a skin disease may be in no stronger sense *in* (ie inside) the organism than are maggots, which are not a disease. They are indeed, a condition *of* the organism; but this wider description will not bear the weight put upon it by Boorse's definition. Being hung in a noose is also a condition *of* the organism; it, likewise, interferes with species-typical contributions to survival and reproduction. The same is true of the condition of being tarred and feathered, and of being bitten by dogs or run over by lorries. None of these is a disease.

The difficulty is not overcome by clause (ii). If to qualify as a disease malaria has to be 'not simply in the nature of the species', then being tarred and feathered satisfies this condition. And if malaria, though typical, counts as a disease because it is due to environmental causes, then so would being hanged. There might be a sense of 'typical' in which malaria was typical but being hanged was not; but this would not help Boorse, because then being hanged would be 'atypical of the species', and so would not be excluded by clause (ii), and so, if it satisfied clause (i), as it does, would be a disease. We shall return in a moment to these problems about what is species-typical, and shall see that the expression 'environmental causes', like 'internal', is too imprecise to bear any weight. A person is tarred and feathered by other people; he is caused to have skin diseases or malaria by fungi or other organisms; but where precisely is the difference? Boorse has not explained either what he means by 'internal' or what he means by 'environmental causes'.

However, as we saw, such difficulties with the definition of 'disease' are not going to affect the question of whether doctors should be professionally concerned with a condition. Whatever the cause of the condition, and whether it is inside or outside the skin, if it is a condition of the organism, and interferes with some species-typical contribution to survival and reproduction, doctors will be professionally concerned with it.

The expression '*state* of the organism' also presents a difficulty, albeit, perhaps, a somewhat pedantic one; are not some diseases processes rather than states? In so-called functional disorders, for example, there may be no state of the organism which causes the malfunction; there may be just the malfunction. But this difficulty I shall not press; it looks fairly easy to surmount.

Looking again at the numbered criteria (i) and (ii) in the definition of 'disease': they both contain the expressions 'species' and 'typical'. These terms have already given us trouble. What is the species, and what is typical of it? Species are subject to mutations; evolutionary changes occur. Some of the mutations give rise to what are called hereditary diseases; others alter the species, or produce a new strain of it, so as to cause that species or strain to multiply at the expense of others. Bacteria develop resistance to penicillin, and rats to the poison, warfarin.

How are we to say which of the changes due to mutations are diseases and which are not? Suppose that the change which makes rats resistant to warfarin is *in itself* (apart from producing this resistance) a minor impediment to reproduction and survival: in an environment free of warfarin, that is, the rats that had not been affected by this change would be more likely to survive than those that had; whereas, of course, if there is warfarin around, the ones that have mutated survive and those that have not are killed by the poison. A somewhat similar situation obtains in the case of sickle-cell anaemia and malaria: if there is malaria around, one is more likely to survive if one has sickle-cell anaemia, but if there is no malaria, those who have sickle-cell anaemia are a bit less likely to survive and reproduce.

Does it depend on the presence or absence of warfarin in the environment whether we say that the rats who have suffered the mutation (if the latter is in itself a minor impediment to reproduction or survival) are the victims of a hereditary disease? In both cases the mutation will be, by definition of 'mutation', atypical of the species. So it will satisfy condition (ii). So if, given the warfarin, the mutation is conducive to

survival, but without the warfarin it is inimical, we might think that it does so depend. However, Boorse can escape this difficulty in the same way as we escaped the difficulty about the soldier with malaria. He can say that the mutation is a disease because *other things being equal* it is inimical to survival and reproduction; but the presence of warfarin makes other things not equal.

Another difficulty with the expression 'species-typical' is this: there are certain diseases which *are* typical of certain species. Only elm trees get Dutch elm disease. So, if Boorse had not put in the phrase 'or, if typical, mainly due to environmental causes', he would have been open to the objection that, on his definition, Dutch elm disease would not be a disease, because it *is* typical of that species, or in the nature of that species.

Actually, however, the phrase does not help him out of the difficulty. For it is hard to say what is or is not due to environmental causes. Ultimately, I suppose, everything is. An individual is literally produced by its environment, including, first of all, its parents, ie their reproductive mechanisms; secondly the other causes, such as nutrition, water, air, warmth and so on, which are necessary for its growth and survival. So everything that happens to it is due to environmental causes. What Boorse seems to mean is that, given an already existing individual at a certain stage of its development, changes which are to be called diseases have to be produced by *new* environmental factors at that stage. But even this will not do to make the distinction. Nearly everything that happens to the organism at a given stage in its development is due to an interaction between the organism and its environment. So Boorse's definition might count as diseases some conditions which are not diseases. It might also exclude some which are. A hereditary disease which became apparent, without any further damage arising from the environment, at a certain age, would not count as a disease.

A further difficulty is raised by the expression 'characteristic of the organism's age'. Boorse's purpose in putting this in must be to avoid the objection that some natural changes, for example the menopause, are inimical to reproduction but are not diseases. He can get over this difficulty by saying that it is not characteristic of ages over fifty to bear children, and therefore the menopause which prevents this is not a disease unless it occurs at an unusually early age – when no doubt it *would be* called some kind of pathological sterility, and any condition which resulted in this would be likely to be called a disease.

The same applies to survival: species have a natural life-span, and to die what is called a 'natural death' after that span is over is not disease. But this might be contested. It might be said that nobody dies literally of old age; we all die of one disease (or injury) or another. So there is no age of which, for example, breathing, which is a natural function, is not characteristic. Yet it might also be said that it is uncharacteristic for someone to be breathing at the age of 120, so that a man who survived to the age of 119 and on his next birthday contracted pneumonia would not, on Boorse's definition, be entitled to call it a disease, since it did not interfere with any natural function characteristic of that organism's age.

Let us, however, waive these subsidiary difficulties in Boorse's definition, some of which, as we have seen, he might overcome, and some of which would affect other definitions besides his – even those which introduced evaluative concepts like 'bad', as I shall later be doing. We must now come to the most difficult phrase, 'natural function'. How are we to tell whether functions are natural or not? Boorse glosses 'some natural function' by the phrase 'some species-typical contribution to survival and reproduction'. But this will hardly do. There are some functions which, though natural enough, do not contribute to survival or reproduction. The growing of hair on the legs seems to be a natural function, and it seems that a condition which prevented it might, if caused by some organism, be called a disease (though in a moment we shall find reason to qualify this suggestion). But how does hair on the legs contribute to survival or reproduction? I do not believe that the ladies who shave it off find it harder to find boy-friends.

It may be that such a condition would be called a disease by analogy with one causing baldness, which would naturally be so called. But baldness too is not inimical to survival or reproduction. The reason why we call conditions causing it diseases is simply that people do not *like* being bald. It is evident from this example that at least part of the differentia between pathological and non-pathological conditions is that the former do, and the latter do not, result in something *bad* for the sufferer.

Suppose that the genetic engineers developed an organism, guaranteed not to spread from one part of the body to another or to other people, which had this effect of preventing hair growth; and suppose that it came to be sold commercially as a depilatory for use on women's legs. Would we then, or would we not, call the condition which it induced a disease? I suspect that, if we did, we should put quotation marks round the word, and would hesitate to say that the skins of the ladies who used it were not healthy. Doctors would probably not concern themselves with this condition if it were thought *harmless*.

If it is true that we would call the condition producing baldness a disease, but would hesitate to use this word of the depilatory-induced condition, this may be an indication that the differentia between pathological and non-pathological conditions is the *badness* of the effects of a condition, and not its interference with survival or reproduction, nor with natural function. For in neither example is there interference with survival or reproduction; and in both there is interference with natural function in the ordinary sense of that expression. It is the fact that the ladies want to get rid of their hair, but balding men want to keep theirs, that makes the difference.

There seems, then, to be missing from Boorse's definition of 'disease' as cited, and thus of 'healthy', an element which he does include in his definition of 'illness': the evaluative element. He is compelled to rely so heavily on the rather wobbly notion of natural function because he wishes to avoid saying that what makes us classify conditions as diseases is that *in general*, though not always in particular cases, they are *bad* things for the patient to have. This in itself is not enough; for otherwise, as we have seen, we should have to call dog-bites diseases. But given that the other criteria are satisfied (and I have not been able to give more than hints as to what they are) we seem to classify conditions as diseases if and only if they are bad things for the patient, in general.

At this point it may strike us that one is perhaps being over-ambitious if one thinks that one will be able to capture our understanding of words like 'health' and 'disease' in cut-and-dried definitions. Wittgenstein has made us familiar with the idea that a word may have a spread of meanings; there are a whole lot of conditions for its use, and perhaps none of them is necessary or sufficient. On a particular occasion the word will be understood although one of these conditions is absent. So although, for example, a word like 'disease' is used of men and of other animals and of plants in the same sense, in a way, yet in another way it is being used in subtly different senses. Understanding its use consists, not in being able to propound a hard-and-fast definition which will work for all cases, but in having learnt to recognise all these conditions, and when they are present or absent in a particular case. Doctors should not need reminding of this, because they will often agree that a patient has, say, dengue, even though one of the common symptoms of that disease is absent, provided that he has the rest.

So I shall not insist that in every case where we call a condition a disease it has to be in general bad for organisms to have it. I shall merely claim that this is one of the standard constituents of the notion: a person who did not know that it was would not understand the notion. And this gives the clue to the importance of the concepts of disease and health, which is more than theoretical or academic.

'Bad' is what moral philosophers call a normative or evaluative word (I myself often use the term 'prescriptive'). To call a thing bad is to imply that it has qualities which, other things being equal, *ought* to be avoided or remedied in things of the kind in question. If I have bad eyesight, for example, I ought to go to the oculist and he ought to prescribe spectacles if they will make my eyesight better. So if 'illness', 'disease' and 'health' involve standardly the notions of 'good' and 'bad', the classification of conditions as diseases is going to have great practical importance. It will determine what actions we think we ought to take with regard to people who have them. If a person has a disease, and we know, and can remove, its cause, or in other ways cure the disease, then, other things being equal, we ought to do so.

This explains the attraction of the expression 'mental illness'. It came into fashion at a time when people began to be more optimistic about *curing* such conditions, because they thought they were on the way to discovering their *causes*. The present reaction against the notion is due to a disillusion, in certain quarters, about both these dreams. The actions which seemed to be called for, once we had classified certain mental conditions as diseases, turned out to be either unsuccessful in curing them or objectionable for various reasons, or both.

We can perhaps begin to understand the point at issue between the two sides in this dispute by considering the following form of argument:

0) A (a person) exhibits observable features $F \ldots F$
So A has a condition C
But C is a disease
So A is not healthy
But T is the treatment most likely to remove C
So A ought to be given T.

This, it might be thought, gives the form of the inference which all doctors make when they decide what to do to their patients. $F \ldots F$ might be, for example, high temperature at two-day intervals, and the presence of a certain organism in the blood; C might be malaria; and T might be the giving of quinine or one of its more up-to-date successors.

The inference then becomes:

1) A has a high temperature at two-day intervals, etc.
So A has malaria
But malaria is a disease
So A is not healthy
But giving quinine etc is the treatment most likely to remove the condition
So A ought to be given quinine.

But now suppose that we use the same form of argument in some cases which are not physical but mental 'diseases'. We then have, for example:

2) A is at recurrent periods intensely dejected, apathetic, wakes early, etc
So A has depression
But depression is a (mental) disease
So A is not (mentally) healthy
But giving amitriptyline is the treatment most likely to remove the condition
So A ought to be given amitriptyline

This looks all right; and one wonders at first sight what Szasz and his supporters find to object to in it. We may perhaps be able to find a clue if we consider, not this example, but some others which look more dubious:

3) A is unable to conform to certain expected patterns of behaviour
So A has schizophrenia
But schizophrenia is a (mental) disease
So A is not (mentally) healthy

But giving ECT is the treatment most likely to remove the condition (assuming for the moment that this is true, though many psychiatrists might doubt it; see below)
So A ought to be given ECT.

4) A is sexually excited only by members of A's own sex
So A is a homosexual
But homosexuality is a (mental) disease
So A is not (mentally) healthy
But aversion therapy is the treatment most likely to remove the condition
So A ought to be given aversion therapy.

And lastly, for good measure:

5) A goes round criticising the regime
So A is a political deviant
But political deviancy is a (mental) disease
So A is not (mentally) healthy
But confinement in a mental hospital with frequent doses of apomorphine is the treatment most likely to remove the condition
So A ought to be confined in a mental hospital and given frequent doses of apomorphine.

Most of us, I suppose, have qualms about 5), and for some of us these qualms extend successively to 4), 3) and even 2). We have here another 'slide'. The trouble is that we cannot find any firm line on which to dig in our heels and stop. Szasz wants to stop the slide right at the beginning, at the transition between physical and mental illnesses. If we find this unacceptable, we shall have to find some other stopping place, and what is much more difficult, give reasons for stopping there.

The earlier part of this paper ought to have suggested to us a factor which, if we pay attention to it, enables us to stop the slide fairly easily and on good grounds. This is the *evaluative* character of the term 'disease' on which I have been insisting. The third line of each of the above inferences says that a certain condition is a disease. Supposing that the condition has been descriptively defined by an enumeration of the observable symptoms which are necessary and/or sufficient conditions for diagnosing it, this third line will be the first value-judgement in the inference. It does not follow in strict logic from the previous lines (which is why I have begun the third line with 'But' and not with 'So'). We are introducing a new, independent, and in this case evaluative, premiss.

The important thing to notice is that, when we introduce an evaluation into an argument, it makes a difference *whose* evaluation it is. In inferences 1), 2) and possibly 3) it is fairly clear that it is going to be an evaluation made by the patient. It is the patient who deems it bad that he should be in the condition in question. So those inferences rely on a third step to which the patient may be presumed to agree, and therefore their conclusions, given the truth of the factual premisses in the first and fifth lines (on which the doctor is the authority) are likely to secure his agreement too.

I say 'are likely to' because the operation of the *ceteris paribus* clauses mentioned earlier has to be allowed for. If the patient is a soldier who, if cured, will be sent back to the battlefront and killed, he may agree that the skin infection he has *is* a disease, because it is *ceteris paribus* and in general bad for people to have; but he may not think the doctors ought to give him whatever would cure it, because this will result in harm to him. In this case, where all are subject to military discipline, it might be held that all have a *military duty* to co-operate in the cure of the disease; but this has nothing to do with the duty of the doctor *qua* doctor, as can be seen by considering a civilian patient with the same disease who for some reason does not want it cured. In that case the doctor would be doing wrong to cure it against the patient's wishes, unless there is a serious danger of harm to others through his or her infecting them.

There is also the possibility, ignored in the above schematic inferences, that the treatment might have side-effects which the patient did not wish to undergo. Mention of these (perhaps by including them in the fifth premiss) would make this premiss evaluative, if they were specified in evaluative terms. If, on the other hand, they were specified in descriptive terms, we should have to add an additional premiss saying that these side-effects were preferable to the continuance of the condition. In either case, we should have an additional evaluative premiss to which, also, the patient would have to agree if the conclusion were going to follow for him. This complication could be dealt with, but in the interests of simplicity I shall ignore it. It is likely to affect the later inferences more than the earlier, and provides an additional reason for a reluctance to follow them. But the main ground for distinguishing them, and thus stopping the slide, is the evaluative character of the third premiss.

Attention to this evaluation will enable us to differentiate clearly between inferences 5) and 1). The 'patient' in 5) will not agree that political deviancy is a disease, because he will not agree with the evaluation of members of the regime who so label it. So the psychiatrists will be doing wrong to try to 'cure' it against the patient's wishes; it will be a breach of *another* principle, that of political freedom, to which we all attach importance. Inference 1) does not breach this principle, simply because the patient agrees with the evaluation in the third line.

This sheds light on inference 4). If the patient agrees that homosexuality is a bad condition to be in, he may agree that it be labelled a disease; and then, if he takes the doctor's word for the fifth premiss, he will agree with the conclusion of the inference, and willingly undergo aversion therapy. But if he does not mind, or even likes, being in that condition, he will not agree, and it will then be an infringement of liberty to make him submit to aversion therapy.

A difficulty is presented by the fact that there are two distinct reasons why he may think it a bad condition to

be in. One is that he would like to fall in love with members of the opposite sex and detests his abnormality as such. The other is that he suffers social or even legal disabilities because of the condition, and, though he does not in the least mind being a homosexual as such, wants to avoid these disabilities. In the second case his predicament could be made tolerable, without altering the condition, by altering the law or social attitudes. It is a political and moral question, not a medical one, whether this ought not rather to be done. Doctors should be grateful to a philosopher who makes this point clear; for he thus relieves them, *qua* doctors, of the responsibility for answering this moral and political question, while, of course, leaving with them the responsibility which they share with all other citizens for answering it.

Now consider 2). Having clarified the evaluative character of the third line, we see that patients are just as likely to agree to it as they are to the corresponding line in 1), and therefore to welcome the treatment. So we can perhaps, in standard cases where such agreement will be forthcoming, classify 2) with 1).

In inference 3), there is often a difficulty in ascertaining the wishes of the schizophrenic patient; and this makes the case more problematic than 2). In the film *Family Life* (8) it was suggested that it was not the patient that made the necessary evaluation, but the patient's parents, backed up by society and its agents, the doctors. If that were so, then the liberty of the patient would be being wrongly infringed. But the makers of the film and the anti-psychiatrists who inspired them were hinting that this is *always* the case where ECT and other strenuous treatments are given. I believe this to be a gross exaggeration. Indeed, from recent articles in *The Times* (9), it looks as if the latest Mental Health Act, which was partly motivated by the sort of thoughts which the film aims at engendering, may have gone too far in the direction of protecting individual liberty. The articles suggest that in some cases schizophrenic patients cannot get the help they need because psychiatrists are too reluctant to do anything which would incur a charge of undue interference.

But the main trouble still is that we do not know enough either about schizophrenia (which may not be a single disease at all but a family of diseases), or about the effects of ECT. If we knew more about both these things, we might be able to be more certain about the first and fifth lines in the inference, and thus form a sound judgement about whether the treatment ought to be used in a particular case; these difficulties are the concern of the medical researcher rather than of the philosopher.

However, one difficulty, already mentioned, would remain. Many mental patients are in no state to give an opinion as to whether their condition is a bad one to be in. In many cases the psychiatrist, if he is to care for the patient at all, cannot avoid judging *on behalf of the patient* whether it is bad. The case resembles that of children. If a child has an incipient but so far not painful disease, his parents and the doctor may rightly begin treatment in the assurance that if the patient knew the facts about what would happen if the treatment were not given, he would agree in accepting the third premiss and therefore the conclusion of the inference.

It is an attraction of the move I have made that it deals with inference 2); but it cannot be extended to inferences 4) and 5), because in those cases, we may presume, the 'patient' already knows all the relevant facts. In case 3), if we were better informed about the causes and cure, (or cures) of schizophrenia, we should at least be able, with more confidence than at present, to set out the prospects for the patient if one or another treatment were used, in factual terms. This would, however, leave us in ignorance as to what the patient would wish done, were he in possession of this information.

I should guess that a great many schizophrenic and other mental patients could, if the information I have postulated were available, give the doctor an idea of what they wanted; and this should be respected. Cases where this is not so have to be assimilated to those of children. If the patient is unable to form a correct factual picture of his own situation and prospects, there is nothing that the doctor can do, if he is going to care for the patient, but judge, in the light of the patient's situation, what the patient *would* wish if he were able to form such a picture. I stress that by 'factual' I mean 'factual'. It is not within the doctor's province to import his own evaluations into the patient's supposed judgement of his situation.

There is obviously a lot more to be said about this. I have tried only to show, from the point of view of a philosopher, how we might *begin* to handle questions like these. I hope I have said enough to indicate why I think that the wholesale rejection of the concept of mental illness, and of psychiatry with it, was too hasty. Mental health and disease have enough in common with physical health and disease to make them proper fields for the exercise of medical skills. But in order to show this I have had to examine the concepts of health and disease in greater depth than might have been thought necessary – though in fact I have only scratched the surface.

Professor R M Hare is Graduate Research Professor of Philosophy, University of Florida, Gainesville USA and White's Professor of Moral Philosophy Emeritus, University of Oxford.

References and notes

(1) Bloch S. The political misuse of psychiatry in the Soviet Union, and references, in Bloch S, Chodoff P, eds. *Psychiatric ethics*. Oxford: Oxford University Press, 1981.

(2) Szasz T. *The myth of mental illness*. New York: Harper and Row, 1961.

(3) Boorse C. Health as a theoretical concept. *Philosophy of science* 1977; 44: 552.

(4) See my article Supervenience. *Proceedings of the Aristotelian Society*, 1984; supp vol 58: 11 ff.

(5) See Sedgwick P. Illness, mental and otherwise. *Hastings Center studies* 1973; 1, 3: 32, citing Mechanic D. Medical sociology: 16. I have profited from other papers in this issue.

(6) What a theory of mental health should be. *Journal for the theory of social behaviour* 1976; 6: 62 ff.

(7) See reference (6) and On the distinction between disease and illness, *Philosophy and public affairs* 1975; 5: 61. I cite Boorse's definitions in these earlier papers because they well illustrate our problem. I shall not have room here to discuss his arguments in full detail, nor his later writings, in which he has developed his views in the direction of treating *both* illness *and* disease as purely descriptive concepts, and has defended them further. See his Health as a theoretical concept (cited above), reprinted revised in Caplan A L, Engelhardt H T, McCartney J J, eds. *Concepts of health and disease*. Reading: Addison-Wesley, 1981: 560, and Concepts of health in Regan T, VandeVeer D, eds. *Border crossings* (forthcoming).

(8) Director, Kenneth Loach. Reviewed by Taylor J. *The Times* 1972 Jan 14: 8 (col 3).

(9) Wallace M. The tragedy of schizophrenia. *The Times* 1985 Dec 16-18: Dec 16: 10 (col 1); Dec 17: 8 (col 1); Dec 18: 8 (col 1); Dec 19: 13 (col 1) [editorial].

[37]

PRAXIS MAKES PERFECT: ILLNESS AS A BRIDGE BETWEEN BIOLOGICAL CONCEPTS OF DISEASE AND SOCIAL CONCEPTIONS OF HEALTH

K.W.M. FULFORD

Research Psychiatrist, Department of Psychiatry, University of Oxford, Warneford Hospital, Oxford OX3 7JX, United Kingdom

ABSTRACT. Analyses of biological concepts of disease and social conceptions of health indicate that they are structurally interdependent. This in turn suggests the need for a bridge theory of illness. The main features of such a theory are an emphasis on the logical properties of value terms, close attention to the features of the experience of illness, and an analysis of this experience as "action failure", drawing directly on the internal structure of action. The practical applications of this theory are outlined for a number of problems in each of the three main practical areas, clinical work, teaching and research. In each case the resources of the theory suggest new models and generate new results. The full practical significance of the theory, however, is shown to consist in the way in which it ties together biological and social theories into an integrated picture of the conceptual structure of medicine as a whole. It is argued, finally, that practical efficiency of this kind is a test of theory not only in the philosophy of medicine but also in general philosophy.

Key words: delusion, disease, medical education, mental illness, psychosis

1. INTRODUCTION

In recent years two broad kinds of theory about the essential conceptual structure of medicine have emerged: biological, focusing on disease concepts defined in terms of disturbances of bodily and mental functioning [1, 2, 3]; and social, concerned with positive conceptions of health related directly or indirectly to social competence [4, 5, 6]. These two kinds of theory have been conceived competitively [7]. In this article, however, it is argued that they are structurally interdependent – that is, the force of either depends on conceptual elements suppressed in the one theory but emphasised in the other. Recognising this leads in turn to the identification of value, illness and action-failure as logical elements of a theory which provides a bridge between biological and social theories.

The integrated picture which emerges from this analysis – disease/illness/health – has a degree of theoretical cogency. It is argued, though, that a crucial test of philosophical theories in this area is their practical ef-

Theoretical Medicine **14**: 305–320, 1993.

306   K.W.M. FULFORD

ficiency. In this respect a bridge theory of illness is shown to increase the resources available for tackling some of the conceptual difficulties which arise in the practice of health care. Specific practical examples of this are described for (1) clinical practice (the relationship between primary health care and hospital medicine; medical ethics, especially the abuse of psychiatry), (2) teaching (the Oxford Practice Skills Project), and (3) research (classification; phenomenology; jurisprudence and neuroimaging). It is suggested, finally, that practical results of this kind provide a test of theory not just in the philosophy of medicine but in philosophy generally. It is in this extended sense, then, as we will see, that praxis does indeed make perfect.

2. DERIVATION OF A BRIDGE THEORY OF ILLNESS

The main features of both biological and social theories are described by Nordenfelt in the Introduction to this issue [7]. Although not always openly hostile to each other, biological theories have been conceived as a defence against the value-relativism of social theories [2], while social theories, as Nordenfelt notes, represent a direct response to the narrowness of purely scientific disease concepts. One consequence of this, however, is that both theories, at least in polar form, fail to encompass important features of what Ryle called the "logical geography" [8]. Biological theories may focus so exclusively on the objective basis of medicine as to neglect altogether the value-laden nature of the loss of agency, or incapacity, by which the actual experience of illness is characterised. Social theories, by contrast, emphasising the experiential aspects of illness, often fail to address the distinction between illness and other kinds of negatively evaluated experience. This is the "demarcation" problem which it is one of the chief claims of biological theories to have resolved.

Less extreme versions of both theories have thus been developed. Boorse's theory, for example, although firmly biological in orientation, incorporates the evaluative element in medicine [2]. The key distinction here is between disease and illness. Disease, for Boorse, is a genuinely scientific concept, defined by disturbances of bodily or mental functioning, the (objective) criteria for which include reduced life and/or reproductive expectations. Illness on the other hand is an evaluative subcategory of disease, it is a disease which is "serious enough to be incapacitating". Similarly, Nordenfelt, although arguing from the value-orientation of theories of health, has tackled the demarcation problem head-on with his action-theoretic approach [4]. Along with social theories he makes the competence of the individual as a social agent central to the notion of health. But he seeks to mark out specifically medical failures of "social competence" from, for example, delinquency, by reference to a particular class of the goals of the *individual*, what he calls their "vital goals."

These less extreme theories gesture towards each other, therefore. Closer examination suggests, however, that the relationship between them is more than gestural, that it is indeed one of mutual dependence. I have described this in detail elsewhere for Boorse's theory [9, Ch. 3]. The essence of Boorse's approach is to exclude value from medical theory by establishing a value-free definition of disease. But his own actual use of the concept remains value-laden – he slips, for example, from the notion of "statistically abnormal functioning" (value-free definition) to that of "reduced functional efficiency" (value-laden use). Following Hare [10], then, this suggests that in defining disease in terms which are value-free, he has written out an element of the meaning of the term (the evaluative element) which is essential. Similar observations though, apply to Nordenfelt's approach to the demarcation problem. As noted a moment ago, the key concept here is that of a "vital goal." In Nordenfelt's account an individual's vital goals are those the satisfaction of which are essential for the individual concerned to achieve a minimal degree of long-term real happiness. The difficulty, though, if this notion is to serve to mark out health from other value-laden concepts, is to establish which of the goals of an individual are in this sense essential. Nordenfelt thus defines a class of basic vital goals, these being those which all human beings must share as a *sine qua non* of whatever particular goals they may individually pursue. Nordenfelt lists a number of such goals [4, p. 91]. Of these, however, only survival (as a *sine qua non*) and (by extension) reproduction really are (in this sense) essential. Nordenfelt emphasises that these are not exhaustive. But he suggests no other examples of basic vital goals which could be considered, in the required sense, essential: that is, goals which, being *sine qua nons*, could in principle serve to resolve the demarcation problem. Moreover Boorse, too, emphasises that survival and reproduction, in their entirely different role in his theory, as biological criteria of disease, are not exhaustive [2].

Boorse's theory is thus not value-free: on the contrary, the cogency of his account of disease depends on the covert presence of a logical element of evaluation emphasised in social theories. Equally, Nordenfelt's theory, to the extent (only) that it is concerned to provide a substantive account of the demarcation problem, rests on criteria which appear in biological theories as criteria of disease.

That these two kinds of theory should turn out to be structurally interdependent to this extent is not, as such, a criticism of either. On the contrary, both represent detailed and comprehensive accounts of the areas of the conceptual structure of medicine with which they are primarily concerned, disease and health respectively. Moreover, that they *are* structurally interdependent points a

308   K.W.M. FULFORD

specific lesson, namely that it could be productive to make the connections between them transparent, to develop a bridge theory. Indeed the two kinds of theory, taken together, suggest what the elements of such a bridge theory are likely to be. From Boorse we should expect one such element to be the experience of illness, and a second to be the properties of this experience specifically as it involves a negative value judgement. From Nordenfelt we should expect a third element to be a focus, not on the goals of action, but on what Austin called the internal "structure of action" [11]. In a bridge theory, then, the experience of illness would be marked out from other negatively evaluated experiences, not (as in biological theories) by reference to underlying disturbances of functioning, nor (as in social theories) by reference to a particular class of the goals of action, but as a particular kind of "failure of action".

A theory of illness of this kind can be shown to have a degree of theoretical cogency in its own terms [9, Ch. 7], especially in the extent to which it explains the features not just of physical illness but of the diverse phenomena by which the experience of mental illness is constituted [12]. In certain of its general features (for example the primacy given to the experience of illness) it has connections with work in the continental philosophical tradition on the phenomenology of illness [13]. Specifically as a bridge theory, moreover, it sits naturally between biological and social theories: illness sits between bodily/mental parts (which become diseased) and social structures (within the values of which standards of health are defined): similarly, the actions of individual agents sit between the functioning of their bodily/mental parts (on which indeed actions are contingently dependent) and the social roles by which (at least in part) the competence of an agent's actions are measured. Rather as with the chemical periodic table of elements, then, an integrated theory, to the extent that it locates illness in the gap between disease and health, has a degree of prima facie validity.

The final test, however, of philosophical analyses in this area is not theoretical cogency but practical efficiency. This is not a matter of cost-effectiveness, of justifying philosophical theory by practical utility. It is, rather, a direct test of theory itself. This is simply because the problems with which philosophy is (specifically) concerned in health care, although conceptual rather than empirical, are *practical* problems. Hence any theory, however internally consistent, however comprehensive, which fails to make at least *some* difference to practice, is necessarily suspect.

3. PRACTICAL COROLLARIES OF A BRIDGE THEORY

The principal effect of filling in the gap between biological and social theories is to produce a more complete picture of the conceptual structure of medicine and thus to increase the resources available for a specifically philosophical contribution, by way of conceptual analysis [14], to the praxis of health care. In this section examples are given of how this works out for each of the three practical areas, clinical work, teaching and research. The focus will be on the conceptual elements – illness, value, action-failure – emphasised in a bridge theory. Nonetheless, as we will see, the practical significance of these elements is not exclusive of that of the elements of biological and social theories. On the contrary, the practical significance of these elements consists, rather, in the way in which they help to knit together the three kinds of theory into an integrated picture of the conceptual structure of health care as a whole.

3.1. Clinical Practice

The competitive stance of biological and social theories is a reflection of territorial disputes, which, as Nordenfelt notes [8], have often led to distortions in the practice of health care. An important weapon in these disputes has been the authority of science. "High-tech", hospital-based medicine has been perceived as the acme of medical practice, as against less "scientific" areas such as primary care (including family medicine and nursing) and psychiatry.

Crucial to this perceived hierarchy is the extent to which the concepts of health and disease employed in these different areas are indeed "scientific". There are hints of this in the way the relationship between hospital medicine and primary care is commonly understood. Primary care is perceived as being concerned with the value-laden concept of illness as against the more objective concerns of hospital medicine with disease [2]. Hence primary care is the scientific poor relation. And this construction has been made fully explicit in the debate about mental illness. As illness is more value-laden than disease, so, within illness, mental illness is more value-laden than physical. Hence, given the scientific self-image of medicine, the very validity of mental illness as a genuinely *medical* concept, has been assumed, by supporters as well as by opponents of the concept, to turn on whether the evaluative element in its meaning can be eliminated [15].

The perspective of biological theory is thus highly prejudicial to the more value-laden areas of health care. Social theories, to the extent that they emphasise the evaluative nature of the medical concepts are not, as such, prejudicial. But, as we have seen, in focusing on substantive questions of value, implicit in the "goals" of the agent, they tend to fall back on the criteria

310   K.W.M. FULFORD

emphasised in biological theories. The dependence on "science" is thus once more reinforced. A bridge theory, on the other hand, in drawing on the logical properties of value terms, is able to avoid this. For there is a property of value terms which suggests a more neutral way of understanding the relationships both between disease and illness and between physical illness and mental. The property in question is that the evaluative connotations of value terms, including such all-purpose value terms as "good" and "bad," varies with context. "Good apple," for example, has mainly factual connotations ("clean-skinned, sweet, etc."), while "good picture" is more overtly value-laden. Hence if "disease" and "illness" are *both* value terms, expressing the same negative-medical-value judgment, disease (with its more factual connotations) could be like "good apple," "illness" (with its more evaluative connotations) could be like "good picture," and similarly for "physical illness" and "mental illness." Hence in a bridge theory all these concepts are seen to be on an equal footing, logically speaking, and it is this which evens up the balance of power between the areas of health care of which they are severally characteristic.

This is an attractive hypothesis from a theoretical point of view to the extent that it is economical. Instead of postulating "scientific" and "nonscientific" concepts according to variations in the strength of their evaluative connotations, the full range of the medical concepts is seen to be consistent with their status (in a bridge theory) as value terms. From a practical point of view, however, the mechanism of this variation takes us even further. For it actually reverses the balance of power between the different areas of health care. Thus, as Hare [10], Urmson [16] and others have argued, the variation with context in the evaluative connotations of value terms reflects (*inter alia*) the extent to which the descriptive criteria for the value judgments they express are settled or agreed upon. The factual connotations of "good apple" reflect the fact (a psychological, not a logical, fact) that most people most of the time take sweet, clean-skinned apples to be good. Conversely there are no such settled criteria for "good picture," the connotations of which thus remain relatively value-laden.

Applying this to the medical concepts, then, suggests, first, that the relationship between illness and disease may be the reverse of that proposed in biological theories. In Boorse's theory, as we saw earlier, illness is an evaluative sub-category of disease: disease is the primary concept, a scientifically established concept, illness the derivative. In a bridge theory, on the other hand, drawing on the mechanism just described, disease, at least in its symptomatic sense, would be a sub-category of illness [9, Ch. 4]. The more value-laden concept of illness would encompass any condition that may be evaluated as an illness: but disease (with its more factual connotations) would be restricted to that sub-category of these conditions which are so evaluated by most people most of the time. Of course, once this symptomatic sense of disease is established, further senses can

PRAXIS MAKES PERFECT 311

become attached to it by way of the processes of generalization and extension described by Wittgenstein [17]. Thus a causal sense of disease would be attached as "any condition that is a cause of a symptomatically defined disease." Moreover, as these causal disease categories become more and more useful, with the growth of medical and biological science, so they will become more and more prominent in medical discourse. For this reason, then, they may *appear* to be logically primary. But it remains nonetheless illness which *is* logically primary. Whatever the development of scientific theories of disease the original flow of meaning, and hence what *counts as* a disease, is from illness to disease, not vice versa.

A good deal more theoretical argument is required to establish this "bridge theory" against the biological model. I have set this out elsewhere [9, Chs. 2–4]. But it is not *prima facie* implausible. And if it is right it reverses at a stroke the prejudicial place of primary care. In the "scientific" medical model, as we have seen, primary care is the scientific poor relation, and this is reflected in the dependent logical place of illness. But in a bridge theory, just as illness is logically primary, so also is primary health care. The primary care worker is in effect selecting those cases for the hospital consultant which are evaluatively uncontentious and hence can be dealt with on a purely empirical basis. In place, then, of an image of empirically difficult cases being "passed up" to the hospital expert, we have an image of conceptually straightforward cases being "passed down" to the medical technician. This is too extreme a picture, of course. But it does show primary care in a quite different light, as the conceptually (as well as empirically) tricky sharp end of health care, rather than as the scientific poor relation of hospital medicine.

In balancing up the relationship between primary care and hospital medicine, then, a bridge theory, drawing on no more than a well-recognised logical property of value terms, has a clear if somewhat global significance for practice. Applied to the relationship between psychiatry and physical medicine, this same property of value terms has a similar balancing-up effect but it also suggests a specific lesson for the organization of clinical work. The balancing-up effect arises from the recognition that, just as illness in being value-laden compared with disease, is not scientifically primitive but conceptually tricky (because evaluatively "open"), so, too, is mental illness conceptually tricky compared with physical. The basis of this is evident by direct inspection: our evaluations of, say, anxiety (a typical symptom of mental illness) are more open and variable than of pain (a typical symptom of physical illness). For this reason alone, therefore, mental illness will be more value-laden than physical illness. But this shows the evaluative connotations of mental illness in a positive light as against the negative light of biological theories. For it shows that mental illness, in being more value-laden than physical, reflects the (logical) properties of

312 K.W.M. FULFORD

phenomena like anxiety as faithfully as physical illness, in being less value-laden than mental, reflects the (logical) properties of phenomena like pain. Indeed to the extent that illness itself is a value term, mental illness, in being overtly value-laden, is actually transparent to an important logical property of illness, a property which the factual connotations of physical illness actually conceal.

Mental illness, then, on this construction, is a valid species of illness, not (as in a biological theory) by assimilation to physical illness, but in its own right. It is this strong claim which balances up the relationship between psychiatry and physical medicine. By the same token, though, mental illness, in *being* a valid species of illness, is inherently, rather than (as in a biological theory) merely contingently, tricky compared with physical illness. It is this corollary of a bridge theory which yields the specific point for practice. For it suggests a quite different explanation for the *de facto* vulnerability of psychiatry to abuse, and hence a quite different approach to prevention.

On the biological theory psychiatry is vulnerable to abuse because its diagnostic concepts are scientifically primitive. Hence the teamwork approach to clinical decision making – the involvement of social workers, relatives, even the courts, in such areas as compulsory psychiatric treatment – is perceived by doctors as a temporary expedient, necessary only so long as the exclusively empirical difficulties involved in psychiatric diagnosis remain unresolved. But in a bridge theory, while empirical difficulties are no less important, a key part of the trickiness of the diagnosis of mental illness is seen to arise from the relatively open nature of the value judgements involved. This trickiness is in itself irreducible, it being a direct reflection of our diversity as human beings. It is also, though, not reducible by future discoveries in the brain sciences. This is because, disease being (in a bridge theory) logically dependent on illness, any ambiguity in the status of a condition as a mental illness, will necessarily be reflected in the status of an underlying causal condition as a mental disease. Hence the biological theory approach to prevention, to the extent that it focuses on the empirical aspects of diagnosis, is looking the wrong way. Far from preventing abuse, therefore, it could actually increase it – there is indeed some evidence of this having happened in the Soviet case [18]. Of course, if we look the other way, towards the evaluative difficulties in psychiatric diagnosis, we have no ready-reckoner method for resolving them. But, at least in a liberal society, a balance of evaluative considerations is recognised to be an important protection against the hegemony of any particular section of opinion, and it is this which teamwork provides. In a bridge theory, then, teamwork is not an unfortunate necessity arising from the primitive state of the brain sciences. It is an essential (*logically* essential) component of good clinical practice.

3.2. Medical Education

Just as a bridge theory makes the evaluative and experiential aspects of illness central to the logic of medicine, and hence to clinical practice, so it brings these same elements into the centre of medical education. There is increasing recognition of the importance in clinical practice both of ethical and legal considerations, and of communication skills (crucial to which is an understanding of the experience of illness). Yet, so dominant is the biological model of disease, these remain marginalised in the curricula of most medical schools. Even social theories, in the UK at least, have had little direct impact in this respect, leading as they do mainly to an increased emphasis on the scientific aspects of preventive medicine. A bridge theory on the other hand suggests a model of medical education in which ethics, law and communication skills (collectively, practice skills) are brought into a fully integrated relationship with the factual and scientific aspects of clinical practice.

The Oxford Practice Skills Course is a conscious attempt to embody this model in the training of medical students [19]. The guiding objective behind the course is to combine the skills required for good clinical practice as fully as possible with the knowledge base of medicine. This means that ethics is not taught separately but alongside medical law and communication skills in a case-based approach to the problems raised by everyday clinical practice. Paradoxically, ethics as such may be less visible with this approach than in conventional ethics courses. But this is because it is so fully embedded in the clinical course rather than because it is marginalised. The focus is on the required clinical skills – in the case of ethics these include awareness, thinking skilss, attitude change, knowledge and behaviour – rather than on ethical argument as such. And this embedding is further reinforced both by the integration of ethics with law and communication skills in the practice skills syllabus, and by a number of important structural features of the course: for example, that it is taught primarily, not by ethicists, lawyers or theologians, but by practitioners; that the seminars are not grouped together as a separate course but spread through the full three years of the clinical training and as an integral part of each clinical attachment (consent, for example, is dealt with *as part of* the surgical attachment); and that the students are appraised on their practice skills not by way of a separate examination but as part of their overall clinical assessment.

Whether or not all this will make any difference at the end of the day only time will tell. The problems involved in assessing the effectiveness of medical education, let alone medical ethics education are formidable. But the approach has so far been well received by a majority of students and it seems to make good sense at a practical level – so good, indeed, that it now seems remarkable that it has not been tried before. After all, it is in a sense no more than an

 Medical Ethics

 K.W.M. FULFORD

extension of the familiar idea that good clinical care is dependent as much on "knowing how" as on "knowing that." Yet the very concept of practice skills, of an integrated package of ethics, law and communication skills, is itself novel; and there appear to be no other training schemes in which these elements are woven together in a seamless syllabus as in the Oxford course. All this *could* have been derived directly from the contingencies of everyday practice, of course. But the fact is that it arose indirectly as the practical counterpart of the abstract analysis of the conceptual framework of medicine summarised here in the notion of a "bridge theory." We will return to the wider significance of this in the penultimate section of this paper.

3.3. Research

Philosophical analysis is often contrasted unfavourably with scientific research as mere "playing with words." To the extent, though, that it is concerned with the concepts which underpin and guide research in other more "practical" disciplines, it may have a significance well beyond the questions of meaning with which it is primarily concerned. In the case of a bridge theory its main effect is to make explicit elements of the conceptual structure of medicine (value, illness and action-failure) which, although generally covert, have profound effects on practice. As we will see in this section, biological theories tend to deny these elements. Social theories, although acknowledging them, are not in general sufficiently fine-grained to bite on specific practical issues. But a bridge theory, in focusing directly on the detailed logical properties of these elements, increases the resources available for tackling the conceptual problems arising in a number of other areas of medical research.

First, then, the element of value. As we have seen, where biological theories aim to eliminate (or at any rate marginalise) the evaluative element in medicine, and where social theories tend to focus on substantive questions of value, a bridge theory seeks to exploit the logical properties which terms like illness and disease share with value terms in general. We have already noted the relevance of this to clinical practice. An important application of the approach in medical research is to classification. Our current exclusively scientific classifications of disease, although highly successful in the context of hospital-based physical medicine, have so far failed to perform satisfactorily in other areas, notably psychiatry and primary care [20]. The essential science-orientation of the dominant biological model suggests that the way to improve matters is by further empirical research. This approach is made explicit by the authors of the latest edition of the influential American classification, the DSM IV [21, 22]. Social theories, as Nordenfelt notes [4, p. 130], have little to offer here, concerned as they are with global questions of the goals of health. But a bridge theory suggests that while empirical research remains vital, conceptual work, concerned in particular with the way in which fact and value are woven together into our classifications of disorder, will be essential as well. As a step towards this I have analysed the problems identified by the authors of DSM-IV themselves as being outstanding [23]. Each of these 39 problems certainly includes an empirical element. But contrary to the exclusively scientific construction placed on them by the authors of DSM-IV, no less than 24 (62%) include an evaluative element as well. Recognising this is not in itself to resolve the problems associated with this element. But it is a step in the right direction. And this is a step which is indeed also proving fruitful in ethics [24] and in a number of other areas of medical research [25].

The emphasis in a bridge theory on the importance of the experience of illness (the second main conceptual element in such theories) is also relevant to classification, though in this case through the understanding it gives of phenomenology. The dependence of illness on disease in a biological model (such as Boorse's) means that attempts to clarify problematic concepts of disorder will always be by way of matching them to the disease concepts which have worked so well in many areas of physical medicine. But in a bridge theory, in which disease rather than illness is the derivative concept, the tendency will be to look the other way, directly at the phenomenology of illness. This simple change of tack can be highly productive. In psychiatry, for example, although the psychotic/non-psychotic distinction remains clinically significant, the key notion of psychotic loss of insight has consistently evaded adequate characterisation [26]. A bridge theory suggests that this is because conventional approaches to understanding this notion are limited to a "disease" model, a model which indeed works well for some forms of loss of insight (as in dementia) but not for psychotic loss of insight [27]. Moreover, there is a particular feature of the experience of illness, a two-way distinction by which illness generally – physical as well as mental – is marked out from other negatively evaluated experiences, in terms of which the notion of psychotic loss of insight can be shown to be immediately transparent. Nor is this merely a general transparency. For the two-way distinction by which the experience of illness is characterised generates a range of detailed differential diagnostic tables (what might be called differential illness-diagnostic tables) for each of the three main classes of psychotic symptom, thought disorder, hallucination and delusion [9, Ch. 10; 27].

The need for a new phenomenology has been emphasised in areas apparently as far from philosophy as neuro-imaging [28]. The third main element of a bridge theory, the analysis of the experience of illness as action-failure, could make an important contribution here by deepening our understanding of the phenomena concerned. Again, psychosis provides a case in point. It is the paradigm case of the jurisprudential notion of mental illness as a legal excuse, and, correspondingly, central to the loss of responsibility which underpins the ethical basis of compulsory psychiatric treatment [9, Ch. 10]. Yet conventional accounts fail to explain why this should be. Boorse himself notes that his "failure of function" account of mental illness makes psychosis a peripheral (rather than as it is central) case of mental illness as an excuse [3]. Similarly, social theories, relying on an internal counterpart to external (i.e., social) compulsion [29], seem to fit disorders such as the addictions or obsessive-compulsive neuroses better than the psychoses. Even in the medical ethics literature, there is a reliance on a mainly cognitive model of rationality, a model which indeed fits cognitive disorders such as dementia and the confusional states, but fails to explain the plain clinical features even of the central psychotic symptom of delusion [30]. A bridge theory, on the other hand, drawing on the internal structure of action, suggests that the relevant model of rationality is one in terms of practical reasoning, of our reasons for action, rather than of cognitive functioning [9, Ch. 10]. This model yields an account of psychosis which is fully consistent with the clinical phenomenology of psychotic symptoms. It also shows why psychotic disorders are the central case of mental illness as an excuse – essentially because in an action-failure account of illness they turn out to involve a constitutive failure of action whereas all other disorders, physical as well as mental, are merely executive. Moreover, this account links medical research – in neuro-imaging as well as in jurisprudence – directly with a rich vein of modern philosophical work in the philosophy of mind on Intentionality [31] and Intentional causation [32].

4. PHILOSOPHY AND PRACTICE

After drifting apart for several decades philosophy and medicine have recently begun to move together again [25]. So much so, indeed, that in relation at least to ethics, it is perhaps no longer contentious to claim that philosophy has a contribution to make to practice. And even in relation to the more self-consciously scientific aspects of medicine, it is increasingly recognised that conceptual and empirical research, far from being antithetical, often go hand-in-hand. This is true in physics, the mother and father of "hard" science, so why not in medicine! In coming closer together, however, philosophy and medicine have sometimes been at risk of merging their identities. In medical ethics, for example, philosophers have been inclined to eschew conceptual analysis in favour of more "practical" questions of substance; and doctors, correspondingly, have sometimes substituted unfocused philosophical speculation for close attention in the details of everyday practice. What is suggested by the results presented here, though, is that it is by preserving their distinct traditions of skills and experience that the two disciplines will move towards a successful working partnership.

On the philosophical side of this partnership, the "bridge" theory of illness from which the practical results described here were all derived, was a product not just of conceptual analysis but of linguistic analytical, or ordinary language, philosophy. This way of doing philosophy – by focusing on actual usage rather than on received definitions [11] – is somewhat unfashionable nowadays. But it is after all in ordinary usage that the problems in a practical area like medicine actually arise. And the increased conceptual resources provided by a bridge concept represents precisely that widening of view which Wittgenstein [17], and in a more positive way Austin [11], regarded as the proper function of philosophy. Again, as a methodology, Austin in particular provides a clear and forceful technique directly related to ordinary usage [11]. This has been our role model here: it is Boorse's use of disease (not his stipulative definition) which shows most decisively its status as a value term; and in the work discussed on insight and psychosis, it was the clinical phenomenology of these symptoms, rather than textbook definitions, which was crucial. Moreover in following up work in these areas Austin's less widely known ideas about the organisation of philosophical research seem apposite. Austin urged a move away from the "sole trader" image of the philosopher to that of a team, or perhaps a community, of researchers, across which a number of connected problems could be distributed, much indeed on the model of scientific research [14]. And this approach seems peculiarly well suited to the wide range of conceptual problems raised within a well-defined area of medical research such as classification.

But the other side to this partnership is that, just as philosophy has a contribution to make to medicine, so medicine has a contribution to make to philosophy. This, too, was anticipated by Austin who pointed to abnormal psychological phenomena as a rich resource for philosophers of action – the ways in which actions fail, he argued (directly foreshadowing the analysis of illness as action-failure) could help us to explore the structure of normal action [11]. Wilkes [33], Glover [34], Braude [35], Gillett [36] and others have recently extended this principle to problems in personal identity. And in my own work [9, Ch. 10], I have shown the significance of the phenomenology of delusions for traditional debates, in ethics and in the philosophy of science, about the relationship between "is" and "ought."

The linking of medicine and philosophy in this way has also a deeper significance, however. Thus we noted earlier that, since the problems with which philosophy is concerned in medicine are practical problems, practical utility is a test of theory. What we see now is that the theory in question is not just theory in the philosophy of medicine but also in general philosophy. Clinical psychopathology is therefore not just a resource. Like the data in

318   K.W.M. FULFORD

science, it is a positive constraint on theory. Within the linguistic analytical tradition, then, there are all the ingredients for a powerful synergy between philosophy and medicine: the skills of philosophical analysis combined with the rich resources of the phenomenology of illness; and philosophy and medicine alike subject to the constraint that they be practically effective.

5. CONCLUSIONS

In this article the practical significance of a theory of illness which bridges between biological concepts of disease and social conceptions of health has been outlined. Although not argued for directly, the components of this bridge theory have been shown to be readily derivable from a demonstration of the mutual interdependence of biological and social theories – both kinds of polar theory depending on elements suppressed in the one and emphasised in the other. By analogy with the chemical periodic table, then, the properties of the bridge theory were inferred from the properties of its neighbours. But the theory gains perhaps greater support from the range of practically useful results to which it leads. These have been reviewed here for each of the three main practical areas, clinical work, teaching and research. In each case the bridge theory of illness provides an enlarged conceptual resource suggesting new models, methods and results. We have seen that this is important, not only practically but also for the justification of philosophy; and for the justification of philosophy, not as a cost-effective contribution to medicine, but as a test of the cogency of its very theories.

We should note finally, though, that although the elements of a bridge theory of illness have been emphasised here, it is, genuinely, an integrated view, rather than the hegemony of any particular theory which is needed. This is no mere hand-waving gesture to eclecticism. We have seen at several points that there is much that a theory of illness on its own cannot do. In relation to insight, for example, as we saw, biological models of disease, alongside a theory of illness, are necessary. But social theories, too, are essential. Indeed in the case of psychotic loss of insight, the central feature of this symptom, that the patient's construction of what is wrong differs radically from everyone else's, is incapable even of being expressed other than in terms which are irreducibly social.

Acknowledgements – I am grateful to Professor Lennart Nordenfelt for his most helpful comments on an early version of this paper.

PRAXIS MAKES PERFECT 319

REFERENCES

1. Kendell RE. The concept of disease and its implications for psychiatry. *British Journal of Psychiatry* 1975;127:305–315.
2. Boorse C. On the distinction between disease and illness. *Philosophy and Public Affairs* 1975;5:49–68.
3. Boorse C. What a theory of mental health should be. *Journal of Theory Social Behaviour* 1976;6:61–84.
4. Nordenfelt L. *On the Nature of Health: An Action-Theoretic Approach.* Dordrecht, Holland: D. Reidel Publishing Company, 1987.
5. Pörn I. Health and adaptedness. This volume, pp. 295–303, 1993.
6. Whitbeck C. A theory of health, in Caplan AL, Engelhardt, HT Jr. McCartney, JJ eds. *Concepts of Health and Disease: Interdisciplinary Perspectives*, Addison-Wesley Publishing Company, Reading, Massachusetts, 1981.
7. Nordenfelt L. Concepts of health and their consequences for health care. This volume, pp. 277–285, 1993.
8. Ryle G. *The Concept of Mind.* England: Penguin Books Ltd, 1980.
9. Fulford KWM. *Moral Theory and Medical Practice.* Cambridge University Press, 1989.
10. Hare RM. Descriptivism. *Proceedings of the British Academy* 1963;49:115–134.
11. Austin JL. A plea for excuses. *Proceedings of the Aristotelian Society* 1956–7;57:1–30.
12. Fulford KWM. *Scandinavian Concepts of Health and the Phenomenology of Mental Illness.* (forthcoming)
13. Sartre JP. *Being and Nothingness.* Tr. Hazel Barnes, London, 1957: 1943.
14. Fulford KWM. Philosophy and medicine: The Oxford connection. *British Journal of Psychiatry* 1990;157:111–115.
15. Fulford KWM. Is medicine a branch of ethics? Ch. 8 in Gillett G, Peacocke A, eds., *Personality and Insanity* Blackwells, 1988.
16. Urmson JO. On grading. *Mind* 1950;59:145–169.
17. Wittgenstein L. *Philosophical Investigations* (second edition). Transl. by Anscombe GEM. Oxford: Basil Blackwell Publisher Ltd, 1958.
18. Fulford KWM, Smirnoff AYU, Snow E. Concepts of disease and the abuse of psychiatry in the USSR *British Journal of Psychiatry* 1993;162:801–810.
19. Hope RA and Fulford KWM. Medical education: patients, principles and practice skills. Gillon R, ed., *Principles of Health Care Ethics*. John Wiley and Sons, 1994.
20. Helman CG. Disease versus illness in general practice. *Journal of the Royal College of Practitioners* 1981;230(3):548–552.
21. Frances A. First MB, Widiger TA, Miele GM, Tilly SM, Davis WW and Pincus HA. An A-Z guide to DSM-IV conundrums. *Journal of Abnormal Psychology* 1991;100(3):407–412.
22. Frances A, Pincus HA, Widiger TA, Davis WW First MB. DSM-IV: work in progress. *American Journal of Psychiatry* 1990;147:1439–1448.
23. Fulford KWM. Closet logics: hidden conceptual elements in the DSM and ICD classifications of mental disorders. In Sadler JZ, Schwartz M, Wiggins O, eds. *Philosophical Perspectives on Psychiatric Diagnostic Classification.* Baltimore, MD: Johns Hopkins University Press (forthcoming).
24. Fulford KWM. The concept of disease. In Bloch S, and Chadoff P, eds. *Psychiatric Ethics* (second edition), Oxford University Press, 1991
25. Fulford KWM. Philosophy and psychiatry: points of contact. *Current Opinion in Psychiatry* 1990;3:668–672.
26. Lewis AJ. The psychopathology of insight. *British Journal of Medical Psychology* 1934;14:332–348.

320   K.W.M. FULFORD

27. Fulford KWM. Thought insertion and insight: disease and illness paradigms of psychotic disorder. In Spitzer M, ed. *Phenomenology, Language and Schizophrenia.* Springer-Verlag, 1993.
28. Mortimer AM. Phenomenology: its place in schizophrenia research. *British Journal of Psychiatry* 1992;161:293–297.
29. Nordenfelt L. *On Crime, Punishment and Psychiatric Care.* Almqvist and Wiksell International, 1992.
30. Fulford KWM and Hope RA. Psychiatric ethics: a bioethical ugly duckling? Gillon R, ed. *Principles of Health Care Ethics,* John Wiley and Sons, 1994.
31. Fulford KWM. Mental illness and the mind-brain problem: delusion, belief and Searle's theory of intentionality. *Theoretical Medicine* 1993;14:181–194.
32. Bolton D and Hill T. *Meaning, Causality and Disorder: Exploration in Psychology and Psychiatry.* Oxford, Oxford University Press (forthcoming).
33. Wilkes KV. *Real People: Personal Identity Without Thought Experiments.* Oxford: Clarendon Press, 1988.
34. Glover J. *I: The Philosophy and Psychology of Personal Identity.* London: The Penguin Press, 1988.
35. Braude SE. *First Person Plural: Multiple Personality and the Philosophy of Mind.* London: Routledge, 1991.
36. Gillett GR. Multiple personality and the concept of a person. *New Ideas in Psychology* 1986;4(2):173–184.

Editorials

Public health medicine – a different kind of ethics?

Medical ethics are generally considered to be that moral code which regulates the clinical relationship. This is because traditional medical ethics have developed in response to the needs of the doctor–patient encounter; and this encounter is one which stretches back into prehistory. Public health is by contrast a much more recent arrival on the scene, reaching roughly its present form during the nineteenth century in Britain[1]. Even if we were to redefine public health in broad terms as the concern of a community with the hygiene of its members – as seen, for example, in ancient Roman civilization – then this is a feature of only *some* societies. There have been many periods of British history (to look no further) when the rulers felt no responsibility for the health of 'the people', and health was seen as entirely a matter for each individual.

There is, I suggest, a sharp difference between the ethics which govern public health compared with those appropriate for clinical specialities. The reason for this difference is related to the 'clinical imperative' which is that when a patient consults their doctor 'something must be done'. This 'something' may be nothing more than the patient telling their story and the doctor responding in an appropriate and helpful fashion[2], or it may involve the whole gamut of modern technology. Nevertheless, something must be done in response to the patient's needs.

But I would argue that the clinical imperative only applies to individual clinical encounters: it does not apply to public health medicine, to medicine applied to the community. For any specific intervention (legislation for clean water, a programme of immunization, a tax upon alcohol or whatever) the necessary precondition is that it will improve the health of the public – and this improvement must be *objectively* demonstrable. Effectiveness must therefore be established by scientific methods *before* widespread action is taken.

In contrast, there is no absolute requirement for clinical medicine to be objectively effective: it is not a science. Although some parts of clinical medicine are of established scientific value (those parts, for example, proven by double-blind, randomized controlled trial) this does not, and never can, extend to the whole of medical practice; nor do the results of even the most rigorous group study ever apply exactly to the infinite individual diversity of clinical experience[3]. Whatever the current state of clinical science with respect to a given problem, nonetheless 'something must be done' to help the patient.

Consequently, we can outline the difference between the ethics of clinical medicine and those governing public health. In one case, the ethics flow from the imperatives of a face-to-face encounter with a sick human being; in the other, they regulate the *optional*
application of scientifically established interventions to improve the health of populations.

However, this does not mean that public health medicine is without an ethical framework – far from it. It is merely that the ethics come at a different point and are of a different kind. If public health is the implementation of scientific measures to enhance the health of *society*; then the ethical constraints concern the effects on the *individual*. For every measure to improve the group, there will inevitably be a price to pay by the individual. That price may be monetary. The administrative cost of a new intervention is one instance: for example, a fee for an item of service, or the salary of a public health professional. Then there is the ethical dimension of whether the money could be better spent, and a consideration of how much it is legitimate to confiscate from the individual (in taxes) to pay for the health of the community.

More often there are individual costs in terms of inconvenience and time. Or there may be a trade-off between a *definite* short-term, mild illness or pain (cow pox, bruising and nausea following inoculation, smoking-withdrawal symptoms) to be set off against a *possible* long-term and serious illness (smallpox, typhoid, lung cancer) – between predictable side-effects and unpredictable benefits in other words. There may even be a more sinister trade-off where some people are actually killed (perhaps by an idiosyncratic anaphylactic reaction, or as the casualty of an industrial accident while building a sewer) in order that many others may survive and flourish: the individual being almost literally 'sacrificed' for the good of the community. All we can say for sure is that there is always some price to pay, and it is one duty of a public health doctor to determine how big a price, and who pays it.

In public health, then, it is generally untrue to say that something *must* be done, because if there is no good scientific evidence of benefit, then it is better that *nothing* be done. Or when slender public benefit is outweighed by great private disadvantage, again it is better that nothing be done. Public health, I would argue, has little place for uncritical zeal. While crusading idealism may usefully promote the placebo effect in clinical encounters, it can seriously distort the scientific evidence and distract attention from individual disadvantage.

Unfortunately, as has been pointed out, such uncritical zeal is a hallmark of the less responsible advocates of preventive medicine[4]. There is a feeling that 'something must be done' about major public health problems such as breast or cervical cancer, and coronary artery disease. Unfortunately there is insufficient scientific backup to support public health interventions in many such areas[5]. For instance, screening for breast and cervical cancer is of unproven benefit, but results in serious and significant disadvantages to numerous individuals. The value for health is scientifically uncertain while the cost of screening in terms of cash, unnecessary operations (just to be safe), worry and pain are all certain.

Journal of the Royal Society of Medicine   Volume 86   April 1993   195

As another example, arteriosclerosis is worsened by regular, heavy smoking (as is well established), but the vast torrent of bogus and inaccurate advice purporting to tell people how to prevent myocardial infarction (and thereby prolong life) by dietary modification causes enormous expense, inconvenience and lost opportunities for enjoyment in countless individuals; as well as resulting in widespread 'victim blaming' for those who choose to ignore the advice[5].

The public health physician must typically steer a middle course between draconian intervention and ignoring a problem entirely. Appropriate action must be devised in response to various degrees of certainty and in the light of the probable consequences. In other words, there are a graded series of possible responses. To take the example of AIDS, there is a conflict between the requirement for public safety at any price, and the serious disadvantages of encroachment upon individual liberty and sheer expense. AIDS cannot, on the one hand, be ignored, but, on the other hand, it is not (yet?) appropriate to act as if *everyone* were a potential HIV carrier. The consequences of assuming universal HIV infectivity would be devastating - morally, financially and in practical terms.

There is a constant temptation for government to be seen to be 'doing something' to tackle illness and disease by making public health interventions despite lacking scientific evidence for efficacy. Public health physicians or health promoters may also be drawn into inappropriate action to increase their public profile, improve status, or simply because they do not have a sceptical and informed attitude to the scientific evidence[6]. The use of personal charisma and enthusiasm is, of course, fine (I would not wish to see a return to the 'grey men' of public health!); but the unscientific exploitation of sensationalist media hype is not.

Naturally, the sharp distinction between public health and clinical medicine is not absolute in all individual doctors - after all some individuals work in both fields. Furthermore, a public health physician is usually responsible for organizing the emergency health response to acute disaster, such as an infectious outbreak or large-scale poisoning. Such situations of immediate urgency share some of the ethical features of a clinical encounter, when compared with the more long-term and strategic role which characterizes the bulk of community-orientated public health. There may even be a version of the clinical imperative, whereby prevention of mass panic or the breakdown of public order become of greater importance than strict adherence to scientific certainties. But, while sometimes necessary, this can only be justifiable in the short-term.

Nevertheless, it is within an ethical framework of balancing community benefit against private disadvantage that the public health physician should operate, acting, if necessary, as a bulwark against political pressure towards interference without good cause[7]. The problem is that, while health benefit is objectively quantifiable using epidemiological techniques; individual disadvantages include a wide range of subjective, qualitative factors such as the anxiety caused by cancer screening programmes, the pain of children suffering injections, or the lost enjoyment of cholesterol-rich fish and chips. So that, as for all ethical systems, we cannot get the answers simply by feeding data into a computer, by following a flowchart, or applying rules-of-thumb. Public health ethics, like all moral systems, are outside the world of quantifiable science, but science must work within the rules of what is morally acceptable.

And this is why it is appropriate that public health be a branch of medicine. It is not *just* an applied science, although all its applications must have a scientific rationale. It must also take into account the qualitative disadvantage of individuals. Such judgement may, of course, be left to personal conscience, but a more reliable way to achieve this is to work from within the ethical framework generated and sustained by traditional professional practice, just as clinical ethics are generated and sustained by good practice as transmitted through personal apprenticeship[3]. All this is part of the medical morality, that relatively cohesive pattern of judgement shared by all good doctors[8]. While epidemiological data can be produced by anyone with sufficient expertise, it is necessary that the practice of public health be informed by the kind of responsible ethos which will encompass an insight into individual disadvantage developed by the process of learning to be a doctor. It is this interaction which turns public health into public health medicine, and which transforms an amoral science into moral human behaviour.

Bruce G Charlton
Department of Epidemiology and Public Health,
University of Newcastle upon Tyne,
Newcastle NE2 4HH

References
1　Acheson RM, Hagard S. *Health, society and medicine.* Oxford: Blackwell, 1984
2　Charlton BG. Stories of sickness (Editorial). *Br J Gen Pract* 1991;**41**:222-3
3　Charlton BG. Medical practice and the double-blind, randomized controlled trial (Editorial). *Br J Gen Pract* 1991;**41**:355-6
4　Skrabanek P. Why is preventive medicine exempted from ethical restraints? *J Med Ethics* 1990;**16**:187-90
5　Skrabanek P, McCormick J. *Follies and Fallacies in Medicine.* Glasgow: Tarragon Press, 1989
6　Kelly MP, Charlton BG. A scientific basis for health promotion: time for a new philosophy? (Editorial). *Br J Gen Pract* 1992;**42**:223-4
7　Charlton B, Kelly M. Profit and loss on the pulse of a nation. *Times Higher Educ Suppl* 7.2.92:19
8　Downie RS, Charlton B. *The making of a doctor: medical education in theory and practice.* Oxford: Oxford University Press, 1992

39

Journal of medical ethics 1993; **19: 135–137**

Symposium

The ethics of medical involvement in torture

R S Downie   *Glasgow University, Scotland*

Author's abstract

The difficulties of establishing a definition of torture are discussed, and a definition is suggested. It is then argued that, irrespective of general ethical questions, doctors in particular should never be involved because of their social role.

If we think of a definition as being a set of necessary and sufficient conditions which uniquely identify what is in question then a definition of torture, as distinct from cruelty or degrading treatment or sustained violence against a person, is not easy to establish. From a practical point of view it does not really matter very much whether a practice is strictly torture or some other form of inhuman treatment; the point would be to get it stopped. But since I have been asked to give a philosophical account of torture then my first task is to try to identify precisely what we ought to mean when we use the term.

As a first attempt we might try the following: Torture is the deliberate infliction of pain on another person or persons. But this will not do. First of all, many medical treatments involve the infliction of pain so we need to add the phrase 'without the consent of the person'. Secondly, it is possible, perhaps all too common, for someone to torture an animal, and it is a moot point whether one animal (for example a cat) can torture another. We can meet these points by simple amendments: Torture is the deliberate infliction of pain on another sentient being without consent. But ordinary assault would fit that definition, so we must add that the victim must be held in captivity. Yet suppose that someone in captivity is systematically beaten up. Is that torture? We might say that it is inhuman and degrading treatment, but not quite torture. True, torture can be used in order to degrade, but not all degrading treatment is torture.

A possible way ahead here might be to suggest that torture always has some objective beyond itself. In other words, whereas degrading treatment need

have no objective beyond degrading, torture must have some objective beyond torturing – such as the extraction of information, the gratification of the torturer, or as a punishment. We could perhaps unify these objectives by saying that torture always involves the infliction of pain with the aim of subjugating a sentient being to the ends of others. Yet sometimes the Inquisition tortured heretics for their *own good*, in order to force them to see the error of their beliefs. Of course, it is true that such an objective might be difficult to distinguish from torture as a punishment for heresy or torture as a gratification for the torturers, but certainly some torture was intended to bring heretics to their senses for their own good. Nevertheless, we can accommodate torture for the victim's own good in the means/end analysis if we say that the pain of the body was used as a means to the end of the soul's repentance. We can now incorporate these points in a revised definition: Torture is the deliberate infliction of pain on another captive sentient being in order to use the being as a means to an end to which he/she has not consented.

There is room for further refinements. First, not all torture involves what is fairly called pain. For example, sensory deprivation might be used in torture and perhaps there can be mental torture which is not exactly pain. But this difficulty is easy to take care of by adding to the definition: 'pain, or other severe distress'. Secondly, can we be said to be able to torture ourselves? This idea is on the margins of the metaphorical. The captivity is that of our own psychological experience, the 'mind-forg'd manacles', as the poet Blake puts it; and the pain or the unpleasantness is that of repeatedly going over in our minds some episodes in which we behaved badly, with the objective of self-punishment. It is clearly no job for Amnesty to deal with self-torture, but there is no doubt that it is sometimes the job of psychiatrists. The final point to note about the definition – it is not a refinement but an attempt to avoid confusion – is that the victims of torture need not be 'innocent'. Those who are entirely justly convicted criminals or terrorists can still be said to be tortured. Indeed, they frequently are. We are left then with the following definition:

Key words

Torture; medical skills; medical role.

136 *Symposium: The ethics of medical involvement in torture*

Torture is the deliberate infliction of pain or other severe distress by one sentient being on another who is in captivity and involves using that being as a means to an end to which the being has not consented.

Moral aspects

The main question I wish to address in this second part of my discussion is whether doctors should ever be involved with torture. Of course, if it could be established that *no one* should ever be involved in torture then it would follow that doctors should not – the greater set would contain the lesser. But it is not easy to establish that no one should ever be involved in torture, and I shall not try to do so in this short paper. Yet even if we cannot establish that no one should ever in any circumstances be involved in torture it may still be possible to establish that *doctors* should never be involved; there may be features of being a doctor that make it always wrong for the doctor *qua* doctor to be involved, even although in rare instances others may legitimately be involved. For example, there may sometimes be cases in which it would be possible by torture to extract information from evil terrorists which would save the lives of thousands of innocent civilians. The fact that examples of this sort are more common in philosophy books than in reality does not really affect the point that it is at least logically possible that in certain circumstances the use of torture to extract life-saving information may be morally legitimate. As I said, I am not arguing for this case but simply noting it as an assumption which lets me proceed to the question of whether, even if it is the case, we can argue that doctors in particular should never be involved.

Before we proceed to this question we must try to dispose of an unattractive possibility which is created by the assumption that in some cases torture may be legitimate. The unattractive possibility is that if we once allow that torture could sometimes be morally legitimate it might be claimed to be morally *obligatory* in some cases for doctors themselves to be the torturers. The argument here is that doctors more than most have the skills necessary to torture with the minimum damage to the victim. Of course, this consideration could not justify a doctor in torturing for just *any* sort of objective, but only for one which was conducive to the good of others. This idea that the skills of the doctor can be used for an end other than healing is an old one. Plato in the *Republic* (333e) notes that the good doctor can also be the good poisoner. Here Plato is thinking of the art of medicine as what he calls a 'techne', a kind of skill which can be used for an end which may be good or bad. Can we reply to this argument?

A reply involves some consideration of the sort of job being a doctor is. Some jobs are basically what we might call 'skill jobs'. For example, the essence of the job of musician is a skill or skills; if you do not have the skills you are no musician. Other jobs are fundamentally 'aim jobs'. For example, the job of 'farmer' is one such. A farmer by definition is one who cultivates fields or animals. Even if he is very unskilful he remains a farmer to the extent that that is what he is aiming to do. Thirdly, some jobs are 'role jobs'. For instance, the job of postman is a 'role job'. If I deliver a letter as a private person, I am only metaphorically a postman, for I am not authorised with official rights and duties. On the other hand, if I am the authorised postman, then, even if I have no skills, for example if I get lost with my mail-bag, and even if I have criminal aims, for example to steal the mail, I am still the postman because I have been authorised in that role. Obviously, these distinctions need much refinement, and many jobs will combine more than one of the characteristics. But medicine has all three. If a person has no *skills* he is no doctor. More controversially, the doctor must be defined as having a certain *aim*, which I suggest is that of relieving suffering or, more ambitiously, that of healing. A doctor also has a role, defined in terms of a set of rights and duties authorised by some sort of governing body, and often strengthened by an official code of ethics. If a doctor fails under any of these aspects of his job he is not acting as a doctor. Let us now apply this analysis of the concept of a doctor to the question of whether the doctor may or must be involved in torture.

The first step requires me to clarify what is meant by the vague phrase I have been using up till now: 'involved in torture'. It can mean at least three things. A doctor may be 'involved in torture' if:

(a) he attempts to heal the victims of torture;
(b) he himself engages in torture either by advising or by actually carrying it out;
(c) he examines possible victims knowing or suspecting that torture will follow.

There seems no problem about (a). It is part of the aim and role of the doctor to heal, and this is the proper purpose of his skills. Turning to (b) I can argue that it follows from my account of what it is to be a doctor that it must always be wrong for the doctor *qua* doctor to engage in torture either by offering advice or by carrying it out. Of course, sometimes a doctor may have the skills to *pretend* that he is engaged in torture but not actually do so. But that situation, a highly unlikely one, is not really a case of the doctor engaging in torture, but only of pretending to do so.

What of case (c)? Should a doctor examine someone with the objective of deciding whether the victim can stand up to torture? It might depend on what was involved. If such an examination would enable the doctor to say that he believes the victim is likely to die of heart-failure if tortured then perhaps this kind of activity is within the role of the doctor and compatible with his intrinsic aim. Perhaps he might even say falsely that the victim would die in order to protect him. But cases of these types must be rare.

What has emerged is that 'doctor' is an evaluative term. I am asserting that it is part of the concept of a doctor that a doctor must aim at relieving suffering or healing and that he also has a certain role in society. I am rejecting the view that the job of doctor can be adequately defined only in terms of the possession of certain skills. The skills of a musician, for example, can be used for a good or bad end, but not those of a doctor. Again, the skills and knowledge of a scientist can be used for good or bad ends. But if a doctor uses his skills for a bad end then he is no doctor. Note that the point is not just that the doctor's skills must be used for a good end. For if torture is sometimes justifiable, for example to prevent a terrorist plot, then torture will be being used for a good end. The point is that the skills of a doctor must be used only for a *certain sort* of good end – healing or relieving suffering. If a person uses them for any other purpose then he has given up being a doctor.

Since this is the central point in my argument it may be worthwhile to expand on it briefly. As I said, the essence of being a musician is the possession of skills. If the musician exercises his skills to soothe a tyrant he is still a musician. Similarly, a scientist has skills and knowledge and remains a scientist even if he puts these to a morally bad end, such as devising chemical weapons. He is a bad scientist if, but only if, he falsifies his results. The doctor can be criticised from three standpoints; if his skills are defective, if the role is not fulfilled adequately (for example when the doctor does not take his/her turn on the rota), and, most relevant here, when the aim is not to relieve suffering or encourage healing.

My argument clearly entails that the profession of medicine has certain values built into it. It is worth noting two implications of this position. First, it prevents a doctor defending himself by saying: 'When in Rome do as the Romans'. For example, the practice of female circumcision is mutilating and a doctor *qua* doctor should never be involved in it, regardless of any local customs. Similarly, it will not do for a doctor to say that torture is endemic in his community so he must go along with it. Medicine stands for something. I am asserting that what it stands for is the ideal of using scientific and other skills by an authorised or legitimated person who has the aim of alleviating suffering or healing. Secondly, it implies 'once a doctor always a doctor'. In other words, it is not open for a doctor to say 'I shall cease acting as a doctor while I engage in torture and then I shall resume the role later'. Being a doctor is more like being a parent than being a postman; resignation is not possible.

The whole argument might have been by-passed by quoting the first clause of the Declaration of Tokyo (adopted by the World Medical Association in 1975) which states unequivocably:

'The doctor shall not countenance, condone or participate in the practice of torture or other forms of cruel, inhuman or degrading procedures, whatever the offence of which the victim of such procedures is suspected, accused or guilty, and whatever the victim's beliefs, or motives, and in all situations including armed conflict and civil strife.'

But however convincing codes are as pieces of deontology it is always philosophically interesting to consider what sort of justification can be given of what is intuitively judged to be binding on doctors.

R S Downie   is Professor of Moral Philosophy at Glasgow University.

This symposium derives from a joint symposium of the Institute of Medical Ethics and The Royal College of Physicians held in 1991.

40

Journal of medical ethics 1993; **19:** 138–141

Symposium

The ethics of medical involvement in torture: commentary

R M Hare   *University of Florida, USA*

Author's abstract

Torture does need to be defined if we are to know exactly what we are seeking to ban; but no single definition will do, because there are many possible ones, and we may want to treat different practices that might be called torture differently. Compare the case of homicide; we do not want to punish manslaughter as severely as murder, and may not want to punish killing in self-defence at all. There are degrees of torture as of murder. Unclarities simply play into the hands of would-be torturers.
Downie is unsuccessful in deriving the duty of doctors not to be involved in torture from an analysis of the word 'doctor'. It may be contrary to the role-duty of doctors to participate in torture; but there might be other duties which overrode this role-duty. The right approach is to ask what principles for the conduct of doctors have the highest acceptance-utility, or, as Kant might have equivalently put it, what the impartial furtherance of everyone's ends demands. This approach yields the result that torture (suitably defined) should be banned absolutely. It also yields prescriptions for the conduct of doctors where, in spite of them, torture is taking place.

Professor Downie's attempt, in his admirably clear and concise paper, to define 'torture' is the best that I have seen so far; but it is necessary to ask what purpose such definitions serve. Some may feel that verbal questions of this kind ought not to occupy our time. But whatever conclusions we reach will have to be expressed in words, and if the words have not been made clear, the conclusions will not be. For example, if we say that torture, or torture in certain specified circumstances, ought to be ruled out, it has to be clear precisely *what* we are saying should be ruled out. Downie says (page 135) 'From a practical point of view it does not really matter very much whether a practice is strictly torture or some other form of inhuman treatment; the point would be to get it stopped'. But we do need to be clear about *what* we want to get stopped.

Key words

Torture; medical skills; medical role.

However, it is probably fruitless, and may be positively confusing, to look for a single definition of 'torture'. There is a great variety of treatments which have been described as torture, ranging from the infliction of the most extreme physical pain for the most wicked purposes to the causing of quite mild mental suffering in pursuit of aims that are in themselves laudable. We may wish to condemn some of these practices and not others, and if we call them all by the same name we may get confused. At least we should try not to beg any substantial moral questions about the rightness or wrongness of certain practices by the way we decide to use words.

It is worth looking at what has in most jurisdictions been done with the words 'murder' and 'homicide'. There are a great many different kinds of homicide (that is, of killing people), and there are even some of these that most people do not wish to condemn (killing in self-defence, for example). So we need at least to distinguish between culpable and non-culpable homicide. But even within the category of culpable homicide we make further distinctions (not the same in all jurisdictions). In English law we distinguish at least between murder and manslaughter (there is also a separate offence of killing by reckless driving and another of infanticide); and it is possible, as some jurisdictions do, to make further distinctions within the class of murders, in terms such as 'first-degree murder', 'second-degree murder', etc.

These distinctions have a purpose. We want to make the punishment, or the degree of condemnation, fit the crime, and do not think all crimes are equally heinous. If we had only one term, 'murder', for all these acts, it would not be easy to frame a clear law that would do this. Some homicides we do not want to condemn at all. So we divide homicides into categories and lay down different penalties, if any, for each of them. The definitions come after, and not before, we have decided how we wish to classify kinds of homicide, for the purpose of directing the courts to treat each category in a different way.

If we followed a similar procedure with torture, we should not start off with a very general, and inevitably vague and unclear, definition of 'torture'.

Rather, we should look at all the various kinds of act that might be called torture, and then decide which of these kinds of acts we wished to condemn, and how severely. Only after that would we give names to the various kinds of act that we wished to condemn, or not condemn. We might end up with a lot of different 'degrees' of torture, and with some other terms (analogous to 'manslaughter') which did not imply so severe condemnation; and there would probably be some classes of acts that we called by names which did not imply condemnation at all.

Past failures to observe these precautions have resulted in the most muddled battles of words. One party calls what another party is doing 'torture'. The other party says that what it is doing is not (or not really) torture – as if it mattered what one calls it. The question rather is: Is this a kind of activity that ought to be banned? When we have decided that (which involves a close factual enquiry into the nature of the activity and its circumstances and aims), we can *then* go on to give it a name, and the name is unlikely to be simply 'torture'. There are certainly practices going on all over the world which ought to be condemned and if possible stopped. We make this more difficult if we use words in such a woolly way that those who are guilty of these practices can always say 'Yes, we use torture; but so do you when you make prisoners suffer as you do'. Since *some* suffering is in practice inseparable from imprisonment, this affords too easy an excuse to torturers. So, although I find Professor Downie's clarifications helpful, I do not think they take us far enough.

I now turn to my other main difficulty with his paper. He thinks that we can get guidance on how doctors should behave by examining the meaning of the word 'doctor'. I do not think he is successful in this. He distinguishes, rightly, between skill jobs, aim jobs and role jobs, and says that the doctor has all three. But it is possible to take on one or more of these jobs without taking on the rest. For example, someone might acquire the skill of a doctor, but not have the aim of healing. Or he (or she) might have both jobs, but not accept the role of doctor; he might *want* to heal people, but not acknowledge any *duty* to heal them. And if it is possible, the question must arise, *ought* a person to take them all on, or only some. This question can arise over a whole career, or on a particular occasion.

Downie says (page 137) 'It is not open for a doctor to say "I shall cease acting as a doctor while I engage in torture and then I shall resume the role later" '. But *if* he thought he had a duty to engage in torture (and we must not beg the question, as Downie seems to be trying to do, of whether he ever could have such a duty), then he might think that this duty required him to override, temporarily, the duties of his doctor-role, in order to perform the more pressing duty. It may be that there is not likely ever to be a duty to torture, but Downie has not shown that there is not.

A parallel may make this clear. It is clearly a role-duty of prison officers not to let prisoners escape. But if a prison officer thought that a certain prisoner had been wrongly convicted and was to be hanged for a crime he had never committed, he might think he ought to let the prisoner escape. He would of course be in breach of his role-duty if he did this; but he might think all the same that he had a moral duty which overrode this role-duty. The question could only be settled by a far-reaching examination of the circumstances of the case. If he let the prisoner escape, and was not detected as the person who did this, he might thereafter resume his duties as a prison officer.

It would be difficult for him to do it with a good conscience; but conscience is not always a reliable guide to duty. Conscience is the product of our upbringing, and gives good guidance in ordinary cases if the upbringing has been sound; but in extra-ordinary cases it may give the wrong answer. It went against Huckleberry Finn's conscience to help the slave to escape.

I am not saying that Downie ought, in his short paper, to have settled the entire question of whether torture is ever justified. But even though he was only asking, less ambitiously, whether, if torture ever is justified, a doctor could ever be right in getting involved in it, he has not settled even this question. For *if* torture were justified on a particular occasion, a doctor could not argue simply that, because he had the role of a doctor, he ought not to be involved in it. He might think that the duty to be involved in the (supposedly) justified torture *overrode* his role-duties as a doctor.

I do not think that either the question of whether torture is ever justified, or the question of whether doctors ought ever to be involved in it, can be settled without a much deeper examination of the 'methods of ethics', as Sidgwick called them. But having found fault with Downie's method, I ought perhaps to give some indication of how I would settle such questions. I am unusual in being both a Kantian and a utilitarian. Many philosophers think this is impossible, but they have not fully understood Kant. On the Kantian side, Downie rightly includes in his definition of torture (page 136) 'using that being as a means to an end to which the being has not consented'. This echoes Kant's dictum 'Act in such a way that you always treat humanity, whether in your own person or in the person of any other, never simply as a means, but always at the same time as an end' (1). Kant explains on the next page that others 'ought always at the same time to be rated as ends, that is, only as beings who must themselves be able to share in the end of the very same action'; and he goes on to say 'For the ends of a subject who is an end in himself must, if this conception is to have its *full* effect in me, be also, as far as possible, *my* ends' (2).

Take now the case of the terrorist who has put a bomb in a litter bin in a crowded place. Is it right to torture him to discover *which* bin? If we did that, we should of course not be treating his ends as our ends; for his ends no doubt include that of having the bomb explode. But what about the ends of all those who will be killed if the bomb explodes? If we treat *their* ends as our own ends, we shall perhaps think it right to torture the terrorist. And if there are a thousand of them and only one terrorist, we might think that we would do better, even according to Kant, to respect their ends rather than his, especially as his end is an immoral one (3). Thus it is possible to argue on Kantian lines for a utilitarian solution to such problems; for the utilitarian also would say that we should maximize preference-satisfaction in such a case, and obviously we shall do this if we use torture to discover the location of the bomb. (For further much needed discussion of the relation between Kantianism and utilitarianism see Hare 1993 (4).)

The same kind of reasoning can be used in the particular case of the doctor who is wondering whether he should get involved in the torture. I have argued that *if* he had a duty to get involved, this duty might override his role-duty as a doctor. Why then do we not only think of torture in itself as morally abhorrent, but think it even more abhorrent for doctors to be involved in it? We can see that it is quite right to think this, if we look at the actual circumstances of the world in which we live. Our moral principles have to be appropriate for everyday use in this actual world. That is why it is wrong to tailor them to extraordinary examples like the one just given.

Many people seem to fall victim to the elementary logical fallacy of thinking the following inference valid:

Torture is justified in some (conceivable) cases;
Therefore it is justified in any case.

If this inference were valid, then we might be led to deny that torture was justified even in the most unusual cases, in order to avoid having to conclude that it was justified in more normal cases. But this is not only fallacious, but practically misleading. What doctors, and all the rest of us, need are sound principles for our conduct in the cases we are likely to encounter. It is hard to believe that the litter bin case would ever occur: that is, a case in which there was no way of locating the bomb except by torture. It is even more unbelievable that the skills of the doctor would be of much use in torturing the terrorist; torture is not all that difficult in such a case; a crude quick and effective means would be what was needed.

I have argued elsewhere (5) that the right rule for police to adopt would be to rule out torture absolutely. The reason is that once it is even contemplated, it will be used, and spread, and the end result will be much worse than the evils that torture was supposed to counter. This is consistent with admitting that cases are *conceivable* in which torture

would be the right course; I gave a highly improbable example in the place cited. In the world as it is, it never will be the right course. Therefore policemen should not even contemplate it; and the same is even more true of doctors.

However, in regimes where, in spite of this, torture is practised by the police, difficult situations can arise where doctors get involved willy nilly. They may find themselves confronted with a prisoner whom they might help medically, and then it is difficult to draw the line between helping the prisoner and helping the regime. For example, if he is patched up, it may be only to be subjected to further torture. Downie misses this point when he says 'Of course, if it could be established that *no one* should ever be involved in torture then it would follow that doctors should not – the greater set would contain the lesser' (page 136). In a regime where torture is practised, a doctor might not be able to avoid being involved in various ways. But he will normally be able to control the extent and the kind of involvement. Doctors living under such regimes will be wise, therefore, to make for themselves some firm rules which they do not depart from, and if possible get them adopted by the governing bodies of their profession. What these rules should be needs further discussion, and has received it. They would probably include a rule not to treat torture victims until they are free, distasteful as this policy may be; for otherwise the doctor will become an ancillary to further torture. And they will certainly include a rule to give only such treatment as is for the good of the victim. However, those with practical experience are better able to suggest and assess such rules than I am.

The main point is that even a utilitarian like me (perhaps especially a utilitarian like me), if he thinks the matter through and looks at the consequences of the adoption or abandonment of such firm rules, will recommend that doctors find the best ones and stick to them. He should not be led astray by considering unusual examples in which involvement in torture in support of the regime might be for the best. Even if there are such cases, principles devised to suit them would not be appropriate to the normal case; and if we are to give ourselves the best chance of acting rightly in all normal cases, we had better have firm rules that suit those normal cases. Hard cases make bad law.

R M Hare is Professor of Philosophy at the University of Florida, Gainesville, Florida, USA.

References

(1) Kant I. *Groundwork of the metaphysic of morals*, BA66=429, in translation by Paton H J. *The moral law*. London: Hutchinson, 1948: 91.
(2) See reference (1): 92
(3) Kant I. *Doctrine of virtue*. A119=449, in translation by Gregor M. Philadelphia: University of Pennsylvania Press, 1964: 117.

(4) Hare R M. Could Kant have been a utilitarian? *Utilitas* 1993; 5: 1–16.

(5) Hare R M. *Freedom and reason*. Oxford: Oxford University Press, 1963.

Name Index

Abercrombie, N. 5
Akhmedzhanov. M. 428, 429
Aleksakhina, R.I. 474
Almond, B. xxi, 269–74
Andrusko, David 213
Angell, M. 377
Annas, George J. 327, 331
Anscombe, G.M.A. 176
Aquinas, Thomas 28, 173–4
Aristotle xviii, xx, 23, 31–2
Auster, Paul 116
Austin, J.L. 470, 479

Bambrough, R. 73–4
Barley, Nigel 112
Barsky, Arthur 214
Baudrillard, J. 139
Beauchamp, T.L. xv, 40, 41, 46–52, 54, 55
Benedict, Ruth 329
Benner, P. 96, 99, 101
Bennett, Jonathan 176–8
Benoliel, J.Q. 99
Bentham, Jeremy 232
Birley, J.L.T. 434
Bloch, S. 427, 430, 431, 432
Blum, L.A. 89
Boorse, C. 429, 430, 459–60, 461–3, 468–70,
    472, 477, 478, 479
Bosk, C.L. 154
Bowsma, W.J. 11
Bradley, F.H. 29
Brahams, D. 272
Braude, S.E. 479
Brock, D.W. xxii, 407–11
Brody, B.A. 104, 337–8
Brody, H. 122
Brooks, D.H.M. 273
Buchanan, A. xxi, 243–68
Buchanan, W. 95
Byar, D.P. 376

Callahan, D. xvii, xviii, xx, 146, 213–20
Callahan, Sidney 331
Calvin, John 4, 11, 13
Caplan, A. 387
Capron, Alexander M. 329
Cassell, C. 134
Chadwick, Ruth 391, 399–400

Chalmers, T.C. 379, 380, 381
Charlton, Bruce xxii, 483–4
Chesler, Phyllis 332, 333
Childress, J.F. xv, 40, 41, 46–52, 54, 55
Chodoff, P. xxii, 401–6, 427, 432
Cicero, M.T. 60
Clare, A. 427, 432
Clouser, K.D. xviii, 39–56
Conkin, P. 12
Conrad, P. 96
Cooke, M. 103
Cornford, F.M. 280, 294
Crowley, Rosemary 370, 371

Daniel, S.L. xix, 159–65
Daniels, N. xvi, xxii, 437–43
Davidovskii, I.V. 428, 429, 430
Davidson, Donald 176
Davies, J. 211
Davis, Alison 395
Dawson, K. xxi, 355–72
Delaney, Samuel R. 330
Derrida, J. 161
De Vries, William 454
Didion, Joan 112
Downie, R.S. xx, 485–7
Dunn, John 12
Dworkin, R. 449

Edwards, Jonathan 6
Edwards, R.G. 275–80 *passim*, 290, 302, 356,
    358
Eisenberg, C. 93
Elliott, Carl xix, xx, xxii, 111–18, 413–25, 453–8
Ellis, J.T. 8–9
Engelhardt, H.T. Jr 104, 120, 144
Ennis, B. 402

Fairbairn, G.J. 209
Fauci, Anthony 373–4
Feinstein, A.R. 383
Fiering, N. 6
Firestone, Shulamith 309
Fischer, J.M. xvii, xx, 195–204
Fletcher, J.F. 25–6, 133
Foot, P. 172, 178–9, 188, 199, 209
Fox, R.C. 143, 144
Frankena, W. 41, 43–6, 55